THE Drug & Natural Medicine ADVISOR

THE Drug & Natural Medicine ADVISOR

THE COMPLETE GUIDE TO
Alternative & Conventional Medications

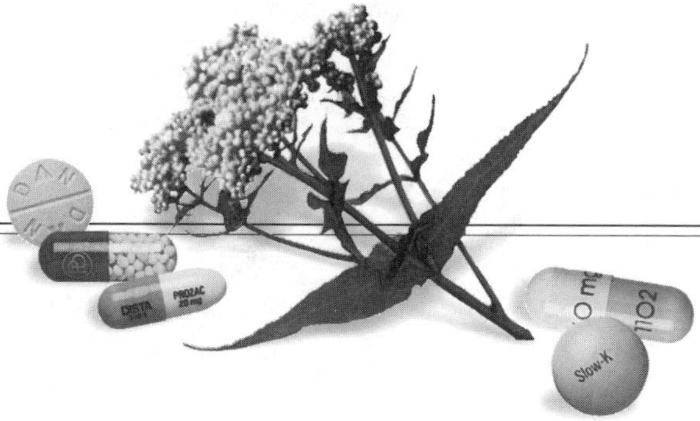

BY THE EDITORS OF TIME-LIFE BOOKS
ALEXANDRIA, VIRGINIA

AROMATHERAPY

CHINESE MEDICINE

HOMEOPATHY

NUTRITIONAL SUPPLEMENTS

OVER-THE-COUNTER DRUGS

PRESCRIPTION DRUGS

VITAMINS AND MINERALS

WESTERN HERBS

Consultants

ZOË BRENNER, LAC, DIPL AC AND DIPL CH (NCCA), FNAAOM, has practiced acupuncture since 1977 and Chinese herbal medicine since 1984. She teaches Oriental medicine and the history and philosophy of Chinese medicine at the Traditional Acupuncture Institute in Columbia, Maryland, and lectures at other schools around the United States.

JOHN G. COLLINS, ND, DHANP, teaches dermatology and homeopathy at the National College of Naturopathic Medicine in Portland, Oregon. He also has a private practice in Gresham, Oregon.

KYLE H. CRONIN, ND, specializes in women's healthcare in her medical practice in Phoenix, Arizona. Dr. Cronin is also cofounder of Southwest College of Naturopathic Medicine and Health Sciences, where she is dean of curricular development.

DAVID E. GOLAN, MD, PHD, is an attending physician at Brigham and Women's Hospital in Boston and an associate professor of biological chemistry and molecular pharmacology at Harvard Medical School. A board-certified internist and hematologist, Dr. Golan directs research on blood cell membranes. He has also created a computer-learning program for pharmacology.

CHERYL HOARD began her three-year term as president of the National Association for Holistic Aromatherapy (NAHA) in January 1997. An expert aromatherapist and herbalist who has studied natural healing throughout the Far East, Ms. Hoard is a member of the BJC Health Systems Complementary Health Care Committee in St. Louis, Missouri. She also owns an international herb business.

KAREN SUE LEVENTHAL, RPH, is a registered pharmacist currently with the Rite Aid Corporation in Beltsville, Maryland, where she is a pharmacy manager. She received her Bachelor of Science in pharmacy from the University of Pittsburgh School of Pharmacy in 1995.

GARY C. ROSENFELD, PHD, is a professor of pharmacology and is the assistant dean for educational programs at the University of Texas at Houston Medical School, where he also teaches in the Graduate School of Biomedical Sciences. In 1996 Dr. Rosenfeld was selected for the Harvard Medical School's Macy Institute Program for Leaders in Medical Education.

JILL M. SIEGFRIED, PHD, is an associate professor in the Department of Pharmacology, School of Medicine, at the University of Pittsburgh. She specializes in cancer pharmacology. She is a member of the American Association for Cancer Research and since 1996 has served as a permanent member of the Environmental Health Sciences Study Section at the National Institutes of Health.

J. JAMISON STARBUCK, JD, ND, practices family medicine in Missoula, Montana. A former practicing attorney, she is past president of the American Association of Naturopathic Physicians and a member of the Homeopathic Academy of Naturopathic Physicians.

S. MARK TANEN, MD, is a board-certified internist and endocrinologist. He is a clinical assistant professor at the Georgetown University School of Medicine and has a private practice in McLean, Virginia.

DICK W. THOM, DDS, ND, teaches clinical and physical diagnosis at the National College of Naturopathic Medicine in Portland, Oregon. He is also a clinic supervisor at the Portland Naturopathic Clinic and maintains a general family practice at Natural Choices Health Clinic in Beaverton, Oregon.

TIME® LIFE BOOKS

TIME-LIFE BOOKS IS A DIVISION OF TIME LIFE INC.

TIME-LIFE CUSTOM PUBLISHING

VICE PRESIDENT AND PUBLISHER: TERRY NEWELL
ASSOCIATE PUBLISHER: TERESA HARTNETT
DIRECTOR OF EDITORIAL DEVELOPMENT: JENNIFER PEARCE
VICE PRESIDENT OF SALES AND MARKETING: NEIL LEVIN
DIRECTOR OF SPECIAL SALES: LIZ ZIEHL
DIRECTOR OF NEW PRODUCT DEVELOPMENT: QUENTIN MCANDREW
MANAGING EDITOR: DONIA ANN STEELE
PRODUCTION MANAGER: CAROLYN M. CLARK
QUALITY ASSURANCE MANAGER: JAMES KING

Books produced by Time-Life Custom Publishing are available at special bulk discount for promotional and premium use. Custom adaptations can also be created to meet your specific marketing goals.
Call 1-800-323-5255.

EDITORIAL STAFF

EDITOR: ROBERT SOMERVILLE
DEPUTY EDITOR: TINA S. MCDOWELL
DESIGN DIRECTOR: TINA TAYLOR
TEXT EDITOR: JIM WATSON
ASSOCIATE EDITORS/RESEARCH AND WRITING: NANCY BLODGETT (PRINCIPAL), STEPHANIE SUMMERS HENKE
SENIOR COPYEDITOR: ANNE FARR
EDITORIAL ASSISTANT: PATRICIA D. WHITEFORD
PICTURE COORDINATORS: RUTH GOLDBERG, KIM GRANDCOLAS

SPECIAL CONTRIBUTORS

DESIGN: JOHN DRUMMOND, SABA SUNGAR, MONIKA THAYER
TEXT: ZOË BRENNER, ANN LEE BRUEN, LINA B. BURTON, DONNA CAREY, JULI DUNCAN, LINDA FERRAGUT, ANNE HEISING, SILVIA HINES, LAURIE JONES, BARBARA L. KLEIN, ELIZABETH SCHLEICHERT, JAYNE R. WOOD
COPYEDITING: CLAUDIA S. BEDWELL, JAYNE R. WOOD
BRAND NAME INDEX: BARBARA L. KLEIN
INDEX: SUNDAY OLIVER
PRESCRIPTION DRUG SECTION OF THE COLOR GUIDE TO PRESCRIPTION DRUGS AND HERBS: KAREN SUE LEVENTHAL, RPH, AND JACK M. SIEGEL, RPH, PD, RITE AID CORPORATION

First printing. Printed in U.S.A. School and library distribution by Time-Life Education
P.O. Box 85026
Richmond, Virginia 23285-5026.

Library of Congress Cataloging-in-Publication Data
The drug & natural medicine advisor: the complete guide to alternative & conventional medications / by the editors of Time-Life Books.
p. cm
Includes bibliographical references and index.
ISBN 0-7835-4938-5
ISBN 0-7835-5300-5
1. Alternative medicine—Encyclopedias.
2. Drugs—Encyclopedias.
I. Time-Life Books.
R733.D77 1997
615'.03—dc21 97-3309 CIP

The descriptions of medical conditions and treatments in this book should be considered as a reference source only; they are not intended to substitute for a healthcare practitioner's diagnosis, advice, and treatment. Always consult your physician or a qualified practitioner for proper medical care.

Before using any drug or natural medicine mentioned in this book, be sure to check the appropriate sections of this book and the product's label for any warnings or cautions. Keep in mind that herbal remedies are not as strictly regulated as drugs.

Be advised that although every effort has been made to ensure accurate reproduction of the prescription drugs in the Color Guide to Prescription Drugs and Herbs, variations in color can result from the printing process, and pills are not shown actual size. Take care not to confuse brand-name drugs with their generic counterparts. Do not depend only on the images in this book to identify a given drug or herb; consult a physician, pharmacist, or qualified healthcare practitioner for proper identification.

CONTENTS

HOW TO USE THIS BOOK

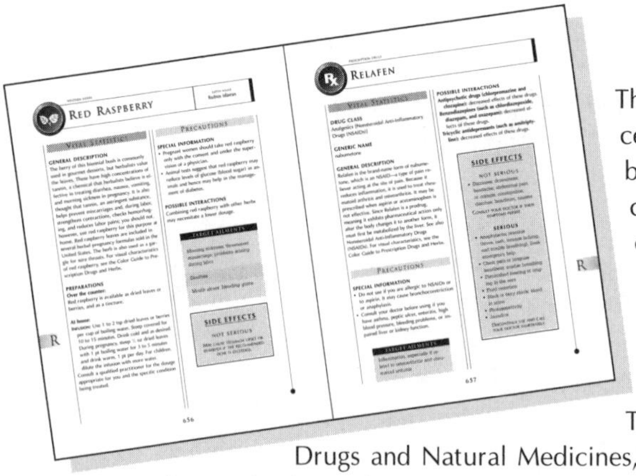

This book is designed to give you quick access to information about a wide range of both conventional and alternative medicines—from prescription and over-the-counter (OTC) drugs to so-called natural remedies such as herbs and homeopathic treatments. There are several ways to use the book's sections to get to what you need to know.

The heart of the book is the A-Z Guide to Drugs and Natural Medicines, an 817-page directory with entries covering nearly 700 healing substances. Each entry is clearly labeled with an icon that identifies which type of remedy it is, such as Chinese Medicine, Aromatherapy, or Prescription Drugs. For conventional medications, you'll find individual entries for drug classes and subclasses, such as Analgesics or Topical Antibiotics; for generic drugs, such as acetaminophen; and for dozens of the most common brand-name drugs, such as Tylenol or Prozac. If you can't find the name of your medication in this section, check the general index at the back of the book; information about your drug may be in an entry for the class or subclass to which it belongs, and the index will tell you where to look. If your brand-name drug doesn't have its own entry, turn to the Brand Name Index on page 853, where you'll find a page reference for the appropriate generic name entry.

For both conventional and natural medicines, each entry in the A-Z Guide provides a broad overview of a given remedy, along with important specifics about its use and effects. The first part of the entry is Vital Statistics, a catalog of basic facts such as a generic drug's class and brand names as well as the names of other generics in its class; natural sources for a vitamin or mineral; the various ways an herbal remedy can be prepared; and the ingredients and alternate names of a Chinese formula.

The General Description is a brief profile of the remedy, covering such topics as its history or origin, how it works, and the types of conditions it is used to treat. At the end of the General Description you may be referred to other entries for more information or, if appropriate, to the Color Guide to Prescription Drugs and Herbs. This gallery of nearly 250 photographs and drawings shows you exactly how a drug or herb should look, allowing you to identify a pill or plant at a glance or distinguish between similar-looking remedies.

To learn which conditions the remedy is used to treat, consult the box labeled Target Ailments. Another box lists "Serious" and "Not Serious" Side Effects, along with clear guidelines on what to do if you experience these symptoms.

Many healing substances can be dangerous, even deadly, if used improperly or by people with certain medical conditions. Such concerns are covered under the heading Precautions. Before using a remedy, be sure to read Special Information, which offers advice and important facts about the substance, including how to recognize symptoms of an overdose. Potentially life-threatening effects and other serious concerns are clearly labeled with a skull-and-crossbones Warning. You should also carefully read the list of Possible Interactions so you can avoid other substances—drugs, natural medicines, or foods—that may interact adversely with the remedy you are using.

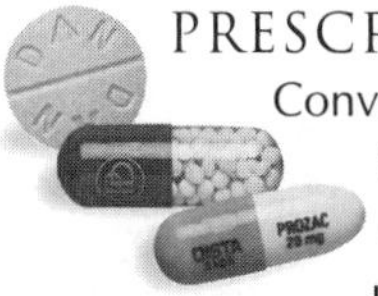

PRESCRIPTION VS. OTC DRUGS

Conventional drugs are classified as either prescription (Rx) or over-the-counter (OTC); some drugs are available in both prescription and OTC forms. Prescription drugs are those that, for reasons of safety, can be dispensed only under a doctor's supervision. The United States Food and Drug Administration (FDA) places such restrictions on drugs that are habit forming or have a high potential for causing harmful effects, and also on medications used for ailments (such as asthma and some vaginal fungal infections) that are not readily self-diagnosed. Over-the-counter drugs can be sold without a prescription if it is determined that consumers, following label instructions, can use them safely without guidance from a healthcare provider.

Pharmaceutical companies spend an average of eight and a half years and more than $360 million in the development of a new drug. Although some OTC drugs are approved as such from the outset, most are introduced only in prescription form so that the FDA can monitor their safety more effectively. Later, the drug may switch to OTC status following review by a panel of experts, or after the FDA has evaluated additional information submitted by the drug's manufacturer.

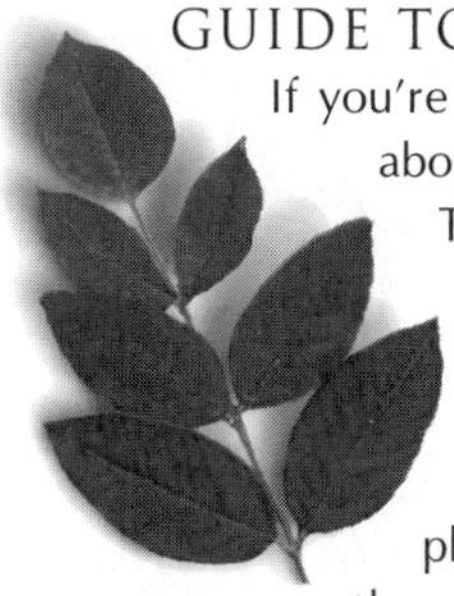

GUIDE TO NATURAL THERAPIES

If you're interested in trying an alternative remedy but first want to learn more about it, turn to the Guide to Natural Therapies, beginning on page 10. This guide offers a brief but detailed look at each of the six natural systems of medicine represented throughout the book: Aromatherapy, Chinese Medicine, Herbal Therapy, Homeopathy, Nutritional Supplements, and Vitamins and Minerals. You can quickly find out which remedies belong to a particular system of therapy by consulting the Alphabetical Index of Natural Remedies, which begins on page 834. All of the natural remedies covered in the book's main section are also listed here, grouped by therapy and accompanied by a list of their target ailments. Glancing through the index for Western herbs, for example, you'll see that chicory can be used to treat caffeine-induced rapid heartbeat, jaundice, and constipation, among other conditions.

GUIDE TO NATURAL THERAPIES

On the following pages you will find brief descriptions of the six forms of so-called natural therapies included in this book. Each of these introductions includes a general description of the therapy and the principles on which it is founded, followed by an explanation of the way each therapy's healing substances are prepared or applied. You should also take note of the Caution paragraph for each therapy. For the first four therapies, a separate box explains the licensing rules for practitioners and whether treatments are covered by insurance.

AROMATHERAPY

Aromatherapy is the therapeutic use of essential oils—concentrated, fragrant extracts of plants—to promote relaxation and help relieve various symptoms. Suppliers of aromatherapy oils extract them from specific parts of plants—the roots, bark, stalks, flowers, leaves, or fruit—by two methods: Distillation uses successive evaporation and condensation to pull the oils from the plants; cold-pressing squeezes rinds or peels through a machine to press out the oils. Users then administer the oils in several ways, generally by applying them to the skin or inhaling their scents.

Some practitioners believe the oils have both physical and ethereal (spiritual) qualities and effects. They assert that the oils work on the emotions because the nerves involved in the sense of smell are directly linked to the brain's limbic system, which governs emotion, and that the active components of the oils give them specific therapeutic value.

PREPARATIONS/TECHNIQUES

Essential oils may be applied externally and used in massage, or incorporated into compresses and ointments. They may also be inhaled or taken internally (orally, rectally, or vaginally). A common aromatherapy technique is to dilute the oils in a vegetable carrier oil, such as safflower or sweet almond oil, for an aromatherapy massage. Another way to use the oils is in an aromatic warm bath. You may also apply hot or cold compresses, creams, or lotions made from the oils directly to the skin.

CAUTION

Oils used in aromatherapy can have potentially serious side effects, including neurotoxicity and inducement of abortion as well as skin reactions, allergies, and liver damage. Overexposure to oils by inhalation can produce headache and fatigue. Consult a qualified healthcare practitioner before taking oils internally. Some oils, such as eucalyptus, lavender, myrrh, peppermint, and thyme, should never be taken internally.

LICENSED & INSURED?

Aromatherapy practitioners are not licensed in the United States today, although licensed healthcare providers may include aromatherapy as one of their techniques.

Chinese Medicine

Chinese medicine is an ancient system of healthcare that uses a variety of techniques, including herbal therapy, to treat disorders by restoring the balance of vital energies in the body. Unlike Western medicine, which tends to focus on specific parts of the body immediately affected by disease or injury, Chinese medicine takes a more global, holistic approach to healthcare, fashioning remedies to treat the entire body rather than just its component parts. Practitioners think of the human body not as a bundle of cells, bones, and tissues but rather as a complex system of interrelated processes. It is, they believe, a microcosm of the grand cosmic order, moved by the same rhythms and cycles that shape the natural world. At the core of Chinese medicine is the belief that disease is the result of disturbances in the flow of a bodily energy called chi or qi (pronounced "chee") or a lack of balance in the complementary states of yin (characterized by darkness and quiet) and yang (characterized by light and activity).

PREPARATIONS/TECHNIQUES

Chinese medicine recognizes more than 6,000 healing substances, although only a few hundred are currently in practical use. Herbs are grouped according to four basic properties, or "essences": hot, cold, warm, and cool. In general, practitioners choose plants for their ability to restore balance in individuals whose conditions are said to show signs of excessive heat or cold. Herbs are further categorized according to their "flavor": pungent, sour, sweet, bitter, or salty. An herb's taste indicates its action in the body, particularly on the movement and direction of chi.

Because many Chinese herbs work best when taken with others, practitioners almost always prescribe herbs in combination. Herbs are prepared in a variety of ways. Many are cooked and made into a soup or tea. In some cases the raw plants are ground into a powder, then combined with a binding agent and pressed into a pill. A number of herbs are cooked and processed into a powder and are then either mixed with warm water and swallowed or taken as capsules. Some herbs are made into pastes that are applied to the skin, while others are extracted in alcohol and used as tinctures.

CAUTION

Mixing herbs is an extremely tricky business. Certain Chinese herbs can be poisonous in large amounts, so you should always check with a qualified practitioner for the proper dosages. Some Chinese herbs, such as safflower flower, should be used with caution during pregnancy. Complex mixtures should be formulated only by a trained practitioner.

Licensed & Insured?

In the United States, practitioners of Chinese medicine usually operate under the title of "licensed" or "certified" acupuncturist. Few insurance providers reimburse patients for the cost of Chinese herbal treatments, although a number do cover acupuncture.

HERBAL THERAPY

Herbal medicines are prepared from a wide variety of plant materials—frequently the leaves, stems, roots, and bark but also the flowers, fruits, twigs, seeds, and exudates (material that oozes out, such as sap). They generally contain several biologically active ingredients and are used primarily for treating chronic or mild conditions, although on occasion they are employed as complementary or supportive therapy for acute and severe diseases.

Across the spectrum of alternative medicine, the use of herbs varies: Western herbology and Chinese medicine, for example, differ in the way practitioners diagnose diseases and prescribe herbal remedies. Naturopathic physicians, or those who use natural remedies rather than synthetic drugs, may use herbs from any of various systems. Entries in this book on herbs listed as Western herbs contain information based on Western herbological practices.

PREPARATIONS/TECHNIQUES

Herbs are available in various forms at health food stores and pharmacies, and many can be ordered by mail. Herbal remedies can be prepared at home in a variety of ways, using either fresh or dried ingredients. Herbal teas, or infusions, can be steeped to varying strengths. Roots, bark, or other plant parts can be simmered into strong solutions called decoctions. Honey or sugar can be added to infusions and decoctions to make syrups. You can also buy many herbal remedies over the counter in the form of pills, capsules, or powders, or in more concentrated liquid forms called extracts and tinctures. Certain herbs can be applied topically as creams or ointments, used as compresses, or applied directly to the skin as poultices.

CAUTION

Be especially careful when using herbs if you have allergies, are sensitive to drugs, are taking drugs for a chronic illness, or are younger than 12 or older than 65. To help minimize any adverse reactions, start with the lowest appropriate dose. Be aware that some herbs are toxic if taken incorrectly; comfrey, for example, can cause liver damage if taken in excessive amounts for too long a time.

In the United States today, herbal remedies are not regulated, and they come in unpredictable strengths because the amount of the active ingredients varies greatly. If you consistently develop nausea, diarrhea, or headache within two hours of taking an herb, discontinue its use immediately. Call your practitioner if the symptoms persist. Women who are pregnant or nursing are advised not to take medicinal amounts of herbs without first consulting a healthcare professional.

LICENSED & INSURED?

Naturopathic physicians are licensed on a state-by-state basis, and in some states their services are covered by medical insurance. However, clinical or medical herbalists are not licensed, and insurance companies usually do not provide coverage for their services.

Homeopathy

Homeopathy is a method of healing based on the idea that like cures like; that is, that substances causing specific symptoms in a healthy person can cure these symptoms in someone who is sick. Also called the law of similars, this principle gives homeopathy its name: "homeo" for similar, "pathy" for disease. The remedies are prepared from plant, mineral, and animal extracts that are highly diluted in a specific way that makes toxicity impossible and, paradoxically, is purported to increase their potential to cure.

Homeopathic treatment, in its principles and procedures, is unlike any other system of medical care. Although a few conventional therapies, such as allergy desensitization and immunization, involve the use of "similars" to some degree, modern medicine relies almost exclusively on counteracting substances; laxatives, for example, are medications that work to counteract constipation.

PREPARATIONS/TECHNIQUES

Remedies come in a variety of forms, including tablets, powders, wafers, and liquids in an alcohol base. Recently, over-the-counter combination remedies have become available for common ailments. These products, labeled according to the name of the ailment, allow self-treatment of such minor conditions as insomnia, flu, sore throat, and headache.

The specific dilution of a remedy is the ratio of active substance to inactive base. Ratios containing an *x* indicate that the remedy consists of 1 part mother tincture (concentrated extract) mixed with 9 parts water-and-alcohol base; ratios containing a *c* consist of 1 part mother tincture and 99 parts base. Further dilutions are represented by a number preceding the *x* or *c*. For example, a remedy labeled 30c has first been mixed 1 part to 99; then, 1 part of the resulting mixture is diluted again with 99 parts of the base, and this process is repeated for a total of 30 times. Modern over-the-counter remedies usually have dilution ratios ranging from 1x to 30c; remedies restricted to professional use generally range from 200c to 1,000,000c.

CAUTION

Although homeopathic remedies are too highly diluted to cause toxicity from overdose, taking them for too long a time can cause symptoms to worsen, and taking ones that are inappropriate may cause new symptoms to appear.

Licensed & Insured?

Licensing varies from state to state for homeopathic practitioners. The pharmaceuticals they prescribe are recognized and regulated by the FDA. Although many homeopathy products can be purchased over the counter, those offered for treating serious conditions must be dispensed under the supervision of a licensed practitioner.

Nutritional Supplements

Nutritional supplements are substances that are rich in essential nutrients or that contain ingredients helpful in the digestion or metabolism of food. In this book, the traditional definition of nutritional supplements as food or food by-products has been expanded to include a broader range of substances—such as hormones, amino acids, and plant or animal products—that are thought to provide certain health benefits.

Most people get all the nutrition they need from their diet. But sometimes the food we eat fails to deliver all the nutrients we require, perhaps as a result of disease, stress, poor eating habits, or a special medical condition. In such cases, supplements can help supply the missing ingredients and restore good health. Some of these products are taken for short periods to combat specific disorders. Others can be used long term—to ward off the effects of aging, for example, or to maintain good health and general wellness.

Because age impairs the body's ability to use nutrients effectively, the elderly often need to balance their diet with supplements. Other groups that may require supplemental nutrients include women who are pregnant, breast-feeding, or have excessive menstrual bleeding; heavy drinkers or smokers; strict vegetarians; and newborns.

PREPARATIONS/TECHNIQUES

Nutritional supplements are available in a variety of shapes and forms, including capsules, tablets, powders, liquids, flakes, gels, creams, wafers, and granules. Most are taken orally, although some are injected or applied to the skin. These products can be purchased at health food stores and at some pharmacies and grocery stores, or ordered through the mail. Potencies vary, and sometimes the potency is affected by temperature or the length of time the supplement sits on the shelf.

CAUTION

Some nutritional supplements can be poisonous if taken in large amounts. In other cases, excess amounts of one nutrient can actually reduce the body's supplies of another. Beware of combinations: Taken together, certain supplements can interact in the body and cause harmful effects. Because the quality of these products may vary considerably, you should always buy from a reputable source.

Be very skeptical of "miracle cures" and other wild claims about the effectiveness of nutritional supplements. Find out all you can about the product before using it, and remember that nothing takes the place of a balanced diet. You should also be aware that the efficacy and safety of some supplements listed in this book—such as EDTA, a synthetic amino acid used in chelation therapy—are under intense debate. Always consult a qualified practitioner before using any nutritional supplement.

VITAMINS AND MINERALS

A balanced diet is an essential part of a healthy lifestyle. Your body requires more than 40 nutrients for energy, growth, and tissue maintenance. In addition to carbohydrates, proteins, fats, and dietary fiber, the food you eat supplies the important micronutrients we call vitamins and minerals. They are needed only in trace amounts, but the absence or deficiency of just one vitamin or mineral can cause major illness.

Vitamin and mineral supplements figure in the dietary recommendations of many therapies. Although some vitamins, such as A and D, are fat soluble and can reach toxic levels in the body if they are not carefully monitored, others, such as vitamin C, are water soluble and are not stored; any bodily excess is usually excreted. Generally, vitamins and minerals are recommended for daily use as a preventive measure only, but some healthcare practitioners also suggest them as a treatment for specific ailments. Some such treatments are considered controversial, so it's best to check with your own practitioner.

PREPARATIONS/TECHNIQUES

Vitamin and mineral supplements often come in tablet form. Doses are measured by weight in milligrams (mg), or thousandths of a gram; in micrograms (mcg), or millionths of a gram; or in a universal standard known as international units (IU). The Food and Nutrition Board of the National Research Council, National Academy of Sciences, has determined a recommended dietary allowance (RDA)—also known as the recommended daily allowance—for many vitamins and minerals. Essential nutrients that do not yet have RDAs are assigned a safe and adequate daily intake or an estimated minimum daily requirement (EMDR). These values are listed in the vitamins and minerals entries in this book.

CAUTION

Always take supplements in moderation; they are safe in doses at or below RDAs, but higher doses may be harmful and should be taken only under the guidance of a doctor or registered dietitian. Be particularly cautious about fat-soluble vitamins such as A and D, excesses of which are harder for the body to handle.

A-Z GUIDE TO

DRUGS & NATURAL MEDICINES

ACARBOSE

A

VITAL STATISTICS

DRUG CLASS
Antidiabetic Drugs

BRAND NAME
Precose

OTHER DRUGS IN THIS CLASS
glipizide, glyburide, insulin, metformin, troglitazone

GENERAL DESCRIPTION
Acarbose is used to treat excess blood sugar in people with non-insulin-dependent diabetes when diet, weight loss, and exercise do not produce sufficient control but insulin is not required. It helps to lower blood sugar but does not cure diabetes.

Introduced in 1996, acarbose is different from other diabetes medications in that it doesn't enhance insulin production or the body's sensitivity to insulin. Rather, it acts by inhibiting the digestion and absorption of dietary sugars (carbohydrates).

Acarbose can be combined with a sulfonylurea drug for more effective blood sugar control.

PRECAUTIONS

WARNING
Acarbose, when used in combination with other antidiabetes agents, can cause symptoms of hypoglycemia, or low blood sugar (unusual weakness, shakiness, stomach pain, nausea or excessive hunger, rapid heartbeat, cold sweats or chills, confusion, anxiety, convulsions, unconsciousness).

For mild symptoms of hypoglycemia, consume something that contains dextrose—not sucrose (table sugar) because of the way the drug acts on it—as soon as possible. For more severe symptoms, contact a poison control center or seek emergency care immediately.

Make sure that you can recognize the symptoms of hypoglycemia before you begin to take a combination of this drug and any other antidiabetes drug. Ask your doctor if you aren't confident.

Avoid driving and other dangerous activities until you see how the drug affects you. Caution is also advised if you participate in heavy exercise, as the blood sugar necessary for the effort may not be present. Consult your doctor.

SPECIAL INFORMATION
- Consult your doctor before beginning to take acarbose if you are allergic to it or to anything else, if you have a chronic health problem, other than diabetes, including kidney or liver dysfunction or any heart or circulatory disease, if you have a history of intestinal disorders, or if you are planning to have surgery under general anesthesia.
- Some weeks may be needed to assess the effectiveness and correct dosage level of acarbose.

ACARBOSE

- Take this medicine at each main meal, after the first bite has been eaten, three times a day. Regular use is essential to help control diabetes, which is a chronic condition.
- The common gastrointestinal side effects of acarbose will often lessen over time and may be limited by lowering dietary sucrose.
- If you develop an illness or infection, undergo surgery, or experience physical trauma, contact your doctor. You may need a temporary change of medication.
- Pregnant women should consult with a physician and decide if the drug's benefits justify the risks to the unborn child. There is no information on the use of acarbose during pregnancy, and insulin is usually used if blood sugar control is required during gestation.
- Acarbose is not recommended for nursing mothers; no data on safety exist.
- The safety and effectiveness of acarbose has not been established for children under 18.
- Diabetes and its treatment are complex, requiring patient participation as well as periodic monitoring. Consult with your doctor regularly to determine the continuing effectiveness and safety of treatment.
- Acarbose may interfere with some lab tests. Inform any practitioner you consult that you are taking this drug.
- It is advisable for you to wear medical identification containing the information that you take acarbose for diabetes management.

TARGET AILMENTS

Diabetes

POSSIBLE INTERACTIONS

Alcohol: no expected interaction with acarbose, but if you also take a sulfonylurea, increased risk of hypoglycemia.

Amylase, beta blockers, bumetanide, calcium channel blockers, corticosteroids, estrogens, furosemide, isoniazid, nicotinic acid, pancreatin, phenothiazines, phenytoin, rifampin, sympathomimetics, theophylline, thiazide diuretics, thyroid hormones: decreased effect of acarbose.

Charcoal, activated, and other intestinal adsorbents: decreased effect of acarbose.

Clofibrate, disopyramide, sulfonamide antibiotics: increased risk of hypoglycemia.

Hyperglycemia-causing medications: increased risk of hyperglycemia.

Metformin: decreased effect of acarbose; increased risk of side effects.

SIDE EFFECTS

NOT SERIOUS

- Gas
- Bloating
- Diarrhea
- Nausea
- Stomach cramps
- Skin rash or itching

CALL YOUR DOCTOR IF THESE EFFECTS PERSIST OR BECOME TROUBLESOME.

SERIOUS

- Yellow eyes or skin (jaundice)

DISCONTINUE USE AND CALL YOUR DOCTOR IMMEDIATELY.

ACCUPRIL

VITAL STATISTICS

DRUG CLASS
Angiotensin-Converting Enzyme (ACE) Inhibitors

GENERIC NAME
quinapril

OTHER DRUGS IN THIS CLASS
benazepril, captopril, enalapril, fosinopril, lisinopril, ramipril

GENERAL DESCRIPTION
Accupril is the brand-name form of the generic drug quinapril, which is prescribed for mild-to-moderate high blood pressure and for congestive heart failure. Like other ACE inhibitors, this drug blocks a body enzyme needed for the production of a substance that causes blood vessels to constrict. As a result, it relaxes the artery walls, thereby lowering blood pressure. For further information, see Angiotensin-Converting Enzyme (ACE) Inhibitors. For visual characteristics, see the Color Guide to Prescription Drugs and Herbs.

PRECAUTIONS

WARNING
Get medical attention immediately if you notice swelling of the face, tongue, or vocal cords or have difficulty swallowing or breathing; this reaction can be life threatening.

This drug should not be taken during pregnancy; it has been associated with death of the fetus and the newborn.

SPECIAL INFORMATION
- Accupril causes an increase in blood levels of potassium. Do not use potassium-rich products, including salt substitutes and low-salt milk, without consulting your doctor. The potassium in your blood could rise to dangerous levels, leading to heart-rhythm problems.
- Do not stop taking this medication abruptly. Your doctor may tell you to reduce the dosage gradually.
- Accupril's high magnesium content may reduce the body's absorption of drugs interacting with magnesium.
- Use caution during hot weather or while exercising; excessive perspiration can lead to dehydration and reduced blood pressure in people taking ACE inhibitors.
- Let your doctor know if you have arthritis or kidney disease, or if you are on a strict low-sodium diet or are taking diuretics.

Accupril

POSSIBLE INTERACTIONS

Alcohol: increased ACE inhibitor effects, leading to much lower blood pressure.

Central nervous system stimulants (including pseudoephedrine, an over-the-counter decongestant): reduced ACE inhibitor effect.

Diuretics: combining these drugs may initially cause a significant drop in blood pressure.

Drugs that interact with magnesium, such as tetracycline and diuretics: because of its high magnesium content, Accupril may reduce the body's absorption of these medications.

Estrogens: fluid retention, possibly raising blood pressure.

Lithium: lithium toxicity, which can lead to stupor, coma, and seizures.

Other medications that lower blood pressure, such as beta-adrenergic blockers, calcium channel blockers, diuretics, levodopa, nitrates, and opioid analgesics: increased hypotensive (blood-pressure-lowering) effect of both combined medications.

Potassium products and diuretics that do not eliminate potassium from the body (such as amiloride, spironolactone, and triamterene): increased blood potassium levels, leading to heart-rhythm problems.

TARGET AILMENTS

High blood pressure

Sometimes congestive heart failure (in conjunction with digitalis preparations and diuretics)

SIDE EFFECTS

NOT SERIOUS

- Dry, persistent cough; fatigue; nausea; diarrhea; temporary skin rash; low blood pressure; dizziness on suddenly rising or changing position

CALL YOUR DOCTOR IF THESE EFFECTS BECOME BOTHERSOME.

SERIOUS

- Fainting; persistent skin rash; joint pain; drowsiness; numbness and tingling; abdominal pain; vomiting; severe diarrhea; signs of infection; chest pain; heart palpitation; jaundice (yellowing of skin or eyes)

CALL YOUR DOCTOR RIGHT AWAY. GET MEDICAL ATTENTION IMMEDIATELY IF YOU NOTICE SWELLING OF YOUR FACE, TONGUE, OR VOCAL CORDS OR HAVE DIFFICULTY SWALLOWING OR BREATHING; THIS REACTION CAN BE LIFE THREATENING.

ACETAMINOPHEN

A

VITAL STATISTICS

DRUG CLASS
Analgesics

BRAND NAMES
Acetaminophen-only brands: Tylenol, Tylenol Extra Strength
Acetaminophen-containing combinations for colds: Chlor-Trimeton Allergy-Sinus Headache Caplets, Comtrex, Contac, Drixoral, TheraFlu, Triaminic Sore Throat Formula, Tylenol in various forms, Vicks DayQuil Liquid or LiquiCaps, Vicks NyQuil
Combinations for pain: Excedrin Extra-Strength, Tylenol in various forms
Combinations for sinus problems: Sinutab
Combinations for sleep: Excedrin PM

OTHER DRUGS IN THIS CLASS
aspirin, caffeine (as an adjunct treatment), methyl salicylate, nonsteroidal anti-inflammatory drugs (NSAIDs), opioid analgesics

GENERAL DESCRIPTION
A pain reliever as well as a fever reducer, acetaminophen is a good alternative to aspirin, particularly for people who are allergic to aspirin. One drawback is that acetaminophen does not reduce inflammation, so it is not effective for such conditions as swelling, redness, or menstrual cramps. If you seek relief from inflammation, try aspirin or a nonsteroidal anti-inflammatory drug.

For the visual characteristics of acetaminophen with codeine, a prescription drug, see the Color Guide to Prescription Drugs and Herbs.

PRECAUTIONS

SPECIAL INFORMATION
- Acetaminophen can cause or exacerbate liver problems, so you should avoid alcoholic beverages when taking this drug. If you are too sick to eat, even moderate overdoses of acetaminophen can cause serious liver damage, possibly leading to convulsions, coma, and death. If you already have liver disease, use acetaminophen with caution, preferably under a doctor's supervision.
- Don't take more than the recommended dose. Persistent pain or high fever may indicate serious illness. If pain persists for more than 10 days or fever lasts for three days, contact your physician.
- If an overdose occurs, seek emergency help. Possible symptoms of overdose include nausea, vomiting, increased sweating, loss of appetite, and abdominal pain, although in some cases there are no symptoms. Treatment must start within 24 hours to prevent severe liver (and possible kidney) damage.
- To avoid involuntary overdose, be careful when combining this drug with other medications that contain acetaminophen. Read labels carefully.

ACETAMINOPHEN

A

POSSIBLE INTERACTIONS

Alcohol: risk of liver damage.

Anticoagulants (oral): if acetaminophen is taken regularly and in high doses, this combination can lead to an increased anticoagulant effect.

Aspartame: possibly hazardous for phenylketonuria patients.

Aspirin: risk of increased side effects of both drugs when combination is taken over a long period.

Barbiturates (except butalbital): reduced acetaminophen effect. Taking too much acetaminophen in combination with barbiturates also increases the risk of liver damage.

Isoniazid: risk of liver damage.

Nonsteroidal anti-inflammatory drugs (NSAIDs): risk of increased side effects of either drug when combination is taken over a long period.

Zidovudine (AZT): increased blood levels of zidovudine and risk of serious side effects.

TARGET AILMENTS

Fever

Headaches, muscle aches, pain, or injuries

SIDE EFFECTS

SERIOUS

- Hypersensitivity reaction (rash, hives, itching)
- Kidney damage (lower-back pain, sudden reduction in urine output)
- Liver damage (pain or swelling in the upper abdominal area) or hepatitis (jaundice)
- Blood disorder (unusual sore throat or fever)
- Anemia (unusual fatigue)
- Platelet disorder (unusual bruising or bleeding; black, tarry stools; bloody or cloudy urine)

(RARE, IF TAKEN IN RECOMMENDED DOSES): IF YOU NOTICE ANY OF THESE SYMPTOMS, DISCONTINUE USE AND CALL YOUR DOCTOR IMMEDIATELY.

ACONITE

LATIN NAME
Aconitum napellus

A

VITAL STATISTICS

GENERAL DESCRIPTION

Native to the mountainous regions of Europe, Russia, and central Asia, aconite has flowers that look like monks' cowls, giving it its common name, monkshood. It was the preferred poison of the ancient Greeks because it is highly toxic. Given in very small doses, it produces mental and physical restlessness and tissue inflammation. Thus, homeopathic physicians prescribe *Aconite* for patients who seem distressed or fearful and complain of thirst and unbearable aches and pains.

For homeopathic use, the whole plant—except the root, which is the most poisonous part—is gathered in full bloom and pounded to a pulp. Juice from the pulp is mixed with alcohol and diluted. When a patient exhibits a set of symptoms that matches the cataloged symptoms brought on by *Aconite,* the homeopathic practitioner then prescribes it in an extremely dilute form. For more information on homeopathic medicine, see page 14.

PREPARATIONS

Aconite is available in various potencies at selected stores and pharmacies. Consult your practitioner for more precise information.

PRECAUTIONS

SPECIAL INFORMATION

- Only the patient should touch the pills. Any spilled tablets should be thrown away.
- The mouth should be clear of flavors 15 minutes before and after taking a remedy, and strong flavors and aromas, such as coffee and heavy perfume, should be avoided for the duration of treatment.

TARGET AILMENTS

- Angina
- Arrhythmia
- Anxiety induced by sudden shock
- Arthritis
- Asthma
- Bronchitis
- Colds and flu
- Croup
- Fevers with rapid onset and chills that may be accompanied by restlessness or thirst
- Eye inflammations with burning pain and sensitivity to light
- Laryngitis
- Sore throat
- Middle ear infections
- Toothaches with a sensitivity to cold water

SIDE EFFECTS

NONE EXPECTED

ACYCLOVIR

A

VITAL STATISTICS

DRUG CLASS
Antiviral Drugs

BRAND NAME
Zovirax

OTHER DRUGS IN THIS CLASS
valacyclovir

GENERAL DESCRIPTION
Introduced in 1979, acyclovir is an antiviral drug used to treat various types of herpes, shingles, and chickenpox infections. It is also used to fight other viral diseases, including mononucleosis and the Epstein-Barr virus.

Acyclovir hinders viral reproduction by inhibiting the expression of genetic material (DNA) in the virus and in infected cells, thus slowing or stopping the organism's spread. Acyclovir may be used in tablet or topical form, depending on the ailment and the patient's condition.

For visual characteristics, see the Color Guide to Prescription Drugs and Herbs.

PRECAUTIONS

SPECIAL INFORMATION
Use caution when taking acyclovir if you are pregnant or are breast-feeding. Although no adverse effects are known to have resulted from its use in such cases, the drug can cross the placenta and affect the fetus, and it can pass to nursing infants through breast milk.

POSSIBLE INTERACTIONS
Zidovudine (AZT): increased toxicity; profound drowsiness and lethargy.

TARGET AILMENTS

Genital herpes

Herpes simplex

Herpes simplex in patients with compromised immune systems (people with cancer or HIV, for example)

Chickenpox in patients with compromised immune systems

Shingles in patients with compromised immune systems

Herpes simplex encephalitis (brain infection)

SIDE EFFECTS

NOT SERIOUS

- Gastrointestinal upsets (such as nausea)
- Lightheadedness
- Headache
- Mild burning, stinging, itching, or skin rash (topical preparation)

CALL YOUR DOCTOR IF THESE SYMPTOMS PERSIST OR BECOME BOTHERSOME.

SERIOUS

NONE EXPECTED FOR SHORT-TERM TREATMENT OUTSIDE A HOSPITAL SETTING.

AGASTACHE

LATIN NAME
Agastache rugosa

VITAL STATISTICS

GENERAL DESCRIPTION

The leaves, stems, and flowers of agastache are most often used to treat disorders that affect the digestive tract. This plant is also known as patchouli or pogostemon. An aromatic herb grown throughout China, agastache is classified in Chinese herbal medicine as acrid and slightly warm. Harvested in June and July, the best-quality agastache has many soft, thick, and fragrant leaves.

Chinese medicine takes a holistic approach to healthcare, fashioning remedies to treat the entire being as well as the specific parts or areas. Single herbs may be used alone or in combination with other herbs to prevent and combat disease, which is thought to arise from disturbances in the flow of a bodily energy called chi (pronounced "chee") and blood, or from a lack of balance in the complementary states of yin and yang.

TARGET AILMENTS
Take internally for:
Nausea and vomiting
Diarrhea and dysentery
Morning sickness
Swelling of the abdomen
Reduced appetite
Colds without fever

PREPARATIONS

Agastache is available in Chinese pharmacies, Asian markets, and Western health food stores, where it is in the form of dried leaves or powder.

COMBINATIONS: The herb, appearing in several preparations with other Chinese herbs, should not be cooked for more than 15 minutes or it will lose its fragrant quality. In combination with pinellia and atractylodes (black), it may be prescribed for nausea and vomiting, bloating of the chest and abdomen, reduced appetite, and diarrhea. A mixture of agastache with coptis and bamboo shavings is used by Chinese herbalists for certain types of vomiting. Practitioners of Chinese medicine also recommend agastache together with grains-of-paradise fruit for morning sickness. Consult a Chinese medicine practitioner for information on dosages and additional herbal combinations.

PRECAUTIONS

WARNING

Do not use agastache when there are what Chinese medicine calls heat signs. These include symptoms such as fever, thirst, and sweating.

SIDE EFFECTS

NONE EXPECTED

AIDS Treatment

Vital Statistics

GENERIC NAMES

Reverse transcriptase inhibitors: cidofovir, didanosine, lamivudine, nevirapine, stavudine, zalcitabine, zidovudine

Protease inhibitors: indinavir, ritonavir, saquinavir

GENERAL DESCRIPTION

These powerful antiviral drugs are used singly and in combination to treat people who are infected with the human immunodeficiency virus (HIV), which causes acquired immunodeficiency syndrome (AIDS). HIV damages the body's ability to produce adequate numbers of the white blood cells called T cells, leaving the immune system unable to fight off invading bacteria or viruses. Eventually, a severely impaired immune system leaves the AIDS sufferer highly susceptible to a whole host of infections and diseases.

Antiviral drugs work to slow down the virus by inhibiting its ability to propagate itself. Reverse transcriptase inhibitors act by restricting the ability of the virus to make copies of itself; protease inhibitors interfere with the proper production of proteins required for the infection of new cells.

None of these drugs will cure AIDS or rid the body of HIV, but they may help stave off the worst symptoms of disease for several years in some people.

A problem with this group of drugs is that the virus often becomes resistant to them within a few years. Also, they can cause serious side effects. Switching from one type of drug to another may help temporarily, but combining drugs is often the most helpful form of treatment. Two reverse transcriptase inhibitors are often combined, with the addition of a protease inhibitor. The drugs may later be given in different combinations, with substitution of one or more, as resistance develops. Protease inhibitors are often active against strains of HIV that become resistant to reverse transcriptase inhibitors.

The best-tolerated of the reverse transcriptase inhibitors is lamivudine; the best-tolerated protease inhibitor is saquinavir.

Among these drugs, zidovudine and lamivudine have shown some effect on viruses other than HIV and on some bacteria as well. Researchers don't yet know if this is clinically significant.

Precautions

WARNING

An overdose of these drugs can be dangerous, causing seizures, loss of coordination, severe nausea and vomiting, or extreme weakness. Contact a poison control center or seek emergency treatment if you have taken more than the prescribed amount.

These drugs can cause dizziness or drowsiness and can impair your ability to concentrate; restrict your activities as necessary and do not drive or operate machinery until you know how these medications affect you. Be especially careful if you take other drugs that have similar effects, such as alcohol, opioid analgesics, or tranquilizers.

Using any of these drugs does not lower the risk of transmitting human immunodeficiency virus to other people through blood contamination or sexual contact. Appropriate precautions must be taken to avoid spreading HIV.

CONTINUED

AIDS Treatment

A

SPECIAL INFORMATION

- Inform your doctor before taking any of these drugs if you are allergic to AIDS/HIV antivirals; if you are currently taking drugs that depress bone marrow or have compromised bone marrow function; if you have a history of alcoholism, folic acid or vitamin B_{12} deficiency, liver or kidney disease, peripheral neuropathy, pancreatitis, phenylketonuria, anemia, gout, or hypertriglyceridemia; or if you restrict sodium intake for any reason.
- The safety and effectiveness of these drugs is still being studied, and their long-term consequences are unknown. They may neither slow the progression of the disease nor prevent other diseases or opportunistic infections. In fact, they may lead to serious disorders such as anemia. Discuss possible benefits and side effects with your physician.
- Take these drugs exactly as prescribed; doses and schedules are usually individualized. Some of these drugs should be taken on an empty stomach; others, with food. Consult your doctor or pharmacist, and make sure that you understand the instructions.
- It is essential that your doctor regularly monitor you while you are taking any of these medications.
- Consult your doctor before you discontinue these drugs, especially if you have been taking them for a long time. They may require gradual reduction, and dosages of your other medications might need adjustment.
- If drugs in this group are combined for treatment, the risk of side effects is increased. Also, the seriousness and frequency of side effects are greater in people with more advanced infection.
- There are many potential interactions between drugs in this group and other medications, both prescription and over-the-counter. The interactions between them also vary. Consult your doctor before taking any other drug while you are undergoing therapy with these antivirals.
- Some of these drugs affect laboratory tests. Inform any doctor you consult that you are taking them.
- If you are pregnant, consult your doctor about possible benefits and risks of these drugs. Zidovudine (AZT) reduces the risk of HIV transference from mother to baby.
- The U.S. Centers for Disease Control and Prevention cautions that women who are infected with HIV should not breast-feed because of the possibility of transferring the virus to the baby.
- When these drugs are used for a child, there is a risk of retinal depigmentation. The patient should be monitored for vision changes.

TARGET AILMENTS
HIV infection
AIDS
HIV prevention in unborn children of pregnant women with AIDS or HIV

POSSIBLE INTERACTIONS

REVERSE TRANSCRIPTASE INHIBITORS INTERACTIONS

Acetaminophen, acyclovir, amphotericin B, aspirin, benzodiazepines, cimetidine, fluconazole, ganciclovir, interferon beta, morphine, NSAIDs, probenecid, ribavirin, sulfonamides: increased risk of zidovudine or zalcitabine toxicity.

Alcohol: increased risk of pancreatitis or peripheral neuropathy.

Amphotericin, foscarnet, aminoglycosides: increased risk of peripheral neuropathy when taken with zalcitabine.

Antacids containing aluminum or magnesium: decreased effect of zalcitabine and didanosine.

Asparaginase, azathioprine, estrogens, furosemide, methyldopa, nitrofurantoin, pentamidine (IV), sulfonamides, sulindac, tetracyclines, thiazide diuretics, valproic acid: increased risk of pancreatitis when taken with didanosine.

Blood medications (for leukemia, hemophilia), bone marrow medications, radiation therapy: bone marrow suppression, resulting in fewer blood cells and platelets, when taken with zidovudine.

Chloramphenicol, cisplatin, dapsone, disulfiram, ethambutol, ethionamide, glytethimide, gold, hydralazine, iodoquinol, isoniazid, lithium, metronidazole, nitrofurantoin, nitrous oxide, phenytoin, ribavirin, stavudine, vincristine, zalcitabine: increased risk of peripheral neuropathy when taken with didanosine or zalcitabine.

Cimetidine: increased effects of zalcitabine and zidovudine.

Clarithromycin: decreased effects of zidovudine.

Contraceptives, oral: combining with nevirapine may decrease the effectiveness of oral contraceptives.

Dapsone, itraconazole, ketoconazole: reduced

SIDE EFFECTS

NOT SERIOUS

REVERSE TRANSCRIPTASE INHIBITORS:

- Indigestion; constipation; diarrhea; nausea
- Headache (mild or severe); dizziness; drowsiness
- Anxiety; restlessness
- Muscle aches
- Mild allergic reactions (fever, sweating, pricking, tingling, or itching sensations)

PROTEASE INHIBITORS:

- Indigestion; constipation; diarrhea; nausea; abdominal pain; vomiting; loss of appetite; altered sense of taste
- Weakness or lack of energy

SERIOUS

THIS IS A GENERAL LIST COVERING MANY DRUGS. CONSULT YOUR DOCTOR ABOUT THE REACTIONS YOU MIGHT EXPECT AND ABOUT ANY SYMPTOMS YOU FIND TROUBLESOME. SOME OF THESE EFFECTS MAY ALSO BE CAUSED BY HIV ITSELF OR OTHER INFECTIONS.

REVERSE TRANSCRIPTASE INHIBITORS:

- Pancreatitis (abdominal pain, nausea, and vomiting)
- Difficulty breathing
- Cardiomyopathy (swollen feet or lower legs, shortness of breath)

CONTINUED

CONTINUED

AIDS TREATMENT

A

SIDE EFFECTS

CONTINUED

- Severe rash or rash with fever, blistering, swelling, muscle or joint aches, malaise, lesions in the mouth, or conjunctivitis
- Bone marrow depression (fatigue, weakness, fever, sore throat, abnormal bleeding or bruising)
- Seizures
- Anemia
- Vision problems, retinal depigmentation
- Extreme weakness, fatigue, loss of coordination, loss of speech, confusion, mania, or mood swings
- Tremors, twitching, involuntary movement of eyes
- Yellow skin and eyes
- Pale skin
- Muscle or joint pain

PROTEASE INHIBITORS:

- Peripheral neuropathy (numbness, tingling, pain, or burning in hands, wrists, feet, or ankles)
- Extreme nausea, vomiting, or diarrhea
- Mouth or throat sores; esophageal ulcers
- Kidney stones

CALL YOUR DOCTOR IMMEDIATELY IF YOU NOTICE ANY OF THESE SYMPTOMS.

absorption of these drugs.

Fluoroquinolones and tetracyclines: decreased effect of antibiotic.

Ganciclovir: increased risk of toxicity of both.

Phenytoin: risk of seizures with zidovudine.

Rifampin, rifabutin: decreased concentrations of zidovudine.

Trimetrexate: risk of toxicity with zidovudine.

PROTEASE INHIBITORS INTERACTIONS

Alcohol: increased risk of pancreatitis or peripheral neuropathy.

Alprazolam, amiodarone, astemizole, bepridil, bupropion, cisapride, clorazepate, clozapine, diazepam, encainide, estazolam, flecainide, flurazepam, meperidine, midazolam, piroxicam, propafenone, propoxyphene, quinidine, rifabutin, terfenadine, triazolam, zolpidem: ritonavir and saquinavir can increase the effects of these drugs, possibly causing adverse effects such as heart arrhythmias, seizures, or respiratory depression.

Carbamazepine, dexamethasone, phenobarbital, phenytoin, rifabutin, rifampin, tobacco (smoking): reduced concentrations of ritonavir.

Clarithromycin: increased concentrations of clarithromycin when taken with ritonavir.

Desipramine: increased concentration when taken with ritonavir.

Rifampin, rifabutin: decreased concentrations of ritonavir and saquinavir.

Terfenadine, astemizole, cisapride: possibly higher concentrations of these drugs when taken with saquinavir.

Theophylline: reduced concentration when taken with ritonavir.

Rx ALBUTEROL

VITAL STATISTICS

DRUG CLASS
Bronchodilators

BRAND NAMES
Proventil, Proventil HFA, Ventolin

OTHER DRUGS IN THIS CLASS
Rx: epinephrine, ipratropium, salmeterol, terbutaline, theophylline
OTC: ephedrine, epinephrine, theophylline

GENERAL DESCRIPTION
Albuterol, an antiasthmatic drug that acts by relaxing the muscles surrounding the bronchial tubes, is commonly prescribed for symptoms of acute bronchial asthma. The drug is also used to reduce the frequency and severity of recurrent asthma attacks and exercise-induced bronchospasms. Albuterol is available as an inhalant and in syrup and tablet form. For more information, see Bronchodilators.

PRECAUTIONS

WARNING
Your body can build up tolerance to bronchodilator inhalants, causing them to become less effective. If this happens, discontinue the drug and tell your doctor. Do not increase the dose. Increasing the dose can lead to serious, perhaps fatal bronchial constriction. Overuse of albuterol can cause heart-rhythm irregularities.

SPECIAL INFORMATION
- Before you use albuterol, tell your doctor if you have cardiovascular disease, narrow-angle glaucoma, prostatic hypertrophy, or difficulty urinating.
- Women who are pregnant or breast-feeding should consult a doctor before using a bronchodilator.

POSSIBLE INTERACTIONS
Beta-adrenergic blockers: decreased effects of both drugs.
See Bronchodilators for other interactions.

TARGET AILMENTS

Bronchial asthma

Exercise-induced bronchospasms

SIDE EFFECTS

NOT SERIOUS
- Mild nausea or weakness
- Nervousness, restlessness, or insomnia

CALL YOUR DOCTOR IF THESE EFFECTS BECOME BOTHERSOME.

SERIOUS
- Changes in blood pressure or heartbeat (irregular or pounding, for example)
- Trembling; anxiety
- Breathing problems
- Dizziness; lightheadedness
- Muscle cramps
- Nausea or vomiting
- Chest pain or discomfort (rare)

LET YOUR DOCTOR KNOW RIGHT AWAY IF YOU EXPERIENCE THESE SIDE EFFECTS.

ALENDRONATE

VITAL STATISTICS

DRUG CLASS
Osteoporosis Treatment

BRAND NAME
Fosamax

OTHER DRUGS IN THIS CLASS
calcitonin

GENERAL DESCRIPTION
Alendronate slows the loss of bone tissue and helps increase bone mass in women who have postmenopausal osteoporosis, a progressive disease in which loss of bone outstrips formation of new bone. Osteoporosis can lead to bone fractures, which can be very serious in older people; taking alendronate can decrease the risk of fractures.

Alendronate can be used to treat women for whom estrogen replacement therapy is inappropriate. In addition to medication, intake of adequate calcium and vitamin D and weight-bearing exercise are essential to preventing bone loss. Your doctor may recommend supplements and a program of exercise. Alendronate is also used to treat Paget's disease, a serious bone disorder.

PRECAUTIONS

WARNING
You should not take this drug if you have hypocalcemia (abnormally low blood levels of calcium), esophageal abnormalities, or a serious kidney disease. Patients with mild to moderate kidney disease can use alendronate. Consult your doctor.

SPECIAL INFORMATION
- Notify your doctor if you have an allergy to alendronate, if you have ulcers or another gastrointestinal problem, or if you have difficulty swallowing before starting to take alendronate.
- You may have to take alendronate for six months or longer before seeing results.
- Take alendronate at the same time every day. If you miss a dose, simply resume your schedule the following day; do not double the dose.
- Swallow alendronate with six to eight ounces of water. To avoid throat irritation and ulceration, don't lie down for at least 30 minutes after you take it. Take alendronate with plain water only; it is extremely important to wait at least 30 minutes before ingesting any other liquids, medicines, or food, any of which can interfere with the body's absorption of alendronate and may irritate the throat. Waiting longer than 30 minutes before eating or drinking will improve the absorption of alendronate.

- Alendronate may affect medical tests; notify any doctor or dentist that you are taking this medicine.
- Alendronate is not normally used or recommended for premenopausal women or for children. It should not be used during pregnancy or by breast-feeding mothers.
- Talk to your doctor before you stop taking alendronate.

POSSIBLE INTERACTIONS

Antacids: antacids can decrease the absorption of alendronate by the body. Take antacids at least 30 minutes after a dose of alendronate.

Aspirin and other salicylates: taken with alendronate, these drugs can increase the risk of stomach irritation.

Calcium supplements: can interfere with the body's absorption of alendronate and should be taken at least 30 minutes after taking alendronate.

Estrogen replacement therapy: the effect of combining alendronate with estrogen therapy is not known; their combination is not recommended.

Vitamin supplements: these can interfere with the absorption of alendronate by the body and should be taken at least 30 minutes after taking alendronate.

TARGET AILMENTS

Osteoporosis

Paget's disease

SIDE EFFECTS

NOT SERIOUS

- Nausea, constipation, diarrhea, gas, or a bloated feeling
- Headache

CALL YOUR DOCTOR IF THESE SYMPTOMS PERSIST.

SERIOUS

- Abdominal pain
- Heartburn
- Irritation, pain, or ulceration of the esophagus
- Difficulty swallowing
- Muscle pain
- Skin rash

CONSULT YOUR DOCTOR IF YOU NOTICE ANY OF THESE SYMPTOMS.

ALFALFA

LATIN NAME
Medicago sativa

VITAL STATISTICS

GENERAL DESCRIPTION

The alfalfa plant is considered a nutritional supplement and a body cleanser. Its leaves are thought to nourish the body by stimulating the appetite, acting as a laxative and diuretic, and providing such nutrients as fiber, protein, calcium, and vitamin A (beta carotene). For visual characteristics, see the Color Guide to Prescription Drugs and Herbs.

PREPARATIONS

Over the counter:

Available as tincture, prepared tea, capsules, dried leaves, powder extract, or sprouts.

At home:

TEA: Steep covered 1 to 2 tsp dried leaves per 1 cup water 5 to 10 minutes. Drink 3 cups a day or consult a practitioner for dosage.

NUTRITION AND DIET: Add sprouts or powdered alfalfa to soups, salads, or sandwiches.

Consult a qualified practitioner for the dosage appropriate for your specific condition.

TARGET AILMENTS

Inflammation of the bladder; bloating or water retention; indigestion; constipation; halitosis

SIDE EFFECTS

NOT SERIOUS

- Stomach upset; diarrhea

STOP USING AND CONSULT YOUR PRACTITIONER.

PRECAUTIONS

WARNING

Avoid eating alfalfa seeds; they contain relatively high levels of the toxic amino acid canavanine. Ingesting large quantities of alfalfa seeds over a long period of time may lead to pancytopenia, a blood disorder that causes the deterioration of both platelets, responsible for blood clotting, and white blood cells, which fight infections.

SPECIAL INFORMATION

- Alfalfa contains saponins, chemicals thought to destroy red blood cells. Consequently, anyone suffering from anemia should use alfalfa only under the direction of an herbalist or a licensed healthcare professional.
- If you are pregnant, check with a practitioner before ingesting this herb. Alfalfa seeds contain stachydrine and homostachydrine, which promote menstruation and in some cases can lead to miscarriage.
- If you have a predisposition to systemic lupus erythematosus, use this herb only in consultation with an herbalist or a healthcare professional. The canavanine in alfalfa is believed to reactivate this disease in some people who are in remission.
- Although scientists have found no direct evidence, some herbalists believe, on the basis of animal studies, that alfalfa can help the body ward off heart disease and strokes by delaying the absorption of cholesterol and dissolving plaque deposits on the arterial walls.

POSSIBLE INTERACTIONS

Combining alfalfa with other herbs may necessitate a lower dosage.

ALLEGRA

VITAL STATISTICS

DRUG CLASS
Antihistamines

GENERIC NAME
fexofenadine

GENERAL DESCRIPTION
Allegra, a brand-name drug, is an antihistamine medication used to treat symptoms of seasonal allergic rhinitis triggered by exposure to allergens such as ragweed pollen. Symptoms affected include sneezing; nasal discharge; red, watery eyes; and itching nose, eyes, and throat.

The beneficial effects of allegra begin about one hour after administration, reach their peak in two to three hours, and have a duration of about 12 hours. Allegra is considered a safer alternative than a related drug, terfenadine (seldane), which the Food and Drug Administration may withdraw from the market because of the risk of dangerous interactions with other drugs. Unlike seldane, allegra appears to be safe to take while the patient is also taking the antibiotic erythromycin or the antifungal medication ketoconazole.

Allegra may have less of a sedative effect than some other antihistamines. Because the drug does not appear to cross the blood-brain barrier, it should have minimal effects on the central nervous system. For more information about this class of drugs, see Antihistamines.

For visual characteristics, see the Color Guide to Prescription Drugs and Herbs.

PRECAUTIONS

SPECIAL INFORMATION
- If you have impaired kidney function, your doctor will likely recommend a reduced dosage of this drug at first.
- Allegra has not been determined safe for use during pregnancy; consult your doctor.
- It is not known whether fexofenadine, the principal ingredient in allegra, passes into breast milk; therefore, this drug is not recommended for use by nursing mothers.
- The safety and efficacy for children under 12 years has not been established.
- Because allegra may cause drowsiness and fatigue, restrict your activities as necessary. Do not drive or operate machinery until you know how allegra affects you.
- Do not take if you are hypersensitive to fexofenadine.
- If you miss a dose, do not double a future dose; take the remaining doses at the originally prescribed, regularly spaced intervals.

TARGET AILMENTS

Seasonal allergic rhinitis

SIDE EFFECTS

NOT SERIOUS
- Drowsiness; fatigue
- Painful menstrual bleeding
- Stomach upset

CALL YOUR DOCTOR IF THESE PROBLEMS PERSIST.

ALLIUM CEPA

LATIN NAME
Allium cepa

A

VITAL STATISTICS

GENERAL DESCRIPTION

Cultivated worldwide, *Allium cepa,* otherwise known as red onion, has been used in folk medicine for centuries. This common garden vegetable has been applied to the skin in poultices for acne, arthritis, and congestion, and used internally to clear worms from the intestines. Modern-day herbalists find onion useful for treating conditions as varied as earaches, hemorrhoids, and high blood pressure. Homeopathic practitioners consider *Allium cepa* a remedy for conditions that are accompanied by the same symptoms as those brought on by exposure to red onions—watering eyes and a burning, runny nose.

For the homeopathic preparation, red onions are harvested in midsummer. The bulbs are pounded to a pulp and then mixed with water and alcohol through several stages of extreme dilution.

Like most homeopathic prescriptions, *Allium cepa* was developed as a remedy by observation of the reactions of healthy individuals to doses of various strengths. The mental, emotional, and physical changes induced by *Allium cepa* were then cataloged. When a patient exhibits a set of symptoms that matches the cataloged symptoms brought on by *Allium cepa,* the homeopathic practitioner then prescribes the remedy in an extremely dilute form. It is presumed that in this highly dilute dosage, *Allium cepa* can counter symptoms that are similar to the ones it induces when it is at full strength. For more information on homeopathic medicine, see page 14.

PREPARATIONS

Allium cepa is available in various potencies, in liquid or tablet form, at selected stores and pharmacies. Consult your homeopathic practitioner for more precise information.

PRECAUTIONS

SPECIAL INFORMATION

- When a remedy is administered, no one but the patient should touch the pills. If tablets are spilled, throw them away.
- The mouth should be clear of flavors 15 minutes before and after taking a remedy, and strong flavors and aromas, such as coffee, camphor, and heavily scented perfumes, should be avoided for the duration of treatment.

TARGET AILMENTS

- Colds with sinus congestion that shifts from side to side in the head
- Coughs that cause a ripping, tearing pain in the throat
- Watery and inflamed eyes
- Hay fever with rawness of the nose and watery eyes
- Neuralgic pains
- Earaches

SIDE EFFECTS

NONE EXPECTED

Allopurinol

Vital Statistics

DRUG CLASS
Antigout Drugs

BRAND NAMES
Alloprin, Apo-Allopurinol, Lopurin, Novopurol, Purinol, Zurinol, Zyloprim

OTHER DRUGS IN THIS CLASS
colchicine

GENERAL DESCRIPTION
Allopurinol, a systemic antigout medication, is one of several drugs administered orally that reduce the body's production of uric acid (a naturally occurring substance in body fluids). It is recommended for those prone to chronic bouts of gouty arthritis due to overproduction of uric acid salts, and for patients who have calcified deposits of these salts (called tophi) or who suffer from impaired kidney function.

Patients with hyperuricemia (excessively high levels of uric acid in the blood) are given this medication when urinary complications lead to an underexcretion of uric acid, or when the condition is secondary to malignancies. The precise action of this drug, when used as an antigout agent, is as an enzyme inhibitor to prevent the production of uric acid and decrease uric acid levels in serum and urine. After several months of therapy with allopurinol, the patient usually experiences less frequent attacks of acute gout. Gout sufferers should note that allopurinol will not, of itself, alleviate the pain, inflammation, or urinary underexcretion of excessive amounts of uric acid in the body. But it can inhibit the overproduction of uric acid, which often leads to gout.

For visual characteristics, see the Color Guide to Prescription Drugs and Herbs.

Precautions

WARNING
Discontinue allopurinol immediately at the first appearance of a skin rash or other allergic reaction. Allergic reactions to allopurinol may be increased in patients also taking thiazide diuretics or ampicillin. These drug combinations should be administered with caution.

SPECIAL INFORMATION
- This drug can cause an increase in acute attacks of gout at first. In such cases, colchicine can be administered to help suppress and manage the gouty attacks.
- Certain adverse effects of allopurinol can mimic natural disease processes, such as viral hepatitis or Stevens-Johnson syndrome (a severe skin disorder).
- Fluid intake should be increased to prevent kidney stones when using antigout drugs.
- Allopurinol should not be taken when breast-feeding and should be taken with caution during pregnancy.
- Taking allopurinol after meals minimizes gastric irritation.
- Cancer patients who exhibit excessively

TARGET AILMENTS
Gout
Gouty arthritis
Recurrent kidney stones
Hyperuricemia
Ulcers of mouth, stomach, intestines during chemotherapy

CONTINUED

ALLOPURINOL

high blood levels of uric acid can experience renal failure when using allopurinol.

POSSIBLE INTERACTIONS

Anticoagulants: decreased blood-clotting ability, or increased anticoagulant effect, in some patients taking allopurinol. Increased monitoring of prothrombin activity is recommended.

Antibiotics: increased frequency of skin rash.

Cancer chemotherapeutic agents cyclophosphamide, mercaptopurine, and vidarabine: possible impaired bone marrow functions and increased marrow toxicity in cancer patients (with the exception of leukemia) leading to bleeding or infection.

Chlorpropamide: increased risk of hypoglycemia in patients with impaired kidneys who take this drug with allopurinol.

Probenecid: reduces activity of allopurinol.

Other antigout drugs: usually, an increase in the antigout effect is achieved with the use of two or more antigout drugs.

Iron preparations: can cause iron to concentrate in the liver.

Alcohol: may impair management of gout.

Vitamin C: large doses of this vitamin can cause kidney stones during use with allopurinol.

Caffeine: decreased allopurinol effect.

SIDE EFFECTS

NOT SERIOUS

- Drowsiness
- Diarrhea; stomach pain
- Nausea or vomiting without other symptoms
- Headache
- Numbness or tingling in hands or feet

CALL YOUR DOCTOR IF THESE SYMPTOMS PERSIST OR BECOME TROUBLESOME.

SERIOUS

- Allergic reactions, such as skin rash, hives, lesions, pus-forming sores
- Permanent liver damage and liver toxicity
- Vasculitis (inflammation in veins and arteries)
- Jaundice or yellowing of skin and eyes
- Fever
- Unusual bleeding
- Kidney failure
- Bone marrow depression
- Increased attacks of acute gout
- Inflammation of nerve ends

CALL YOUR DOCTOR IMMEDIATELY.

ALOE

LATIN NAME
Aloe barbadensis

VITAL STATISTICS

GENERAL DESCRIPTION

This tropical herb yields two therapeutic substances. The first, a translucent gel, works externally to relieve minor burns, skin irritations, and infections; taken internally, aloe gel relieves stomach disorders. It is used as a beauty aid and moisturizer because it contains polysaccharides, which act as emollients to soothe, soften, and protect the skin.

The second remedy contained in the aloe plant is a bitter yellow juice known as latex, which acts as a powerful laxative.

For visual characteristics, see the Color Guide to Prescription Drugs and Herbs.

PREPARATIONS

Over the counter:

Available as powder, fluidextract, powdered capsules, bottled gel, or latex tablets.

At home:

EYEWASH: Dissolve ½ tsp powdered aloe gel in 1 cup water. Add 1 tsp boric acid to accelerate healing. Pour the solution through a coffee filter before applying to the eyes.

BATH: Add 1 to 2 cups aloe gel to a warm bath to relieve sunburn or skin lesions.

COMBINATIONS: Use aloe gel with wheat-germ oil and safflower flower to reduce bruising.

Consult a practitioner for the dosage appropriate for you and the ailment being treated.

PRECAUTIONS

WARNING

Do not exceed the recommended dose of aloe latex. Pregnant and nursing women should not take aloe internally.

SPECIAL INFORMATION

If you have a gastrointestinal illness, take aloe internally only in consultation with an herbalist or a licensed healthcare professional.

POSSIBLE INTERACTIONS

Combining aloe with other herbs may necessitate a lower dosage.

SIDE EFFECTS

NOT SERIOUS

- Allergic dermatitis
- Intestinal cramps
- Diarrhea

TRY A LOWER DOSAGE OR STOP USING THE PRODUCT.

TARGET AILMENTS

Take aloe gel internally for:

Digestive disorders
Gastritis
Stomach ulcers

Use aloe latex internally for:

Constipation

Use aloe gel externally for:

Minor burns; sunburn
Infection in wounds
Insect bites
Acne; skin irritations
Bruising
Chickenpox
Poison ivy
Irritated eyes

Rx ALPHA1-ADRENERGIC BLOCKERS

VITAL STATISTICS

GENERIC NAMES
doxazosin, terazosin

GENERAL DESCRIPTION
Members of a general category of medicines known as antihypertensives, $alpha_1$-adrenergic blockers are used primarily to treat high blood pressure (hypertension). They work by selectively blocking nerve endings called alpha receptors; the blockage allows the blood vessels to relax and expand, which enables blood to pass through more easily and lowers blood pressure.

$Alpha_1$-adrenergic blockers can be used alone or in conjunction with other drugs, such as beta-adrenergic blockers or diuretics. These drugs do not cure high blood pressure, but they do help control it.

Doxazosin and terazosin are also used to relax the muscles in the prostate gland and increase urine flow. They will not, however, shrink an enlarged prostate.

Other antihypertensive medications include diuretics, beta-adrenergic blockers, calcium channel blockers, angiotensin-converting enzyme (ACE) inhibitors, and sympathetic nerve inhibitors, which act either centrally (in the brain) or peripherally (in the blood vessels) to block signals from the brain that tell the arteries to constrict.

For information on a centrally acting antihypertensive drug used in the control of mild-to-moderate high blood pressure, see Guanfacine. Also see Angiotensin-Converting Enzyme (ACE) Inhibitors, Beta-Adrenergic Blockers, Calcium Channel Blockers, and Diuretics.

PRECAUTIONS

SPECIAL INFORMATION
- Avoid driving and hazardous tasks for 24 hours after the first dose, after a dosage increase, or after resumption of treatment.
- The effects of $alpha_1$-adrenergic blockers on pregnant women, nursing mothers, and children under 12 years of age are not yet known. Use only if directed by your physician.
- Before taking these drugs, tell your doctor if you have previously experienced an unusual or allergic reaction to any of the alpha blockers or have encountered dizziness, faintness, or lightheadedness with other drugs. Inform your doctor if you have a history of mental depression, stroke, or impaired circulation to the brain; coronary artery disease; impaired liver function or active liver disease; impaired kidney function; or any plans to undergo surgery in the near future.
- To minimize dizziness, take the first dose at bedtime. Dosages must be adjusted on an individual basis.
- $Alpha_1$-adrenergic blockers may affect some laboratory tests. Effects may include a mild decrease in white blood cell counts, certain cholesterol ratios, and blood sugar levels.
- The symptoms of prostate cancer are similar to those of benign prostate enlargement. Ask your doctor to test for prostate cancer before starting $alpha_1$-adrenergic treatment.
- You should not take doxazosin or terazosin if you have ever had an allergic or unusual reaction to either of these medications or to prazosin.

ALPHA1-ADRENERGIC BLOCKERS

A

POSSIBLE INTERACTIONS

Alcohol: can intensify the blood-pressure-lowering actions of alpha1-adrenergic blockers and increase the chances of fainting or dizziness.

Drugs that lower blood pressure, such as beta-adrenergic blockers and diuretics: may increase the effects of the alpha1-adrenergic blockers, possibly affecting the duration and severity of the first-dose (low blood pressure) symptoms.

Estrogens and indomethacin: may reduce the blood-pressure-lowering effect.

TARGET AILMENTS
High blood pressure
Benign prostatic hyperplasia (benign enlargement of the prostate)

SIDE EFFECTS

NOT SERIOUS

- Nasal congestion
- Headache
- Fatigue; weakness
- Nausea
- Indigestion
- Nervousness; irritability
- Skin rash
- Blurred vision
- Drowsiness

THESE EFFECTS SHOULD SUBSIDE AS YOU ADJUST TO THE DRUG. CHECK WITH YOUR DOCTOR IF THESE OR OTHER SYMPTOMS PERSIST OR ARE BOTHERSOME: YOU MAY NEED A DOSAGE ADJUSTMENT.

SERIOUS

- Lightheadedness
- Dizziness; vertigo
- Palpitations
- Fainting

THESE FIRST-DOSE EFFECTS ARE COMMON SYMPTOMS OF MARKED LOW BLOOD PRESSURE CAUSED BY ALPHA1-ADRENERGIC BLOCKERS. YOU ARE MOST LIKELY TO EXPERIENCE THESE SYMPTOMS IF, WHEN YOU FIRST START TAKING THE DRUG, YOU RISE TOO QUICKLY FROM A SITTING OR PRONE POSITION, DRINK ALCOHOL, EXERCISE STRENUOUSLY, OR STAND FOR LONG PERIODS OF TIME, ESPECIALLY IN HOT WEATHER. CHECK WITH YOUR DOCTOR IMMEDIATELY.

ALPRAZOLAM

VITAL STATISTICS

DRUG CLASS
Antianxiety Drugs [Benzodiazepines]

BRAND NAME
Xanax

OTHER DRUGS IN THIS SUBCLASS
clonazepam, diazepam, lorazepam, temazepam, triazolam

GENERAL DESCRIPTION
Alprazolam is used for short-term management of anxiety disorders and anxiety associated with depression. It is also used to treat panic disorders. Since this drug can become habit forming, it is not used to treat the anxiety and stress of everyday living. The effects of alprazolam start working after the first dose. For visual characteristics of alprazolam and the brand-name drug Xanax, see the Color Guide to Prescription Drugs and Herbs.

PRECAUTIONS

WARNING
Never combine alcohol with alprazolam; the combination can cause dangerous central nervous system and respiratory depression.

Do not abruptly stop taking alprazolam. Sudden cessation can provoke withdrawal symptoms, including seizures; irritability; insomnia; confusion; mental depression; hypersensitivity to pain, noise, or light; and feelings of suspicion and distrust. Slowly reduce the dosage under your doctor's guidance.

SPECIAL INFORMATION
- Be careful not to confuse the brand names Xanax and Zantac. Zantac is the brand name for ranitidine, a drug used to treat ulcers.
- Alprazolam can impair your alertness, judgment, and coordination. Avoid driving and performing hazardous activities until you know how the drug affects you.
- Let your doctor know if you have narrow-angle glaucoma, a liver or kidney impairment, chronic respiratory disease, myasthenia gravis, depression, sleep apnea, or a history of drug abuse or addiction. Alprazolam may exacerbate these conditions.
- This drug can cause sleep apnea in people with chronic respiratory disease, such as emphysema.
- Alprazolam can cause physical and psychological dependence, sometimes after only one or two weeks, but usually after prolonged use.
- People with a history of drug or alcohol abuse are at a greater risk of psychological dependence on alprazolam.
- Tolerance may increase with prolonged use; as your body adjusts to alprazolam, the drug becomes less effective. Never increase the dose without consulting your doctor, because the risk of alprazolam dependence increases with higher doses.
- Do not take alprazolam if you are pregnant or breast-feeding.

ALPRAZOLAM

A

POSSIBLE INTERACTIONS

Alcohol, anticonvulsants, antihistamines that cause drowsiness (clemastine, diphenhydramine), barbiturates, MAO inhibitors, opioids, tricyclic antidepressants: increased sedative effects, such as excessive mental (central nervous system) depression, sleepiness, and slow or shallow breathing. It is very important that you avoid taking alprazolam in combination with any of these drugs.

Beta blockers, cimetidine, disulfiram, erythromycin, fluvoxamine, fluoxetine, ketoconazole, nefazodone, omeprazole, oral contraceptives, probenecid: may prolong the amount of time alprazolam remains in your body, leading to increased alprazolam effects and possible toxicity.

Clozapine: risk of profound hypotension (low blood pressure), slow or shallow breathing, cessation of breathing, and cardiac arrest leading to death.

Isoniazid: increased effect and possible toxicity of alprazolam.

Levodopa: decreased levodopa effect.

Phenytoin: increased effects and possible alprazolam toxicity.

Rifampin: decreased alprazolam effect.

Tobacco (smoking): decreased alprazolam effects.

Valproic acid: combination may cause behavioral changes.

Zidovudine: risk of zidovudine toxicity.

TARGET AILMENTS
Anxiety
Panic disorders

SIDE EFFECTS

NOT SERIOUS

- Clumsiness or unsteadiness
- Lethargy
- Dry mouth, nausea, or change in bowel habits
- Temporary amnesia (especially "travelers' amnesia") when taken to treat insomnia associated with jet lag

TELL YOUR DOCTOR IF THESE SYMPTOMS PERSIST OR BECOME BOTHERSOME. CONTACT YOUR DOCTOR IF YOU ARE HAVING DIFFICULTY WITH YOUR MEMORY.

SERIOUS

- Drowsiness, dizziness, or blurred vision
- Persistent or severe headache
- Confusion or depression
- Changes in behavior (outbursts of anger, difficulty concentrating)
- Hallucinations
- Uncontrolled movement of body or eyes
- Muscle weakness
- Chills, fever, or sore throat
- Allergic reaction (rash or itching) (rare)
- Low blood pressure (rare)
- Jaundice, anemia, or low platelet count (unusual bruising or bleeding) (rare)

TELL YOUR DOCTOR ABOUT THESE SYMPTOMS RIGHT AWAY.

Aluminum Hydroxide

Vital Statistics

DRUG CLASS
Antacids

BRAND NAMES
Gaviscon; some types of Maalox and Mylanta

OTHER DRUGS IN THIS CLASS
calcium carbonate, magnesium carbonate, magnesium hydroxide, sodium bicarbonate and citric acid

GENERAL DESCRIPTION
Aluminum hydroxide is an aluminum-containing antacid used to relieve upset and sour stomach, heartburn, acid indigestion, and some types of ulcers. It is most effective when taken on an empty stomach. The most common adverse effect of aluminum hydroxide is constipation. See Antacids for more information, including facts about possible drug interactions and additional special information.

Precautions

SPECIAL INFORMATION

- Check with your doctor before taking aluminum hydroxide if you are on kidney dialysis; aluminum toxicity could result.
- Because they can affect the rate of absorption of other drugs, antacids should not be taken within one to two hours of many other oral medications. Ask your doctor or pharmacist for guidance.
- Notify your doctor if you develop symptoms such as black, tarry stools or vomit the consistency of coffee grounds. These are indications of bleeding in the stomach or intestines.

Target Ailments

Upset stomach; heartburn

Acid indigestion; sour stomach

Ulcers

Side Effects

Not Serious

- Mild constipation
- Laxative effect or diarrhea
- Chalky taste in the mouth
- Stomach cramps, nausea, or vomiting
- Belching
- Flatulence
- White specks in the stool

CALL YOUR DOCTOR IF THESE PROBLEMS PERSIST.

Serious

- Swelling of the wrist, foot, or lower leg
- Bone pain
- Severe constipation
- Dizziness
- Mood changes
- Muscle pain, weakness, or twitching
- Nervousness or restlessness
- Slow breathing
- Irregular heartbeat
- Fatigue
- Pain upon urinating or frequent need to urinate
- Change in appetite

CONTACT YOUR DOCTOR IMMEDIATELY.

Rx AMBIEN

VITAL STATISTICS

DRUG CLASS
Anti-Insomnia Drugs

GENERIC NAME
zolpidem

OTHER DRUGS IN THIS CLASS
Antihistamines: diphenhydramine, doxylamine
Benzodiazepines: lorazepam, temazepam, triazolam

GENERAL DESCRIPTION
Ambien, introduced in 1993, is the brand name for zolpidem, the most commonly prescribed drug for the short-term (seven to 10 days) management of sleeping problems in adults. Its major advantages include a low incidence of adverse effects, rapid absorption and elimination, and minimal interference with normal sleep patterns, which includes the rapid eye movement (REM) stage.

A nonbenzodiazepine medication, Ambien works by binding to a specific receptor in the brain to simulate normal sleep processes. Most users report few side effects, and little or no hangover effects, memory loss, or "rebound" insomnia when not using the drug.

The anti-insomnia drug class (sometimes called the sedative-hypnotic class) includes a large number of drugs used in the treatment of sleeping problems. Since insomnia is often related to psychological or physical disorders, the choice of medication will depend on the underlying condition. Certain benzodiazepines, a subclass of antianxiety drugs, are often prescribed for people in acute distress. Milder alternatives include the antihistamine drugs diphenhydramine and doxylamine, which are prescribed for short-term treatment of insomnia. Antipsychotic and antidepressant drugs with sedative effects are also used if warranted. For visual characteristics, see the Color Guide to Prescription Drugs and Herbs.

TARGET AILMENTS

Insomnia (short-term)

SIDE EFFECTS

NOT SERIOUS

- Daytime drowsiness
- Dizziness or blurred vision
- Dry mouth
- Memory problems
- Abdominal or gastric pain
- Diarrhea
- Nausea
- Headache
- Unusual dreams
- Malaise

SEE YOUR DOCTOR IF THESE SYMPTOMS PERSIST OR BECOME BOTHERSOME.

SERIOUS

- Clumsiness
- Confusion
- Unsteadiness and falling
- Mental depression
- Skin rash
- Agitation or irritability
- Wheezing or difficulty in breathing
- Hallucinations
- Increased insomnia

CONTACT YOUR DOCTOR AS SOON AS POSSIBLE.

CONTINUED

Ambien

Precautions

SPECIAL INFORMATION

- Do not take Ambien if you have had an allergic reaction to this drug in the past.
- Before taking this drug, tell your doctor if any of the following conditions apply: You are pregnant, plan to become pregnant, or are nursing; you have a kidney or liver disease; you have sleep apnea; you have asthma, bronchitis, emphysema, or other chronic lung disease; you have a history of mental depression or disorder; you have a history of alcoholism or drug dependence.
- Ambien is most rapidly absorbed when taken on an empty stomach (at least two hours after eating).
- Because Ambien works so fast, it should be taken just before bedtime.
- Take Ambien only if you have time to get a full night's sleep (seven or eight hours). Otherwise, the drug will not have time to wear off, and you may experience hangover effects, including drowsiness and memory problems.
- Some people experience carryover effects from Ambien the next day. If you haven't taken this drug before, wait to see how it affects you the next day before driving, operating heavy machinery, or doing anything requiring unimpaired coordination and clear vision.
- Long-term use of Ambien may result in dependence. Withdrawal symptoms may occur when you stop taking the drug.
- Older adults may be more sensitive to the drug's effects and side effects and may require a smaller dosage.

POSSIBLE INTERACTIONS

Alcohol and other central nervous system depressants [anesthetics, antidepressants, antihistamines, barbiturates, benzodiazepines, monoamine oxidase (MAO) inhibitors, muscle relaxants, narcotics or prescription pain medicines, tranquilizers]: increased anti-insomniac and depressant effect.

Caffeine and nicotine: these are stimulants that can interfere with Ambien's anti-insomniac effects.

Amiloride

Vital Statistics

DRUG CLASS
Diuretics

BRAND NAMES
Midamor, Moduretic

OTHER DRUGS IN THIS CLASS
bumetanide, furosemide, hydrochlorothiazide, indapamide, potassium chloride (adjunct therapy), spironolactone, triamterene

GENERAL DESCRIPTION
Like other diuretics, amiloride is used to remove excess fluid from the body by increasing urine production, thereby lowering blood pressure. Amiloride is among the group of medicines called potassium-sparing diuretics; it prevents the excess loss of potassium, a frequent consequence of the excretion of body fluids. This drug is usually used in combination with a non-potassium-sparing diuretic, such as hydrochlorothiazide. For more information, see Diuretics and Hydrochlorothiazide.

Precautions

SPECIAL INFORMATION

- Because amiloride inhibits potassium excretion, you should not take potassium supplements (including salt substitutes, which often contain potassium) or eat large quantities of potassium-rich foods (such as bananas) while on this medication. Excess potassium can lead to heart-rhythm problems.
- Do not use amiloride if you have kidney disease or if your kidneys are impaired.
- Because diuretics have both known and suspected effects on glucose (blood sugar) levels, people with diabetes or who have received a diagnosis of borderline diabetes should have their blood sugar levels monitored closely.

TARGET AILMENTS

General edema (swelling caused by water retention), especially of the ankles and feet

Edema associated with various medical conditions, including congestive heart failure and cirrhosis of the liver

High blood pressure (hypertension)

CONTINUED

AMILORIDE

POSSIBLE INTERACTIONS

Alcohol: increased action of amiloride.

Angiotensin-converting enzyme (ACE) inhibitors: increased risk of hyperkalemia (excessively high levels of potassium in the blood).

Foods high in potassium (such as bananas and low-salt milk), salt substitutes, potassium supplements: may lead to potassium toxicity if ingested in sufficient amounts while taking a potassium-sparing diuretic.

Lithium: amiloride may increase the risk of lithium toxicity.

Nonsteroidal anti-inflammatory drugs (NSAIDs): reduced effectiveness of diuretics and increased risk of kidney failure.

Oral antidiabetic drugs, insulin: in rare cases, diuretics may interfere with these medicines or raise blood glucose levels.

Other blood pressure drugs, especially angiotensin-converting enzyme (ACE) inhibitors: though diuretics are frequently taken with medications to lower blood pressure, caution should be exercised to ensure that blood pressure does not go too low.

SIDE EFFECTS

NOT SERIOUS

- Headache
- Blurred vision
- Diarrhea
- Dizziness or lightheadedness when getting up (orthostatic hypotension)
- Increased risk of sunburn

SERIOUS

- Nausea or vomiting
- Fatigue or weakness
- Irregular or weak pulse
- Increased thirst
- Dry mouth
- Muscle pain or cramps
- Mood changes
- Mental confusion
- Bleeding in urine or stools
- Unusual bruising
- Skin rash

CALL YOUR DOCTOR AT ONCE.

AMITRIPTYLINE

VITAL STATISTICS

DRUG CLASS
Antidepressants [Tricyclic Antidepressants (TCAs)]

BRAND NAME
Elavil

OTHER DRUGS IN THIS SUBCLASS
doxepin, nortriptyline

GENERAL DESCRIPTION
Since 1961, the tricyclic antidepressant amitriptyline has been used in the treatment of depression. The drug acts on the nervous system by restoring levels of the vital brain chemicals serotonin and norepinephrine. Amitriptyline may also be used to prevent migraine, to treat bulimia, and, when combined with other medications, to alleviate chronic pain, including neuropathy. See Antidepressants for information about side effects and other possible drug interactions. For visual characteristics of amitriptyline and the brand-name drug Elavil, see the Color Guide to Prescription Drugs and Herbs.

PRECAUTIONS

SPECIAL INFORMATION
- Before taking amitriptyline, let your doctor know if you are suffering from glaucoma, urinary retention, epilepsy, heart disease, hyperthyroidism, or schizophrenia.
- This drug may cause drowsiness. When taking amitriptyline, use care while driving, operating machinery, or performing tasks that require mental alertness.
- Amitriptyline can trigger manic attacks in individuals with manic-depression. Be sure to tell your doctor if you have manic-depression.
- Amitriptyline can affect blood sugar (glucose tolerance) tests by causing fluctuation in blood sugar levels.
- The full effects of this drug may not occur for several weeks.
- If you are pregnant, nursing, or planning a pregnancy, check with your doctor before taking amitriptyline.

POSSIBLE INTERACTIONS
Anticoagulant drugs (such as warfarin): amitriptyline may increase the anticlotting activity.

Barbiturates: decreased effectiveness of amitriptyline.

Cimetidine (antiulcer): increased amitriptyline effects.

Clonidine (blood pressure medication): may cause a dangerous increase in blood pressure.

Haloperidol (antipsychotic), oral contraceptives, phenothiazines (antipsychotic), levodopa (anti-Parkinsonism): increased levels of amitriptyline.

Thyroid medications: combining amitriptyline with thyroid drugs may increase the effects, including side effects, of both medications.

Tobacco (smoking): increased elimination of amitriptyline from the body, lessening its effectiveness.

TARGET AILMENTS
Major depressive disorders
Bulimia
Chronic pain
Migraine

AMLODIPINE

VITAL STATISTICS

DRUG CLASS
Calcium Channel Blockers

BRAND NAME
Norvasc

OTHER DRUGS IN THIS CLASS
diltiazem, isradipine, nifedipine, verapamil

GENERAL DESCRIPTION
Amlodipine, introduced in 1986, is a calcium channel blocker used to treat hypertension and angina. Like other drugs in its class, amlodipine inhibits the passage of calcium into vascular smooth muscle cells, thus dilating the arteries and lowering blood pressure. These actions also reduce the strain on the heart and open the coronary arteries—blocking spasms of the coronary arteries and thus lessening angina. Amlodipine is used alone or in carefully selected combinations with other heart and blood pressure medications. For information on possible drug interactions, see Calcium Channel Blockers. For visual characteristics of the brand-name drug Norvasc, see the Color Guide to Prescription Drugs and Herbs.

PRECAUTIONS

WARNING
Rarely, people with advanced coronary artery disease have experienced increased angina (chest pain) or myocardial infarction (heart attack) on beginning treatment with a calcium channel blocker. Contact your doctor immediately if this occurs.

SPECIAL INFORMATION
- Recent findings have prompted warnings about the safety of calcium channel blockers. Before using amlodipine, be sure to discuss this matter thoroughly with your doctor. If you are already taking this drug, do not stop the medication without first consulting your doctor.
- Let your doctor know if you are suffering from low blood pressure, heart or liver disease, congestive heart failure, or sever obstruction of the coronary arteries.

TARGET AILMENTS

Angina (chest pain)

High blood pressure

SIDE EFFECTS

NOT SERIOUS
- Gastrointestinal upset
- Drowsiness; fatigue
- Lightheadedness; dizziness
- Headache; flushing
- Weight gain; increased appetite; muscle cramps (rare)

CALL YOUR DOCTOR IF THESE EFFECTS BECOME TROUBLESOME.

SERIOUS
- Edema (swelling)
- Heart problems, such as congestive heart failure, heart-rhythm irregularities, or increased angina (rare)
- Shortness of breath (rare)
- Allergic reactions, such as skin rash (rare)

CONTACT YOUR DOCTOR AT ONCE.

AMOXICILLIN

VITAL STATISTICS

DRUG CLASS
Antibiotics [Penicillins]

BRAND NAMES
Amoxil, Polymox, Trimox, Wymox

OTHER DRUGS IN THIS SUBCLASS
amoxicillin and clavulanate, ampicillin, penicillin V

GENERAL DESCRIPTION
Introduced in 1969, amoxicillin is an antibiotic used to treat genitourinary tract infections, gonorrhea, otitis media, sinusitis, pharyngitis, and other bacterial infections caused by certain strains of staph, strep, and *E. coli*. For more information, see Penicillins. For visual characteristics of amoxicillin and the brand-name drugs Amoxil and Trimox, see the Color Guide to Prescription Drugs and Herbs.

PRECAUTIONS

SPECIAL INFORMATION
- Taking amoxicillin when you have mononucleosis may produce a skin rash.
- Take the full course of your prescription, even if you feel better before finishing it; otherwise, the infection may return.
- If possible, avoid taking this drug if you are pregnant or breast-feeding.

POSSIBLE INTERACTIONS
Allopurinol: may cause a skin rash.
Bacteriostatic drugs (chloramphenicol, erythromycins, sulfonamides, tetracyclines): may decrease amoxicillin's effectiveness.
Oral contraceptives: effectiveness may be decreased.
Probenecid: decreases the kidneys' ability to excrete amoxicillin; possible amoxicillin toxicity.

TARGET AILMENTS
Genitourinary tract infections
Gonorrhea
Otitis media
Sinusitis
Pharyngitis

SIDE EFFECTS

NOT SERIOUS
- Mild nausea or diarrhea
- Oral or vaginal candidiasis

TELL YOUR DOCTOR WHEN CONVENIENT.

SERIOUS
- Allergic reaction (skin rash, hives, intense itching, or difficulty breathing)
- Severe allergic reactions (anaphylactic shock) can be life threatening; call your doctor, 911, or your emergency number immediately.
- Unusual bruising or bleeding, sore throat with fever
- Severe abdominal pain with diarrhea
- Seizures

CALL YOUR DOCTOR IMMEDIATELY.

Amoxicillin and Clavulanate

A

Vital Statistics

DRUG CLASS
Antibiotics [Penicillins]

BRAND NAME
Augmentin

OTHER DRUGS IN THIS SUBCLASS
amoxicillin, ampicillin, penicillin V

GENERAL DESCRIPTION
Introduced in 1982, amoxicillin and clavulanate is a combination antibiotic drug. Clavulanate reinforces amoxicillin's ability to destroy bacteria. This combination and the single drug amoxicillin are used to treat some of the same bacterial infections. For more information, see Penicillins.

Precautions

SPECIAL INFORMATION
- Take the full course of your prescription, even if you feel better before finishing it; otherwise, the infection may return.
- Amoxicillin and clavulanate works equally well whether taken on a full or on an empty stomach.
- Tell your doctor if you are allergic to cephalosporins; you may also be allergic to amoxicillin and clavulanate.
- Penicillins also kill "good" intestinal bacteria that keep harmful fungi and intestinal bacteria in check. Eating yogurt containing *Lactobacillus acidophilus* culture or taking acidophilus tablets may help restore the body's normal bacteria.
- If possible, avoid taking penicillins if you are pregnant or breast-feeding.

POSSIBLE INTERACTIONS
Disulfiram: do not take this drug with amoxicillin and clavulanate.

TARGET AILMENTS

Otitis media

Sinusitis and other infections of the respiratory tract

Infections of the skin and urinary tract

Side Effects

Not Serious
- Mild nausea
- Mild diarrhea
- Oral candidiasis (sore mouth or tongue)
- Vaginal candidiasis

Tell your doctor when convenient.

Serious
- Allergic reaction (skin rash, hives, intense itching, or difficulty breathing)
- Severe allergic reactions (anaphylactic shock) can be life threatening; call your doctor, 911, or your emergency number immediately.
- Sore throat with fever
- Severe abdominal pain

Call your doctor immediately.

Amoxil

Vital Statistics

DRUG CLASS
Antibiotics [Penicillins]

GENERIC NAME
amoxicillin

OTHER DRUGS IN THIS SUBCLASS
amoxicillin and clavulanate, ampicillin, penicillin V

GENERAL DESCRIPTION
Amoxil is a brand name for the generic drug amoxicillin, a penicillin antibiotic commonly used to treat bacterial infections caused by certain strains of staph, strep, and *E. coli*. For more information, see entries Amoxicillin and Penicillins. For visual characteristics, see the Color Guide to Prescription Drugs and Herbs.

Precautions

SPECIAL INFORMATION
- Taking Amoxil when you have mononucleosis may produce a skin rash.
- Take the full course of your prescription, even if you feel better before finishing it; otherwise, the infection may return.
- Tell your doctor if you are allergic to cephalosporins; you may also be allergic to penicillins.
- If possible, avoid taking this drug if you are pregnant or breast-feeding.

POSSIBLE INTERACTIONS
Allopurinol: may cause a skin rash.
Bacteriostatic drugs (chloramphenicol, erythromycins, sulfonamides, tetracyclines): these medicines can interfere with the bacteria-killing action of Amoxil.
Probenecid: decreases the kidneys' ability to excrete penicillins, possibly leading to penicillin toxicity.

TARGET AILMENTS
- Genitourinary tract infections
- Gonorrhea
- Otitis media
- Sinusitis
- Pharyngitis

SIDE EFFECTS

NOT SERIOUS
- Mild nausea or diarrhea
- Oral candidiasis (sore mouth or tongue)
- Vaginal candidiasis

TELL YOUR DOCTOR WHEN CONVENIENT.

SERIOUS
- Allergic reaction (skin rash, hives, intense itching, or difficulty breathing)
- Severe allergic reactions (anaphylactic shock) can be life threatening; call your doctor or your emergency number immediately.
- Sore throat with fever
- Severe abdominal pain with diarrhea

CALL YOUR DOCTOR IMMEDIATELY.

Ampicillin

Vital Statistics

DRUG CLASS
Antibiotics [Penicillins]

BRAND NAMES
Omnipen, Polycillin, Principen, Totacillin

OTHER DRUGS IN THIS SUBCLASS
amoxicillin, amoxicillin and clavulanate, penicillin V

GENERAL DESCRIPTION
Ampicillin, like the other penicillin antibiotics, destroys sensitive strains of bacteria that cause infections. Generally, ampicillin is used to treat infections of the skin, soft tissues, and the urinary, respiratory, and gastrointestinal tracts, and is used also in the treatment of meningitis. See Penicillins for more information. For visual characteristics, see the Color Guide to Prescription Drugs and Herbs.

Precautions

SPECIAL INFORMATION
- Tell your doctor before taking this drug if you have allergies, mononucleosis, a history of blood disorders, or kidney disease.
- Inform your doctor if you notice no improvement within a few days of beginning this medicine.

POSSIBLE INTERACTIONS
Aminoglycosides: reduced effectiveness of both combined drugs.
Antacids: reduced absorption of ampicillin; separate doses by at least two hours.
Atenolol: reduced effects of atenolol.
Food: may inhibit ampicillin absorption. Take one hour before or two hours after eating.
Methotrexate: large doses of ampicillin may lead to toxic levels of methotrexate.
Oral contraceptives: ampicillin may decrease the effectiveness of oral contraceptives; possible breakthrough bleeding.
Probenecid: although these drugs are sometimes prescribed together, probenecid may slow the secretion of ampicillin and increase the risk of toxic effects.

TARGET AILMENTS
Bacterial infections

SIDE EFFECTS

NOT SERIOUS
- Mild nausea or diarrhea
- Headache; dizziness
- Oral candidiasis
- Muscle aches
- Yeast infection

SERIOUS
- Breathing difficulties or swelling around the face.

SEEK EMERGENCY TREATMENT.

- Severe nausea or vomiting
- Severe abdominal pain
- Fever
- Swollen and painful joints
- Skin rash or itching
- Sore throat

CONTACT YOUR DOCTOR IF YOU NOTICE ANY OF THESE SYMPTOMS.

ANALGESICS

A

VITAL STATISTICS

GENERIC NAMES

acetaminophen, aspirin; caffeine (adjunct therapy); methyl salicylate (topical analgesic)

Nonsteroidal Anti-Inflammatory Drugs (NSAIDs): diclofenac, etodolac, flurbiprofen, ibuprofen, ketoprofen, ketorolac, nabumetone, naproxen, oxaprozin

Opioid Analgesics: codeine, hydrocodone, oxycodone, propoxyphene, tramadol

GENERAL DESCRIPTION

Analgesics are drugs that relieve pain. Some, such as the opioid analgesics, offer relief by affecting the brain and nervous system; these drugs are sometimes called narcotics because they can cause physical and psychological dependence. Nonnarcotic pain relievers, on the other hand, act at the site of the pain, usually by relieving inflammation. Sometimes two or more analgesics are combined to increase the effectiveness or the range of their action.

Aspirin, among the most popular of all over-the-counter pain relievers, is used to treat headache, arthritis, muscle aches, and minor injuries. It is also taken to suppress fever, reduce inflammation, and lower the risk of heart attack. Acetaminophen, widely used to relieve pain and reduce fever, is a good alternative to aspirin, although acetaminophen does not reduce inflammation. The opioid analgesic codeine helps control coughing and is often prescribed along with aspirin or acetaminophen for moderate pain relief. Ibuprofen, an over-the-counter drug used to relieve the pain of headaches, menstrual cramps, muscle aches, and certain types of arthritis, also reduces inflammation and fever.

Analgesics have side effects that depend on their mode of action and also on individual response. Some can cause drowsiness or a severe allergic reaction, while others may affect the digestive system or blood vessels. For more information, including possible drug interactions, see entries for the individual drugs listed at left.

PRECAUTIONS

WARNING

Do not give aspirin to children or teenagers with fevers. Aspirin can provoke a potentially fatal liver inflammation called Reye's syndrome in young people if the drug is used to treat a fever or viral infection such as chickenpox or influenza.

TARGET AILMENTS
Fever
Headaches
Muscle and joint aches
Pain, especially from injuries or surgery
Inflammation associated with menstrual cramps, arthritis, bursitis, and other conditions

SIDE EFFECTS

SEE ENTRIES FOR THE INDIVIDUAL ANALGESICS LISTED ABOVE, LEFT.

ANEMARRHENA

LATIN NAME
Anemarrhena asphodeloides

VITAL STATISTICS

GENERAL DESCRIPTION

Anemarrhena, a plant that grows in China's Hebei province, is classified in traditional Chinese medicine as an herb with bitter and cold properties. The rhizome is used to treat fever and other ailments that practitioners associate with yin deficiency, a disorder distinguished by "heat" symptoms such as afternoon fevers, night sweats, hot hands and feet, and a red tongue. Used by practitioners of Chinese medicine to treat infection, anemarrhena has demonstrated possible antibiotic effects in laboratory tests. A high-quality specimen of this herb appears large, thick, and hard, and has a white cross section.

Chinese medicine takes a holistic approach to healthcare, fashioning remedies to treat the entire being as well as the specific parts or areas. Single herbs may be used alone or in combination with other herbs to prevent and combat disease, which is thought to arise from disturbances in the flow of a bodily energy called chi (pronounced "chee") and blood, or from a lack of balance in the complementary states of yin and yang.

PREPARATIONS

Anemarrhena is available in bulk at Chinese pharmacies. Practitioners sometimes recommend a preparation of the herb cooked in salt water to treat the kidneys.

COMBINATIONS: In a mixture with phellodendron, anemarrhena is used to treat night sweating, dizziness, and vertigo. The herb is also combined with fritillaria to treat coughing. Chinese herbalists mix anemarrhena with scrophularia and Chinese foxglove root for ulcers in the mouth.

Check with a practitioner of Chinese medicine for information on appropriate dosages and other herbal combinations.

TARGET AILMENTS
Take internally for:
High fever and thirst accompanied by a rapid pulse
Coughing that brings up thick, yellow phlegm
Abnormally high sex drive and nocturnal emission
Night sweats
Low-grade fever
Afternoon fever
Certain types of dizziness and vertigo
Ulcers in the mouth
Bleeding gums

SIDE EFFECTS

NONE EXPECTED

ANESTHETICS

VITAL STATISTICS

GENERIC NAMES
benzocaine, dyclonine, pramoxine

GENERAL DESCRIPTION
Over-the-counter anesthetics are topical drugs used to relieve pain and discomfort by blocking the initiation and conduction of nerve impulses to the brain. They are used on all body surfaces and in easily accessible areas inside the body, such as the mouth and esophagus.

Although the most commonly used over-the-counter anesthetics are for mouth pain, the drugs are also found in preparations used to treat minor burns, sunburn, and rectal pain (from hemorrhoids), and to aid in medical examinations and minor surgical procedures. These medications have relatively few side effects except when used excessively, which results in their absorption into the bloodstream, or when they trigger an allergic or hypersensitivity reaction. For more information, see the entries for the generic drugs listed above.

PRECAUTIONS

SPECIAL INFORMATION
- Before using dyclonine or pramoxine, consult your doctor if you are pregnant or nursing or have heart disease, high blood pressure, thyroid disease, or diabetes.
- Some anesthetic preparations can be applied to the mouth or throat; others, including those that contain pramoxine, are for external application only. Read labels carefully.

TARGET AILMENTS

Canker sores (benzocaine, dyclonine)

Mouth or gum injury (benzocaine, dyclonine)

Toothache (benzocaine, dyclonine)

Cold sores; minor burns (pramoxine)

Uncomplicated hemorrhoidal itching and pain (pramoxine)

SIDE EFFECTS

NOT SERIOUS
- Burning sensation in the eyes (pramoxine)
- Irritation or stinging of mucous membranes

CALL YOUR DOCTOR IF THESE EFFECTS CONTINUE.

SERIOUS
- Allergic skin reactions, burning, stinging, or hive-like swelling
- Cardiovascular effects including irregular heartbeat, low blood pressure, fainting
- Overdose effects, including nervousness, dizziness, tremors, seizures, blurred vision, ringing in the ears, respiratory depression

CALL YOUR DOCTOR RIGHT AWAY.

Angelica Root

LATIN NAME
Angelica pubescens

A

Vital Statistics

GENERAL DESCRIPTION
Angelica root, an aromatic herb with thick, glistening roots, is frequently prescribed by practitioners of Chinese medicine as a pain reliever. Remedies made from the plant's root are used to alleviate the pain and numbness in joints and muscles (especially of the lower body) that are attributed to cold, damp weather conditions. The herb angelica root is classified as acrid, bitter, and warm according to the tenets of traditional Chinese medicine.

Chinese medicine takes a holistic approach to healthcare, fashioning remedies to treat the entire being as well as the specific parts or areas. Single herbs may be used alone or in combination with other herbs to prevent and combat disease, which is thought to arise from disturbances in the flow of a bodily energy called chi (pronounced "chee") and blood, or from a lack of balance in the complementary states of yin and yang.

PREPARATIONS
Angelica root is available in bulk at Chinese pharmacies, Asian food markets, and some Western health food stores.

COMBINATIONS: A mixture of angelica root with Chinese wild ginger and gentiana macrophylla root is prescribed for pain and numbness in the neck, back, and legs. When combined with ephedra stem, angelica root is used for body aches with colds and flu if the patient is not perspiring. The herb is also mixed with a root known as siler in a remedy for numbness in the legs.

Angelica root is related to notopterygium root, which is regarded as a better treatment for pain in the upper back and shoulders. Chinese herbalists often use these two herbs together. For example, a traditional headache remedy is made by combining angelica root with notopterygium, a root called cnidium *(Ligusticum chuanxiong),* and a fruit known as vitex.

Consult a Chinese medicine practitioner for information on specific dosages and additional herbal combinations.

Precautions

WARNING
Do not use angelica root if you have what Chinese practitioners refer to as heat signs, which include fever with no chills, thirst, and a rapid pulse.

TARGET AILMENTS

Take internally for:

Acute and chronic pain in the lower back and legs that is sensitive to cold and damp weather

Mild headache and toothache that respond to changes in the weather

ANGIOTENSIN-CONVERTING ENZYME (ACE) INHIBITORS

VITAL STATISTICS

GENERIC NAMES

benazepril, captopril, enalapril, fosinopril, lisinopril, quinapril, ramipril

GENERAL DESCRIPTION

Angiotensin-converting enzyme (ACE) inhibitors block an enzyme in the body that is essential for the production of a substance, called angiotensin II, that causes blood vessels to constrict. As a result, these drugs relax blood vessels, thereby lowering blood pressure and decreasing the work load on the heart. For increased effectiveness in lowering blood pressure, ACE inhibitors are sometimes combined with a diuretic such as hydrochlorothiazide. For more information, see entries for the generic drugs listed above.

TARGET AILMENTS
High blood pressure
Sometimes congestive heart failure (often used in conjunction with digitalis preparations and diuretics)
Heart attacks (prevention)
Diabetes (to slow or prevent kidney failure)

PRECAUTIONS

WARNING

Get medical attention immediately if you notice swelling of the face, tongue, or vocal cords or have difficulty swallowing or breathing; this reaction can be life threatening.

These drugs should not be taken during pregnancy because they have been associated with malformations and death of the fetus and newborn baby.

SPECIAL INFORMATION

- ACE inhibitors can cause an increase in blood levels of potassium. Do not use salt substitutes (which contain potassium) or other products rich in potassium, including low-salt milk, without first consulting your doctor. Such products could increase the potassium in your blood to dangerous levels, leading to heart-rhythm problems.
- Because your first dose of an ACE inhibitor may cause a sudden drop in blood pressure, your doctor may recommend that you take the first dose at bedtime; you may also need to increase your dose gradually.
- Do not abruptly stop taking these drugs. Your doctor may tell you to reduce the dosage gradually.
- Some of these drugs, especially captopril, may cause photosensitivity, an increased sensitivity to the sun that may result in serious, unexpected sunburn.
- Use caution during hot weather or while exercising; excessive perspiration can lead to dehydration and reduced blood pressure in people taking ACE inhibitors.
- Let your doctor know if you have arthritis or kidney disease, or if you are on a strict low-sodium diet or are taking diuretics.

CONTINUED

Angiotensin-Converting Enzyme (ACE) Inhibitors

POSSIBLE INTERACTIONS

Alcohol: increased ACE inhibitor effects, leading to much lower blood pressure.

Central nervous system stimulants (including pseudoephedrine, an over-the-counter decongestant): reduced ACE inhibitor effect.

Diuretics: combining these drugs may initially cause a significant drop in blood pressure.

Drugs that interact with magnesium, such as tetracycline and diuretics: because of its high magnesium content, quinapril may reduce the body's absorption of these medications.

Estrogens: fluid retention, possibly raising blood pressure.

Indomethacin, NSAIDs, salicylates (such as aspirin): may decrease the effects of ACE inhibitors (especially captopril) and prevent the drugs from lowering blood pressure.

Lithium: lithium toxicity, which can lead to stupor, coma, and seizures.

Other medications that lower blood pressure, such as beta-adrenergic blockers, calcium channel blockers, diuretics, levodopa, nitrates, and opioid analgesics: increased hypotensive (blood-pressure-lowering) effect of both combined medications.

Potassium products and diuretics that do not eliminate potassium from the body (such as amiloride, spironolactone, and triamterene): increased potassium blood levels, leading to heart-rhythm problems.

SIDE EFFECTS

NOT SERIOUS

- Dry, persistent cough
- Headache or fatigue
- Nausea, diarrhea, loss of sense of taste
- Temporary skin rash
- Low blood pressure or dizziness on suddenly rising or changing position

CALL YOUR DOCTOR IF THESE EFFECTS BECOME BOTHERSOME.

SERIOUS

- Fainting
- Joint pain
- Persistent skin rash
- Drowsiness; numbness and tingling
- Abdominal pain; vomiting; diarrhea
- Excessive perspiration; fever; chills
- Chest pain; heart palpitation
- Jaundice (yellowing of skin or eyes)

CALL YOUR DOCTOR RIGHT AWAY.

ANISE

LATIN NAME
Pimpinella anisum

VITAL STATISTICS

GENERAL DESCRIPTION

Anise, an annual plant growing to a height of about two feet, carries tufts of small yellow or white blossoms and bears sweet-tasting seeds traditionally used for tea. Today herbalists recommend anise to relieve cough and promote digestion; the herb can also be found in many standard cough syrups and lozenges. Two chemicals, creosol and alpha-pinene, may account for the herb's effectiveness as an expectorant and cough suppressant.

Anise can help ease breathing and relieve nasal congestion, and it can be used to treat bronchitis. The herbal tea is often taken as a remedy for flatulence. Anise has a mild estrogenic effect and is sometimes recommended to help relieve morning sickness and to treat the symptoms of menopause.

PREPARATIONS

Over the counter:

Available in bulk or as tincture or essential oil.

At home:

TEA: Pour 1 cup boiling water over 1 to 2 tsp crushed seeds; steep covered 5 to 10 minutes. Drink 1 cup three times a day.

TINCTURE: Take ¼ to 1 tsp as often as but no more than three times a day.

COMBINATIONS: To ease cough, prepare a tea using 1 part anise, 2 parts coltsfoot, 2 parts marsh mallow, 2 parts hyssop, and 1 part licorice; add to 1 cup boiling water, steep covered for 20 minutes, and drink hot. For bronchitis, combine with coltsfoot, lobelia, or horehound. To help relieve flatulence, mix with equal parts fennel and caraway.

Consult a qualified practitioner for the dosage appropriate for you and the specific condition being treated.

PRECAUTIONS

WARNING

Do not mistake the poisonous Japanese anise *(Illicium lanceolatum)* for this herb.

SPECIAL INFORMATION

- Anise prepared as a mild tea may be helpful for treating infant colic; use a low-strength solution only.
- If taking anise for flatulence, drink the tea before meals.

POSSIBLE INTERACTIONS

Combining anise with other herbs may necessitate a lower dosage.

TARGET AILMENTS
Cough
Bronchitis
Indigestion
Flatulence

SIDE EFFECTS

NOT SERIOUS

Anise oil:

- Upset stomach
- Diarrhea
- Nausea
- Vomiting

DISCONTINUE USE AND CONSULT YOUR DOCTOR.

ANTACIDS

VITAL STATISTICS

GENERIC NAMES
aluminum hydroxide, calcium carbonate, magnesium carbonate, magnesium hydroxide, sodium bicarbonate and citric acid

GENERAL DESCRIPTION
Antacids relieve the occasional unpleasant symptoms that accompany heartburn, acid indigestion, and "sour" stomach. The drugs work to neutralize excess gastric acid in the stomach, and as a result they help to heal and reduce the pain of ulcers. Antacids are most effective when taken on an empty stomach.

Many popular antacid preparations are combinations of different generic drugs. These combination antacids, such as aluminum and magnesium or calcium and magnesium, have the advantage of offsetting either constipation or diarrhea.

Taken regularly over a long period of time, some calcium-containing antacids may help prevent osteoporosis and other conditions associated with calcium deficiency. For more information, see entries for the generic drugs listed above.

PRECAUTIONS

SPECIAL INFORMATION
- Except under special circumstances determined by your doctor, antacids should not be used if you have impaired renal function or if you have high levels of calcium in your blood, a condition known as hypercalcemia.
- If you have any of the following conditions, you and your doctor will have to weigh the benefits and risks of taking the different types of antacids: symptoms of appendicitis; gastrointestinal or rectal bleeding of undiagnosed cause; intestinal obstruction; sensitivity to aluminum, calcium, magnesium, simethicone, or sodium bicarbonate medications.
- Before taking antacids, check with your doctor if you have had a colostomy or ileostomy, or if you have any of the following: cirrhosis, congestive heart failure, edema, colitis, diverticulitis, diarrhea, constipation or fecal impaction, hemorrhoids, sarcoidosis (a rare disease manifested by lesions in the skin, eyes, lungs, and lymph nodes), or hypophosphatemia (abnormally low concentrations of phosphates in the blood).

ANTACIDS

A

- Children under the age of six should not take antacids without a doctor's approval.
- Notify your doctor if you develop symptoms such as black, tarry stools or vomit the consistency of coffee grounds. These are indications of bleeding in the stomach or intestines.
- Although antacids are considered safe if taken in low doses and for short periods (under two weeks), pregnant and nursing women should consult a doctor first; antacids containing sodium may increase fluid retention.
- Any long-term antacid therapy—such as the treatment of ulcers—should be administered by a doctor.
- Because they can affect the rate of absorption of other drugs, antacids should not be taken within one to two hours of many other oral medications. Ask your doctor or pharmacist for guidance.
- If taken for any length of time, antacids can have a rebound effect that worsens your symptoms when you stop taking the medication.
- Calcium carbonate and sodium bicarbonate antacids can cause milk-alkali syndrome, which is characterized by headaches, nausea, irritability, and weakness. In time, milk-alkali syndrome can lead to kidney disease or failure.

POSSIBLE INTERACTIONS

Staggering medication times is one way to avoid undesirable drug interactions.

Anticholinergics, digoxin, phenothiazines, quinidine, warfarin: antacids are known to interfere with the effectiveness of these drugs.

Aspirin and other salicylates: antacids may increase excretion of these drugs, lessening their effectiveness. Do not take aspirin or other salicylates within three to four hours of antacids.

Cellulose sodium phosphate: the ability of this drug to reduce hypercalciuria (excretion of abnormally large amounts of calcium in the urine) may be lessened when it is taken with calcium antacids.

Enteric-coated medications: antacids may cause the enteric coating to dissolve too rapidly, resulting in gastric irritation. Do not take these medications within one to two hours of antacids.

Iron: decreased iron absorption. Space doses of iron and antacids as far apart as possible (12 hours).

Isoniazid (oral): absorption of this antituber-

TARGET AILMENTS
Upset stomach
Heartburn
Acid indigestion
Sour stomach
Ulcers
Calcium deficiency (calcium carbonate)

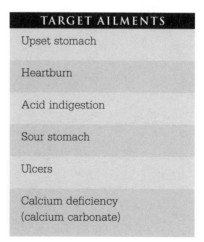

CONTINUED

ANTACIDS

A

cular drug may be delayed and decreased when taken with antacids.

Ketoconazole (antifungal drug): absorption of ketoconazole may be reduced when taken within three hours of antacids.

Mecamylamine: antacids may prolong the effects of this high blood pressure drug. Do not take mecamylamine with antacids.

Methenamine: this drug, used to treat urinary tract infections, may be less effective when taken with antacids.

Phenytoin should not be taken within two to three hours of antacids, since antacids may decrease absorption of this seizure-control drug.

Quinolones: reduced effectiveness of quinolones and fluoroquinolones.

Sodium polystyrene sulfonate (a cholesterol-reducing drug): risk of kidney failure and alkalosis.

Tetracycline (antibiotic): decreased absorption of tetracycline; do not take this drug within three to four hours of antacids.

Vitamin D: if taken concurrently with antacids containing either magnesium or calcium, vitamin D can result in abnormally large amounts of either mineral in the blood.

SIDE EFFECTS

NOT SERIOUS

- Mild constipation
- Laxative effect or diarrhea
- Chalky taste in the mouth
- Stomach cramps, nausea, or vomiting
- Belching
- Flatulence
- White specks in the stool

CALL YOUR DOCTOR IF THESE PROBLEMS PERSIST.

SERIOUS

- Swelling of the wrist, foot, or lower leg
- Bone pain
- Severe constipation
- Dizziness
- Mood changes
- Muscle pain, weakness, or twitching
- Nervousness or restlessness
- Slow breathing
- Irregular heartbeat
- Fatigue
- Pain upon urinating or frequent need to urinate

CONTACT YOUR DOCTOR IMMEDIATELY.

Rx Antiacne Drugs

Vital Statistics

GENERIC NAMES

Rx: erythromycin, isotretinoin, tetracycline, tretinoin
OTC: benzoyl peroxide, resorcinol, salicylic acid, sulfur

GENERAL DESCRIPTION

The antiacne drug class includes a number of prescription and over-the-counter medicines commonly advertised to treat acne and oily skin. These drugs, most of which are applied topically as creams, gels, lotions, or solutions, may work in several ways. Some affect the skin itself, acting as drying agents to reduce oiliness, or as agents that promote cell growth and sloughing or peeling of skin. Others may have antiseptic or antibacterial action, or a combination of actions.

The antibiotics erythromycin and tetracycline and the vitamin A derivatives isotretinoin and tretinoin are prescribed for the treatment of serious cases of acne. For further information about side effects and interactions of these drugs, see the entries for erythromycin, tetracycline, and tretinoin.

Isotretinoin, a chemical cousin of vitamin A, is a powerful drug prescribed for the treatment of severe, disfiguring cystic acne that has not responded to milder medications, including antibiotics. This drug shrinks oil glands and diminishes their output. Isotretinoin is taken by mouth for several months, followed by a two-month rest period.

Resorcinol, salicylic acid, and sulfur are over-the-counter drugs considered safe and effective for the treatment of acne. Benzoyl peroxide is considered effective but has not been proved safe for use in all cases. All over-the-counter acne medications are for external use only. None are to be taken by mouth. Use of more than one topical acne product at a time may increase dryness or skin irritation, although a combination of drugs may be used under the direction of a physician. These products are effective only if you adhere strictly to the treatment plan, which may require weeks or even months.

Resorcinol is a skin-peeling agent and is most effective in combination with sulfur. It should be applied to affected skin areas only.

Salicylic acid is a skin-peeling agent, chemically related to aspirin, that is particularly effective against inflammatory pimples, whiteheads, and blackheads.

Sulfur is believed to cause the outer layer of dead and dying skin to peel away, and it may kill microorganisms that cause acne.

Benzoyl peroxide causes peeling by mildly irritating the blemished outer layer of skin; it also kills underlying acne-causing microorganisms. This drug can be used alone or in combination with systemic antibiotics and products that contain retinoic acid, sulfur, or salicylic acid. The FDA has declared benzoyl peroxide effective in the treatment of acne in adults and children over the age of 12, but has ordered additional safety studies.

Precautions

WARNING

Isotretinoin can cause severe birth defects and must not be taken by pregnant women. To avoid passing the drug on to the baby, do not use isotretinoin if you are breast-feeding.

When taking isotretinoin, be alert to a possible sudden decrease in night vision.

SPECIAL INFORMATION

- Most antiacne drugs cause local irritation and reddening of the skin, which effects

CONTINUED

Antiacne Drugs

may lessen with time. These drugs should not be used if skin is inflamed by sunburn, windburn, cuts, or abrasions. Keep all antiacne medications away from the eyes, nose, and mouth. Consult a doctor if excessive skin irritation occurs.

- Consult your physician if you experience headache, nausea, and visual disturbances when taking isotretinoin along with tetracycline.
- Do not take isotretinoin if you are allergic to parabens, the preservative used in the capsules.
- Benzoyl peroxide may cause severe skin irritation, in which case you should discontinue its use and consult a doctor.
- Do not use benzoyl peroxide or tetracycline if you are pregnant or breast-feeding. (Use of tetracycline during pregnancy, infancy, and in childhood up to age eight can cause permanent discoloration of teeth.)
- Do not use benzoyl peroxide if you are sensitive to compounds derived from benzoic acid or to cinnamon.
- Do not use benzoyl peroxide if you have sensitive skin.

POSSIBLE INTERACTIONS

Alcohol: avoid alcohol consumption when taking isotretinoin.

Sunscreens containing PABA (para-aminobenzoic acid): use with benzoyl peroxide may cause temporary skin discoloration.

Vitamin A: To avoid a possible overdose, do not take vitamin A supplements while taking isotretinoin.

TARGET AILMENTS

Acne

SIDE EFFECTS

NOT SERIOUS

- Conjunctivitis (isotretinoin)
- Dry or fragile skin (isotretinoin)
- Dry mouth (isotretinoin)
- Dry nose (isotretinoin)
- Itching (isotretinoin and benzoyl peroxide)
- Joint pains (isotretinoin)
- Nosebleed (isotretinoin)
- Allergic rash (benzoyl peroxide)
- Excessive drying (red and peeling skin and possible swelling) (benzoyl peroxide)

Call your doctor if these effects become bothersome.

SERIOUS

- Abdominal pain
- Dizziness
- Dry, cracked, inflamed lips
- Facial flushing
- Headache
- Rectal bleeding
- Severe diarrhea
- Vomiting

Call your doctor immediately.

Rx ANTIANXIETY DRUGS

VITAL STATISTICS

GENERIC NAMES
alprazolam, buspirone, diazepam, lorazepam

GENERAL DESCRIPTION
Drugs in this class are prescribed to manage anxiety disorders and relieve symptoms of anxiety. They may also be used to treat panic disorder. Antianxiety drugs are potentially habit forming (addictive). These medications also vary in the amount of time they take to start working and in their duration of action: For example, the effects of alprazolam and other drugs in its subclass (benzodiazepines) start after the first dose, while those of buspirone (a nonbenzodiazepine) can take as long as two weeks.

For more information, including possible drug interactions, see the entries for the generic drugs listed above.

PRECAUTIONS

SPECIAL INFORMATION
- Be careful not to confuse the brand names Xanax (alprazolam) and Zantac. Zantac is the brand name for ranitidine, used to treat ulcers.
- Buspirone has milder sedative effects than other antianxiety drugs and produces no withdrawal symptoms. However, you should not use buspirone unless it is clearly needed. Prolonged periods of use may increase the likelihood of serious side effects.
- Antianxiety drugs should not be used for the stress and anxiety associated with everyday living. They are potentially habit forming, especially when used for extended periods of time or at high dosages.

TARGET AILMENTS

Anxiety and panic disorders (alprazolam, diazepam, lorazepam)

Insomnia (lorazepam)

Convulsions or seizures (diazepam as an adjunct)

Skeletal muscle pain and spasticity (diazepam as an adjunct)

Alcohol withdrawal (diazepam)

Presurgery anxiety (diazepam, lorazepam). Used as an adjunct to anesthesia.

Anxiety disorders or short-term treatment of anxiety symptoms (buspirone)

SIDE EFFECTS

SEE ENTRIES FOR THE INDIVIDUAL GENERIC DRUGS LISTED ABOVE.

Rx ANTIBIOTICS

VITAL STATISTICS

GENERIC NAMES
clindamycin, nitrofurantoin
Carbacephems: loracarbef
Cephalosporins: cefaclor, cefadroxil, cefalexin hydrochloride, cefixime, cefprozil, ceftibuten, cefuroxime, cephalexin
Erythromycins: azithromycin, clarithromycin, erythromycin
Fluoroquinolones: ciprofloxacin, ofloxacin
Ophthalmic Antibiotics: erythromycin, tobramycin
Penicillins: amoxicillin, amoxicillin and clavulanate, ampicillin, penicillin V
Sulfonamides in Combination: sulfamethoxazole and trimethoprim
Tetracyclines: doxycycline, tetracycline
Topical Antibiotics: bacitracin, chlorhexidine, mupirocin, neomycin, polymyxin B

TARGET AILMENTS

Bacterial infections, including those of the respiratory tract, urinary tract, skin, and eyes

SIDE EFFECTS

SEE ENTRIES FOR THE SUBCLASSES LISTED ABOVE.

GENERAL DESCRIPTION
Antibiotics are a large class of drugs used against bacterial infections, such as strep throat, otitis media, and other infections of the respiratory tract, eyes, skin, and other organs. Bactericidal antibiotics kill bacteria by attacking bacterial cell walls. Bacteriostatic antibiotics prevent bacteria from reproducing, thus enabling the body's defenses to overcome the infection. Antibiotics are not effective against fungal infections or against viruses, such as those that cause colds.

Because antibiotics target bacteria and not fungi, the drugs can disturb the body's normal balance of fungi and bacteria. This imbalance may be manifested as a fungal superinfection, such as a yeast infection, or in symptoms of diarrhea or gastrointestinal disturbance. To help restore your body's normal bacteria, some doctors recommend eating yogurt that contains *Lactobacillus acidophilus* culture or taking acidophilus tablets during antibiotic therapy and for a week afterward. For more information, including possible drug interactions, see the entries for the generic drugs and their subclasses listed at left.

PRECAUTIONS

SPECIAL INFORMATION
To prevent reinfection, take the full course of your prescription, even if you feel better before you've taken all the medicine.

Rx ANTICANCER DRUGS

VITAL STATISTICS

GENERIC NAMES
bleomycin, cyclophosphamide, daunorubicin, doxorubicin, fluorouracil, goserelin, hydroxyurea, leuprolide, methotrexate, mitotane, mitoxantrone, procarbazine, tamoxifen, vincristine

GENERAL DESCRIPTION
Medications in the anticancer drug class are used against the various forms of cancer, such as leukemia, lymphoma, and cancers of the prostate, colon, ovaries, and breasts. The drugs, used in treatment regimens known as chemotherapy, generally work by preventing the growth of abnormal, tumor-forming cells. Some drugs in this class are thought to block the effects of hormones that may stimulate cancer cell growth. For side effects and other information about a specific drug used to treat breast cancer, see Tamoxifen.

PRECAUTIONS

SPECIAL INFORMATION
Tell your doctor if you have ever had thrombophlebitis, pulmonary embolism, impaired liver function, cataracts, a blood cell or bone-marrow disorder, or abnormally high blood calcium levels. Your doctor may lower your dose or prescribe a different drug.

POSSIBLE INTERACTIONS
Anticancer drugs can interact adversely with a wide range of other medicines. Be sure to tell your doctor about any medications you may already be taking, including anti-inflammatory drugs and other anticancer medicine.

TARGET AILMENTS

Various types of cancer, including cancer of the breast, ovaries, skin, lung, prostate, testicles, lymph nodes, colon, bone marrow, and liver

SIDE EFFECTS

NOT SERIOUS

- Loss of appetite
- Nausea
- Vomiting
- Diarrhea
- Temporary hair loss
- Skin rash
- Itching
- Darkening of the skin and fingernails
- Unusual fatigue

CALL YOUR DOCTOR IF THESE EFFECTS PERSIST OR ARE BOTHERSOME.

SERIOUS

- Fever
- Chills
- Abnormal bleeding
- Easy bruising

CALL YOUR DOCTOR IMMEDIATELY.

ANTICOAGULANT AND ANTIPLATELET DRUGS

VITAL STATISTICS

GENERIC NAMES

Rx: dalteparin, dipyridamole, heparin, warfarin
OTC: aspirin

GENERAL DESCRIPTION

Anticoagulants and antiplatelet drugs decrease the blood's clotting ability. They are generally used as a secondary form of prevention for diseases in which the formation of harmful blood clots may cause serious problems. Although sometimes called blood thinners, these drugs do not really thin the blood or dissolve existing blood clots. They stop clots from growing larger and prevent new clots from forming in the blood vessels.

Antiplatelet drugs (aspirin, dipyridamole) and anticoagulants (dalteparin, heparin, warfarin) can be used alone or in combination. The drugs and dosages must be carefully balanced for each patient. See also entries for the generic drugs listed above.

PRECAUTIONS

☠ *WARNING*

Do not use these drugs without telling your physician if you have had a heart attack, uncontrolled high blood pressure, ulcers, internal bleeding, or a stroke.

SPECIAL INFORMATION

- Pregnant and nursing women should check with a physician before taking dalteparin, dipyridamole, or heparin. If you are pregnant or nursing, you should not take aspirin. Warfarin may cause birth defects.
- These medications must be taken as directed by your physician.

TARGET AILMENTS

These drugs are prescribed as prophylaxis to reduce the risk of:

- Blood clot formation in the veins (phlebitis)
- Blood clot formation in the lungs (pulmonary thromboembolism)
- Blood clot formation in the brain (cerebral thrombosis)
- Heart attack and stroke
- Blood-clotting complications during or after surgery
- Blood clot formation in the heart chambers due to atrial fibrillation or a prosthetic heart valve

Anticoagulant and Antiplatelet Drugs

- Do not use a given drug if you have had an allergic reaction to it in the past.
- Tell your doctor if you have or have had low blood pressure, an impaired kidney or liver, a bleeding disease or disorder, chest pains, allergies, asthma, colitis, diabetes, active tuberculosis, a recent childbirth, medical or dental surgery, spinal anesthesia, x-rays, a bad fall, heavy bleeding or menstrual periods, diarrhea, or any other medical problem. Also, tell your doctor if you are using an intrauterine device (IUD) for birth control or a catheter.
- Antiplatelet drugs and anticoagulants may affect some lab tests. Before undergoing a lab test, be sure to advise the practitioner administering the test that you are taking the drug.
- Tell your pharmacist, dentist, and physician that you are taking the medicine. You may be advised to carry a medication identification card.
- Avoid dangerous activities that might cause injuries. Be sure to report all falls and blows to your doctor. Internal bleeding may occur without symptoms.

POSSIBLE INTERACTIONS

Anticoagulant drugs seem to be involved in more interactions than any other class of drug. Be sure to let your healthcare professional know if you are taking any other medicine (prescription or over-the-counter) including aspirin, vitamins, laxatives, and antacids.

SIDE EFFECTS

NOT SERIOUS

SEE INDIVIDUAL ENTRIES FOR THE GENERIC DRUGS LISTED OPPOSITE.

SERIOUS

- Unexplained bruising or purplish areas on the skin
- Bleeding from gums
- Heavy bleeding from cuts or wounds
- Unusually heavy nosebleeds or menstrual periods

CALL YOUR DOCTOR IMMEDIATELY IF YOU EXPERIENCE ANY OF THESE EARLY SIGNS OF TOO MUCH BLEEDING (EXCESS ANTICOAGULATION, OR OVERDOSE). THIS COULD BE A RESULT OF THESE DRUGS BEING USED ALONE OR IN COMBINATION.

- Headache, visual disturbances, muscle weakness, or sensory changes
- Backache or back pain
- Abdominal swelling or pain
- Blood in urine
- Tarry or bloody stools
- Constipation
- Coughing up or vomiting blood
- Joint stiffness, pain, or swelling

CALL YOUR DOCTOR IMMEDIATELY IF YOU EXPERIENCE ANY OF THESE SIGNS OF INTERNAL BLEEDING. THIS COULD BE A RESULT OF THESE DRUGS BEING USED ALONE OR IN COMBINATION.

ANTICONVULSANT DRUGS

A

VITAL STATISTICS

GENERIC NAMES
carbamazepine, phenytoin, valproic acid

GENERAL DESCRIPTION
The anticonvulsant drug class contains a number of medications used in the treatment of epilepsy. Although the exact mechanisms by which these drugs work are unknown, anticonvulsants appear to inhibit the sudden spread of excessive or abnormal electrical impulses in the brain, thereby limiting or preventing epileptic convulsions.

Anticonvulsants are not curatives, but they can reduce the possibility of seizure-related brain damage. They are usually prescribed, either alone or in combination, to control specific types of epileptic seizures. Since every case of epilepsy is unique and all anticonvulsants have toxic effects when taken in large dosages, a period of trial and error is usually needed to determine the appropriate drug and dosage. For more information, including serious side effects, see entries for the generic drugs listed above. See also Benzodiazepines, Clonazepam, and Diazepam.

PRECAUTIONS

SPECIAL INFORMATION
- Driving and hazardous activities should be avoided.
- You may be advised to wear a bracelet or carry an identification card stating which anticonvulsant drug you are taking.

TARGET AILMENTS

Epilepsy

SIDE EFFECTS

NOT SERIOUS
- Skin rashes
- Headache
- Nausea
- Dizziness
- Confusion
- Unsteadiness

CALL YOUR DOCTOR IF THESE EFFECTS PERSIST OR ARE BOTHERSOME.

Rx ANTIDEPRESSANTS

A

VITAL STATISTICS

GENERIC NAMES

Monoamine Oxidase (MAO) Inhibitors: isocarboxazid, phenelzine, tranylcypromine
Selective Serotonin Reuptake Inhibitors (SSRIs): fluoxetine, paroxetine, sertraline, venlafaxine
Tricyclic Antidepressants (TCAs): amitriptyline, doxepin, nortriptyline

GENERAL DESCRIPTION

Antidepressants are a class of nonnarcotic drugs that restore the normal levels of neurotransmitters such as serotonin and norepinephrine in the brain. Subclasses of antidepressants include tricyclic antidepressants (amitriptyline, doxepin, and nortriptyline) and selective serotonin reuptake inhibitors such as fluoxetine. Although the drugs in each subclass are somewhat distinct in structure and mode of action, they have similar uses and side effects. A few appear to be effective for nondepressive diseases such as phobias. For more information, see entries for the individual generic drugs listed above. Also see the entries for the individual subclasses and generic drugs listed above.

PRECAUTIONS

☠ *WARNING*

On rare occasions, antidepressant drugs may cause the following effects: allergic reactions, skin rash or spots, bruising or bleeding, jaundice, sore throat, fever, ringing in the ears. Call your doctor immediately if you notice these symptoms.

SPECIAL INFORMATION

- Antidepressants may cause drowsiness. When taking these drugs, use care while driving, operating machinery, or performing tasks that require mental alertness.
- These drugs, especially fluoxetine, can trigger manic attacks in individuals with manic-depression. Be sure to tell your doctor if you have manic-depression.
- Antidepressants can affect blood sugar (glucose tolerance) tests by causing fluctuation in blood sugar levels.
- Fluoxetine may exacerbate suicidal tendencies in some individuals. Be sure to tell your healthcare provider if you have experienced thoughts of suicide or believe you may be susceptible to such thoughts. The doctor may want to prescribe a different drug.
- The full effects of an antidepressant drug may not occur for several weeks.
- If you are pregnant, nursing, or planning a pregnancy, check with your doctor before taking antidepressants.

TARGET AILMENTS
Major depressive disorders
Obsessive-compulsive disorders
Phobias
Eating disorders
Chronic severe pain, especially in migraine headaches, cancer, and severe arthritis (TCAs)

CONTINUED

ANTIDEPRESSANTS

POSSIBLE INTERACTIONS

Alcohol and other drugs that depress the central nervous system: increased antidepressant effects, leading to problems such as respiratory depression or very low blood pressure.

Anticoagulant drugs (such as warfarin): Tricyclic antidepressants may increase the anticlotting activity.

Anticonvulsants: decreased effectiveness of anticonvulsants, making seizures more likely.

Antihistamines: increased antihistamine action, including any side effects; antihistamines may also increase the action of antidepressants, including any side effects.

Barbiturates: decreased effectiveness of tricyclic antidepressants.

Digitalis preparations: using fluoxetine or sertraline with heart medications may increase blood levels of both the antidepressant and the heart drugs, increasing the risk of side effects.

Lithium: taking fluoxetine or sertraline with lithium could increase blood levels of lithium, leading to toxicity.

MAO inhibitors: severe, possibly fatal reactions such as seizures, tremor, and coma because of additive effects of the drugs.

Other antidepressants: combining antidepressants will likely increase the action of one or both drugs, leading to increased side effects.

Thyroid medications: combining tricyclic antidepressants with thyroid drugs may increase the effects, including side effects, of both medications.

SIDE EFFECTS

NOT SERIOUS

- Dizziness on changing position
- Drowsiness
- Mild fatigue or weakness
- Dry mouth
- Headache
- Increased appetite or food cravings
- Weight gain
- Nausea or, less frequently, diarrhea
- Increased sweating or insomnia
- Photosensitivity

CALL YOUR DOCTOR IF THESE SYMPTOMS PERSIST.

SERIOUS

- Blurred vision, confusion, delirium, or hallucinations
- Paralytic ileus (blockage of intestines, possibly indicated by abdominal pain or swelling, difficulty in breathing, and severe constipation)
- Difficulty in urination
- Eye pain from aggravated glaucoma
- Tremors
- Changes in heartbeat
- Nervousness or restlessness
- Parkinson's-like symptoms (shuffling walk, stiffness in the extremities)

CALL YOUR DOCTOR IMMEDIATELY.

Rx ANTIDIABETIC DRUGS

VITAL STATISTICS

GENERIC NAMES
insulin; glipizide, glyburide (Oral Hypoglycemics); acarbose, metformin, troglitazone (Oral Antihyperglycemics)

GENERAL DESCRIPTION
The specific medication used to treat diabetes depends on which type of the disease you have. Oral drugs are prescribed for non-insulin-dependent diabetes, commonly known as Type 2 diabetes. Insulin-dependent diabetes (Type 1) can be controlled only through injections of insulin, a hormone normally produced by the pancreas. A program of diet and exercise, used in conjunction with antidiabetic drugs, is vital to controlling both types of the disease.

Oral hypoglycemic drugs, such as glipizide and glyburide, stimulate the release of existing insulin in people whose bodies are capable of producing insulin. Also known as sulfonylureas, these drugs do not lower blood sugar on their own but must be combined with a prescribed regimen of diet and exercise to perform effectively.

The newer oral antihyperglycemic drugs work by several different mechanisms and may be used alone or in combination with oral hypoglycemic drugs.

Injected insulin provides necessary amounts of insulin in people whose bodies are not capable of producing the hormone. Insulin does lower blood sugar by itself, although it works most effectively in combination with a prescribed program of diet and exercise. For more information, including side effects and possible interactions with other medications, see entries for the generic drugs listed above and Oral Hypoglycemics.

PRECAUTIONS

WARNING
An overdose of these drugs can result in hypoglycemia (abnormally small concentrations of sugar in the blood). Signs of hypoglycemia include excessive hunger, cold sweats, shakiness, nervousness or anxiety, rapid pulse, headache, drowsiness, confusion, nausea, and cool, pale skin. Keep hard candy, fruit juice, or glucose tablets handy to raise your blood sugar level and counteract hypoglycemia. Call your doctor immediately.

SPECIAL INFORMATION
- People who are elderly, debilitated, or malnourished, as well as those with adrenal, thyroid, pituitary, kidney, or liver problems, have an increased susceptibility to the hypoglycemic action of antidiabetic drugs and should use them with caution.
- It is important to self-monitor your glucose level when taking these drugs.

TARGET AILMENTS
Type 1 diabetes (insulin only)
Type 2 diabetes (oral drugs or insulin)
Gestational (pregnancy) diabetes (temporary insulin therapy)
Severe blood sugar imbalances occurring in nondiabetics as a result of surgery, acute stress, or shock (temporary insulin therapy)

ANTIDIARRHEAL DRUGS

A

VITAL STATISTICS

GENERIC NAMES

attapulgite, bismuth subsalicylate, loperamide

GENERAL DESCRIPTION

Over-the-counter antidiarrheal drugs are used for the short-term control and symptomatic relief of diarrhea. Diarrhea can vary in intensity from mild (three to four loose, watery stools a day) to severe (10 or more per day) and may be accompanied by weakness, flatulence, pain, fever, or vomiting.

Antidiarrheal drugs have different functions. Some combat the symptoms of diarrhea; some are directed against the cause; and others try to counter some of the effects of the ailment. Attapulgite, a claylike substance, binds and inactivates the intestinal irritants that are causing the problem. Bismuth subsalicylate and loperamide seem to stop diarrhea and cramps by slowing down the movements and contractions of the intestinal tract. For more information, see entries for the generic drugs listed above.

A number of antidiarrheal drugs are available only by prescription. If over-the-counter medications do not solve the problem, see your doctor.

PRECAUTIONS

SPECIAL INFORMATION

- It is possible to take too much over-the-counter medication. Symptoms of bismuth subsalicylate overdose include anxiety, confusion, depression, fast or deep breathing, headache, sweating, muscle spasms or weakness, nausea, vomiting, stomach pain, ringing in the ears, and trembling. Check with your doctor immediately.
- Diarrhea can cause excessive fluid loss. Call your doctor as soon as possible if you have any signs of dehydration, including decreased urination, lightheadedness and dizziness, wrinkled skin, dryness of mouth, or increased thirst.
- When you use antidiarrheal drugs, it is vitally important that you replace lost fluids by drinking large quantities of water and other clear liquids (such as decaffeinated colas and tea, ginger ale, and broth). Eat only gelatin for the first 24 hours. The next day you may eat bland foods, such as bread, crackers, cooked cereals, and applesauce. Other beverages and foods may make the condition worse.
- Antidiarrheals are not recommended for children under three years of age or for geriatric patients. If used, follow your doctor's instructions.
- Do not use antidiarrheals if you have a fever or your stool contains blood or mucus: These are symptoms of dysentery, an infection of the lower intestinal tract. Contact your doctor.

POSSIBLE INTERACTIONS

Alcohol, sleeping pills, and tranquilizers: may increase depressant and sedative effects.

Antibiotics and narcotic pain medicine: may cause severe constipation if taken with antidiarrheals.

TARGET AILMENTS

Acute diarrhea:
the sudden onset of loose stools in an otherwise healthy person. The cause may be infectious, toxic, dietary, drug induced, or the result of various ailments. Infectious diarrhea, especially in children in the United States, is usually viral in origin.

Traveler's diarrhea:
a form of acute infectious diarrhea afflicting tourists in foreign lands. It is usually caused by various bacteria found in contaminated food or water.

Chronic diarrhea:
persistent or recurrent bouts of diarrhea associated with inflammatory bowel disease

SIDE EFFECTS

WHEN USED AT THE RECOMMENDED DOSAGE FOR NO MORE THAN TWO DAYS, THESE DRUGS RARELY CAUSE SIDE EFFECTS. BUT IF THE DIARRHEA DOES NOT DECREASE WITHIN ONE OR TWO DAYS, CHECK WITH YOUR DOCTOR.

NOT SERIOUS

- Fever
- Mild constipation
- Grayish black stool and darkened tongue (bismuth subsalicylate)

THESE EFFECTS ARE HARMLESS, BUT CHECK WITH YOUR DOCTOR IF THE CONSTIPATION CONTINUES OR IS TROUBLESOME.

SERIOUS

- Bismuth subsalicylate can be toxic if taken in very large doses.

SEE OVERDOSE SYMPTOMS OPPOSITE.

- Constipation, bloating, loss of appetite, and stomach pain with vomiting and nausea (loperamide)

VERY RARE BUT MIGHT INDICATE A MORE DANGEROUS BOWEL PROBLEM. CALL YOUR DOCTOR PROMPTLY IF THESE SYMPTOMS DEVELOP, OR IF YOU DEVELOP A RASH.

ANTIFUNGAL DRUGS

A

VITAL STATISTICS

GENERIC NAMES
Rx: clotrimazole, fluconazole, ketoconazole, miconazole, terconazole
OTC: clotrimazole, miconazole, tolnaftate, undecylenate

GENERAL DESCRIPTION
Antifungal drugs are used to treat a wide variety of conditions, including fungal infections of the skin, lungs, mouth, groin, hands, feet, and nails. Ringworm infections, including athlete's foot and jock itch, are among the best-known groups of skin disorders for which these drugs are used. Some antifungal medications are also used to treat yeast infections of the mouth (oral thrush); skin folds and hands; urethra, penis and foreskin (balanitis); and vagina.

Antifungal drugs work in different ways to interfere with the growth and reproduction of fungal cells or, in strong concentrations, to destroy fungal cells. These medications can be topical, vaginal, or systemic (acting throughout the body) and are available as creams, suppositories, lotions, powders, sprays, shampoos, lozenges, and oral tablets.

Topical lotions, creams, powders, and sprays are applied directly to the skin to treat fungal skin infections. Because they are massaged into the skin, creams and ointments are more effective than sprays and powders for the treatment of skin infections. Spray and powder forms of antifungal medications are effective in preventing fungal skin infections.

Vaginal antifungal creams and suppositories are inserted directly into the vagina, usually at bedtime, for a period of three to seven days.

Systemic antifungal medications (ketoconazole) are available in oral suspension and tablet form. They are used to treat a variety of disorders, including pneumonia and urinary tract infections.

For more information, see entries for the generic drugs listed at left. Also see Vaginal Antifungal Drugs for information about a subclass of medications commonly used to treat vaginal yeast infections.

TARGET AILMENTS
Yeast infections (candidiasis) of the vulva and vagina, mouth, skin, hands, and internal organs
Ringworm (tinea) of the body, scalp, nails, hands, feet (athlete's foot), and groin (jock itch)
Tinea versicolor, a ringworm infection that produces white-brown patches on the skin
Fungal diseases of the lungs
Fungal skin infections (topical)
Seborrheic dermatitis
Dandruff

Antifungal Drugs

A

Precautions

SPECIAL INFORMATION

- Do not use any topical antifungal medications if you have had an allergic reaction to another drug of this type. Check first with your physician or pharmacist.
- Although ringworm medications are available in over-the-counter form, be sure your condition has been correctly diagnosed before treating it yourself.
- Be sure to wash and thoroughly dry the infected area before using creams and ointments to treat skin infections.
- It is very important to medicate the entire area when treating an active fungal infection. If you have athlete's foot, for example, you need to apply the medication between all toes, to the skin around each toenail, and to the sole of the foot. Both feet should be treated with the same thorough care.
- Pregnant and nursing women should avoid antifungal medications, unless administered under a doctor's care.
- Because fungi thrive in moist conditions, avoid tight-fitting shoes and underwear made with synthetic fibers during treatment; wear cotton underwear instead.

POSSIBLE INTERACTIONS

No interactions are expected with most topical and vaginal forms of antifungal drugs. See Ketoconazole for a list of drugs and other substances you should avoid while taking systemic antifungal medications.

SIDE EFFECTS

NOT SERIOUS

- Mild skin irritation in the infected area
- Headache
- Drowsiness
- Dizziness
- Nausea or vomiting
- Stomach pain
- Constipation or diarrhea

CALL YOUR DOCTOR IF THESE SIDE EFFECTS PERSIST OR BECOME BOTHERSOME.

SERIOUS

- Allergic skin reactions, such as a rash or hives (topical preparations)
- Redness, stinging, burning, or itching of the genitals; abdominal cramps or menstrual irregularities; or itching and burning of a sexual partner's penis (vaginal preparations)

CALL YOUR DOCTOR IF YOU EXPERIENCE ANY OF THESE SIDE EFFECTS.

ANTIGASTROESOPHAGEAL REFLUX DRUGS

VITAL STATISTICS

GENERIC NAME
cisapride

GENERAL DESCRIPTION
Drugs in this class target gastroesophageal reflux disease, a digestive disorder affecting the lower esophageal sphincter, the muscle that separates the esophagus from the stomach. The condition results when stomach contents back up into the esophagus, causing the unpleasant sensations known as heartburn and acid indigestion. The problem, which often occurs during pregnancy and is more common in middle age, can usually be corrected through alterations in your diet and meal schedule. Eating shortly before bedtime, for example, is more likely to produce the disorder than eating several hours earlier.

Antigastroesophageal reflux drugs act by strengthening the lower esophageal sphincter to inhibit backflow, and by speeding up the emptying of stomach contents into the intestines. For information about a specific generic drug used to treat this disorder, see Cisapride. Medications known as histamine H_2 blockers, a subclass of antiulcer drugs, are also used to treat chronic gastroesophageal reflux. For information about these drugs, see Histamine H_2 Blockers, as well as individual entries for Cimetidine, Famotidine, Nizatidine, and Ranitidine.

PRECAUTIONS

SPECIAL INFORMATION
- Do not take antigastroesophageal reflux drugs if you have intestinal or stomach bleeding, obstruction of the bowel, or any other gastrointestinal problem.
- Do not take these drugs if you have epilepsy or a history of seizures.
- Weigh the benefit-to-risk ratio with your doctor if you are pregnant or considering pregnancy. If you are nursing, discuss use of antigastroesophageal reflux drugs with your doctor, since low levels of these drugs pass into breast milk.
- Inform your doctor if you have a history of liver, kidney, or heart problems.
- Do not take antigastroesophageal reflux drugs if you are taking ketoconazole, troleandomycin, or itraconazole.
- Take these medications at least 15 minutes before meals and at bedtime.

TARGET AILMENTS

Heartburn and acid indigestion caused by gastroesophageal reflux disease

Antigastroesophageal Reflux Drugs

A

POSSIBLE INTERACTIONS

Alcohol and benzodiazepines: antigastroesophageal reflux drugs increase the absorption rate of these drugs, thus increasing their sedating effects. Use these medications with caution if you are taking antigastroesophageal reflux drugs.

Anticholinergic drugs: decreased antigastroesophageal reflux drug effect.

Anticoagulants, cimetidine, ranitidine: increased effects of these drugs.

Ketoconazole, troleandomycin, itraconazole: these drugs inhibit the metabolism of antigastroesophageal reflux drugs, thereby greatly increasing their effects. Do not take these drugs concurrently with antigastroesophageal reflux drugs.

Sleeping pills: use these drugs with caution if you are taking antigastroesophageal reflux drugs.

SIDE EFFECTS

NOT SERIOUS

- Diarrhea or constipation
- Abdominal discomfort
- Runny nose (rhinitis)
- Nausea
- Fatigue
- Headache
- Flatulence
- Dizziness
- Drowsiness
- Rash
- Dry mouth
- Coughing
- Sore throat
- Upper respiratory infection
- Muscle or joint pain
- Nervousness
- Frequent urination
- Vaginal irritation

CONSULT YOUR DOCTOR IF THESE SYMPTOMS PERSIST OR BECOME BOTHERSOME.

SERIOUS

- Seizures in patients with a history of seizures
- Tremors
- Heart palpitations
- Liver inflammation
- Hepatitis
- Migraines
- Swelling of the legs or feet
- Uncontrolled muscle movements

CONSULT YOUR DOCTOR PROMPTLY IF ANY OF THESE SYMPTOMS ARISE.

Antigout Drugs

A

Vital Statistics

GENERIC NAMES
Rx: allopurinol, colchicine, prednisone (corticosteroid)
OTC: nonsteroidal anti-inflammatory drugs (NSAIDs)

GENERAL DESCRIPTION
Antigout drugs are used to reduce high levels of uric acid in the urine or in the blood, a condition called hyperuricemia, or to relieve the pain and inflammation associated with acute attacks of gouty arthritis, or crystal arthritis. OTC drugs, such as oral analgesics, are often used concurrently with antigout drugs to alleviate the pain and swelling in the affected joints.

Gout, a form of arthritis, occurs when the body is unable to rid the blood of excess uric acid. Crystals of the chemical accumulate between the bones of joints, resulting in inflammation, sudden and severe pain, and in severe cases, joint deformity. Gout can be caused by injuries, surgery, stress, infections, kidney disorders, enzyme deficiencies, anemia, drug or alcohol reactions, and cancer. Hyperuricemia may also be caused by an inherited defect in metabolism, but often the cause is unknown.

Along with a purine-reduced diet (e.g., eliminating such foods as organ meats, shellfish, fatty fish, dried beans, and spinach), early use of antigout drugs can often prevent future gout attacks. A trial-and-error process is often necessary to determine the most effective drug therapy.

Low-dose colchicine is the drug of choice for treating and preventing acute attacks of gouty arthritis, although nonsteroidal anti-inflammatory drugs like indomethacin or naproxen are also effective. In chronic gout, allopurinol, probenecid, and sulfinpyrazone assist with the elimination of excess uric acid in the urine. These drugs are also useful for treating crystalline deposits, called tophi, which can form over time in the soft tissue of the hands, feet, or earlobes, causing aching, stiffness, and hard protrusions.

OTC anti-inflammatory agents such as ibuprofen or analgesics such as acetaminophen can alleviate the symptoms of disease until the uric acid level in the blood is properly balanced.

Depending on the patient, long-term drug therapy may be necessary. Once long-term treatment is started, it may need to be continued for life to prevent damage to bone and cartilage or deterioration of the kidneys, where the excess uric acid crystallizes and forms kidney stones. The drug of choice for long-term use is allopurinol.

For more specific information, see the individual entries for the prescription and OTC drugs listed above, left.

Antigout Drugs

A

Precautions

☠ ***WARNING***

Indomethacin and other nonsteroidal anti-inflammatory drugs should be avoided if you have peptic ulcer disease. Use these drugs with caution if you have hypertension or congestive heart failure.

Do not use probenecid if you have kidney disease.

SPECIAL INFORMATION

- Because of the potency of many antigout medications, patients with serious or chronic gout conditions should remain under close medical supervision and undergo periodic diagnostic blood tests. This is especially true for pregnant women who may also be taking thiazide diuretics to lower the body's water retention.
- Drink plenty of fluids (two to three quarts daily) while taking antigout drugs regularly.
- Susceptible individuals can develop gout or hyperuricemia as a result of drug therapy for other conditions, such as diuretic therapy.
- Avoid taking aspirin and other salicylates if you suspect that you have gout. These drugs can retard uric acid excretion.
- Avoid alcohol, acetazolamide, antineoplastic (antitumor) drugs, nicotinic acid, and thiazide diuretics if you have gout. These drugs can raise the blood level of uric acid and thereby encourage the onset of acute gouty arthritis.

TARGET AILMENTS

Gout

Gouty arthritis

Hyperuricemia

Tophaceous gout

SIDE EFFECTS

NOT SERIOUS

- Headache
- Abdominal pain
- Diarrhea, vomiting, or nausea
- Fever
- Hair loss (colchicine)

DISCONTINUE USE AND CALL YOUR DOCTOR FOR GUIDANCE.

SERIOUS

- Skin rash or hives, indicating an allergic reaction (anaphylaxis)
- Bloody diarrhea
- Fever; fatigue; abnormal bleeding or bruising (bone marrow depression)
- Numbness, tingling, or pain in hands or feet
- Ptosis (drooping of the eyes)

DISCONTINUE USE AND CALL YOUR DOCTOR IMMEDIATELY. IN THE CASE OF A SEVERE ALLERGIC REACTION, SEEK EMERGENCY TREATMENT.

Antihistamines

Vital Statistics

GENERIC NAMES

Rx: astemizole, cetirizine, diphenhydramine, fexofenadine, loratadine, promethazine, terfenadine

OTC: brompheniramine, chlorpheniramine, clemastine, dexbrompheniramine, diphenhydramine, doxylamine, triprolidine

BRAND NAMES

Rx brands:

Allegra (fexofenadine); Benadryl (diphenhydramine); Claritin, Claritin-D 12 Hour (loratadine); Hismanal (astemizole); Phenergan (promethazine); Seldane, Seldane-D (terfenadine); Zyrtec (cetirizine)

OTC brands:

- Dimetapp (brompheniramine)
- Alka-Seltzer Plus Cold Medicine, Children's Tylenol Cold Multi-Symptom, Children's Tylenol Cold Plus Cough, Chlor-Trimeton, Comtrex Multi-Symptom Cold Reliever, TheraFlu, Triaminic Nite Light, Triaminic Syrup, Triaminicol Multi-Symptom Relief, Tylenol Allergy Sinus, Tylenol Cold Multi-Symptom Formula (chlorpheniramine)
- Tavist-D (clemastine)
- Drixoral Cold and Flu, Drixoral Cold and Allergy (dexbrompheniramine)
- Benadryl, Excedrin PM, Tylenol Allergy Sinus Night Time Medication, Tylenol Cold Night Time Medication Liquid, Tylenol Flu Night Time, Tylenol PM, Unisom (diphenhydramine)
- NyQuil (doxylamine)
- Actifed (triprolidine)

GENERAL DESCRIPTION

Antihistamines block the action of histamine, a natural substance the body releases when fighting infection and in allergic reactions; histamine causes the runny nose, watery eyes, congestion, and hives or itching associated with allergies. Antihistamines are used primarily to relieve the symptoms of allergies and colds, although they cannot cure the underlying conditions. Since a common side effect of the older antihistamines is drowsiness, some are used as sleeping aids. The newer antihistamines—astemizole, fexofenadine, loratadine, and terfenadine—are less likely to cause drowsiness.

PRECAUTIONS

SPECIAL INFORMATION

- Antihistamines are considered unsafe for women who are pregnant or nursing.
- Many antihistamines are considered unsafe for children under the age of 12. Some are appropriate if the child's dosage is determined by a physician or, in the case of OTC drugs, printed on the label. Children may be more susceptible to side effects than adults. Their reactions to a high dose are different too; while adults may experience sedation and lethargy, children are more likely to become jittery and nervous, and may have trouble sleeping.
- To avoid drowsiness, take less of the drug or try another antihistamine. Some antihistamines, such as loratadine, do not cause drowsiness, and over time you may develop a partial tolerance to the drugs that do.
- If you are taking an antihistamine that causes drowsiness, avoid driving or operating machinery until you know how the drug affects you.
- Some antihistamines, especially astemizole, loratadine, and terfenadine, may cause palpitations, fainting, cardiac arrest, or other serious heart disorders if taken in dosages higher than those recommended. Follow the dosage instructions carefully.
- If antihistamines give you an upset stomach, nausea, diarrhea, or other gastrointestinal problems, take the pills with meals or with milk.
- Check with your doctor before using antihistamines if you have asthma, narrow-angle glaucoma, an enlarged prostate, a stomach ulcer, a bladder obstruction, heart disease, or liver disease; the drugs may exacerbate these conditions.
- The Food and Drug Administration recently announced its intention to withdraw approval of terfenadine; it considers the drug fexofenadine to be a safer alternative, with essentially the same benefits. Talk with your doctor about the best medication for you.

TARGET AILMENTS

Nasal and respiratory allergies (seasonal and nonseasonal), including hay fever

Common cold (although antihistamines alone are not effective for most cold symptoms)

Allergic skin reactions (to poison ivy and insect bites, for example)

Insomnia (except astemizole, fexofenadine, loratadine, and terfenadine)

Motion sickness (diphenhydramine and promethazine)

CONTINUED

ANTIHISTAMINES

POSSIBLE INTERACTIONS

Alcohol: likely to increase the sedative effects of certain antihistamines; do not drink when you take these drugs.

Antianxiety drugs; barbiturates or other sedatives: do not take with antihistamines, as the combination may result in excessive sedation.

Clarithromycin, erythromycin, itraconazole, and ketoconazole: may interfere with the body's metabolism of astemizole, loratadine, or terfenadine and cause life-threatening cardiac problems. WARNING: Do not combine these drugs with astemizole, loratadine, or terfenadine.

MAO inhibitors: can cause hypotension and dryness of the respiratory passages when taken with antihistamines. Do not combine these drugs with antihistamines.

SIDE EFFECTS

NOT SERIOUS

- Drowsiness in varying degrees—avoid driving or operating machinery until you know how the antihistamine you are taking affects you
- Dizziness, weakness, and slower movement and reaction time
- Dryness of the mouth, nose, or throat
- Nervousness, restlessness, and insomnia, especially in children
- Upset stomach, nausea, and change in bowel habits

CALL YOUR DOCTOR IF THESE SYMPTOMS CONTINUE OR BECOME BOTHERSOME.

SERIOUS

- Fainting or irregular heart rhythms caused by astemizole, loratadine, and terfenadine (rare)

CALL YOUR DOCTOR IMMEDIATELY IF YOU NOTICE ANY CHANGE IN YOUR HEARTBEAT.

- Itchiness, rash, or inflammation caused by topical antihistamines (uncommon)

IF YOU THINK ANTIHISTAMINES ARE CAUSING THESE SYMPTOMS, DISCONTINUE USE AND TELL YOUR DOCTOR.

ANTIHYPERTENSIVE DRUGS

VITAL STATISTICS

SUBCLASSES AND RELATED CLASSES

Alpha$_1$-Adrenergic Blockers, Angiotensin-Converting Enzyme (ACE) Inhibitors, Beta-Adrenergic Blockers, Calcium Channel Blockers, Diuretics, Angiotensin II Antagonists (see Losartan)

GENERIC NAME

guanfacine

GENERAL DESCRIPTION

Antihypertensives are drugs used to control high blood pressure (hypertension), which affects some 40 million Americans. The particular antihypertensive drug prescribed for a given person depends, in part, on the severity of the condition.

Antihypertensive medications include diuretics, calcium channel blockers, angiotensin-converting enzyme (ACE) inhibitors, and sympathetic nervous system inhibitors, which act either centrally (in the brain) or peripherally (in the blood vessels) to block signals from the brain that tell the arteries to constrict.

The information here applies specifically to a centrally acting antihypertensive drug (guanfacine) used in the control of mild-to-moderate high blood pressure. For more information on other forms of antihypertensive medication, see the entries Alpha$_1$-Adrenergic Blockers, Angiotensin-Converting Enzyme (ACE) Inhibitors, Beta-Adrenergic Blockers, Calcium Channel Blockers, and Diuretics and the entry for the generic drug losartan.

PRECAUTIONS

SPECIAL INFORMATION

- Do not take guanfacine if you have had an allergic reaction to this drug in the past.
- Tell your doctor if you are pregnant or planning a pregnancy; are nursing; have heart, kidney, or liver disease; have coronary insufficiency or cerebrovascular disease; or are suffering from depression.
- Tell your doctor if you are taking sedatives, hypnotics, or antidepressants, or are planning surgery requiring general anesthesia.
- Be sure to check with your doctor before taking any other medications, especially over-the-counter antihistamines; appetite-control pills; medicines for colds, coughs, sinus, or hay fever; pain pills; or muscle relaxants. Some of these medications may increase your blood pressure; others will result in excessive drowsiness.
- Because guanfacine can act as a sedative, it may impair your mental alertness, judgment, and coordination. Until you know how the drug will affect you, be cautious about driving, using machines, or engaging in any potentially dangerous activity. To reduce daytime drowsiness, take the drug at bedtime.
- Be sure you always have an adequate supply of antihypertensive medication to tide you over during holidays and vacations. You may want to carry a backup prescription for emergency use.

CONTINUED

ANTIHYPERTENSIVE DRUGS

- Pay special attention to dental hygiene when taking guanfacine. It can cause mouth dryness, which may increase the likelihood of dental disease. Check with your dentist or doctor if dry mouth continues for more than two weeks.
- It usually takes four to six weeks to know if guanfacine will control your high blood pressure. Do not abruptly stop taking the drug: You may experience severe withdrawal effects.

POSSIBLE INTERACTIONS

Alcohol and other central nervous system depressants, such as antihistamines and muscle relaxants: may increase drowsiness and guanfacine's blood-pressure-lowering effect.

Food: avoid excessive salt.

TARGET AILMENTS

High blood pressure (hypertension)

SIDE EFFECTS

NOT SERIOUS

- Drowsiness
- Dry mouth and nose
- Constipation
- Headache
- Dizziness
- Fatigue
- Insomnia
- Decreased sex drive
- Dry, itching, or burning eyes
- Nausea or vomiting

CALL YOUR DOCTOR IF THESE SYMPTOMS PERSIST OR ARE BOTHERSOME.

SERIOUS

- Confusion
- Mental depression

CONTACT YOUR DOCTOR AS SOON AS POSSIBLE.

ANTIMONIUM TARTARICUM

LATIN NAME
Antimonium tartaricum

VITAL STATISTICS

GENERAL DESCRIPTION

Antimonium tartaricum, a powerful poison, was sometimes used in the 1700s to clean open, festering wounds. It was not known then that the poison could enter the bloodstream in this way, and the effect of this treatment was often fatal. Sometimes called tartar emetic, *Antimonium tartaricum* was also used as an emetic, or substance that causes vomiting. In fact, it was known as the Prince of Evacuants because even tiny doses could cause severe vomiting and profuse sweating.

Homeopathic practitioners consider the remedy *Antimonium tartaricum,* or *Antimonium tart,* helpful for persons with a rattling, persistent cough and mucus in the chest. It can be particularly effective among the very young or elderly who are in the latter stages of a worsening cough, when they have difficulty coughing up phlegm. Children with chickenpox or measles may experience these symptoms. The patient is often pale and cold, with a bluish hue around the lips—symptoms that require medical evaluation.

Antimonium tart is prepared by mixing, then heating together, oxide of antimony and acid potassium tartrate. Once the mixture is cooled and dried, crystals form. These crystals are then dissolved in distilled water. When a patient exhibits a set of symptoms that matches the cataloged symptoms brought on by *Antimonium tart,* the homeopathic practitioner then prescribes it in an extremely dilute form. For more information on homeopathic medicine, see page 14.

PREPARATIONS

Antimonium tart is available in various potencies at selected stores and pharmacies. Consult your practitioner for more information.

PRECAUTIONS

SPECIAL INFORMATION

- Only the patient should touch the pills. Any spilled tablets should be thrown away.
- The mouth should be clear of flavors 15 minutes before and after taking a remedy, and strong flavors and aromas, such as coffee and heavy perfume, should be avoided for the duration of treatment.

TARGET AILMENTS
Cold sweat, especially at night; pale, sunken face; blue hue around the lips
Bronchitis
Chickenpox, with symptoms of cough
Measles, with symptoms of cough
Difficulty breathing
Nausea
Pneumonia
Rattling cough, with difficulty expectorating
Thirstlessness

SIDE EFFECTS

NONE EXPECTED

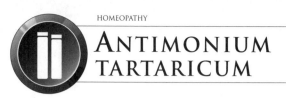

Antinausea Drugs

Vital Statistics

GENERIC NAMES
prochlorperazine, scopolamine

GENERAL DESCRIPTION
The antinausea drug class (sometimes called the antiemetic class) includes a large number of drugs used in the control of nausea and vomiting. These symptoms may be caused by or associated with a number of factors, ranging from motion sickness to psychosis. For information about specific antinausea medications, including additional special information and possible interactions, see the entries for the generic drugs listed above.

Precautions

SPECIAL INFORMATION
- Tell your doctor if you are planning surgery within two months; have diabetes, asthma, glaucoma, emphysema, or heart disease; have a history of lupus erythematosus, prostate problems, or seizure disorders; or are pregnant or nursing.
- These drugs have many different side effects. Report any unusual symptoms to your physician.
- Do not drive or operate machinery until you know how the antinausea drug you are taking affects you.

POSSIBLE INTERACTIONS
Antinausea drugs interact unfavorably with many OTC cold, cough, and allergy medications, and with many prescription drugs. Ask your pharmacist or physician for assistance.

Alcohol, barbiturates, tranquilizers, narcotics, sedatives: increased sedative and depressive effects.

Target Ailments

Nausea and vomiting

Side Effects

Not Serious

- Drowsiness
- Blurred vision
- Dry mouth
- Impaired urination

Call your doctor if these effects persist or are bothersome.

Serious

- Extreme restlessness or agitation
- Fainting
- Skin rashes

Call your doctor immediately.

ANTIULCER DRUGS

VITAL STATISTICS

GENERIC NAMES
lansoprazole, omeprazole, sucralfate
Histamine H_2 blockers: cimetidine, famotidine, nizatidine, ranitidine

GENERAL DESCRIPTION
Antiulcer drugs are used to treat disorders associated with the overproduction of stomach acid, such as gastritis, gastroesophageal reflux, multiple endocrine neoplasia, Zollinger-Ellison syndrome, and, most commonly, ulcers of the stomach and duodenum (first portion of the small intestine). In general, antiulcer drugs work by inhibiting the production of the stomach's digestive juices, most notably hydrochloric acid and the digestive enzyme pepsin. Individual drugs achieve this effect in different ways.

Medications among the subclass of antiulcer drugs known as histamine H_2 blockers (including cimetidine, famotidine, nizatidine, and ranitidine) block the stomach's response to the chemical compound histamine, thereby reducing the secretion of hydrochloric acid. The drugs lansoprazole and omeprazole reduce the production of hydrochloric acid by inhibiting the action of enzymes in the acid-producing cells of the stomach lining. The exact mechanism of sucralfate is not completely understood, but the drug is believed to inhibit the digestive action of pepsin. It may also form a coating over stomach and duodenal ulcers, protecting them from the erosive effect of hydrochloric acid.

Antacids and antibiotics may also be used to treat ulcers.

PRECAUTIONS

WARNING
Rare or infrequent side effects that are not serious include dizziness, lightheadedness, constipation, mild drowsiness, headache, mild diarrhea, skin rash, itching or other skin problems, muscle or joint pain, hair loss, temporary impotence and decreased libido, breast enlargement and tenderness (in women or men), abdominal pain, heartburn, indigestion, nausea, gas, appetite loss, dry mouth or skin, insomnia, depression, and anxiety. Call your doctor if these effects persist or become bothersome.

TARGET AILMENTS
Duodenal ulcer
Gastric ulcer
Upper gastrointestinal bleeding associated with gastric ulcer or duodenal ulcer, or with gastritis
Zollinger-Ellison syndrome, multiple endocrine neoplasia, and other conditions characterized by an overproduction of stomach acid
Gastroesophageal reflux
Gastrointestinal symptoms associated with the use of nonsteroidal anti-inflammatory drugs (NSAIDs) and aspirin
Heartburn or acid indigestion (OTC formulas)

CONTINUED

ANTIULCER DRUGS

A

SPECIAL INFORMATION

- Do not take these medications if you have had an allergic reaction or any unusual reactions to an antiulcer drug in the past.
- The side effects of the various antiulcer medications differ from drug to drug; see individual entries for the drugs listed above, left.
- Avoid antiulcer drugs if you are pregnant or nursing.
- Be sure to inform your doctor if you have any other medical problems, especially kidney or liver disease or any disease that causes obstruction of the gastrointestinal tract.
- Antiulcer drugs can interfere with the accuracy of some laboratory tests. Be sure to tell the person giving you a lab test that you are taking one of these drugs.
- Remember that some medications—such as aspirin and nonsteroidal anti-inflammatory drugs (NSAIDs)—and certain foods and drinks, including citrus products and beverages that are carbonated, alcoholic, or caffeinated, may irritate your stomach and make your problem worse.
- Check with your doctor before using antacids concurrently with an antiulcer drug.

POSSIBLE INTERACTIONS

Antiulcer drugs interact with many prescription and over-the-counter medications, some of which are listed below. Be sure to inform your doctor of any other drugs you may be taking.

Alcohol, caffeine, carbonated drinks, citrus foods, tobacco: may stimulate secretion of stomach acid and slow ulcer recovery rate; drinking alcoholic beverages while taking a histamine H_2 blocker may also increase blood levels of alcohol.

Alprazolam, carbamazepine, diazepam, digitalis preparations, glipizide, metoprolol, oral anticoagulants (including aspirin, dipyridamole, heparin): histamine H_2 blockers may increase the effects and possibly the toxicity of these drugs.

Aluminum-containing antidiarrheal drugs, aspirin buffered with aluminum, and aluminum-containing vaginal douches: sucralfate may increase the absorption of aluminum into the body, possibly to toxic levels.

Antacids: reduced effects of antiulcer drugs. Sometimes switching to another type of antacid or taking the antacid and the antiulcer drug at different times of the day can eliminate this problem. Consult your doctor. Avoid aluminum-containing antacids while taking sucralfate; the combination may lead to weakening of the bones and other symptoms of aluminum toxicity.

Aspirin: stomach irritation; increased effect of aspirin if large doses of aspirin are taken with nizatidine.

Cimetidine, ciprofloxacin, digoxin, ofloxacin, phenytoin, ranitidine, tetracycline, theophylline, warfarin: sucralfate may decrease the effectiveness of these drugs; omeprazole may increase the effects of phenytoin and warfarin.

Enteric-coated tablets: changes in stomach acidity may cause these drugs to dissolve prematurely in the stomach; avoid taking enteric-coated medications with cimetidine, famotidine, and nizatidine.

Iron: absorption of iron into the body may be inhibited by omeprazole.

Itraconazole and ketoconazole: omeprazole and histamine H_2 blockers may inhibit the absorption of these drugs into the body.

Vitamins A, D, E, and K: sucralfate may decrease the absorption of these vitamins.

SIDE EFFECTS

NOT SERIOUS

NOT SERIOUS SIDE EFFECTS ARE RARE OR INFREQUENT.
SEE WARNING, PAGE 91.

SERIOUS

- Unusual bruising, bleeding, or fatigue
- Rapid or irregular heartbeat
- Confusion, delirium, or hallucinations
- Shortness of breath
- Bronchospasm (tightness in the chest)
- Vomiting
- Vomit the consistency of coffee grounds
- Mouth ulcers
- Numbness or tingling in the fingers or toes
- Jaundice
- Severe abdominal pain accompanied by vomiting or fever (inflammation of the pancreas)
- Black, tarry stools (internal bleeding)
- Combined weakness, fever, and sore throat (bone marrow depression)

CONTACT YOUR DOCTOR IMMEDIATELY.

ANTIVIRAL DRUGS

A

VITAL STATISTICS

GENERIC NAMES
acyclovir, valacyclovir

RELATED CLASS
AIDS Treatment

GENERAL DESCRIPTION
Antivirals, a class of drugs introduced in recent decades, are used to treat viral infections ranging from the flu to herpes and AIDS. Each antiviral medication is usually effective against only one virus, although in some cases a single antiviral drug is useful against several organisms in a viral class. (Because viruses differ greatly from bacteria, antibiotics do not work against viral diseases.)

Antiviral drugs work in several different ways. Some suppress a virus's ability to reproduce by stopping the formation or duplication of its genetic material. Others work by keeping the virus (or its genetic material) from penetrating body cells. No serious side effects are expected for short-term treatment outside a hospital setting. For more information, see AIDS Treatment and the entries for the generic drugs acyclovir and valacyclovir.

PRECAUTIONS

SPECIAL INFORMATION
- Use caution when taking an antiviral drug if you are pregnant or breast-feeding. Drugs such as acyclovir can cross the placenta and affect the fetus, and they can pass to nursing infants through breast milk.

POSSIBLE INTERACTIONS
Antiviral drugs may interact with each other, and with drugs of other classes, in undesirable ways. Acyclovir, for example, should not be taken in conjunction with the AIDS treatment zidovudine (AZT) because the combination produces increased toxicity; it also causes profound drowsiness and lethargy.

TARGET AILMENTS
Genital herpes
Herpes simplex
Chickenpox
Flu
Shingles
Herpes simplex encephalitis (brain infection)
HIV infection

SIDE EFFECTS

NOT SERIOUS
- Gastrointestinal upsets (such as nausea)
- Lightheadedness
- Headache
- Mild burning, stinging, itching, or skin rash (topical preparations)

CALL YOUR DOCTOR IF THESE SYMPTOMS PERSIST OR BECOME BOTHERSOME.

Apis

LATIN NAME
Apis mellifica

Vital Statistics

GENERAL DESCRIPTION

The medicinal value of *Apis,* the scientific name for the honeybee, may date to ancient Egypt, where bees were a symbol of power, wealth, and health. Egyptian doctors revered honey over all other healing substances, and extensive methods of beekeeping were already in practice in 4000 BC. It is not the honey but the bee itself, however, that is used in homeopathic medicine.

This remedy is made from the body of the honeybee; it is used to treat those patients whose ailments are accompanied by symptoms similar to the results of a bee sting—for example, redness and swelling—and also patients who express behavior considered bee-like, such as restlessness or irritability. To prepare this remedy, the entire live honeybee is crushed and highly diluted by mixing it into a water-alcohol base.

Like most homeopathic prescriptions, *Apis* was developed as a remedy by observation of the reactions of healthy individuals to doses of various strengths. The mental, emotional, and physical changes induced by *Apis* were then cataloged. When a patient exhibits a set of symptoms that matches the cataloged symptoms brought on by *Apis,* the homeopathic practitioner then prescribes it in an extremely dilute form. It is presumed that in this highly dilute dosage, *Apis* can counter the symptoms that are similar to the ones it induces when it is at full strength. For more information on homeopathic medicine, see page 14.

TARGET AILMENTS
Bites and stings, especially those that burn, itch, or swell
Conjunctivitis
Edema (accumulation of fluids in body tissues) and conditions of general swelling such as hives and food allergies
Headaches that include sudden, stabbing pains
Red, swollen joints
Mumps

SIDE EFFECTS

None expected

PREPARATIONS

Apis is available in various potencies, in both liquid and tablet form, at selected stores and pharmacies or from your homeopathic practitioner. Consult your practitioner for more precise dosage information.

Precautions

SPECIAL INFORMATION

- When a remedy is administered, no one but the patient should touch the pills. If tablets are spilled, throw them away.
- The mouth should be clear of flavors 15 minutes before and after taking a remedy, and strong flavors and aromas, such as coffee, camphor, and heavily scented perfumes, should be avoided for the duration of treatment.

Appetite Suppressants

A

Vital Statistics

GENERIC NAMES
fenfluramine, phentermine

GENERAL DESCRIPTION
Appetite suppressant drugs are to be used as part of a weight-reduction plan that includes calorie restriction, exercise, and behavior modification. They are appropriate only for obese people in whom there is no physiological basis for the disorder and for whom there are no contraindications. Intended for short-term use only, these drugs generally lose their effectiveness within a few weeks. When that happens, they should be stopped; the recommended dosage should never be exceeded.

It is believed that these medications work by stimulating the hypothalamus, the part of the brain that controls appetite. The effects of most of these drugs are similar to the actions of amphetamines, which stimulate the central nervous system and elevate blood pressure. These drugs generally begin to have an effect about one hour after they are taken, and their actions last from four to 14 hours, depending on whether they are long- or short-acting forms.

Appetite suppressants are controlled substances, meaning they have been identified as having the potential for abuse. They can produce tolerance and severe psychological dependence. Because of these and other problems, such as their ability to produce drowsiness, to cause mental depression (fenfluramine), or to act as a stimulant (phentermine), these drugs are considered to have limited usefulness, and their benefits should be weighed against the risk factors involved in their use. For more information about specific drugs in this class, see the entries Fenfluramine and Phentermine.

Precautions

☠ ***WARNING***
Do not take an appetite suppressant if you are allergic to any drug classified as a sympathomimetic, such as phenylpropanolamine.

These drugs should not be taken, except under special circumstances, by people who have glaucoma, hyperthyroidism, diabetes, moderate or severe hypertension, or a history of alcoholism, psychotic illness, or drug abuse.

SPECIAL INFORMATION
- Appetite suppressant drugs have not been determined to be safe to take during pregnancy or when nursing.
- Appetite suppressants are not established to be safe or effective in children under 12.
- If you have cardiovascular disease (including arrhythmias), high blood pressure, an overactive thyroid gland, epilepsy, chronic anxiety, a tendency to be agitated, or mental depression, check with your doctor before taking any of these drugs.
- Discuss with your doctor the need for special examinations or laboratory tests if you take one of these drugs for longer than a few weeks.
- Tell your doctor about any over-the-counter medication you take or plan to take.
- Because appetite suppressants may impair your driving ability or your ability to engage in other potentially hazardous activities, refrain from such activities until you know how the drug will affect you.
- Do not stop taking one of these drugs on your own. Your doctor may tell you to reduce the dosage gradually or even change the doses of other drugs you are taking.

- Discuss with your doctor any plans to have surgery or dental treatment that will require general or spinal anesthesia within two months of taking an appetite suppressant.

POSSIBLE INTERACTIONS

Alcohol: may cause confusion, dizziness, fainting.

Anesthetics: may cause irregular heart rhythms, which can be serious or even fatal.

Caffeine: increases the stimulant effect.

Chlorpromazine (and other phenothiazines): may reduce the effect of the appetite suppressant.

Clonidine, methyldopa, guanadrel, rauwolfia, guanethidine (and other drugs for hypertension): may reduce effect of blood pressure medications; in the case of fenfluramine, may increase effect.

Furazolidone: may cause severe increase in blood pressure.

Insulin or oral drugs for diabetes: may change blood sugar concentrations, requiring dosage adjustment of the insulin or oral drug.

MAO inhibitors: may result in hypertensive crisis. Appetite suppressants should not be taken within 14 days following the use of these drugs. To do so can cause a dangerous rise in blood pressure.

Thyroid hormones: may stimulate the nervous system, with effects such as rapid heart rate, increased appetite, insomnia, and anxiety (not true of fenfluramine, however).

TARGET AILMENTS

Obesity with no physiological basis

SIDE EFFECTS

NOT SERIOUS

- Euphoria; irritability; restlessness; insomnia; nervousness
- Fatigue; drowsiness
- Blurred vision
- Dry mouth; unpleasant taste in mouth
- Diarrhea; constipation
- Cramps; vomiting; nausea
- Altered sex drive
- Increased sweating
- Headache; weakness

CALL YOUR DOCTOR IF THESE PROBLEMS PERSIST.

SERIOUS

- Raised blood pressure (unlikely for fenfluramine)
- Hives
- Psychotic behavior; confusion; depression
- Shortness of breath (a sign of pulmonary hypertension, which is a risk with fenfluramine)
- Irregular heartbeat
- Urgency or difficulty urinating
- Difficulty breathing

CONTACT YOUR DOCTOR IMMEDIATELY.

APRICOT SEED

LATIN NAME
Prunus armeniaca

A

VITAL STATISTICS

GENERAL DESCRIPTION

Practitioners of Chinese medicine frequently use the inner kernel of apricots to relieve bronchial ailments. These seeds are believed to serve as an expectorant, expelling mucus from the lungs, and also as an agent to stop coughing. Apricot seeds are also prescribed as a laxative. In traditional Chinese medicine, apricot seeds are classified as bitter and slightly warm.

Chinese medicine takes a holistic approach to healthcare, fashioning remedies to treat the entire being as well as the specific parts or areas. Single herbs may be used alone or in combination with other herbs to prevent and combat disease.

PREPARATIONS

Apricot seeds or decoctions such as cough syrups are available at Chinese pharmacies, Asian markets, and Western health food stores.

COMBINATIONS: Chinese medicine practitioners recommend treating dry coughs with apricot seed and either white mulberry leaf or a tuber known as ophiopogon. The choice, depending on the nature of the cough, and dosages should be made in consultation with a herbalist.

TARGET AILMENTS
Take internally for:
Coughing and wheezing
Bronchitis or emphysema
Asthma
Constipation

PRECAUTIONS

WARNING

Patients should use extreme caution with this herb, since it includes a poisonous substance. In the human body, the components of apricot seed break down into several products, including prussic acid, which is highly toxic. Chinese herbalists have reported that a dose of 50 to 60 kernels of apricot seed can kill adults, while just 10 kernels can be fatal in children. Activated charcoal and syrup of ipecac are recommended as antidotes to overdoses.

SPECIAL INFORMATION

Chinese medicine practitioners advise caution in using apricot seed to treat children or to treat patients with diarrhea.

POSSIBLE INTERACTIONS

Some Chinese medicine practitioners believe that apricot seeds should not be taken in combination with astragalus, skullcap, or kudzu root.

SIDE EFFECTS

SERIOUS

- Dizziness
- Nausea or vomiting
- Headache
- Spasms
- Dilated pupils
- Erratic heartbeat

RESULTING FROM EXCESSIVE DOSES; CALL YOUR DOCTOR AT ONCE IF YOU EXPERIENCE ANY OF THESE EFFECTS. COMA OR DEATH MAY RESULT.

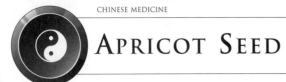

ARNICA

LATIN NAME
Arnica montana

A

VITAL STATISTICS

GENERAL DESCRIPTION

Arnica, sometimes called mountain daisy, grows wild across the higher elevations of Europe, northern Asia, and parts of the United States. Mountain climbers in the Alps have traditionally chewed arnica after a long day's hike to relieve muscle aches. Homeopathic practitioners prescribe *Arnica* for bruises, sprains, strains, and other types of accidents that are sudden and may induce shock. The flowers, leaves, stem, and root of arnica are crushed to a pulp and soaked in alcohol before undergoing the homeopathic dilution process, which renders the substance nontoxic.

Like most homeopathic prescriptions, *Arnica* was developed as a remedy by observation of reactions of healthy individuals to doses of various strengths. The mental, emotional, and physical changes induced by *Arnica* were then cataloged. When a patient exhibits a set of symptoms that matches the cataloged symptoms brought on by *Arnica,* the homeopathic practitioner then prescribes it in an extremely dilute form. It is presumed that in this highly dilute dosage, *Arnica* can counter the symptoms that are similar to the ones it induces when it is at full strength. For more information on homeopathic medicine, see page 14.

PREPARATIONS

Arnica is available over the counter in various potencies, in both tablet and liquid form, at selected stores and pharmacies. Consult your practitioner for more precise information.

PRECAUTIONS

SPECIAL INFORMATION

- Only the patient should touch the pills. If tablets are spilled, throw them away.
- The mouth should be clear of flavors 15 minutes before and after taking a remedy, and strong flavors and aromas, such as coffee, camphor, and heavy perfume, should be avoided for the duration of treatment.

TARGET AILMENTS

Blood blisters caused by a blow to the affected area

Broken bones, sprains, strains, and other sudden injuries with swelling, tenderness, and pain, where posttraumatic shock is a threat

Bruises, especially if *Arnica* is given before the skin begins to turn black and blue

Sore and swollen joints, as in rheumatism

Head pain

Toothache, pain from dental work

Groin strain

SIDE EFFECTS

NONE EXPECTED

Arsenicum Album

LATIN NAME
Arsenicum album

Vital Statistics

GENERAL DESCRIPTION

This remedy, also called *Ars alb* by homeopathic practitioners, is an extremely dilute form of arsenic, a metallic poison derived from the chemical element of the same name. Weak preparations of arsenic have had a history of medicinal use; but slow accumulation of the element in body tissues can cause chronic poisoning, leading to gastrointestinal disorders, nausea, dehydration, and even paralysis and death. In step with the homeopathic theory that like cures like, *Ars alb* is preferred by practitioners to treat patients with various digestive complaints that are accompanied by signs of dehydration and burning pains, the same symptoms that are induced by *Ars alb.*

In its homeopathic form, arsenic is separated from other metals like iron, cobalt, and nickel by baking at high temperatures. The extracted powder is then finely ground and weakened by mixing successively greater amounts of milk sugar with the poison. When a patient exhibits a set of symptoms that matches the cataloged symptoms brought on by *Ars alb,* the homeopathic practitioner then prescribes it in an extremely dilute form. It is presumed that in this highly dilute dosage, *Ars alb* can counter the symptoms that are similar to the ones it induces when it is at full strength. For more information on homeopathic medicine, see page 14.

PREPARATIONS

Ars alb is available in various potencies, in both liquid and tablet form, at selected stores and pharmacies. Consult your practitioner for more precise information.

Precautions

SPECIAL INFORMATION

- When a remedy is administered, no one but the patient should touch the pills. If tablets are spilled, throw them away.
- The mouth should be clear of flavors 15 minutes before and after taking a remedy, and strong flavors and aromas, such as coffee, camphor, and heavy perfume, should be avoided for the duration of treatment.

TARGET AILMENTS

Angina
Anxiety disorders and panic attacks
Asthma
Hay fever; burns that form blisters
Chronic skin problems
High fevers accompanied by chills
Recurrent headaches
Dry, hacking coughs
Colds accompanied by excessive watery nasal discharge and frequent sneezing
Colitis
Indigestion
Food poisoning
Crohn's disease
Influenza
Insomnia; exhaustion brought on by an illness and coupled with restlessness

SIDE EFFECTS

NONE EXPECTED

ASHWAGANDA

LATIN NAME
Withania somnifera

VITAL STATISTICS

GENERAL DESCRIPTION

Identified by clusters of tiny green-and-yellow flowers, this small shrub from India is believed to strengthen the body and to serve as a source of energy. Sought after for its roots, leaves, and berries, ashwaganda is thought to aid in restoring muscles, body tissues, and bone marrow. It is commonly prescribed as a medicinal supplement for people recovering from an illness or suffering from excessive fatigue. Ashwaganda also has a reputation as an aphrodisiac, and according to tradition, it is believed to help prevent male sterility and other sexual ailments.

PREPARATIONS

Over the counter:
Available as tincture, dried roots and leaves, or powder.

At home:

Tea: Boil covered 1 oz ashwaganda root in 1 cup water for 15 to 20 minutes. Drink up to 2 cups a day.

Milk decoction: Combine 1 oz ashwaganda root, 1 cup milk, and 4 cups water. Heat over low flame for 30 minutes to 2 hours, until water evaporates. Drink 2 cups daily. Add honey, raw sugar, or syrup to sweeten.

Medicated oil: Combine 2 oz crushed ashwaganda leaves, 1 cup castor oil, and 4 cups water. Heat over low flame for 4 to 8 hours, until water is evaporated.

Compress: Soak a clean cloth in the tea and apply directly to the affected area. Consult a qualified practitioner for the dosage appropriate for you and the specific condition being treated.

PRECAUTIONS

WARNING

Do not eat ashwaganda berries. They may cause severe gastrointestinal pain. This herb should not be used with children unless it is specifically prescribed by a healthcare practitioner knowledgeable about herbs.

POSSIBLE INTERACTIONS

Combining ashwaganda with other herbs may necessitate a lower dosage.

TARGET AILMENTS

Take internally for:

Loss of muscular strength
Multiple sclerosis
Rheumatism
Fatigue
Infertility; male sterility
Sexual debility
Indigestion
Heart disease
Hay fever

Apply medicated oil externally for:

Carbuncles; sores
Inflammations; swelling

Apply compress to affected area for:

Ringworm

SIDE EFFECTS

None expected

ASPIRIN

A

VITAL STATISTICS

DRUG CLASSES
Analgesics; Anticoagulant and Antiplatelet Drugs

BRAND NAMES
Alka-Seltzer Plus Cold Medicine, Anacin Caplets, Bayer (various forms), Bufferin (various forms), Ecotrin, Excedrin Extra-Strength

GENERAL DESCRIPTION
Since its introduction in 1899, aspirin has become one of the most popular over-the-counter pain relievers, used for headache, arthritis, muscle aches, and minor injuries. Aspirin also suppresses fever and reduces the inflammation associated with menstrual cramps, arthritis, bursitis, and other conditions. It may be combined with other analgesics to increase the effectiveness or range of its action.

As an antiplatelet drug, aspirin is used once a day in very low dosages to reduce the risk of heart attack, stroke, and postsurgical problems that can develop when a blood vessel is obstructed by blood clots. It may be used alone or in combination with dipyridamole or an anticoagulant. Aspirin works by preventing the production of thromboxane, a powerful stimulator of platelet activation. For more information, see Analgesics and Anticoagulant and Antiplatelet Drugs.

PRECAUTIONS

WARNING
Do not give aspirin to children or teenagers with fevers. Aspirin can provoke a potentially fatal liver inflammation called Reye's syndrome in young people if the drug is used to treat a fever or viral infection such as chickenpox or influenza.

SPECIAL INFORMATION
- Aspirin may increase the chance of excessive bleeding in some people. Do not take aspirin to prevent stroke, heart attack, or blood clots unless prescribed by your doctor.
- Pregnant and nursing women should not use aspirin.
- Before any surgery, let your doctor or dentist know if you use aspirin regularly. You may be told to discontinue it for a week or two before surgery.

TARGET AILMENTS

- Fever
- Pain
- Inflammation
- Heart attack or stroke (preventive treatment)

SIDE EFFECTS

NOT SERIOUS
- Stomach irritation

SERIOUS
- Gastric ulceration (black or bloody stools, stomach pain, vomiting of blood)
- Ringing in the ears, hearing loss, headache, dizziness, and nausea (may occur with large doses of aspirin)

DISCONTINUE USE AND CALL YOUR DOCTOR.

Astemizole

Vital Statistics

DRUG CLASS
Antihistamines

BRAND NAME
Hismanal

GENERAL DESCRIPTION
A newer, nonsedating antihistamine, astemizole is commonly prescribed for seasonal allergies or hives. By blocking the action of histamine—a natural substance the body releases in allergic reactions—astemizole prevents the runny nose, watery eyes, congestion, itching, and hives associated with allergy. Astemizole is taken for long-term treatment of symptoms, not for immediate relief. See Antihistamines for additional side effects and interaction information. For visual characteristics of the brand-name drug Hismanal, see the Color Guide to Prescription Drugs and Herbs.

Precautions

WARNING
Astemizole is slow to take effect. It usually starts working in two to three days and reaches peak effect in nine to 12 days. Never try to speed up the drug's action by increasing the dose. Larger amounts won't make the drug work faster and may lead to life-threatening heart problems.

SPECIAL INFORMATION
- If your liver is impaired, astemizole can build up in your body and provoke life-threatening heart problems.
- Let your doctor know if you are pregnant or breast-feeding. Your doctor may advise you to discontinue the drug.

POSSIBLE INTERACTIONS
Azithromycin, clarithromycin, erythromycin, itraconazole, ketoconazole, troleandomycin: may cause life-threatening heart problems. Do not take astemizole in combination with these drugs.
Food: decreases the drug's effectiveness. Take astemizole on an empty stomach and don't eat for at least an hour afterward.

TARGET AILMENTS

Nasal and respiratory allergies, including hay fever

Chronic hives

Asthma (adjunct treatment)

SIDE EFFECTS

NOT SERIOUS
- Headache
- Increased appetite
- Weight gain

CALL YOUR DOCTOR IF THESE SYMPTOMS CONTINUE OR BECOME BOTHERSOME.

SERIOUS
- Fainting
- Heart palpitations or change in heartbeat
- Cardiac arrest

CALL YOUR DOCTOR RIGHT AWAY. THESE EFFECTS ARE RARE BUT MAY OCCUR IF YOUR DOSE IS TOO HIGH OR IF YOU HAVE LIVER DAMAGE.

Asthma Therapy

A

Vital Statistics

RELATED CLASSES
bronchodilators, corticosteroids, leukotriene modifiers

GENERIC NAMES
Anti-inflammatory drugs: cromolyn, nedocromil
Bronchodilators: albuterol, epinephrine, ipratropium, terbutaline, theophylline, salmeterol
Corticosteroids: beclomethasone, fluticasone, triamcinolone
Leukotriene modifiers: zafirlukast, zileuton

GENERAL DESCRIPTION
Asthma therapy involves the use of several classes of prescription and over-the-counter drugs to relieve the symptoms associated with asthma. While none of these drugs represents a cure, each can be effective in alleviating symptoms that interfere with normal breathing. Some of these drugs are used for acute asthma attacks, while others are taken for long-term therapy.

Two of the newest long-term asthma drugs, zafirlukast and zileuton, come in pill form. They work against leukotrienes, a class of chemicals released by the body's immune system in response to allergens and other stimuli. Zafirlukast blocks the inflammatory action of two such leukotrienes, whereas zileuton prevents the production of several different leukotrienes.

Anti-inflammatory drugs such as cromolyn and nedocromil are also used long term and are inhaled. Long-term therapy drugs must be taken every day, even when there are no symptoms. These drugs should never be used to control an acute asthma attack. They frequently are used in combination with a bronchodilator or corticosteroid drug.

Bronchodilators relax the muscles surrounding the bronchial tubes in the lungs by inhibiting certain body chemicals. This relieves bronchial muscle spasm and improves lung capacity, thereby alleviating the symptoms of bronchial asthma and bronchitis. Bronchodilators are the main drugs used to treat an acute asthma attack.

Orally inhaled corticosteroids are potent drugs used to reduce chronic bronchial inflammation and control the symptoms of bronchial asthma, but not to relieve an acute asthma attack. This class of drugs is often prescribed when asthma cannot be controlled by bronchodilators and/or the anti-inflammatory drugs cromolyn and nedocromil.

For more information, see the class entries for Bronchodilators and Corticosteroids, as well as the individual entries for cromolyn and the corticosteroid drugs beclomethasone, fluticasone, and triamcinolone.

Precautions

WARNING
Your body can build up tolerance to bronchodilators used as inhalants, causing them to become less effective. If this happens, discontinue the drug and tell your doctor. Do not increase the dose. Increasing the dose can lead to serious, perhaps fatal bronchial constriction. Zileuton can cause liver dysfunction. If you take this medication, your doctor may perform periodic blood screenings to check your liver enzymes. Nobody with active liver disease should use zileuton.

SPECIAL INFORMATION
- Women who are pregnant or are breast-feeding should consult a doctor before using any asthma therapy drug. Zafirlukast is

not recommended during breast-feeding.
- If you have a history of heart arrhythmias or coronary artery disease, let your doctor know; cromolyn inhalants may affect your condition.
- Bronchodilators (especially epinephrine) can cause adverse effects in individuals with high blood pressure, diabetes, heart disease, seizures, peptic ulcers, or thyroid problems. Before you use bronchodilators, let your doctor know if you have any of these conditions.

POSSIBLE INTERACTIONS

Zafirlukast and zileuton interact with a number of drugs, including astemizole, cisapride, cyclosporine, certain calcium channel blockers, and warfarin. Zafirlukast also interacts with carbamazepine, phenytoin, and tolbutamide. Ask your doctor about drug interactions when taking zafirlukast or zileuton.

Beta blockers (noncardioselective): provoke asthma attacks in some people. Increased effects when combined with zileuton.

Corticosteroids: increased steroid effect. Your doctor may decrease your dosage.

Ipratropium (asthma inhalant): increased cromolyn effect.

Terfenadine: do not take terfenadine in combination with zileuton.

Theophylline: interacts with many drugs, including zileuton. See the theophylline entry.

See also Bronchodilators, Corticosteroids.

TARGET AILMENTS

Bronchial asthma

Bronchospasm from all sources (including environmental irritants and exercise)

SIDE EFFECTS

NOT SERIOUS

- Abdominal pain, upset stomach, nausea (zafirlukast, zileuton)
- Headache
- Mild nausea, weakness, insomnia, nervousness or restlessness (bronchodilators)
- Dry mouth or throat, throat irritation, cough, or nausea (cromolyn, nedocromil)

CALL YOUR DOCTOR IF THESE EFFECTS BECOME TROUBLESOME.

- A bad taste in the mouth (cromolyn, nedocromil)

THIS IS A HARMLESS SIDE EFFECT.

SERIOUS

- Increased bronchospasm (more wheezing, chest tightness, trouble breathing)
- Anaphylactic reaction (skin rash; hives; swelling of the face, lips, eyelids, hands, feet, inside of mouth)
- Liver dysfunction (fatigue, jaundice, itching, flulike symptoms, pain in upper right abdomen) (zileuton)
- Pneumonia

THESE EFFECTS ARE UNCOMMON, BUT CALL YOUR DOCTOR IMMEDIATELY IF YOU EXPERIENCE THEM.

ASTRAGALUS

LATIN NAME
Astragalus membranaceus

VITAL STATISTICS

GENERAL DESCRIPTION

The perennial plant astragalus, or milk-vetch root, has sprawling stems and pale yellow blooms. In traditional Chinese medicine astragalus is regarded as sweet and slightly warm. Astragalus has been used for centuries in *fu-zheng* therapy, the treatment of ailments by strengthening the body's natural defense mechanisms. The concept of fu-zheng therapy was recently acknowledged by Western medical researchers who examined astragalus's effect on the immune system of cancer patients undergoing chemotherapy and radiation. Although not conclusive, the results of these studies suggest that astragalus had a positive effect on these cancer patients. Check with your doctor before using astragalus in this capacity.

Chinese medicine takes a holistic approach to healthcare, fashioning remedies to treat the entire being as well as the specific parts or areas. Single herbs may be used alone or in combination with other herbs to prevent and combat disease, which is thought to arise from disturbances in the flow of a bodily energy called chi (pronounced "chee") and blood, or from a lack of balance in the complementary states of yin and yang.

PREPARATIONS

Over the counter:
Astragalus is available as prepared tea, fluidextract, capsules, and dried root.

At home:
Combine 1 part honey, 4 parts dried root, and a small amount of water in a wok. Allow mixture to simmer until the water evaporates and the herbs are slightly brown.

COMBINATIONS: For spontaneous perspiration, astragalus is mixed with Asian ginseng. As an immune system stimulant, the herb is combined with siler. Blood abnormalities are treated with a mix of astragalus and dong quai. Herbalists combine astragalus and atractylodes (white) for diarrhea. Astragalus with rhubarb root and bupleurum is aimed at uterine disorders.

PRECAUTIONS

SPECIAL INFORMATION

Pregnant women should check with their practitioners before using.

TARGET AILMENTS
General weakness and fatigue
Loss of appetite
Spontaneous perspiration
Diarrhea
Blood abnormalities or deficiencies resulting from excessive bleeding

SIDE EFFECTS
NONE EXPECTED

ASTRAGALUS

LATIN NAME
Astragalus membranaceus

VITAL STATISTICS

GENERAL DESCRIPTION

The perennial plant astragalus, or milk-vetch root, has sprawling stems and pale yellow blooms. Western herbalists believe that substances known as polysaccharides in this herb stimulate the immune system and generally strengthen the body by speeding metabolism, promoting tissue regeneration, and increasing energy.

PREPARATIONS

Over the counter:
Astragalus is available as prepared tea, fluidextract, capsules, and dried root.

At home:
TINCTURE: Take 1/8 to 1/2 tsp three times per day.

Consult a qualified practitioner for the dosage appropriate for you and the specific condition being treated.

PRECAUTIONS

SPECIAL INFORMATION

- Pregnant women should check with their practitioners before using.
- Use of this herb by children for more than seven to 10 days should be done in conjunction with a healthcare practitioner.

POSSIBLE INTERACTIONS

Combining astragalus with other herbs may necessitate a lower dosage.

TARGET AILMENTS

Take internally in conjunction with conventional medical treatment for:

Chronic colds and flu

AIDS

Cancer

Chronic fatigue

SIDE EFFECTS

NONE EXPECTED

ATENOLOL

A

VITAL STATISTICS

DRUG CLASS
Beta-Adrenergic Blockers

BRAND NAME
Tenormin

OTHER DRUGS IN THIS CLASS
bisoprolol, metoprolol, nadolol, propranolol, timolol

GENERAL DESCRIPTION
Introduced in 1973, atenolol is a beta-blocking drug prescribed to help manage angina, high blood pressure (hypertension), and heart attack (myocardial infarction). By blocking the action of major body chemicals in the heart, blood vessels, and certain muscles, the drug reduces the oxygen requirement of the heart and relaxes blood vessels. These actions result in lower blood pressure and decreased angina.

Atenolol is a cardioselective beta blocker, meaning it primarily affects the muscles in the heart. See Beta-Adrenergic Blockers for more special information and possible drug interactions. For visual characteristics of atenolol and the brand-name drug Tenormin, see the Color Guide to Prescription Drugs and Herbs.

TARGET AILMENTS

Heart disease, especially angina (pain), heart attack (myocardial infarction), and abnormal heart rhythms

High blood pressure

Alcohol withdrawal

PRECAUTIONS

SPECIAL INFORMATION
- Do not use beta blockers if you have a bronchospastic disease, bronchial asthma, or a severe chronic obstructive pulmonary disease.
- Suddenly stopping atenolol may cause or increase heart problems. Reduce dosage gradually under your doctor's supervision.

SIDE EFFECTS

NOT SERIOUS
- Drowsiness or weakness
- Decreased sexual ability
- Trouble sleeping
- Upset stomach
- Change in bowel habits
- Nervousness

CONSULT YOUR DOCTOR IF THESE EFFECTS CONTINUE OR ARE BOTHERSOME.

SERIOUS
- Bronchospasm (trouble breathing)
- Dizziness
- Mental depression
- Chest pain
- Fast or irregular heartbeat
- Prolonged reduced circulation (cold hands and feet)
- Congestive heart failure (swelling of feet or lower legs, shortness of breath)
- Sudden shortness of breath
- Sweating and trembling

CALL YOUR DOCTOR IMMEDIATELY.

ATRACTYLODES (WHITE)

LATIN NAME
Atractylodes macrocephala

VITAL STATISTICS

GENERAL DESCRIPTION

The aromatic rhizome of the herb known as atractylodes (white) is primarily a tonic. In several experiments on animals, the herb has indicated a strong diuretic effect, while tests on humans have shown mixed results. Animal experiments have also shown a lowering of blood glucose as a result of taking atractylodes. Classified in traditional Chinese medicine as bitter, sweet, and warm, it is believed to improve digestion and counter fatigue. A good specimen is large, firm, and fragrant, with a yellowish white cross section.

Chinese medicine takes a holistic approach to healthcare, fashioning remedies to treat the entire being as well as the specific parts or areas. Single herbs may be used alone or in combination with other herbs to prevent and combat disease, which is thought to arise from disturbances in the flow of a bodily energy called chi (pronounced "chee") and blood, or from a lack of balance in the complementary states of yin and yang.

PREPARATIONS

Over the counter:

The herb is available fresh and in dried form from Chinese pharmacies, Asian markets, and some Western health food stores.

At home:

Dried atractylodes is used to increase urination. To stop diarrhea, the dried herb is stir-fried before it is decocted.

COMBINATIONS: A mixture with unripened bitter oranges is prescribed for loss of appetite. Vaginal discharges are treated with a preparation containing both white and black atractylodes. Poria, cinnamon twig, and atractylodes make a preparation for chest congestion. Combined with astragalus and wheat grain, the herb is believed to provide relief from spontaneous sweating.

Consult a Chinese herbalist for information on specific dosages and other herbal combinations.

TARGET AILMENTS

Take internally for:

- Diarrhea
- Fatigue
- Lack of appetite
- Vomiting
- Chronic gastroenteritis
- Spontaneous sweating
- Abdominal pain and bleeding during pregnancy
- Edema (the accumulation of fluid in the body)
- Reduced urination

SIDE EFFECTS

NONE EXPECTED

ATTAPULGITE

A

VITAL STATISTICS

DRUG CLASS
Antidiarrheal Drugs

BRAND NAME
Kaopectate

OTHER DRUGS IN THIS CLASS
bismuth subsalicylate, loperamide

GENERAL DESCRIPTION
Attapulgite is taken after each loose bowel movement to treat acute diarrhea that is mild to moderate. For chronic diarrhea, attapulgite should be used only for temporary relief of symptoms until the cause can be determined. See Antidiarrheal Drugs for more information.

PRECAUTIONS

SPECIAL INFORMATION

- Since attapulgite is not absorbed into the body, it should not cause problems during pregnancy or breast-feeding.
- Diarrhea can cause excessive fluid loss. Call your doctor as soon as possible if you have any signs of dehydration, including decreased urination, lightheadedness and dizziness, wrinkled skin, dryness of mouth, or increased thirst.
- When you use antidiarrheal drugs, it is vitally important that you replace lost fluids by drinking large quantities of water and other clear liquids (such as decaffeinated colas and tea, ginger ale, and broth). Eat only gelatin for the first 24 hours. The next day you may eat bland foods, such as bread, crackers, cooked cereals, and applesauce. Other beverages and foods may make the condition worse.
- Do not use antidiarrheals if you have a fever or if your stool contains blood or mucus: These are symptoms of dysentery, an infection of the lower intestinal tract. Call your doctor.
- Antidiarrheal drugs have different functions. Some combat the symptoms of diarrhea; others are directed against the cause. A number of antidiarrheal drugs are available only by prescription. If over-the-counter medications do not help, see your doctor.

POSSIBLE INTERACTIONS
The presence of attapulgite in your body might prevent the absorption of other medications. Avoid taking other medications within two to three hours of taking attapulgite.

TARGET AILMENTS
Mild-to-moderate acute diarrhea
Traveler's diarrhea

SIDE EFFECTS

WHEN USED AT THE RECOMMENDED DOSAGE FOR NO MORE THAN TWO DAYS, ATTAPULGITE AND OTHER ANTIDIARRHEAL DRUGS RARELY CAUSE SIDE EFFECTS. BUT IF THE DIARRHEA DOES NOT DECREASE WITHIN ONE OR TWO DAYS, CHECK WITH YOUR DOCTOR.

NOT SERIOUS

- Mild constipation

CHECK WITH YOUR DOCTOR IF THE CONSTIPATION CONTINUES OR IF YOU DEVELOP A FEVER.

AUCKLANDIA

LATIN NAME
Aucklandia lappa

VITAL STATISTICS

GENERAL DESCRIPTION

Aucklandia root is used for several abdominal disorders. Its Chinese name literally means "wood fragrance"; in English it is sometimes known as costus root or saussurea. In laboratory studies using guinea pigs, extracts of the herb have shown some ability to clear out the bronchial tubes and reduce blood pressure. Classified by Chinese medicine practitioners as acrid, bitter, and warm, it is grown mainly in China's Yunnan province, although it also appears in Sichuan and Tibet.

Chinese medicine takes a holistic approach to healthcare, fashioning remedies to treat the entire being as well as the specific parts or areas. Single herbs may be used alone or in combination with other herbs to prevent and combat disease, which is thought to arise from disturbances in the flow of a bodily energy called chi (pronounced "chee") and blood, or from a lack of balance in the complementary states of yin and yang.

PREPARATIONS

Over the counter:

Aucklandia is available in bulk at Chinese pharmacies, Asian food markets, and some Western health food stores.

At home:

FOR TREATMENT OF DIARRHEA: Aucklandia should be toasted for greater effectiveness and is usually added to a mixture of herbs during the last 5 minutes of cooking.

COMBINATIONS: When mixed with green tangerine peel, aucklandia is given to patients suffering from indigestion or pain and swelling in the abdomen. Chinese herbalists recommend a preparation of aucklandia and coptis to treat the type of diarrhea that feels burning and explosive. Another mixture, with grains-of-paradise fruit, is prescribed for abdominal pain, loss of appetite, nausea, vomiting, morning sickness, and diarrhea. In combination with rhubarb root and betel nut, aucklandia is used to treat swelling of the abdomen accompanied by diarrhea.

Consult a Chinese herbalist for information on specific dosages and additional herbal combinations.

PRECAUTIONS

SPECIAL INFORMATION

Aucklandia is not recommended for use alone when patients suffer either from a loss of body fluids or from what Chinese medicine practitioners call heat signs, such as fever or thirst.

TARGET AILMENTS
Take internally for:
Diarrhea
Lack of appetite
Abdominal pain or distention
Nausea
Vomiting

SIDE EFFECTS

NONE EXPECTED

Augmentin

Vital Statistics

DRUG CLASS
Antibiotics [Penicillins]

GENERIC NAME
amoxicillin and clavulanate

OTHER DRUGS IN THIS SUBCLASS
amoxicillin, ampicillin, penicillin V

GENERAL DESCRIPTION
Augmentin is a brand name for the generic drug amoxicillin and clavulanate, a combination antibiotic drug introduced in 1982. Clavulanate reinforces amoxicillin's ability to destroy bacteria. This combination and the single drug amoxicillin (a penicillin antibiotic) are used to treat some of the same bacterial infections, including otitis media, sinusitis and other infections of the respiratory tract, and infections of the skin and urinary tract. For more information, including side effects and additional drug interactions, see Penicillins.

For visual characteristics, see the Color Guide to Prescription Drugs and Herbs.

Precautions

SPECIAL INFORMATION
- Take the full course of your prescription, even if you feel better before finishing the medicine; otherwise, the infection may return.
- Most penicillins are better absorbed if taken on an empty stomach. However, Augmentin works equally well whether taken on a full or an empty stomach.
- Tell your doctor if you are allergic to cephalosporins; you may also be allergic to the penicillin drug Augmentin.
- Let your doctor know if you have impaired kidneys, gastrointestinal disease, or a history of bleeding disorders. Your doctor may need to adjust your dosage, monitor you more closely, or prescribe a different drug.
- Penicillins also kill "good" intestinal bacteria that keep harmful fungi and intestinal bacteria in check. Eating yogurt containing *Lactobacillus acidophilus* culture or taking acidophilus tablets may help restore the body's normal bacteria.
- Prolonged use of any antibiotic drug can lead to fungal infections, including candidiasis, or to bacterial infections such as pseudomembranous colitis.
- Taking amoxicillin when you have mononucleosis may produce a skin rash.
- If possible, avoid taking Augmentin if you are pregnant or breast-feeding.

POSSIBLE INTERACTIONS
Disulfiram: do not take this drug with Augmentin. See Penicillins for additional interactions.

TARGET AILMENTS
Otitis media
Sinusitis and other infections of the respiratory tract
Infections of the skin and urinary tract

SIDE EFFECTS
See Penicillins.

Azithromycin

Vital Statistics

DRUG CLASS
Antibiotics [Erythromycins]

BRAND NAME
Zithromax

OTHER DRUGS IN THIS SUBCLASS
clarithromycin, erythromycin

GENERAL DESCRIPTION
Azithromycin, an antibiotic introduced in 1991, is a derivative of erythromycin. The drug's action varies with the type of bacteria it is being used to fight. Azithromycin kills some bacteria outright and stops the growth and reproduction of others. For more information, see Penicillins. For visual characteristics of the brand-name drug Zithromax, see the Color Guide to Prescription Drugs and Herbs.

Precautions

SPECIAL INFORMATION
- Let your doctor know if you have impaired kidneys or liver, allergies to another antibiotic, or a history of drug-induced colitis.
- Don't use azithromycin during pregnancy unless your doctor prescribes it. Avoid this drug if you are nursing.

POSSIBLE INTERACTIONS
Antacids containing aluminum, calcium, or magnesium: decreased azithromycin effect. Take azithromycin one hour before or two hours after taking antacids.
Anticoagulants: increased anticoagulant effect, risk of bleeding.
Astemizole, terfenadine: WARNING: There is a risk of life-threatening heart problems. Do not take astemizole or terfenadine if you are also taking azithromycin.
Carbamazepine, cyclosporine, digoxin, ergotamine, phenytoin, theophylline, triazolam: increased effects of these drugs, possible toxicity.

TARGET AILMENTS

Respiratory tract infections (including pharyngitis and sinusitis caused by strep); bronchitis; some types of pneumonia

Skin and soft-tissue infections

Chlamydial infections

SIDE EFFECTS

NOT SERIOUS
- Yeast infections
- Abdominal pain; mild diarrhea; nausea
- Dizziness; headache; fatigue

CONSULT YOUR DOCTOR IF THESE EFFECTS PERSIST.

SERIOUS
- Inflammation of the colon (diarrhea, cramps, vomiting, and fever)
- Kidney inflammation (fever, joint pain, rash)
- Anaphylactic reaction
- Swelling of the face, mouth, neck, hands, and feet

DISCONTINUE USE AND CONTACT YOUR DOCTOR IMMEDIATELY.

BACITRACIN

B

VITAL STATISTICS

DRUG CLASS
Antibiotics [Topical Antibiotics]

BRAND NAME
Neosporin

OTHER DRUGS IN THIS SUBCLASS
Rx: chlorhexidine (for gums); mupirocin (for skin); combination of neomycin, polymyxin B, and hydrocortisone (antibiotic-corticosteroid for ears)
OTC: neomycin, polymyxin B

GENERAL DESCRIPTION
Bacitracin is available by itself and in combination with neomycin and polymyxin B as an over-the-counter topical antibiotic. This combination and other over-the-counter topical antibiotics are available in an ointment base that helps close and soothe wounds. In general, though, the primary purpose of such OTC drugs is to guard against possible infections in minor cuts, scrapes, and burns. Once a skin infection is under way, your doctor may prescribe a stronger medication.

PRECAUTIONS

SPECIAL INFORMATION
- Check with your doctor if you notice no improvement after using these medications for two or three days.
- The use of topical antibiotics increases the risk of kidney damage or hearing loss in people with impaired kidney function who are already taking nephrotoxic medicines.
- If you are pregnant or nursing, check with your doctor before using.

POSSIBLE INTERACTIONS
None expected.

TARGET AILMENTS
Minor cuts, scrapes, and burns

SIDE EFFECTS

NOT SERIOUS
- Itching, stinging, rash, redness, or swelling at the application site

CALL YOUR DOCTOR IF THESE SYMPTOMS PERSIST OR ARE BOTHERSOME.

Rx BACTRIM

VITAL STATISTICS

DRUG CLASS
Antibiotics [Sulfonamides in Combination]

GENERIC NAME
sulfamethoxazole and trimethoprim

OTHER BRANDS
Cotrim, Cotrim D.S.

GENERAL DESCRIPTION
Bactrim is a brand name for the combination drug sulfamethoxazole (a sulfonamide antibiotic) and trimethoprim (a generic antibiotic); the combination of these two antibiotics increases the effectiveness of both medications. This combination is sometimes known as cotrimoxazole or TMP-SMZ.

Drugs in the antibiotic class are used against a wide variety of bacterial infections and are of two types. Bactericidal antibiotics kill bacteria by attacking bacterial cell walls. Bacteriostatic antibiotics prevent bacteria from reproducing, thus enabling the body's defenses to overcome the infection. Both component drugs in Bactrim, a bacteriostatic drug, work by interfering with the ability of certain disease-causing bacteria to synthesize folic acid, thereby inhibiting the organisms' growth.

Antibiotics are not effective against fungal infections or against viruses, such as those that cause colds. But some illnesses with symptoms similar to colds and the flu, such as sinusitis or bronchitis, may be bacterial in origin and will respond to antibiotic treatment.

Because antibiotics target bacteria and not fungi, the drugs in this class can disturb the body's normal balance of fungi and bacteria. This imbalance may be manifested as a fungal superinfection, such as a yeast infection, or in symptoms of diarrhea or gastrointestinal disturbances. See Special Information *(below)* for advice on how to restore your body's normal balance of bacteria and fungi.

For visual characteristics, see the Color Guide to Prescription Drugs and Herbs.

PRECAUTIONS

SPECIAL INFORMATION

- Antibiotics kill not only harmful bacteria, but also "good" bacteria that keep unwanted fungi and intestinal organisms in check. Eating yogurt containing *Lactobacillus acidophilus* culture or taking acidophilus tablets may help restore the body's normal bacteria.
- Prolonged use of any antibiotic drug can lead to fungal infections, including candidiasis, or to bacterial infections such as pseudomembranous colitis.
- Pregnant and nursing women should avoid using this combination since it may interfere with folic acid metabolism in the fetus and infant, especially near birth.
- Bactrim may cause sensitivity to the sun or to sunlamps. Limit your exposure while on this drug.
- Cross-sensitivity reactions: If you are sensitive to thiazide diuretics, PABA, local anesthetics (benzocaine), or oral antidiabetic medicines, you may also have sensitivity to Bactrim. Advise your doctor of your sensitivity.
- Many people are sensitive to these drugs, so be sure to tell your doctor if you have severe allergies or bronchial asthma.
- To prevent reinfection, complete the full course of your prescription, even if you feel better before you've taken all the medicine.
- When taking these drugs, drink plenty of fluids to prevent formation of crystals in the urine.

CONTINUED

BACTRIM

B

POSSIBLE INTERACTIONS

This combination can interact with a number of drugs, especially those that affect the liver or blood. Consult your doctor before taking any other medication.

Anticoagulants (warfarin), anticonvulsants (hydantoin), oral antidiabetics, phenylbutazone (NSAID), or sulfinpyrazone (antigout): may interfere with action or metabolism of these drugs and could result in increased effects or toxicity. Your doctor may need to adjust the dosage.

Birth-control pills containing estrogen: may result in decreased contraceptive effectiveness and increased breakthrough bleeding.

Cyclosporine: decreased effectiveness of cyclosporine.

Digoxin: decreased digoxin effects.

Methotrexate: increased methotrexate effects.

TARGET AILMENTS
Bronchitis
Urinary tract infections
Enterocolitis (caused by certain species of *Shigella*)
Acute otitis media (in children)
Prevention and treatment of pneumonia *(Pneumocystis carinii)* in people with compromised immune systems (including AIDS patients)
Traveler's diarrhea
Numerous other infections

SIDE EFFECTS

NOT SERIOUS

- Gastrointestinal problems (including diarrhea and nausea)
- Headache
- Dizziness
- Photosensitivity

LET YOUR DOCTOR KNOW IF THESE SYMPTOMS BECOME TROUBLESOME.

SERIOUS

- Allergic reactions (fever, itching skin rash)
- Blood abnormalities causing fever, sore throat, unusual bleeding, bruising, fatigue, or weakness
- Liver problems, including jaundice
- Stevens-Johnson syndrome (fever, skin blisters or blisters and open sores on mucous membranes and genitals, weakness, joint pain)
- Urinary problems resulting in burning with urination, back pain
- Goiter
- Bluish fingernails, skin, or lips
- Difficulty in breathing

CALL YOUR DOCTOR IMMEDIATELY.

BARBERRY

LATIN NAME
Berberis vulgaris

VITAL STATISTICS

GENERAL DESCRIPTION

The root bark of barberry is prescribed for several liver ailments. Herbalists also use the herb to reduce blood pressure, aid digestion, and fight infection. These effects on the body are attributed to the herb's active ingredients, isoquinoline alkaloids, which include berberine, berbamine, and oxyacanthine.

PREPARATIONS

Over the counter:
Available as root, fluidextract, and powder.

At home:

TEA: Boil 1 oz barberry root in 1 cup water for 15 to 20 minutes; let cool. Drink up to 1 cup a day. Add honey to sweeten.

COMPRESS: Soak a clean cloth in barberry tea and apply it directly to the infected area.

COMBINATIONS: To cleanse the liver, combine 1 part barberry root, 1 part wild yam, 1 part dandelion, and ½ part licorice root. Simmer covered 1 oz in 1 pt water for 10 minutes. Strain through a coffee filter. Drink 2 oz three or four times daily.

Consult a qualified practitioner for the dosage appropriate for your specific condition.

PRECAUTIONS

WARNING

Do not take barberry if you are pregnant, because of its stimulant effect on the uterus.

Use only in consultation with an herbalist or licensed healthcare professional if you have heart disease or chronic respiratory problems.

Use of this herb by children for more than seven to 10 days should be done in conjunction with a healthcare practitioner.

POSSIBLE INTERACTIONS

Combining barberry with other herbs may necessitate a lower dosage.

TARGET AILMENTS

Take internally for:

Jaundice; hepatitis
Anemia
Indigestion; heartburn; hangover
Constipation
Swollen spleen; gallstones

Gargle with barberry tea for:

Sore throat

Use as a compress for:

Inflamed eyelids; conjunctivitis
Skin infection

SIDE EFFECTS

NOT SERIOUS

- Upset stomach; diarrhea
- Nausea; vomiting
- Dizziness; faintness

CHECK WITH A PRACTITIONER.

SERIOUS

- Convulsions
- Drastic lowering of blood pressure
- Drastic slowing of heart rate, respiration

STOP USING AT ONCE AND INFORM YOUR PRACTITIONER.

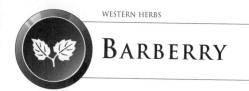

BASIL

LATIN NAME
Ocimum basilicum

B

VITAL STATISTICS

GENERAL DESCRIPTION

Basil comes in more than 100 varieties and is native to India. It is now cultivated in the Mediterranean, in Florida, and in Morocco. The common herb has dark green leaves that give off an aromatic scent when rubbed between the fingers. The plant's white flowers are crowded at the base of leafy stalks.

The plant is also known as the royal herb, because its name derives from *basilicum,* the Latin for royal.

PREPARATIONS

The colorless to yellow oil is distilled from the flower tops, shoots, and leaves. It has a very strong aroma, similar to that of tarragon. It is a popular cooking herb, a good digestive aid, and is useful as a nerve tonic and antispasmodic. Basil also has antidepressant properties and is noted for its ability to help the mind focus and concentrate, as well as being effective against migraine headaches.

Basil can be used in the bath, inhaled to clear the sinuses, or diffused to purify the air. If you want to mask its smell, use it with a citrus-based oil or rose oil.

BATH: Add 5 to 10 drops to bathwater.

MASSAGE: Mix 10 to 15 drops basil oil with 2 tbsp aloe gel or a carrier oil. Apply to aching joints or muscles. Rub on the chest to relieve respiratory problems.

DIFFUSED OIL: Use essential oil in a diffuser or place a few drops on a handkerchief to help relieve anxiety, stress, fatigue, and respiratory complaints.

STEAM: Add 6 drops basil oil to a bowl of water just off the boil. Hold a towel over the bowl and your head and inhale the steam for up to 5 minutes. This method is used to relieve hay fever and respiratory discomfort.

PRECAUTIONS

WARNING

Avoid basil during pregnancy.

SPECIAL INFORMATION

Basil may cause skin sensitization in some people.

TARGET AILMENTS
Menopausal symptoms
Anxiety and stress
Mental and physical fatigue
Colds and flu
Hay fever
Insect bites
Muscular aches and pains
Rheumatism
Menstrual cramps
Bronchitis
Sinusitis

SIDE EFFECTS

BASIL IS NONIRRITATING AND NONTOXIC.

BAYBERRY

LATIN NAME
Myrica spp.

VITAL STATISTICS

GENERAL DESCRIPTION

In the 19th century bayberry was used to treat colds, flu, fever, and diarrhea. The bark of the bayberry tree contains myricitrin, an antibiotic that promotes sweating, which in turn can reduce fever; it also stimulates the flow of bile. The herb is therefore prescribed today to relieve fever and diarrhea. Myricitrin is also an expectorant. And some herbalists regard bayberry as a stimulant for the circulatory system. Two commonly used species are *Myrica cerifera* and *Myrica pensylvanica.*

PREPARATIONS

Over the counter:
Available as tincture, fluidextract, capsules, and root bark.

At home:
DECOCTION: In 1 pt water, boil 1 tsp powdered root bark for 10 to 15 minutes. Add a little milk and drink it cool, up to 2 cups a day.
GARGLE: Use the same preparation as a gargle.
FOMENTATION: Soak a cotton towel in a hot herbal tea or decoction and apply to the affected area. To retain the heat, place a layer of plastic over the towel, then cover with a heating pad or a cloth soaked in hot water.
Consult a qualified practitioner for the dosage appropriate for you and your specific condition.

PRECAUTIONS

WARNING

The herb affects the body's electrolyte balance, retaining sodium but depleting potassium. This in turn can lead to high blood pressure and edema. Consult your practitioner for advice. Individuals with high blood pressure, edema, kidney disease, congestive heart failure, gastrointestinal conditions, or any type of imbalance between sodium and potassium should consult a doctor before using bayberry.

Use of this herb by children for more than seven to 10 days should be done in conjunction with a healthcare practitioner.

SPECIAL INFORMATION

Do not use this herb if you have a history of cancer. Bayberry contains a high proportion of tannins, chemicals that in laboratory studies seemed to promote cancer.

POSSIBLE INTERACTIONS

Combining bayberry with other herbs may necessitate a lower dosage.

TARGET AILMENTS

Take internally for:

Dysentery; diarrhea
Fever
Nasal congestion; sore throat

Apply externally for:

Poor circulation; varicose veins
Hemorrhoids

SIDE EFFECTS

NOT SERIOUS

- Nausea
- Vomiting

THESE EFFECTS MAY OCCUR IF TOO LARGE A DOSE IS TAKEN. IF THEY PERSIST, CALL YOUR DOCTOR.

Bay Laurel

LATIN NAME
Laurus nobilis

Vital Statistics

GENERAL DESCRIPTION

Native to the Mediterranean, this hardy evergreen shrub or tree has dark green leaves and a dark green trunk. Only the female tree produces the black berries. Its oil is greenish yellow and has a powerful, spicy scent. Bay laurel is an overall strengthener. It can be used as an antiseptic, a diuretic, or a sedative, and it may help to expel gas and clear the lungs.

PREPARATIONS

The essential oil comes from a distillation of the leaves and twigs. To apply to the skin and scalp for various purposes, mix 10 drops in 2 tbsp vegetable or nut oil or aloe gel. Baths can be taken with 3 to 5 drops mixed into the bathwater. For inhalation, place a few drops on a cloth or tissue and hold up to your nose and mouth. You can also use a diffuser to spread the fragrance in the air.

Precautions

SPECIAL INFORMATION

- Avoid bay laurel if you are pregnant.
- Because of its possible narcotic properties, use bay laurel in moderation.

TARGET AILMENTS

- Digestive problems and appetite loss
- Bronchitis
- Colds and flu
- Tonsillitis
- Scabies
- Lice
- Rheumatic aches
- Muscular and joint pain
- Arthritis
- Swollen lymph nodes

SIDE EFFECTS

NOT SERIOUS

- Can cause drowsiness in some individuals
- May be slightly irritating to skin and mucous membranes

BA ZHEN WAN

VITAL STATISTICS

ENGLISH NAME
Eight Treasure Pills

ALSO SOLD AS
Precious Pills or Women's Precious Pills

GENERAL DESCRIPTION
Ba Zhen Wan (Eight Treasure Pills) is a tonic specially formulated to correct deficiencies in chi (bodily energy) and blood. According to Chinese medicine, when these vital substances are depleted, a person will feel tired, appear pale, and have a pale tongue. Eight Treasure Pills are often prescribed by practitioners of Chinese medicine when a patient has lost blood as a result of disease, an accident, heavy menstrual flow, or childbirth. They are also sometimes used to treat lightheadedness or dizziness.

Chinese medicine takes a holistic approach to healthcare, fashioning remedies to treat the entire being as well as specific parts or areas. Precise combinations of herbs are used to prevent and combat disease, which is thought to arise from disturbances in the flow of a bodily energy called chi or qi (pronounced "chee") and blood, or from a lack of balance in the complementary states of yin and yang. A patent formula, *Ba Zhen Wan* is made by using a standardized combination of herbs and method of preparation.

INGREDIENTS
ginseng, white atractylodes, poria, honey-fried licorice, rehmannia, white peony root, dong quai, ligusticum

PREPARATIONS
This formula is sold in pill form at many Chinese pharmacies and Oriental grocery stores.

TARGET AILMENTS

- Fatigue with pale complexion
- Weakness following blood loss
- Dizziness or lightheadedness
- Postpartum fatigue
- Lack of menstruation
- Irregular menstruation

SIDE EFFECTS

NONE EXPECTED

Beclomethasone

B

Vital Statistics

DRUG CLASS
Corticosteroids

BRAND NAMES
Inhalant: Beclovent, Vanceril
Nasal: Beconase, Beconase AQ, Vancenase, Vancenase AQ, Vanceril

OTHER DRUGS IN THIS CLASS
Rx: betamethasone, fluticasone, methylprednisolone, mometasone furoate, prednisone, triamcinolone
OTC: hydrocortisone

GENERAL DESCRIPTION
Beclomethasone is a potent adrenal corticosteroid, available in nasal spray and oral inhalant forms, which acts to inhibit inflammation. Introduced in 1976, this drug is normally prescribed when a person does not respond to other treatments. Oral inhalant forms are used to treat bronchial asthma. They are intended to prevent, not relieve, acute asthma attacks. Concurrent use of bronchodilators in tablet, nasal spray, or oral inhalant form may increase the effects of beclomethasone.

As a nasal spray, beclomethasone is used to treat severe seasonal or perennial hay fever (allergic rhinitis) when decongestants are inadequate (although clearing your nasal passages with a decongestant spray before using beclomethasone may improve the drug's effect). For more information, see Corticosteroids.

Precautions

SPECIAL INFORMATION
- Beclomethasone should not be used for nonasthmatic lung diseases without the advice of your physician.
- Use with caution if you have a nasal disease; consult your doctor.
- Rinse your mouth after oral use to decrease the possibility of a fungal infection.
- Beclomethasone should be avoided by individuals who are hypersensitive to medication.
- Corticosteroid nasal and oral sprays or inhalers may be absorbed into your system after prolonged use. Tell your doctor if you are taking any other medication, and watch for any significant side effects or possible drug interactions.
- Ask your doctor about the risks and benefits of corticosteroid treatment if you have or have had any of the following conditions: HIV infection or AIDS, heart disease, hypertension, ulcerative colitis, diabetes, diverticulitis, gastritis or peptic ulcers, recent chickenpox or measles, candidiasis or other fungal infections, glaucoma, herpes simplex, liver or kidney disease, myasthenia gravis, osteoporosis, anastomoses, lupus, tuberculosis, recent intestinal problems, or any infection, such as a cold or flu.
- Prolonged use of corticosteroids can cause birth defects. Pregnant and nursing women should avoid these drugs.

Beclomethasone

- One of the actions of corticosteroids is to suppress your immune system, which can make you more susceptible to opportunistic infections. Corticosteroids can also mask symptoms of infection that occur while you are taking the drugs; because the symptoms will not appear, an infection may worsen without your being aware of it.
- Prolonged use of corticosteroids increases the risk of osteoporosis, cataracts, glaucoma, Cushing's syndrome (moon face), and diabetes. It can also reactivate tuberculosis.

POSSIBLE INTERACTIONS

Aspirin and other salicylates: may increase gastrointestinal irritation.

Diuretics: decreased effectiveness of both combined drugs.

Growth hormones, isoniazid, potassium supplements, and salicylates: beclomethasone may decrease the effectiveness of these drugs.

Oral anticoagulants: beclomethasone may increase or decrease the effectiveness of oral anticoagulants.

Vaccines (live virus, other immunizations): beclomethasone may make you more susceptible to the injected virus.

TARGET AILMENTS

Nasal inflammation, including hay fever (allergic rhinitis)

Nonallergic inflammation of the nasal passages

Respiratory ailments such as severe asthma

SIDE EFFECTS

NOT SERIOUS

- White patches in the mouth, throat, or nose
- Throat irritation
- Stuffy or runny nose
- Burning or dryness inside the nose

SEE YOUR DOCTOR IF THESE SYMPTOMS PERSIST OR IF THERE IS NO IMPROVEMENT IN YOUR CONDITION IN THREE WEEKS.

SERIOUS

NONE EXPECTED WITH LOW-DOSE, SHORT-TERM USE

B

BEE POLLEN

B

VITAL STATISTICS

GENERAL DESCRIPTION

The nutritional components of bee pollen, which is extracted by professional methods from hives, include vitamin C, B-complex vitamins, amino acids, carotene, calcium, copper, iron, magnesium, and potassium. Although its benefits have not been scientifically proved, bee pollen is said to boost physical energy and endurance, and athletes sometimes take it to improve their performance. It may also relieve stress, fatigue, and depression, and aid in weight-loss efforts. Although it is reputed to help with respiratory allergies, it should not be taken by anyone allergic to bee stings.

Bee pollen has a germ-killing effect, and ailments for which it may be beneficial include bowel problems, cancer, heart ailments, and arthritis, although no scientific studies support such claims. It thus remains somewhat controversial as a health promoter.

NATURAL SOURCES

Flowering plants

PREPARATIONS

Available in capsules and by injection.

PRECAUTIONS

WARNING

Do not use bee pollen if you are allergic to bee stings. Do not use if you have gout or kidney disease. Do not give to children under the age of two.

Do not use if you are pregnant or planning a pregnancy. If you are breast-feeding, do not use except under the advice of your healthcare practitioner.

SPECIAL INFORMATION

- Standard dosages and possible side effects of bee pollen have not been determined thoroughly. Begin with small amounts and discontinue if any allergic reactions occur.
- Those who are allergic to airborne pollen may wish to avoid taking bee pollen as a supplement, although the effects are not necessarily the same.
- Some commercial flower-pollen preparations do not contain pollen collected from bees. They are similar to bee pollen and may provide health benefits, although these too have yet to be proved.

TARGET AILMENTS

See General Description *(left)*.

SIDE EFFECTS

NOT SERIOUS

- Rash
- Itching
- Pain at injection site
- Swelling

DISCONTINUE USE AND CALL YOUR DOCTOR.

SERIOUS

- Anaphylactic shock (a severe allergic reaction indicated by extreme itching, swelling, loss of breath, lowered blood pressure, and loss of consciousness)

STAY WITH THE VICTIM, ADMINISTER CPR, AND HAVE SOMEONE CALL 911 OR YOUR EMERGENCY NUMBER.

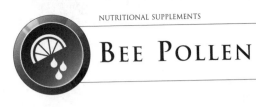

BELLADONNA

LATIN NAME
Belladonna

VITAL STATISTICS

GENERAL DESCRIPTION

Belladonna, a highly toxic plant also known as deadly nightshade, grows wild across Europe, producing yellow flowers in July and dark red berries in late summer. Its name, meaning "beautiful woman" in Italian, dates from the Renaissance, when ladies of Italy dilated their pupils with belladonna eye drops for a doe-eyed appearance. Belladonna poisoning brings on a range of symptoms, including a dry mouth and hot, flushed skin, nausea, convulsive movements, and delirium. Homeopathic practitioners prescribe the remedy *Belladonna* for illnesses that are accompanied by these same symptoms. All parts of the belladonna plant are gathered for use in the homeopathic remedy. The plant is crushed and pressed, and the extracted juice is mixed with alcohol in an extremely dilute preparation.

Like most homeopathic prescriptions, *Belladonna* was developed as a remedy by observation of the reactions of healthy individuals to doses of various strengths. The mental, emotional, and physical changes induced by *Belladonna* were then cataloged. When a homeopathic practitioner encounters a patient with symptoms that match the cataloged symptoms brought on by *Belladonna,* the practitioner then prescribes it in an extremely dilute form. It is presumed that in this highly dilute dosage, *Belladonna* can counter symptoms that are similar to the ones it induces when it is at full strength. For more information on homeopathic medicine, see page 14.

PREPARATIONS

Belladonna is available in various potencies, in both liquid and tablet form. Consult your practitioner for more precise dosage information.

PRECAUTIONS

SPECIAL INFORMATION

- When a remedy is administered, no one but the patient should touch the pills. If tablets are spilled, throw them away.
- The mouth should be clear of flavors 15 minutes before and after taking a remedy, and strong flavors and aromas, such as coffee, camphor, and heavily scented perfumes, should be avoided for the duration of treatment.

TARGET AILMENTS

Cold; flu; sore throat; earache with excruciating pain; high fever accompanied by chills but with no signs of thirst

Acute inflammatory arthritis or bursitis; gallstones; acute diverticulitis

Colic; measles; mumps

Neuralgia; sunstroke; acutely inflamed varicose veins

Toothache; teething pains

Painful menstrual periods

Breast-feeding complications, especially when the breasts are engorged and inflamed

SIDE EFFECTS

NONE EXPECTED

BENAZEPRIL

B

VITAL STATISTICS

DRUG CLASS
Angiotensin-Converting Enzyme (ACE) Inhibitors

BRAND NAME
Lotensin

OTHER DRUGS IN THIS CLASS
captopril, enalapril, fosinopril, lisinopril, quinapril, ramipril

GENERAL DESCRIPTION
Introduced in 1991, the ACE inhibitor benazepril is prescribed for control of high blood pressure. It works by blocking a body enzyme that is essential for the production of a substance that causes blood vessels to constrict. This action relaxes arterial walls, lowering blood pressure. For further information see Angiotensin-Converting Enzyme (ACE) Inhibitors.

PRECAUTIONS

WARNING
Get medical attention immediately if you notice swelling of your face, tongue, or vocal cords or have difficulty swallowing or breathing; this reaction can be life threatening.

This drug should not be taken during pregnancy because it has been associated with malformations and death of the fetus and newborn baby.

SPECIAL INFORMATION
- Benazepril causes an increase in blood levels of potassium. Do not use potassium-rich products, including salt substitutes and low-salt milk, without first consulting your doctor. The potassium in your blood could rise to dangerous levels, leading to heart-rhythm problems.
- Do not abruptly stop taking this drug. Your doctor may tell you to reduce the dosage gradually.

TARGET AILMENTS
High blood pressure

SIDE EFFECTS

NOT SERIOUS
- Dry, persistent cough
- Headache
- Fatigue
- Nausea or diarrhea
- Loss of sense of taste
- Temporary skin rash
- Low blood pressure or dizziness on suddenly rising or changing position

CALL YOUR DOCTOR IF THESE SIDE EFFECTS BECOME BOTHERSOME.

SERIOUS
- Fainting
- Persistent skin rash
- Joint pain
- Drowsiness
- Numbness and tingling
- Abdominal pain; vomiting; severe diarrhea; fever; chills
- Chest pain; heart palpitation
- Jaundice (yellowing of skin or eyes)

CALL YOUR DOCTOR RIGHT AWAY.

BENZOCAINE

VITAL STATISTICS

DRUG CLASS
Anesthetics

BRAND NAMES
Anbesol, Orajel

OTHER DRUGS IN THIS CLASS
dyclonine, pramoxine

GENERAL DESCRIPTION
Benzocaine is an over-the-counter local anesthetic (derived from the same source as the sunscreen preparation PABA) that is frequently used to relieve pain and discomfort in the mouth and on the skin or mucous membranes. The drug works by deadening nerve endings so that they do not transmit pain messages to the brain. Most side effects associated with local anesthetics are caused by excessive applications or by individual sensitivity to the anesthetic. Benzocaine is more likely to cause sensitivity reactions than most other anesthetics.

PRECAUTIONS

SPECIAL INFORMATION
- Benzocaine should not be used on areas where irritation, infection, or bleeding is present unless your doctor directs you to do so. Benzocaine can cause excess irritation or become absorbed into the bloodstream, leading to overdose symptoms.
- Do not use benzocaine if you are sensitive or allergic to PABA, since the two are chemically similar.

POSSIBLE INTERACTIONS
None expected.

TARGET AILMENTS

Canker sores

Mouth or gum injury

Toothache

Pain from dental procedures or appliances

Pain associated with other minor skin and mouth problems

SIDE EFFECTS

SERIOUS

- Allergic reactions such as skin rash, hives, redness, and itching at the site of application
- Large hivelike swellings on the skin or in the mouth or throat
- Burning, stinging, and swelling not present before application

THESE SYMPTOMS ARE RARE. CALL YOUR DOCTOR TO DETERMINE WHETHER YOU USED TOO MUCH MEDICATION OR ARE SENSITIVE TO BENZOCAINE.

- Overdose symptoms including dizziness, headache, tiredness, blurred vision, irregular heartbeat, or ringing in the ears

CALL YOUR DOCTOR IMMEDIATELY.

Rx BENZODIAZEPINES

B

VITAL STATISTICS

DRUG CLASS
Antianxiety Drugs

GENERIC NAMES
alprazolam, clonazepam, diazepam, lorazepam, temazepam, triazolam

GENERAL DESCRIPTION
Benzodiazepines are used to treat anxiety, insomnia, muscle spasms, and convulsions. Drugs in this class work by enhancing the action of a natural chemical in the brain that acts to depress certain areas of the central nervous system. The effects of benzodiazepines start after the first dose.

Some benzodiazepines can be used to treat any of the conditions listed below, but most have one or two primary uses. For example, alprazolam is used mainly for anxiety, clonazepam for convulsions, temazepam and triazolam for insomnia. Though benzodiazepines can cause physical and psychological dependence, they are considered particularly useful because they have fewer toxicity problems, fewer side effects, and less abuse potential than other drugs used for the same purposes. For more information, see the entries for the generic drugs listed above.

PRECAUTIONS

☠ ***WARNING***
Never combine alcohol with benzodiazepines; the combination can cause dangerous central nervous system and respiratory depression.

Do not abruptly stop taking these drugs. Sudden cessation can provoke withdrawal symptoms including seizures; irritability; insomnia; confusion; mental depression; hypersensitivity to pain, noise, or light; and feelings of suspicion and distrust. Slowly reduce the dosage under your doctor's guidance.

SPECIAL INFORMATION
- Benzodiazepines can impair your alertness, judgment, and coordination. Avoid driving and performing hazardous activities until you know how the drug affects you.
- Let your doctor know if you have narrow-angle glaucoma, a liver or kidney impairment, chronic respiratory disease, myasthenia gravis, depression, sleep apnea, or a history of drug abuse or addiction. Benzodiazepines may exacerbate these conditions.

Benzodiazepines

- These drugs can cause sleep apnea in people with chronic respiratory disease, such as emphysema.
- Benzodiazepines can cause physical and psychological dependence, sometimes after only one or two weeks but usually after prolonged use.
- People with a history of drug or alcohol abuse are at a greater risk of psychological dependence on benzodiazepines.
- Tolerance may increase with prolonged use; as your body adjusts to the benzodiazepine, the drug becomes less effective. Never increase the dose without consulting your doctor, because the risk of benzodiazepine dependence increases with higher doses.
- Do not take benzodiazepines if you are pregnant or breast-feeding.

POSSIBLE INTERACTIONS

Alcohol, anticonvulsants, antihistamines that cause drowsiness (clemastine, diphenhydramine), barbiturates, MAO inhibitors, opioids, tricyclic antidepressants: increased sedative effects, such as excessive mental (central nervous system) depression, sleepiness, and slow or shallow breathing. It is very important that you avoid taking benzodiazepines in combination with any of these drugs.

Antacids: may slow the absorption of benzodiazepines. Separate from benzodiazepine dose by an hour.

Beta blockers, cimetidine, disulfiram, erythromycin, ketoconazole, omeprazole, oral contraceptives, probenecid: may prolong the amount of time benzodiazepines remain in your body, leading to increased benzodiazepine effects and possible toxicity.

TARGET AILMENTS
Anxiety and panic disorders (alprazolam, diazepam, lorazepam)
Insomnia (lorazepam, temazepam, triazolam)
Convulsions or seizures (clonazepam, diazepam as an adjunct)
Skeletal muscle pain and spasticity (diazepam as an adjunct)
Alcohol withdrawal (diazepam)
Presurgery anxiety (diazepam, lorazepam as an adjunct to anesthesia)

CONTINUED

BENZODIAZEPINES

B

Clozapine: risk of profound hypotension (low blood pressure), slow or shallow breathing, cessation of breathing, and cardiac arrest leading to death.

Isoniazid: increased effect and possible toxicity of diazepam and triazolam. This interaction may also occur with other benzodiazepines.

Levodopa: decreased levodopa effect.

Rifampin: decreased effect of diazepam and possibly of other benzodiazepines.

Tobacco (smoking): decreased benzodiazepine effects.

Valproic acid: increased benzodiazepine effects, including mental depression; risk of certain types of seizures if taken with clonazepam.

Zidovudine: risk of zidovudine toxicity.

SIDE EFFECTS

NOT SERIOUS

- Clumsiness or unsteadiness
- Lethargy
- Dry mouth
- Nausea
- Change in bowel habits
- Temporary amnesia (especially "traveler's amnesia" when taken to treat insomnia associated with jet lag)

TELL YOUR DOCTOR IF THESE SYMPTOMS PERSIST OR BECOME BOTHERSOME. CONTACT YOUR DOCTOR IF YOU ARE HAVING DIFFICULTY WITH YOUR MEMORY.

SERIOUS

- Slurred speech
- Dizziness or blurred vision
- Persistent or severe headache
- Confusion
- Depression
- Changes in behavior (outbursts of anger, difficulty concentrating)
- Hallucinations
- Uncontrolled movement of body or eyes
- Muscle weakness
- Chills or fever
- Sore throat
- Jaundice (rare)
- Low blood pressure (rare)
- Low platelet count (unusual bruising or bleeding) (rare)

TELL YOUR DOCTOR ABOUT THESE SYMPTOMS RIGHT AWAY.

BERGAMOT

LATIN NAME
Citrus bergamia

B

VITAL STATISTICS

GENERAL DESCRIPTION

This small fruit-bearing citrus tree is native to tropical Asia and is cultivated extensively in southern Italy. Its name derives from the Italian city of Bergamo, in Lombardy, where the oil was first sold. Recent research has shown bergamot oil to be useful in healing infections of the skin, mouth, respiratory tract, and urinary tract. It is also used as an analgesic, antidepressant, and antispasmodic and as a digestive aid. In the home, bergamot vapor can help eliminate airborne bacteria and help balance the emotions when inhaled.

PREPARATIONS

Bergamot oil comes from the peel of the nearly ripe fruit. It is light greenish yellow to emerald in color and it has a sweet, fruity, slightly spicy scent.

Inhalation: Add a few drops of bergamot oil to a bowl of warm water and let stand, or place several drops on a tissue and inhale.

Bath: Use 5 drops bergamot oil mixed in bathwater or in a sitz bath.

Gargle: Mix 3 drops bergamot oil in ½ cup of water. Do not swallow.

SIDE EFFECTS

NOT SERIOUS

- Skin irritation

DISCONTINUE USE.

PRECAUTIONS

☠ *WARNING*

Bergamot can gradually increase the skin's sensitivity to the sun. Avoid using undiluted bergamot oil on the skin. Do not apply before long periods of exposure to the sun or before entering a tanning booth. Avoid using if you have a tendency toward skin cancer. Photosensitivity can last several days after use.

SPECIAL INFORMATION

When used as directed, bergamot is relatively nontoxic and nonirritating.

TARGET AILMENTS
Mouth infections (gargle)
Sore throat (gargle)
Tonsillitis (gargle)
Flatulence; loss of appetite (baths, inhalation)
Cystitis (baths, sitz baths)
Colds and flu (baths, inhalation)
Fever (baths, inhalation)
Depression (baths, inhalation)
Anxiety and stress (baths, inhalation)

Beta-Adrenergic Blockers

B

Vital Statistics

GENERIC NAMES
atenolol, bisoprolol, metoprolol, nadolol, propranolol, timolol (oral and ophthalmic)

GENERAL DESCRIPTION
Also known as beta blockers, these drugs interfere with the action of certain parts of the nervous system, thereby slowing the heart rate and the nerve impulses to the heart and other organs. This in turn results in lowered blood pressure and decreased angina. The first of the beta-blocking drugs to be developed (including nadolol, propranolol, and timolol) are called nonselective agents because they work in the whole body and can be used to treat a variety of medical conditions.

The newer beta blockers, among them atenolol, bisoprolol, and metoprolol, are called cardioselective because they primarily target beta receptors in the muscles of the heart. These drugs are particularly useful for treating heart disorders such as angina and arrhythmia. For more information, see the individual entries for the generic drugs listed above.

Precautions

SPECIAL INFORMATION
- Beta-adrenergic blockers can make you drowsy, dizzy, and lightheaded.
- Tell your doctor if you are planning surgery or have any of the following conditions, which beta blockers may complicate: allergies, bronchial asthma, or emphysema; congestive heart failure; diabetes mellitus; hyperthyroidism; impaired liver or kidneys; mental depression; myasthenia gravis; poor circulation or circulatory disease.
- Do not use beta blockers if you have a bronchospastic disease, bronchial asthma, or a severe chronic obstructive pulmonary disease.
- These drugs can both mask symptoms of low blood sugar and boost blood sugar levels in patients with diabetes mellitus.
- Beta-adrenergic blockers can increase the severity of allergic reactions to drugs, food, or insect stings. Contact your doctor immediately if a severe allergic reaction occurs.
- Suddenly stopping these drugs may cause or increase heart problems. Dosage must be reduced gradually under your doctor's supervision.
- Before taking these drugs, let your doctor know if you are pregnant or nursing.

TARGET AILMENTS
Heart disease, especially angina (pain), heart attack (myocardial infarction), and abnormal heart rhythms
High blood pressure (hypertension)
Migraine headaches (propranolol, timolol)
Tremors (propranolol)
Schizophrenic and anxiety disorders (propranolol, timolol)
Alcohol withdrawal (atenolol, propranolol)
Glaucoma (timolol)

BETA-ADRENERGIC BLOCKERS

B

POSSIBLE INTERACTIONS
Beta blockers may interact with many over-the-counter and prescription medications, including the following:

Aminophylline, theophylline: decreased clearance of these drugs and possible toxicity.

Antacids (aluminum hydroxide or magnesium): decreased beta blocker absorption. Take antacid four hours before or two hours after taking beta blocker.

Antidiabetic drugs, insulin: increased risk of high blood sugar and impaired recovery from hypoglycemia.

Antihypertensive drugs (including calcium channel blockers, clonidine, and guanabenz): increased antihypertensive effect.

Antipsychotic drugs (thioridazine, chlorpromazine): increased effects of both combined drugs, producing excessively low blood pressure, slowed heart rate, and difficulty breathing.

Cimetidine: increased beta blocker effect.

Ephedrine, epinephrine, and isoproterenol: decreased effects of these drugs; risk of increased blood pressure.

Estrogens: decreased antihypertensive effect of beta blockers.

MAO inhibitors: combination can cause hypertension. Do not take beta blockers until 14 days after discontinuing MAO inhibitors.

Nonsteroidal anti-inflammatory drugs (NSAIDs), such as ibuprofen: reduced beta blocker effect.

Phenothiazines: increased effects of both combined drugs.

SIDE EFFECTS

NOT SERIOUS

- Decreased sexual ability
- Drowsiness or weakness
- Trouble sleeping
- Upset stomach
- Change in bowel habits
- Nervousness

CONSULT YOUR DOCTOR IF THESE EFFECTS CONTINUE OR ARE BOTHERSOME.

SERIOUS

- Bronchospasm (trouble breathing)
- Dizziness
- Mental depression
- Chest pain
- Fast or irregular heartbeat
- Prolonged reduced circulation (cold hands and feet)
- Congestive heart failure (swelling of feet or lower legs, shortness of breath)
- Sudden shortness of breath
- Sweating, trembling, and weakness

CALL YOUR DOCTOR IMMEDIATELY. SEE TIMOLOL FOR SIDE EFFECTS OF AN OPHTHALMIC (EYE DROP) FORM OF A BETA-ADRENERGIC BLOCKER.

Rx BETAMETHASONE

B

VITAL STATISTICS

DRUG CLASS
Corticosteroids

BRAND NAME
Lotrisone (with clotrimazole)

OTHER DRUGS IN THIS CLASS
Rx: beclomethasone, fluticasone, methylprednisolone, mometasone furoate, prednisone, triamcinolone
OTC: hydrocortisone

GENERAL DESCRIPTION
Lotrisone, a combination of the corticosteroid drug betamethasone and the antifungal medication clotrimazole, is a topical preparation used to destroy fungi and relieve any accompanying skin inflammation. It is important to note that betamethasone treats only the inflammation and does not kill fungi. (Other forms of the drug are used systemically to decrease the body's inflammatory response.)

See Corticosteroids for more information about this class of medications. For information about specific corticosteroid medications, see the entries for the individual generic drugs listed above. Also see Antifungal Drugs and Clotrimazole.

PRECAUTIONS

SPECIAL INFORMATION
- Betamethasone should be used with caution if you are allergic to other corticosteroids; if you have an infection or thin skin at the treatment site; or if you have or have had cataracts, glaucoma, diabetes, or tuberculosis.
- Corticosteroid topical creams may be absorbed into your system after prolonged use. Tell your doctor if you are taking any other medication, and watch for any significant side effects or possible drug interactions.
- Ask your doctor about the risks and benefits of corticosteroid treatment if you have or have had any of the following conditions: HIV infection or AIDS, heart disease, hypertension, ulcerative colitis, diabetes, diverticulitis, gastritis or peptic ulcers, recent chickenpox or measles, glaucoma, herpes simplex, liver or kidney disease, myasthenia gravis, osteoporosis, anastomoses, lupus, tuberculosis, recent intestinal problems, or any infection, such as a cold or flu.

TARGET AILMENTS

Athlete's foot

Jock itch

Yeast infections

SIDE EFFECTS

NONE EXPECTED

Bezoar Antidotal Tablets

Vital Statistics

PINYIN NAME
Niu Huang Jie Du Pian

GENERAL DESCRIPTION
Bezoar Antidotal Tablets are used to treat certain acute inflammatory conditions such as an inflamed throat, earache, mouth sores, and conjunctivitis (pinkeye). Sometimes the formula is used for boils and other skin infections. The herbs in Bezoar Antidotal Tablets help the body rid itself of the infection causing the inflammation.

Chinese medicine takes a holistic approach to healthcare, fashioning remedies to treat the entire being as well as the specific parts or areas. Precise combinations of herbs are used to prevent and combat disease, which is thought to arise from disturbances in the flow of a bodily energy called chi (pronounced "chee") and blood, or from a lack of balance in the complementary states of yin and yang. A patent formula, Bezoar Antodotal Tablets are made by using a standardized combination of herbs and method of preparation.

INGREDIENTS
coptis, borneol, forsythia, mint, scute, angelica, gardenia, rhubarb root, cow's gallstones, ligusticum

PREPARATIONS
This formula is often available in pill form at Chinese pharmacies and Oriental grocery stores.

Precautions

WARNING
Do not use Bezoar Antidotal Tablets if you are pregnant.

Do not use this formula if you have loose stools or diarrhea.

Use only with acute conditions where there is inflammation.

TARGET AILMENTS
Sore throat
Tongue or mouth ulcers
Toothache
Tonsillitis or pharyngitis with fever
Earache with fever
Conjunctivitis
Sores, carbuncles, and boils

SIDE EFFECTS

NOT SERIOUS
- Loose stools

Biaxin

Vital Statistics

DRUG CLASS
Antibiotics [Erythromycins]

GENERIC NAME
clarithromycin

GENERAL DESCRIPTION
Biaxin is a brand name for the generic drug clarithromycin, an antibiotic introduced in 1991. Clarithromycin is a type of erythromycin but has fewer side effects than other drugs in that class. Its action varies with the type of bacteria it is used to fight; the drug kills some and stops the growth and reproduction of others. This drug may be used to treat respiratory tract infections, including sinusitis, pharyngitis due to strep, tonsillitis, bronchitis, and some types of pneumonia, as well as some types of skin infections and AIDS-related infections due to *Mycobacterium avium* or *Mycobacterium intracellulare.* For visual characteristics of Biaxin, see the Color Guide to Prescription Drugs and Herbs.

Precautions

SPECIAL INFORMATION
- Some infections may require 14 days of treatment. Take the full course to prevent the infection from returning.
- Tell your doctor if your kidneys or liver is impaired. You may need to have your dose adjusted.
- Tell your doctor if you are allergic to erythromycin, azithromycin, or troleandomycin, because you may also be allergic to this drug.
- Avoid using Biaxin if you are pregnant or nursing a baby.

POSSIBLE INTERACTIONS
See Erythromycin for other possible drug interactions.
Astemizole: WARNING: risk of life-threatening heart problems. Do not take astemizole with Biaxin.
Terfenadine: WARNING: risk of life-threatening heart problems. Do not take terfenadine with Biaxin.
Zidovudine: decreased zidovudine effect.

TARGET AILMENTS

Respiratory tract infections

Infections of the skin and soft tissue

SIDE EFFECTS

NOT SERIOUS
- An unusual taste in the mouth
- Abdominal pain; headache
- Mild diarrhea; nausea
- Yeast infections

CONSULT YOUR DOCTOR IF THESE SYMPTOMS ARE PROLONGED OR BOTHERSOME.

SERIOUS
- Unusual bleeding or bruising
- Rash; vomiting
- Inflammation of the colon (diarrhea lasting more than 24 hours, cramps, fever)

DISCONTINUE USE AND CALL YOUR DOCTOR IMMEDIATELY.

Bilberry

LATIN NAME
Vaccinium myrtillus

Vital Statistics

GENERAL DESCRIPTION

Herbalists have long valued the berries and leaves of the bilberry, a wild shrub that grows in Europe and North America. To enhance their night vision, British pilots in World War II ate bilberry jam before flying night missions. Small laboratory studies since then have indicated that the berries are useful for treating other eye problems, including glaucoma, cataracts, and macular degeneration (a common cause of blindness in adults). Bilberry's healing effects probably stem from chemicals in the berries known as anthocyanosides.

Some European herbalists claim that bilberry anthocyanosides may protect the arteries by reducing deposits that can lead to heart attacks, strokes, and high blood pressure. Dried berries work directly on the small intestine and are used to treat diarrhea. Herbalists have also prescribed bilberry leaves to lower blood sugar in diabetics.

PREPARATIONS

Over the counter:

Available as tinctures, fluidextract, dried leaves, and dried berries.

At home:

Fruit: Eat dried berries alone or mixed with apple powder to treat diarrhea.

Tea: Boil covered 2 to 3 tsp leaves in 1 cup water. Drink 1 cup per day for vomiting and stomach cramps. Use externally as a wash for skin problems and burns.

Decoction: Use 1 cup water with 1 tsp dried berries and simmer covered for 10 to 15 minutes. Drink 1 to 2 cups a day, cold.

Consult a qualified practitioner for the dosage appropriate for you and the specific condition being treated.

Precautions

WARNING

If consumed over a long period of time, the leaves can be poisonous. Do not exceed the recommended dose.

POSSIBLE INTERACTIONS

Combining bilberry with other herbs may necessitate a lower dosage.

TARGET AILMENTS

Take internally for:

Eyestrain; cataracts; night blindness

Constipation; diarrhea; vomiting

Apply externally for:

Varicose veins; spider veins

Hemorrhoids

Skin problems; burns

SIDE EFFECTS

NOT SERIOUS

- Eating fresh bilberries can cause diarrhea.
- Eating fresh or dried bilberries may irritate the intestines.

BIOFLAVONOIDS

B

VITAL STATISTICS

OTHER NAME
vitamin P

DAILY DOSAGE
For staph infection: 300 mg to 2,000 mg
For otitis media: child's age times 50 mg, with 250 mg as maximum
For sinusitis: 1 gram

GENERAL DESCRIPTION
Bioflavonoids are compounds abundant in the white pith of citrus fruits and other foods containing vitamin C. Their most important function is to help maximize the benefits of vitamin C by inhibiting its breakdown in the body. (A normal, healthful diet usually provides all the bioflavonoids a person needs.)

Supplements are sometimes recommended for patients with weak capillaries, a problem that manifests itself in abnormal bleeding such as that associated with diabetes, bleeding gums, nosebleeds, and menorrhagia. Bioflavonoids are thought to boost the immune system and help limit histamine reactions, and they are sometimes used to treat allergies. The chemical rutin in bioflavonoids may help improve nearsightedness, sharpen night vision, and prevent cataracts.

NATURAL SOURCES
Good sources are citrus fruits (white pith), peppers, buckwheat, blueberries, black currants, grapes, and cherries.

PREPARATIONS
Available in vitamin and mineral supplements. Also sold separately.

PRECAUTIONS

WARNING
Do not take bioflavonoid supplements if you have a blood-clotting disorder or other blood problem.

SPECIAL INFORMATION
- Consult your doctor for dosages.
- Do not take bioflavonoid supplements with other medications or herbal therapies except under the advice of your doctor.
- If you are pregnant or breast-feeding, consult a doctor before taking bioflavonoids.

TARGET AILMENTS
Abnormal bruising
Inflammation
Allergy
Eye disorders
Asthma

SIDE EFFECTS

NOT SERIOUS
- Diarrhea (if excessive amounts are ingested)

DECREASE INTAKE AND CONSULT YOUR DOCTOR.

BIOTA

LATIN NAME
Biota orientalis

VITAL STATISTICS

GENERAL DESCRIPTION

Biota is derived from the leafy twig of the arborvitae shrub. Among its various uses, the herb is prescribed to control bleeding and to heal burns. Laboratory experiments with animals suggest that preparations of biota may be effective as expectorants. Low concentrations of the herb in alcohol extractions also appeared to inhibit the growth of tuberculosis and streptococcus bacteria. In human tests, oral preparations containing the herb slightly reduced the time it took to stop bleeding from gastric and duodenal ulcers, compared with standard therapy.

Chinese medicine takes a holistic approach to healthcare, fashioning remedies to treat the entire being as well as the specific parts or areas. Single herbs may be used alone or in combination with other herbs to prevent and combat disease, which is thought to arise from disturbances in the flow of a bodily energy called chi (pronounced "chee") and blood, or from a lack of balance in the complementary states of yin and yang. According to the principles of traditional Chinese medicine, this herb is astringent, bitter, and slightly cold.

PREPARATIONS

Biota leaves are available in bulk and can be purchased in dried form in Chinese pharmacies, Asian markets, and some Western health food stores. A powdered form is available for treatment of burns.

COMBINATIONS: Two mixtures that contain biota may be prescribed to prevent bleeding. In one, the fresh herb is combined with the leaves of fresh lotus and fresh mugwort; in the other, biota is mixed with mugwort leaf and dried ginger. A blend of biota and cattail pollen is recommended for excessive uterine bleeding. A mixture of biota and Chinese dates is used to treat chronic dry coughs.

TARGET AILMENTS

Take internally for:

Bleeding disorders such as vomiting or coughing up blood

Coughing that fails to bring up phlegm

Bleeding gums

Blood in the stool or urine

Uterine bleeding

Apply powdered form externally for:

Burns

SIDE EFFECTS

SERIOUS

- Dizziness
- Nausea or vomiting

CALL YOUR DOCTOR. THESE EFFECTS MAY BE CAUSED BY LARGE DOSES OR BY PROLONGED USE OF THE HERB.

BIOTIN

B

VITAL STATISTICS

OTHER NAMES
vitamin B_7, vitamin H

GENERAL DESCRIPTION
Along with other B vitamins, biotin helps convert food to energy and is required for the synthesis of carbohydrates, proteins, and fatty acids. Biotin is especially important for healthy hair, skin, and nails.

Biotin deficiency is rare, and supplements are unnecessary.

EMDR
30 mcg to 100 mcg

NATURAL SOURCES
Among the types of food that are good dietary sources of biotin are cheese, kidneys, salmon, soybeans, sunflower seeds, nuts, broccoli, and sweet potatoes.

PRECAUTIONS

SPECIAL INFORMATION
- Because breast milk contains little biotin, infants who are breast-fed can suffer biotin deficiency, although this is uncommon.
- Signs of biotin deficiency include dry, grayish skin; hair loss; nausea; vomiting; muscle pain; loss of appetite; a pale, smooth tongue; and fatigue.
- People can become biotin deficient through long-term use of antibiotics or by regularly eating raw egg whites, which contain avidin, a protein that blocks the body's absorption of biotin. Research has not revealed a toxic level for biotin.

TARGET AILMENTS
Immune problems

Skin problems

SIDE EFFECTS
NONE EXPECTED

Bismuth Subsalicylate

Vital Statistics

DRUG CLASS
Antidiarrheal Drugs

BRAND NAME
Pepto-Bismol

OTHER DRUGS IN THIS CLASS
attapulgite, loperamide

GENERAL DESCRIPTION
Bismuth subsalicylate is used to treat diarrhea. Because it appears to inhibit intestinal secretions, it is also effective in preventing symptoms of traveler's (infectious) diarrhea and can be taken regularly during the first two weeks of travel. This drug is also used to treat symptoms of gastric distress or upset stomach, including heartburn, acid indigestion, and nausea; it is also used in combination with antibiotics to treat duodenal ulcers. For more information, see Antidiarrheal Drugs.

Precautions

SPECIAL INFORMATION
- Advise your healthcare professional if you have had allergic reactions to other salicylates, including aspirin.
- Do not give this drug to children without the approval of a doctor.
- If taken in higher doses and for longer periods to prevent traveler's diarrhea, bismuth subsalicylate may intensify some of the symptoms of dysentery, gout, kidney disease, stomach ulcers, and hemophilia and other bleeding problems. If you have any of these conditions, consult your doctor first before taking the drug.
- Bismuth subsalicylate may have an effect on some laboratory tests. Be sure to tell the healthcare practitioner performing the test that you are taking the medication.

POSSIBLE INTERACTIONS
Antidiabetic drugs (oral): may reduce blood sugar levels.
Tetracycline: reduced tetracycline absorption.

TARGET AILMENTS

Diarrhea, especially traveler's (infectious) diarrhea

Upset stomach

Heartburn; acid indigestion; nausea

SIDE EFFECTS

WHEN USED AT THE RECOMMENDED DOSAGE FOR NO MORE THAN TWO DAYS, THIS DRUG RARELY CAUSES SIDE EFFECTS. BUT IF THE DIARRHEA DOES NOT SUBSIDE WITHIN ONE OR TWO DAYS, CHECK WITH YOUR DOCTOR.

NOT SERIOUS
- Mild constipation
- Grayish black stools and darkened tongue

THESE EFFECTS ARE HARMLESS, BUT CHECK WITH YOUR DOCTOR IF THE CONSTIPATION CONTINUES OR YOU DEVELOP A FEVER.

BISOPROLOL

VITAL STATISTICS

DRUG CLASS
Beta-Adrenergic Blockers

BRAND NAMES
Ziac, Zebeta

OTHER DRUGS IN THIS CLASS
atenolol, metoprolol, nadolol, propranolol, timolol

GENERAL DESCRIPTION
Bisoprolol is a beta-adrenergic-blocking agent, a class of drugs that interfere with particular actions of the nervous system. The effects of beta blockers, as these drugs are often called, include slowing of the heart rate and of nerve impulses to the heart and other organs; this results in lowered blood pressure. Bisoprolol is a newer drug that is called cardioselective because it specifically targets nerves that stimulate the heart.

Bisoprolol, whether used alone or in combination with other drugs, is primarily used to treat high blood pressure. The brand-name medication Ziac, for example, contains two active ingredients, bisoprolol and the diuretic drug hydrochlorothiazide. A reduction in blood pressure may occur within the first week of treatment, but the maximum effect may not be apparent for two or three weeks. Some people may require an increased dose to achieve the maximum effect.

Bisoprolol is also used to treat abnormal heart rhythms and angina pectoris, which is chest pain due to inadequate blood and oxygen supply to the heart. For more information about this class of drugs, see Beta-Adrenergic Blockers. For visual characteristics, see the Color Guide to Prescription Drugs and Herbs.

PRECAUTIONS

WARNING
Do not take bisoprolol if you have cardiogenic shock, heart failure, second- or third-degree atrioventricular (A-V) block, or a type of slowed heart rhythm called sinus bradycardia.

An overdose of this drug may cause slowed heartbeat, reduced blood pressure, congestive heart failure, reduced blood sugar level, and bronchospasm. Stop taking the drug and seek medical treatment immediately.

Call your doctor if you experience any difficulty breathing or show any signs or symptoms of heart failure or slowed heart rate.

SPECIAL INFORMATION
- Use this drug with caution if you have liver or kidney disease. Your body may not be able to eliminate it properly, and it may be necessary to decrease the dose.
- Bisoprolol should be used with caution in patients who have peripheral vascular disease, bronchospastic disease, controlled congestive heart failure, diabetes mellitus, and hyperthyroidism.
- If you have surgery planned, this drug should be stopped gradually by two days before the scheduled date.
- Unless your doctor considers it essential, avoid using this drug if you are pregnant or may become pregnant while taking it.
- Do not discontinue this drug abruptly. To do so may cause severe symptoms such as chest pain and difficulty breathing. Consult your doctor.
- Because bisoprolol may lower the blood sugar level, it may interfere with glucose or insulin tolerance tests. If you have diabetes, it is important to know that this drug may also mask some signs of lowered blood sugar, especially rapid heartbeat.

Bisoprolol

- Check with your doctor or pharmacist before using any over-the-counter medications while taking bisoprolol.
- Bisoprolol may pass into breast milk. Use caution if you are nursing a baby while taking this drug, and observe your infant for possible side effects.
- If you are receiving therapy with the drugs clonidine and bisoprolol and are planning to stop taking the clonidine, do so only after you have discontinued the bisoprolol for several days.
- If you have a history of severe allergic reaction to a variety of allergens, be especially cautious in taking any beta blocker.
- Do not take this drug within two weeks of taking a monoamine oxidase (MAO) inhibitor type of antidepressant.
- If you stop smoking while taking bisoprolol, check with your doctor about a possible dose reduction because of changes in your body's ability to break down this drug.

POSSIBLE INTERACTIONS

Calcium channel blockers, flecainide, hydralazine, oral contraceptives, propafenone, haloperidol, phenothiazine tranquilizers, quinolones, quinidine: may increase the effect of bisoprolol.

Clonidine, nifedipine, guanabenz, reserpine, and other blood-pressure-lowering agents: may lower blood pressure excessively.

Ergots (used for migraine): may worsen cold hands and feet, possibly causing gangrene.

Other beta blockers: may produce excessive effects. Do not combine these drugs.

Phenytoin, digitalis: may slow the heart excessively.

Theophylline, antiasthma drugs: reduced effect of these drugs.

Thyroid hormones: bisoprolol counteracts the effects of thyroid hormones.

TARGET AILMENTS

High blood pressure

Angina pectoris

Abnormal heart rhythms

SIDE EFFECTS

NOT SERIOUS

- Dizziness; diarrhea, nausea, or vomiting; sexual impotence; stuffed nose; itching; trouble sleeping; fatigue or weakness

CALL YOUR DOCTOR IF THESE PROBLEMS PERSIST.

SERIOUS

- Difficulty breathing; depression; confusion; changes in heart rhythm; chest pain; skin rash; cold hands or feet; swelling of legs or feet; bronchospasm

CONTACT YOUR DOCTOR IMMEDIATELY.

Bi Yan Pian

B

Vital Statistics

ENGLISH NAME
Nose Inflammation Pills

GENERAL DESCRIPTION
As suggested by the name, Nose Inflammation Pills help the body rid itself of inflammation or infection affecting the nose and sinuses. This formula is used to treat all sorts of runny, stuffy nose problems, particularly when the mucus is thick and yellow or greenish. It is prescribed for acute problems, such as colds and the flu, as well as for allergies and other chronic conditions, sometimes in combination with other formulas.

Chinese medicine takes a holistic approach to healthcare, fashioning remedies to treat the entire being as well as the specific parts or areas. Precise combinations of herbs are used to prevent and combat disease, which is thought to arise from disturbances in the flow of a bodily energy called chi (pronounced "chee") and blood, or from a lack of balance in the complementary states of yin and yang. A patent formula, *Bi Yan Pian* is made by using a standardized combination of herbs and method of preparation.

INGREDIENTS
xanthium, magnolia flower, licorice, phellodendron, platycodon root, schisandra, forsythia, angelica, chrysanthemum, ledebouriella, schizonepeta

PREPARATIONS
This formula is available in pill form at many Chinese pharmacies and Oriental grocery stores.

TARGET AILMENTS

- Chronic or acute rhinitis
- Nasal sinusitis
- Hay fever and other allergies
- Pain in the forehead or cheekbones with congestion

SIDE EFFECTS
None expected

BLACK COHOSH

LATIN NAME
Cimicifuga racemosa

VITAL STATISTICS

GENERAL DESCRIPTION

Black cohosh, whose rhizome and root contain substances that act like the female hormone estrogen, is prescribed for several menstrual and menopausal conditions. The herb also acts as a sedative and is believed to promote urination and aid in expelling mucus from the lungs. For visual characteristics, see the Color Guide to Prescription Drugs and Herbs.

PREPARATIONS

Over the counter:
Available as tincture, syrup, capsules, fluidextract, and also as dried root and rhizome.

At home:

DECOCTION: Boil covered ½ tsp powdered rootstock per cup of water for 30 minutes and let cool. Take as much as a cup per day, 2 tbsp at a time. Add lemon and honey to taste.

COMBINATIONS: Mix the dried herb with skullcap, wood betony, passionflower, and valerian to make a mild tranquilizer.

PRECAUTIONS

WARNING

Black cohosh can cause serious side effects; use this herb only under medical supervision.

Individuals suffering from congestive heart failure or any other type of heart disease should not use black cohosh.

SPECIAL INFORMATION

- Do not use this herb if you are pregnant.
- Children should not use black cohosh unless it is specifically prescribed by a healthcare practitioner familiar with herbs.
- The herb's estrogen-like compound can contribute to abnormal blood clotting and liver problems, and encourage breast tumors. If symptoms of any of these conditions develop, or if any side effects listed below as Serious develop, stop using black cohosh and call your doctor immediately.

TARGET AILMENTS

Take internally for:

Menstrual discomfort; amenorrhea

Menopausal disorders

Headache; spasmodic coughs

Rheumatic pains

Apply externally for:

Sciatica; neuralgia

Muscle spasms; rheumatism

SIDE EFFECTS

NOT SERIOUS

- Irritation of the uterus

SERIOUS

- Diarrhea; abdominal pain
- Nausea
- Joint pains
- Headaches
- Lowered heart rate
- Lowered blood pressure

STOP USING AND CALL YOUR DOCTOR IMMEDIATELY.

Black Walnut

LATIN NAME
Juglans nigra

B

Vital Statistics

GENERAL DESCRIPTION

Native Americans used the bark of the black walnut, a tree that grows in the eastern United States, to treat skin problems such as ringworm. They drank a tea made from the bark as a laxative, and they chewed on the bark to relieve headache pain. Today, the bark, leaves, fruit rind, and liquid extracts of black walnut are prescribed by herbalists for constipation, fungal and parasitic infections, and mouth sores. Black walnut is rich in tannins and contains a large amount of iodine, which makes it a good antiseptic. Also, the herb is believed to relieve toxic blood conditions.

PREPARATIONS

Over the counter:
Available as tinctures, extract, dried bark, leaves, and fruit rind.

At home:

Decoction: Simmer the bark in boiling water for 10 to 15 minutes. Take 1 tbsp three or four times a day.

Gargle: Use the decoction as a mouthwash or gargle to treat mouth sores.

Extract: Rub on the affected area twice a day.

Poultice: Make a poultice from the green rind of black walnut; apply to sites of ringworm.

SIDE EFFECTS

NOT SERIOUS

- Mild laxative effect

CALL YOUR DOCTOR IF THIS PROBLEM PERSISTS.

Precautions

SPECIAL INFORMATION

Use of this herb by children for more than seven to 10 days should be done in conjunction with a healthcare practitioner.

POSSIBLE INTERACTIONS

Combining with other herbs may necessitate a lower dosage.

TARGET AILMENTS

Take internally for:

Constipation

Intestinal worms and parasites

Warts

Mouth sores

Apply externally for:

Ringworm

Scabies

Eczema

Herpes; cold sores

Psoriasis

Sores

Pimples

Athlete's foot; jock itch

Blessed Thistle

LATIN NAME
Cnicus benedictus

Vital Statistics

GENERAL DESCRIPTION

During the Middle Ages, blessed thistle was used to treat bubonic plague. Modern herbalists consider the aboveground parts of this annual plant a remedy for a range of problems. A component of blessed thistle is the chemical cnicin, an anti-inflammatory agent that also stops bleeding. In addition, extracts from the plant contain more than a dozen antibacterial compounds. Blessed thistle is also used to induce vomiting in individuals who have taken poisons, and to regulate menstrual cycles. This bitter-tasting herb is used in the liqueur Benedictine.

PREPARATIONS

Over the counter:

Available as a tincture, extract, and dried herb.

At home:

Tea: Steep covered 1 tsp dried herb in ½ cup boiling water. Drink 1 cup to 1½ cups a day, unsweetened, for problems with digestion.

Poultice: Mash leaves and other parts, and apply to chilblains, wounds, and sores.

Combinations: Use with cramp bark, blue cohosh root, and ginger to treat menstrual difficulties.

Consult a qualified practitioner for the dosage appropriate for your specific condition.

SIDE EFFECTS

- Overdoses of this herb can cause vomiting.

Discontinue use.

Precautions

WARNING

Use recommended amounts and only under a doctor's supervision. Blessed thistle is a strong emetic and induces vomiting very effectively.

SPECIAL INFORMATION

- During pregnancy, avoid blessed thistle and any compounds that include the herb.
- Because this herb stimulates gastric activity, avoid using it if you have an ulcer.
- Use of this herb by children for more than seven to 10 days should be done in conjunction with a healthcare practitioner.

POSSIBLE INTERACTIONS

Combining blessed thistle with other herbs may necessitate a lower dosage.

TARGET AILMENTS

Take internally for:

- Poor digestion; diarrhea; flatulence
- Fever; headache
- Anorexia
- Colic
- Liver and gallbladder disorders

Apply externally for:

- Cuts and wounds
- Fever
- Shingles

BLOODROOT

LATIN NAME
Sanguinaria canadensis

B

VITAL STATISTICS

GENERAL DESCRIPTION

Named for the crimson extract made from its root, bloodroot is potentially toxic and can cause severe side effects if ingested in excess. For this reason, herbalists prescribe the root primarily as an external remedy to relieve eczema, venereal blisters, rashes, and other skin disorders. Only rarely is it taken internally, and that is when herbalists recommend it for respiratory disorders. Bloodroot is a major ingredient in many mouthwashes and toothpastes because of its ability to kill the bacteria that can lead to gingivitis. Its key components are the antibacterial isoquinoline alkaloids.

Bloodroot has a long folk history in the treatment of cancer and is currently the subject of research. It contains sanguinarine, a constituent thought to impede tumor formation.

PREPARATIONS

Available as tincture and dried root; it is also an ingredient in several dental products.

SIDE EFFECTS

NOT SERIOUS

- Contact dermatitis

SERIOUS

- Burning in the stomach
- Nausea; intense thirst
- Slowed, irregular heart rate
- Impaired vision; dizziness

LARGE DOSES MAY PRODUCE THESE SYMPTOMS. STOP USING AT ONCE AND CONSULT YOUR PRACTITIONER.

PRECAUTIONS

☠ WARNING

Bloodroot is potentially toxic. Take it internally only under the supervision of a herbalist or licensed healthcare professional.

This herb should not be used with children unless it is specifically prescribed by a healthcare practitioner who is knowledgeable about herbs.

SPECIAL INFORMATION

Avoid using internally during pregnancy.

POSSIBLE INTERACTIONS

Combining bloodroot with other herbs may necessitate a lower dosage.

TARGET AILMENTS
Use as toothpaste and mouthwash for:
Gingivitis
Take internally for:
Lung congestion; bronchitis
Asthma
Fever; head colds
Apply externally for:
Fungus
Ringworm; athlete's foot
Venereal blisters
Rashes; eczema; warts

BLUE-GREEN ALGAE

B

VITAL STATISTICS

OTHER NAME
spirulina

GENERAL DESCRIPTION
Blue-green algae is widely promoted as a tonic supplement that can be taken regularly for general health. It contains iron and vitamin B_{12} as well as amino acids; its nutritive value is sometimes compared to that of the soybean. Blue-green algae is said to have a blood-cleansing, rejuvenating effect, and it is touted as a low-fat, high-protein supplement that can increase energy levels, enhance mental alertness, and help curb the appetite. The broad claims associated with blue-green algae include its ability to boost the immune system, treat AIDS, and control Alzheimer's disease and diabetes mellitus.

Although anecdotal accounts suggest that some people benefit from these supplements, no scientific studies support claims of its curative powers. Some nutritionists describe blue-green algae as mere "pond scum" that has no medicinal value, contains only minuscule amounts of protein, and tastes horrible. The most widely known commercial product is spirulina, a type of blue-green algae packaged in Mexico, Japan, Thailand, and California.

NATURAL SOURCES
alkaline ponds and lakes

PREPARATIONS
Available as a tablet or a capsule.

PRECAUTIONS

WARNING
Do not take blue-green algae if you are pregnant, planning a pregnancy, or breast-feeding. Do not give to children under the age of two.

SPECIAL INFORMATION
- Thoroughly research the product you intend to buy. Some preparations contain toxins, and others may be labeled as containing spirulina when in fact they do not.
- No standard recommended dosage has been determined for blue-green algae. Consult your doctor for dosages.

POSSIBLE INTERACTIONS
None expected for spirulina, considered the safest type of blue-green algae.

TARGET AILMENTS
Obesity
Fatigue

SIDE EFFECTS

SERIOUS
- Nausea
- Vomiting
- Diarrhea

DISCONTINUE USE AND CONSULT YOUR DOCTOR.

BONESET

LATIN NAME
Eupatorium perfoliatum

B

VITAL STATISTICS

GENERAL DESCRIPTION

Boneset has nothing to do with setting bones; it is used to treat fever. Introduced to the herb by Native Americans, the colonists used it for this purpose. Today herbalists still recommend boneset for the aches and pains that accompany fever, especially during bouts of flu. Boneset also helps clear mucus from the respiratory tract, and is often used for arthritis and rheumatism. For visual characteristics, see the Color Guide to Prescription Drugs and Herbs.

PREPARATIONS

Over the counter:

Available in health food stores as dried leaves and flowers, and as tincture.

At home:

INFUSION: Pour 1 cup boiling water onto 2 to 3 tsp dried herb and let steep covered for 10 to 15 minutes. Drink as hot as possible. For fever or flu, drink a cup every hour up to 4 cups in 6 hours, and only 6 cups in a 24-hour period. Add honey and lemon to mask the bitterness, if desired.

Consult a qualified practitioner for the dosage appropriate for you and the specific condition being treated.

TARGET AILMENTS
Fever
Colds; flu; coughs
Upper respiratory tract congestion
Arthritis; rheumatism

PRECAUTIONS

WARNING

Do not use fresh boneset. It contains a toxic chemical, called tremerol, that can cause vomiting, rapid breathing, and at high doses, possibly coma and death. Drying boneset reduces the tremerol.

Use of this herb by children for more than seven to 10 days should be done in conjunction with a healthcare practitioner.

SPECIAL INFORMATION

- If you have a history of alcoholism, liver disease, or liver cancer, consult your herbalist before taking boneset; it contains pyrrolizidine alkaloids, which are toxic to the liver.
- Because of its toxic effects, you should not take boneset for more than two weeks at a time.

POSSIBLE INTERACTIONS

Combining boneset with other herbs may necessitate a lower dosage.

SIDE EFFECTS

SERIOUS

- Respiratory changes
- Coma
- Nausea
- Vomiting
- Diarrhea

LARGE DOSES MAY CAUSE THESE EFFECTS. DO NOT EXCEED THE RECOMMENDED DOSAGE; CALL YOUR DOCTOR IMMEDIATELY IF YOU EXPERIENCE ANY ADVERSE REACTIONS.

BREWER'S YEAST

VITAL STATISTICS

OTHER NAME
nutritional yeast

GENERAL DESCRIPTION
Brewer's yeast, a nonleavening yeast grown from hops, is valued as a source of protein, phosphorus, chromium, and B vitamins (it does not contain B_{12}, however). In small doses, the supplement is considered safe for growing children and older adults. Sold as a powder or in tablets or flakes, it is easily incorporated into cooked dishes, and it can be added to beverages or taken between meals for a quick energy boost.

The supplement contains trace amounts of the mineral chromium, which helps regulate blood sugar in diabetics. One to two teaspoons of brewer's yeast a day may help aid in weight loss by reducing cravings for sweets. The supplement is often recommended for skin problems such as eczema, and as a bulking agent it can be an effective remedy for constipation. Brewer's yeast is said to have an immune-building effect, and, although its effectiveness has not been determined, some practitioners recommend it to help treat diabetes, high cholesterol, and cancer.

NATURAL SOURCES
hops

PREPARATIONS
Available as a powder, tablets, or flakes.

PRECAUTIONS

WARNING
Do not use brewer's yeast if you have candidiasis.

SPECIAL INFORMATION
No standard recommended dosage has been determined for brewer's yeast. Consult your doctor for dosages.

POSSIBLE INTERACTIONS
Do not combine brewer's yeast with other medications or herbal therapies except under the advice of your doctor.

TARGET AILMENTS
Eczema
Nervousness
Fatigue
Heart problems
Diabetes
Constipation

SIDE EFFECTS

NOT SERIOUS
- Headache
- Upset stomach; nausea
- Diarrhea

DISCONTINUE USE AND CALL YOUR DOCTOR.

BROMELAIN

B

VITAL STATISTICS

DAILY DOSAGE
250 mg to 500 mg

GENERAL DESCRIPTION
Bromelain is a natural protein-digesting (or proteolytic) enzyme found in the pineapple fruit. Studies suggest that bromelain enhances blood circulation while reducing inflammation. Specifically, it is thought to reduce platelet stickiness and to dissolve fibrin, a protein active in the formation of blood clots. Its anti-inflammatory action can help reduce bruising and inflammation caused by cuts, scratches, and small wounds. Bromelain may also be helpful in treating rheumatoid arthritis.

In controlled studies, bromelain has been shown to reduce the headache, nasal discharge, inflammation, and breathing difficulties associated with sinusitis. It can also act as a muscle relaxant to help relieve menstrual cramps. On a regular basis, bromelain is beneficial for improving digestion. A small dish of pineapple after a meal provides a light dessert as well as a healthy stimulus for the digestive tract. Because of its blood-thinning effect, bromelain may also be useful in helping to prevent heart attack and stroke.

NATURAL SOURCES
pineapple

PREPARATIONS
Available in capsules and tablets.

PRECAUTIONS

SPECIAL INFORMATION
- Do not take if you have a clotting disorder, if you are pregnant, or if you are taking blood-thinning drugs (including aspirin).
- Bromelain should be taken with meals or between meals, depending on the ailment. To improve digestion, take with meals. To help with inflammatory conditions, take between meals.

TARGET AILMENTS
Back pain
Arthritis
Inflammation
Sinusitis
Menstrual cramps
Poor digestion

SIDE EFFECTS
NONE EXPECTED

Rx BRONCHODILATORS

VITAL STATISTICS

GENERIC NAMES
Rx: albuterol, epinephrine, ipratropium, salmeterol, terbutaline, theophylline
OTC: ephedrine, epinephrine, theophylline

GENERAL DESCRIPTION
Bronchodilators relax the muscles surrounding the bronchial tubes in the lungs by stimulating or inhibiting certain body chemicals. This relieves spasm and improves lung capacity, thereby alleviating the symptoms of bronchial asthma and bronchitis.

Theophylline (found naturally in commercial tea and related to the caffeine found in coffee) acts mainly on the muscles of the respiratory tract. Other bronchodilators act on the sinuses and upper respiratory tract as well. All of these drugs may act on the heart, arteries, and veins, especially if taken in large doses. For this reason, bronchodilators can affect blood pressure and heart function.

PRECAUTIONS

WARNING
Your body can build up tolerance to bronchodilators used as inhalants, causing them to become less effective. If this happens, discontinue the drug and tell your doctor. Do not increase the dose, since this can lead to serious, perhaps fatal bronchial constriction.

SPECIAL INFORMATION
- These drugs (especially ephedrine and epinephrine) can cause adverse effects in individuals with high blood pressure, diabetes, heart disease, seizures, peptic ulcers, or thyroid or prostate problems. If you have any of these conditions do not use bronchodilators—even in their over-the-counter forms—without your doctor's permission.
- Women who are pregnant or breast-feeding should consult a doctor before using these drugs.

TARGET AILMENTS
Anaphylactic shock from severe allergic reactions
Acute bronchial asthma
Chronic, recurrent bronchial asthma
Bronchitis
Emphysema
Hay fever and cold symptoms (ephedrine)
Other chronic obstructive pulmonary diseases
Heart-rhythm problems and cardiac arrest (epinephrine)
Exercise-induced bronchospasm

CONTINUED

BRONCHODILATORS

POSSIBLE INTERACTIONS

Alcohol: increased effect of theophylline, possibly causing theophylline toxicity.

Alpha and beta blockers: these drugs decrease the action of bronchodilators, especially ephedrine and epinephrine.

Blood pressure medicines, including diuretics: bronchodilators may decrease the actions of these medicines.

Caffeine and other central nervous system stimulants: increased nervousness and insomnia.

Diabetes medications, including insulin: decreased effectiveness of diabetes medications.

Heart medications (such as digoxin): heart-rhythm problems.

Levodopa: increased heart-rhythm problems. Your doctor may need to adjust your dosage.

Lithium: theophylline may decrease the effectiveness of lithium.

MAO inhibitors: possible effects on the heart or blood vessels.

Nitrates: decreased effectiveness of nitrates in relieving angina.

Other antiasthmatic drugs: do not combine these drugs unless your doctor directs you to do so or unless your prescription contains a combination. Using two bronchodilators may increase the side effects, especially on the heart.

Phenytoin: serious cardiovascular effects, such as heart-rhythm problems or very low blood pressure.

Thyroid medications: increased bronchodilator effect.

Tricyclic antidepressants and maprotiline: increased effects of bronchodilators on the cardiovascular system.

SIDE EFFECTS

NOT SERIOUS

- Mild nausea
- Mild weakness
- Insomnia
- Mild nervousness
- Restlessness

CALL YOUR DOCTOR IF THESE EFFECTS BECOME BOTHERSOME.

SERIOUS

- Change in blood pressure, change in heartbeat (irregular or pounding, for example)
- Trembling
- Breathing problems
- Weakness
- Anxiety; nervousness
- Dizziness; lightheadedness
- Muscle cramps
- Nausea or vomiting
- Chest pain or discomfort (rare)

LET YOUR DOCTOR KNOW RIGHT AWAY IF YOU EXPERIENCE THESE SIDE EFFECTS.

BRYONIA

LATIN NAME
Bryonia alba

VITAL STATISTICS

GENERAL DESCRIPTION

Bryonia, or wild hops, is a creeping vine commonly found along hedgerows and in forests across southern Europe. Its medicinal value was known to the Greeks, who used the root as a purgative and may have given the plant its name, derived from *bryo,* meaning "to thrust or sprout," a reference to the speed with which the vine grows. Accidental ingestion of the root can cause tissue inflammation, severe vomiting, and diarrhea violent enough to cause death. Homeopathic physicians prescribe their dilute solutions of *Bryonia* for illnesses that are accompanied by similar symptoms. The homeopathic remedy is prepared from the root, which is harvested in early spring. An extract pressed from the root pulp is mixed with alcohol into an extremely dilute solution. For more information on homeopathic medicine, see page 14.

PREPARATIONS

Bryonia is available in various potencies, in both liquid and tablet form. Consult your practitioner for more precise information.

PRECAUTIONS

SPECIAL INFORMATION

- When a remedy is administered, no one but the patient should touch the pills. If tablets are spilled, throw them away.
- The mouth should be clear of flavors 15 minutes before and after taking a remedy, and strong flavors and aromas, such as coffee, camphor, and heavily scented perfumes, should be avoided for the duration of treatment.

TARGET AILMENTS

- Arthritis with sharp pains
- Backaches centered in the small of the back; bursitis
- Colds with chest congestion
- Painful coughs
- Sore throat, with pain upon swallowing
- Influenza
- Severe headaches made worse by light, sound, or any motion
- Dizziness
- Nausea
- Vomiting
- Constipation
- Gastritis
- Acute diverticulitis
- Stomach flu
- Inflammation during breast-feeding

SIDE EFFECTS

NONE EXPECTED

BUCHU

LATIN NAME
Agathosma spp.

VITAL STATISTICS

GENERAL DESCRIPTION

The leaves of this southern African shrub contain an oil that increases the production of urine. African people used it for urinary problems long before they had contact with Europeans. In the 17th century, Dutch settlers in South Africa used it to treat urinary tract infections and kidney stones. In 1847, buchu was introduced in the United States and hailed as a cure-all. Today Western herbalists continue the tradition, prescribing buchu for urinary tract infections and for use as a diuretic, and also for treating premenstrual syndrome. Buchu has a mintlike smell and taste.

PREPARATIONS

Over the counter:

Available dried and as a tincture at health food stores. The herb is also found in Fluidex and Odrinil, two commercial diuretics used to treat premenstrual syndrome.

At home:

INFUSION: Add 1 to 2 tsp dried, crumbled leaves to 1 cup boiling water and let steep covered for 10 minutes. Drink up to 3 cups a day.

COMBINATIONS: Mix buchu with uva ursi, yarrow, or couch grass to treat cystitis (bladder inflammation). Combine buchu with corn silk or marsh mallow for dysuria (painful or difficult urination).

Consult a qualified practitioner for the dosage appropriate for you and the specific condition being treated.

PRECAUTIONS

WARNING

Diuretics such as buchu may deplete the body's potassium levels, so be sure to eat more potassium-rich foods, such as bananas and fresh vegetables, while taking buchu.

Use of this herb by children for more than seven to 10 days should be done in conjunction with a healthcare practitioner.

SPECIAL INFORMATION

- If you are pregnant, consult your doctor before taking buchu or any other diuretic.
- Avoid buchu if you have a history of kidney disease; its oil content may be too irritating.

POSSIBLE INTERACTIONS

Combining buchu with other herbs may necessitate a lower dosage.

TARGET AILMENTS

Bloating caused by premenstrual syndrome

Urinary tract disorders

SIDE EFFECTS

NOT SERIOUS
- Upset stomach
- Diarrhea

THESE SIDE EFFECTS ARE MORE LIKELY TO OCCUR WITH LARGE DOSES.

BUCKTHORN

LATIN NAME
Rhamnus purshiana

B

VITAL STATISTICS

GENERAL DESCRIPTION
The bark and the black pea-sized berries of the buckthorn tree act as a laxative so strong that Western herbalists advise using it only as a last resort, after other laxatives have failed. Its effectiveness stems from chemicals known as anthraquinones; these substances exert an extremely powerful purgative effect. You should use the herb only in consultation with your doctor.

PREPARATIONS
Over the counter:
Available as a tincture and in dried form. It is a component of the commercial laxative Movicol.

At home:
DECOCTION: Boil 1 tsp dried buckthorn in 3 cups water and steep covered 30 minutes. Drink cool, 1 tbsp at a time, before bed.
TINCTURE: Take ½ tsp before bed.
COMBINATIONS: Mix ½ tsp each of dried buckthorn bark, chamomile, and fennel seed, and steep covered in 1 cup boiling water for 10 minutes. Drink at bedtime.
Consult a qualified practitioner for the dosage appropriate for you and the specific condition being treated.

TARGET AILMENTS

Take internally, with care, for:

Constipation

PRECAUTIONS

WARNING
Do not take fresh buckthorn. Dry both the berries and the bark for a year or two before using. For faster drying, put the berries or bark in an oven at 250°F for several hours.

Do not use buckthorn for more than two weeks at a time. It can cause lazy bowel syndrome, in which the stool cannot be moved without chemical stimulation. If this occurs, consult a doctor.

Do not use buckthorn if you are pregnant or nursing, or if you have chronic gastrointestinal problems like hemorrhoids, ulcers, or colitis.

This herb should not be used with children unless it is specifically prescribed by a healthcare practitioner who is knowledgeable about herbs.

SPECIAL INFORMATION
Do not use buckthorn with any other laxatives.

POSSIBLE INTERACTIONS
Combining buckthorn with other herbs may necessitate a lower dosage.

SIDE EFFECTS

SERIOUS
- Vomiting
- Violent diarrhea
- Stomach cramps

FRESH BUCKTHORN CAN CAUSE THESE SYMPTOMS. CONSULT A DOCTOR IMMEDIATELY.

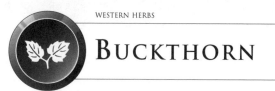

BUMETANIDE

B

VITAL STATISTICS

DRUG CLASS
Diuretics

BRAND NAME
Bumex

OTHER DRUGS IN THIS CLASS
amiloride, furosemide, hydrochlorothiazide, indapamide, potassium chloride (adjunct therapy), spironolactone, triamterene

GENERAL DESCRIPTION
Bumetanide, a fast-acting and powerful diuretic, is prescribed to eliminate excess body fluid and to treat high blood pressure (hypertension). Introduced in 1983, the drug acts by increasing urine production, thereby removing water from the body and helping to reduce swelling and blood volume. However, because this medication belongs to a group known as nonpotassium-sparing diuretics, minerals such as sodium, potassium, calcium, and magnesium are also eliminated; this can sometimes lead to muscle cramps and serious cardiovascular side effects.

Because of the potential effects on the heart of potassium loss due to nonpotassium-sparing diuretics, doctors sometimes also prescribe newer, potassium-sparing diuretics such as amiloride or triamterene, which are designed to lessen the excretion of potassium. In some cases, supplements of potassium chloride are prescribed to restore supplies of that mineral lost through the use of diuretics.

For more information, see entries for the class Diuretics and for the other generic forms listed above.

PRECAUTIONS

SPECIAL INFORMATION

- Taking diuretics in hot weather or while engaged in heavy exertion can cause a dangerous loss of fluids or minerals. Watch for signs of dehydration (fatigue, dizziness, headache, nausea).
- Your doctor will closely monitor your potassium levels to prevent heart-rhythm problems. If you are not also taking a potassium-sparing diuretic, you may be given a potassium supplement (such as potassium chloride). If you are currently taking a potassium-sparing diuretic in conjunction with bumetanide, you should talk with your doctor about the advisability of avoiding potassium supplements, salt substitutes (which are high in potassium), and potassium-rich foods such as bananas.
- Because diuretics have both known and suspected effects on glucose (blood sugar) levels, people with diabetes or who have been diagnosed with borderline diabetes should have their blood sugar levels monitored closely.

BUMETANIDE

B

POSSIBLE INTERACTIONS

Alcohol: increased action of diuretics.

Antigout medications (including probenecid): reduced diuretic effect of bumetanide.

Digitalis and other heart drugs: increased risk of potassium loss and additional heart-rhythm problems. Your doctor will closely monitor your progress.

Lithium: increased risk of lithium toxicity.

Nonsteroidal anti-inflammatory drugs (NSAIDs), especially indomethacin: reduced effectiveness of bumetanide.

Oral antidiabetic drugs, insulin: in rare cases, diuretics may interfere with these medicines or raise blood glucose levels.

Other blood pressure drugs, including angiotensin-converting enzyme (ACE) inhibitors: although diuretics are frequently taken with medications to lower blood pressure, caution should be exercised to ensure that blood pressure does not go too low.

TARGET AILMENTS

General edema (swelling caused by water retention)

Edema associated with various medical conditions, including congestive heart failure and cirrhosis of the liver

High blood pressure (hypertension)

SIDE EFFECTS

NOT SERIOUS

- Problems with sexual performance

CALL YOUR DOCTOR IF THIS CONTINUES OR BECOMES BOTHERSOME.

SERIOUS

- Headache
- Dizziness or lightheadedness when getting up (orthostatic hypotension)
- Nausea or vomiting
- Fatigue or weakness
- Irregular or weak pulse
- Increased thirst
- Dry mouth
- Muscle pain or cramps
- Mood changes
- Mental confusion
- Bleeding in urine or stools
- Unusual bruising
- Skin rash

TELL YOUR DOCTOR IMMEDIATELY IF YOU EXPERIENCE ANY OF THESE SYMPTOMS. YOU MAY BE ADVISED TO LOWER YOUR DOSAGE AND INCREASE YOUR INTAKE OF FLUIDS AND MINERALS.

Bupleurum

LATIN NAME
Bupleurum chinense

B

Vital Statistics

GENERAL DESCRIPTION

The long, coarse root known as bupleurum is often used in Chinese medicine to reduce certain types of fever and to treat irritability and feelings of frustration. Clinical experiments have indicated that the herb may be able to reduce fever resulting from infections of the upper respiratory tract. And in test-tube studies, preparations of bupleurum seem to have inhibited the growth of tuberculosis bacteria, as well as influenza and polio viruses. Sometimes called hare's ear root or thorowax root, it is characterized in traditional Chinese medicine as bitter, acrid, and cool.

Chinese medicine takes a holistic approach to healthcare, fashioning remedies to treat the entire being as well as the specific parts or areas. Single herbs may be used alone or in combination with other herbs to prevent and combat disease, which is thought to arise from disturbances in the flow of a bodily energy called chi (pronounced "chee") and blood, or from a lack of balance in the complementary states of yin and yang.

PREPARATIONS

The root is available in bulk in Chinese pharmacies, Asian markets, and some Western health food stores. Chinese pharmacies also offer mixtures containing the root.

Combinations: White peony root mixed with bupleurum is prescribed for vertigo, dizziness, chest pain, and painful menstrual periods. Irregular menstruation, premenstrual syndrome, and certain kinds of depression may be treated with a blend of bupleurum and field mint. Bupleurum is often combined with bitter orange fruit to alleviate pressure in the chest, abdominal pain, poor appetite, and irregular bowel movements. Chinese herbalists sometimes mix licorice with bupleurum to treat hepatitis. For information on specific dosages and additional herbal combinations, consult a Chinese medicine practitioner.

Precautions

WARNING

Too large a dose of the herb can cause nausea or vomiting.

TARGET AILMENTS

Take internally for:

- Low-grade fevers
- Malaria and malaria-like disorders
- Alternating chills and fever, typically accompanied by a bitter taste in the mouth, pain in the side, irritability, vomiting, or difficulty in breathing
- Prolapse of the uterus
- Dizziness and vertigo combined with pain in the chest, and tenderness in the side or breast, often accompanied by irritability
- Nausea; indigestion

SIDE EFFECTS

See warning.

Burdock

LATIN NAME
Arctium lappa

Vital Statistics

GENERAL DESCRIPTION

For several centuries, herbalists have prescribed burdock root to cure a wide range of illnesses. Today, some practitioners use burdock to treat urinary tract infections, arthritic conditions, external wounds, and skin ulcers. Laboratory trials on animals indicate that burdock has possible antitumor activity. This herb works best in conjunction with professional medical treatment. The root has brown bark and a white, spongy interior that hardens when dried. Burdock got its name from its tenacious burrs and from *dock,* the Old English word for plant.

For visual characteristics, see the Color Guide to Prescription Drugs and Herbs.

PREPARATIONS

Over the counter:

Available as dried powder, slices of root, and tinctures. You can find the fresh root in the vegetable sections of health food stores.

At home:

Decoction: Add 2 tbsp burdock root to 3 cups water and boil for 10 minutes. Drink up to 3 cups a day to treat genital and urinary tract irritations.

Compress: Soak a clean cloth in burdock tea and place it on the skin to speed healing of wounds and skin ulcers.

Combinations: Burdock can be mixed with yellow dock, red clover, or cleavers and taken orally for skin disorders.

Consult a qualified practitioner for the dosage appropriate for you and the specific condition being treated.

Precautions

SPECIAL INFORMATION

If you are pregnant, you should take burdock only under the supervision of a qualified healthcare practitioner.

Do not give burdock to children younger than two years of age. Older children and people over 65 should start with lower-strength doses, increasing them if needed.

POSSIBLE INTERACTIONS

Combining burdock with other herbs may necessitate a lower dosage.

TARGET AILMENTS

Take internally for:

Fungal and bacterial infections

Skin disorders, such as eczema and psoriasis, which cause dry, scaly skin

Urinary tract infections

Rheumatism; arthritis

Apply externally for:

Wounds and skin conditions

SIDE EFFECTS

- Stomach discomfort

May occur with large doses. Do not exceed recommended dosages.

Rx BUSPIRONE

B

VITAL STATISTICS

DRUG CLASS
Antianxiety Drugs

BRAND NAME
BuSpar

GENERAL DESCRIPTION
Buspirone is a nonbenzodiazepine antianxiety drug whose actions on the body appear to be complex and are not clearly understood. Compared with other antianxiety drugs, buspirone may be slow to take action; its effects generally begin after two weeks, and the total treatment time may be three to four weeks. Among its advantages, buspirone produces milder side effects, as well as less sedation. Since it does not appear to be addicting, buspirone can be used in patients who may be prone to addiction, such as alcoholics. See Antianxiety Drugs for more information.

For the visual characteristics of the brand-name drug BuSpar, see the Color Guide to Prescription Drugs and Herbs.

PRECAUTIONS

SPECIAL INFORMATION
- Avoid driving and working near heavy machinery until you learn how this drug affects you.
- Buspirone has milder sedative effects than other antianxiety drugs and no reported withdrawal symptoms. But do not use unless clearly needed. Prolonged use may increase the likelihood of serious side effects.
- Do not use this drug if your liver or kidneys are impaired.
- Do not use buspirone if you are pregnant or breast-feeding.

POSSIBLE INTERACTIONS
Alcohol, anticonvulsants, antihistamines, barbiturates, benzodiazepines, muscle relaxants, opioid analgesics, sedatives, tricyclic antidepressants: possible excessive sedation.
Digoxin: possible increased digoxin effect.
Haloperidol: possible increased haloperidol effect.
MAO inhibitors: significantly increased blood pressure. Do not combine these drugs with buspirone.

TARGET AILMENTS

Anxiety disorders or short-term treatment of anxiety symptoms

SIDE EFFECTS

NOT SERIOUS
- Nausea; sore throat; nasal congestion

CALL YOUR DOCTOR IF SYMPTOMS CONTINUE OR ARE BOTHERSOME.

SERIOUS
- Dizziness, lightheadedness, drowsiness, nervousness, excitement; blurred vision, persistent or severe headache, ringing in the ears, chest pain, shortness of breath, fainting, confusion; muscle weakness, uncontrolled movements of the body, numbness or tingling in the hands or feet

CONTACT YOUR DOCTOR IMMEDIATELY.

BUTCHER'S-BROOM

LATIN NAME
Ruscus aculeatus

VITAL STATISTICS

GENERAL DESCRIPTION

Butcher's-broom acquired its name because ancient Mediterranean butchers used the scrubby stems and leaves of the tough plant to sweep meat scraps off their cutting boards. Its medicinal use dates to classical Greece, when physicians applied its roots and rhizomes to swellings and prescribed it as a laxative and diuretic. Today herbalists believe its rhizomes have anti-inflammatory properties, and they use it to treat disorders of the veins. Butcher's-broom is an astringent that puckers up the insides of veins. Among its active ingredients are two steroidal components called ruscogenin and neuroscogenin, which appear to narrow blood vessels.

PREPARATIONS

Over the counter:

Available in dry bulk, capsules, ointment, and tincture.

At home:

TEA: Put 2 tsp powdered root in 1½ pt boiling water. Simmer slowly in a covered container for about 30 minutes. Drink cold, 2 to 3 tbsp, six times a day.

COMPRESS: Soak a clean cloth in tea and apply.

OINTMENT: Apply small amounts to hemorrhoids until inflammation is cleared.

Consult a qualified practitioner for the dosage appropriate for you and the specific condition being treated.

PRECAUTIONS

☠ ***WARNING***

Use of this herb by children for more than seven to 10 days should be done in conjunction with a healthcare practitioner.

SPECIAL INFORMATION

Consult your doctor for a diagnosis of circulatory problems before using any remedy.

POSSIBLE INTERACTIONS

Combining butcher's-broom with other herbs may necessitate a lower dosage.

TARGET AILMENTS

Use internally or externally for:

Circulation disorders of the legs, such as varicose veins

Hemorrhoids and other rectal inflammation and bleeding

SIDE EFFECTS

NONE EXPECTED

Bu Zhong Yi Qi Wan

B

Vital Statistics

ENGLISH NAME
Tonify the Middle and Augment the Qi Pills

GENERAL DESCRIPTION
This herbal formula, a combination of 10 different herbs and other natural ingredients, is described as supporting or lifting the vital bodily energy known as chi (pronounced "chee"), or qi. According to Chinese medicine, it helps treat problems that involve some kind of falling or falling down—from depression (fallen spirits) and fatigue (a feeling of not being able to get up) to drooping eyelids.

This formula is also prescribed for some kinds of diarrhea, and for a feeling of the inner organs pressing downward, as well as for people who feel cold easily and have shortness of breath. Studies in China have recorded success in the use of this remedy to treat prolapsed stomach and uterine prolapse.

INGREDIENTS
astragalus, codonopsis, licorice, white atractylodes, dong quai, citrus peel, cimicifuga, bupleurum, raw ginger, black dates

PREPARATIONS
This formula comes in pill form and is often available at Chinese pharmacies and Oriental grocery stores.

Precautions

SPECIAL INFORMATION
Each of the target ailments listed below can have various "causes" according to the principles of Chinese medicine. This remedy is particularly suited for treating these problems when the cause is a deficiency in the so-called raising-up-and-holding-in-place quality of the vital energy chi, or qi. Symptoms that would suggest use of this remedy also include a general sensitivity to cold and a pale tongue.

TARGET AILMENTS
Fatigue
Chronic fatigue
Chronic bronchitis or shortness of breath
Prolapses of uterus, rectum, or stomach
Urinary incontinence
Some kinds of chronic diarrhea
Some instances of excessive menstrual periods or spotting between periods

SIDE EFFECTS
NONE EXPECTED

CAFFEINE

C

VITAL STATISTICS

BRAND NAMES

Vivarin; Anacin, Excedrin Extra-Strength (combined with aspirin)

GENERAL DESCRIPTION

Caffeine, obtained from both natural and synthetic sources, has been used for centuries as a mild central nervous system stimulant. It works by stimulating all parts of the central nervous system, affecting the heart, lungs, other organs, and muscles. Caffeine also affects the blood vessels by temporarily increasing the heart's rate, contraction force, and output. While these effects usually produce no change in blood pressure for healthy individuals, you should avoid caffeine if you have high blood pressure.

Some over-the-counter analgesic drugs combine aspirin or acetaminophen with caffeine to enhance the painkilling effects of the analgesic.

Caffeine increases the production of stomach acids. Other effects include a slight diuretic action, a decrease in uterine contractions, and a temporary increase in blood sugar. Some people develop a tolerance to caffeine. When caffeine is used for a long period, abrupt discontinuation can produce withdrawal symptoms such as headache, irritability, dizziness, and unusual tiredness.

PRECAUTIONS

SPECIAL INFORMATION

- There has been some controversy regarding the use of caffeine by pregnant or nursing women. Although no proof of birth defects has been found, caffeine does cross the placenta, and small amounts also pass into breast milk. Caffeine can cause hyperactivity and insomnia in infants. For this reason, pregnant and nursing women should use caution and limit their intake of caffeine.
- Caffeine's effects on children have not been studied.

POSSIBLE INTERACTIONS

There is some evidence of interactions between caffeine and the following drugs: barbiturates, ulcer medications, antacids and supplements containing calcium, erythromycin, troleandomycin, and oral contraceptives. However, the effects of caffeine on the metabolizing of these medications are not well characterized in research studies and may not be clinically signficant.

TARGET AILMENTS
Fatigue
Pain (when used as an adjunctive, or additive, treatment in combination with analgesics such as aspirin)
Migraine and other vascular headaches (used with ergot preparations)

CONTINUED

CAFFEINE

C

Beta blockers: combining these drugs may decrease the action of both.

Bronchodilators: taking caffeine with these may increase stimulation and other side effects.

Disulfiram (for alcohol dependency): may decrease the elimination of caffeine, thus intensifying its effects.

Grapefruit juice: possible increased caffeine effect.

Iron supplements: decreased iron absorption.

Lithium: may increase lithium elimination, decreasing lithium's effectiveness.

MAO inhibitors: combining with large amounts of caffeine may produce heart arrhythmias or severe hypertension.

Other central nervous system stimulants (amphetamines, pseudoephedrine): may add to stimulation and other adverse effects.

Other sources of caffeine or theobromines (related to caffeine) such as tea, coffee, chocolate: may produce an additive effect, making side effects more likely.

SIDE EFFECTS

NOT SERIOUS

- Mild stimulation of the central nervous system (jitters)
- Mild digestive upset or nausea
- Insomnia

CALL YOUR DOCTOR IF THESE SYMPTOMS BECOME BOTHERSOME.

SERIOUS

- Dizziness, increased heart rate, nervousness or tremors
- Digestive upsets such as nausea, vomiting, diarrhea

LET YOUR DOCTOR KNOW IF YOU HAVE THESE EFFECTS. YOU MAY HAVE TAKEN TOO MUCH CAFFEINE. OVERDOSE SYMPTOMS INCLUDE THOSE ABOVE PLUS HEADACHE, VISION DISTURBANCES SUCH AS SEEING FLASHES OR LIGHTS, DELIRIUM, FEVER, INCREASED SENSITIVITY TO PAIN, RINGING IN EARS.

CALCAREA CARBONICA

LATIN NAME
Calcarea carbonica

VITAL STATISTICS

GENERAL DESCRIPTION

Calcarea carbonica, or calcium carbonate, is a source of calcium, one of the most abundant natural elements in the human body. Essential to cell structure and bone strength, calcium is found in many materials, including chalk, coral, and limestone. Perhaps as a reflection of its body-building properties, the remedy *Calcarea carbonica,* also called *Calc carb,* is used by homeopathic physicians for conditions that are accompanied by symptoms of exhaustion, depression, and anxiety. Calcium carbonate prepared for homeopathic use is ground from oyster shells and used at full strength. For more information on homeopathic medicine, see page 14.

PREPARATIONS

Calcarea carbonica is available in various potencies, in both liquid and tablet form, at selected stores and pharmacies. Consult your practitioner for more precise instructions.

PRECAUTIONS

SPECIAL INFORMATION

- When a remedy is administered, no one but the patient should touch the pills. If tablets are spilled, throw them away.
- The mouth should be clear of flavors 15 minutes before and after taking a remedy, and strong flavors and aromas, such as coffee and heavy perfume, should be avoided for the duration of treatment.

TARGET AILMENTS

- Lower-back pain
- Broken bones that are slow to heal
- Sprains from overexertion
- Muscle cramps
- Constipation
- Chronic ear infections
- Eye inflammations
- Headaches
- Insomnia brought on by anxiety
- Eczema
- Allergies; asthma
- Teething problems
- Gastritis
- Gallstones
- Childhood diarrhea
- Menstrual problems
- Palpitations
- Arthritis

SIDE EFFECTS

NONE EXPECTED

C

CALCAREA PHOSPHORICA

LATIN NAME
Calcarea phosphorica

VITAL STATISTICS

GENERAL DESCRIPTION

Calcarea phosphorica, also known as calcium phosphate, is the principal mineral in bones and teeth. It is also essential to the growth and maintenance of blood cells and connective tissue. Calcium phosphate is a mineral salt with many commercial uses, including the manufacture of fertilizers, plastics, and glass.

One obvious homeopathic use for the remedy *Calcarea phosphorica,* or *Calc phos,* is in accelerating the healing of bone fractures. Homeopathic practitioners also find it can be effective in treating anemia, exhaustion, sluggishness, or restlessness. The remedy works especially well for children who are slow to teethe or who have gone through a growth spurt and have become exhausted and pale.

For more information on homeopathic medicine, see page 14.

PREPARATIONS

Calcarea phosphorica is available in various potencies at selected stores and pharmacies. Consult your homeopathic practitioner for more information.

PRECAUTIONS

SPECIAL INFORMATION

- When a remedy is administered, only the patient should touch the pills. If tablets are spilled, throw them away.
- The mouth should be clear of flavors 15 minutes before and after taking a remedy, and strong flavors and aromas, such as coffee, camphor, and heavily scented perfumes, should be avoided for the duration of treatment.

TARGET AILMENTS
Anemia
Broken bones
Colds
Cough with yellow mucus
Exhaustion
Headache made worse by change in the weather, with pain in the skull bones
Painful teething in children
Joint pain with stiffness, coldness, or numbness of the parts
Menstrual cramps with backache

SIDE EFFECTS

NONE EXPECTED

CALCITONIN

VITAL STATISTICS

DRUG CLASS
Osteoporosis Treatment

BRAND NAMES
Calcimar, Cibacalcin, Miacalcin

OTHER DRUGS IN THIS CLASS
alendronate

GENERAL DESCRIPTION
Calcitonin, a naturally occurring hormone that inhibits bone loss, is available as a nasal spray or an injectable preparation. It is generally prescribed for women who have postmenopausal osteoporosis but cannot undergo estrogen replacement therapy.

Osteoporosis is a progressive disease in which bone loss outstrips formation of new bone. The disease can lead to bone fractures, most commonly of the vertebrae, hip, and wrist. Spinal and hip fractures can be very serious in older people. Prevention of bone loss requires proper medication, regular weight-bearing exercise, and adequate intake of calcium and vitamin D. Your doctor may recommend supplements and an exercise program.

You may have to take calcitonin for six months or longer before noticing results. Calcitonin is also used to treat Paget's disease of bone, a serious disorder of bone formation.

SIDE EFFECTS

NOT SERIOUS

- Back or joint pain; headache; itching; nausea; dizziness; loss of appetite; vomiting, diarrhea; increased urination; shivering

THESE ARE RARE SIDE EFFECTS OF THE INJECTABLE DRUG. CALL YOUR DOCTOR IF THEY PERSIST.

- Nasal inflammation, dryness, crusting, sores, irritation, itching, or redness; runny or stuffy nose; mild nasal bleeding, discomfort, or tenderness; salty or metallic taste in the mouth

THESE ARE SIDE EFFECTS OF THE NASAL SPRAY ONLY. CALL YOUR DOCTOR IF THEY PERSIST.

SERIOUS

- Breathing difficulty
- Swelling of hands, feet, face, mouth, or neck
- Skin rash or hives

SEEK EMERGENCY TREATMENT.

- Ulceration of the nose (nasal spray only)

CALL YOUR DOCTOR IMMEDIATELY.

CONTINUED

CALCITONIN

C

PRECAUTIONS

WARNING

Calcitonin is not used or recommended for premenopausal, pregnant, or nursing women, or for children.

SPECIAL INFORMATION

- Consult your doctor or pharmacist about the proper dosing schedule and what to do if you miss a dose.
- Before beginning to take calcitonin, notify your doctor if you are allergic to any medication or other substance, or if you have blocked kidneys.
- Taking calcitonin may affect some medical tests; notify any doctor or dentist you consult that you are taking this medicine.
- Visit your doctor regularly to monitor bone loss (and your nasal condition if you are using calcitonin nasal spray), and consult your doctor before deciding to stop using this medication.
- A skin test is recommended before beginning therapy with calcitonin if you are allergic to any protein.

POSSIBLE INTERACTIONS

Calcium-containing preparations or vitamin D: may interfere with the absorption of calcitonin; take at least four hours after taking calcitonin.

Plicamycin: this drug taken with calcitonin will cause additive reduction of blood calcium levels (hypocalcemia).

TARGET AILMENTS
Osteoporosis
Paget's disease of bone
Hypercalcemia (abnormally high blood levels of calcium)

CALCIUM

VITAL STATISTICS

GENERAL DESCRIPTION

Calcium, the most abundant mineral in the body, is essential for the growth and maintenance of bones and teeth. It enables muscles, including your heart, to contract; it is necessary for normal blood clotting, proper nerve-impulse transmission, and connective-tissue maintenance. It helps keep blood pressure normal and may reduce the risk of heart disease; taken with vitamin D, it may help lessen the risk of colorectal cancer. (*Caution:* Because vitamin D is toxic in high doses, this combination should be taken only if prescribed by a doctor.) It helps prevent rickets in children and osteoporosis in adults.

Different people need calcium in varying amounts. Supplemental calcium is available in many forms; the form that is best absorbed by the body is calcium citrate-malate.

RDA

Adults: 800 mg
Pregnant women and young adults: 1,200 mg

NATURAL SOURCES

Good sources of calcium include dairy products, dark green leafy vegetables, sardines, salmon, soy, and almonds.

PRECAUTIONS

WARNING

Too much calcium can lead to constipation and to calcium deposits in soft tissue, causing damage to the heart, liver, or kidneys.

SPECIAL INFORMATION

- A sedentary lifestyle and consuming too much alcohol, dietary fiber, and fat can interfere with calcium absorption; too much protein and caffeine results in calcium being excreted in urine.
- For calcium to be properly absorbed, the body must have sufficient levels of vitamin D and of hydrochloric acid in the stomach, and a balance of other minerals, including magnesium and phosphorus.

TARGET AILMENTS
Osteoporosis in adults
Rickets in children
Colorectal cancer (when taken with vitamin D and if prescribed by a doctor)
Calcium helps regulate blood pressure and may reduce the risk of heart disease

SIDE EFFECTS

NONE EXPECTED

CALCIUM CARBONATE

C

VITAL STATISTICS

DRUG CLASS
Antacids

BRAND NAMES
Rolaids, Tums

OTHER DRUGS IN THIS CLASS
aluminum hydroxide, magnesium carbonate, magnesium hydroxide, sodium bicarbonate and citric acid

GENERAL DESCRIPTION
Calcium carbonate is a calcium-containing antacid drug that relieves symptoms of upset and sour stomach, heartburn, acid indigestion, and ulcers. Calcium carbonate is most effective when taken on an empty stomach. This medication is also used to help prevent calcium-deficiency diseases such as osteoporosis. See Antacids for more information, including possible drug interactions.

PRECAUTIONS

SPECIAL INFORMATION
- Except under special circumstances determined by your doctor, antacids should not be used if you have impaired renal function or high levels of calcium in your blood, a condition known as hypercalcemia.
- Notify your doctor if you develop symptoms such as black, tarry stools or vomit the consistency of coffee grounds. These are indications of bleeding in the stomach or intestines.
- Calcium carbonate can cause milk-alkali syndrome, which is characterized by headaches, nausea, irritability, and weakness. In time, milk-alkali syndrome can lead to kidney disease or kidney failure.

TARGET AILMENTS

Upset stomach; heartburn; acid indigestion; sour stomach

Ulcers

Calcium deficiency

SIDE EFFECTS

NOT SERIOUS
- Mild constipation
- Laxative effect or diarrhea
- Chalky taste in the mouth
- Stomach cramps; nausea
- Belching
- Flatulence
- White specks in the stool

CALL YOUR DOCTOR IF THESE PROBLEMS PERSIST.

SERIOUS
- Swelling of the wrist, foot, or lower leg
- Bone pain
- Severe constipation
- Dizziness
- Mood changes
- Muscle pain, weakness, or twitching
- Slow breathing
- Irregular heartbeat
- Fatigue
- Pain upon urinating or frequent need to urinate
- Change in appetite

CONTACT YOUR DOCTOR IMMEDIATELY.

Calcium Channel Blockers

Vital Statistics

GENERIC NAMES

amlodipine, diltiazem, isradipine, nifedipine, verapamil

GENERAL DESCRIPTION

Calcium channel blockers inhibit the flow of calcium into certain muscle cells. This action helps dilate the arteries, lower blood pressure, and prevent some heart-rhythm abnormalities and coronary artery spasms. These drugs are used alone or in carefully selected combinations with other heart and blood pressure medications.

Precautions

SPECIAL INFORMATION

- Recent findings have prompted warnings from some healthcare professionals about the safety of calcium channel blockers, particularly large doses of the short-acting form of nifedipine. Before using any of these drugs, be sure to discuss this matter thoroughly with your doctor. If you are already taking a calcium channel blocker, do not stop the medication without first consulting your doctor.
- Pregnant and nursing women should use these drugs only if clearly needed.
- Let your doctor know if you are suffering from low blood pressure (hypotension); heart, liver, or kidney disease; or pulmonary congestion.

POSSIBLE INTERACTIONS

All heart drugs, including digoxin, nitroglycerin, beta blockers, and angiotensin-converting enzyme (ACE) inhibitors: calcium channel blockers taken in combination with a heart medication may increase the effect of any of the drugs. However, it is not uncommon for these drugs to be prescribed together. If you are taking more than one of these medications, your doctor will want to monitor your reactions closely.

Alcohol: increased effect of calcium channel blockers, leading to dangerously low blood pressure; increased blood levels of alcohol. Do not drink alcohol while being treated with these drugs.

Anti-inflammatory drugs, including nonsteroidal anti-inflammatory drugs (NSAIDs): decreased calcium channel blocker effect.

Blood pressure drugs: can interact with calcium channel blockers, increasing the effect of any of the combined drugs and leading to excessive lowering of blood pressure.

Calcium supplements: may decrease the action of calcium channel blockers.

Carbamazepine, theophylline: increased blood levels of these medications when taken with certain calcium channel blockers.

Cimetidine: may increase the effects of some calcium channel blockers by interfering with their metabolism by the liver.

Cyclosporine: certain calcium channel blockers may cause toxic levels of cyclosporine to accumulate in the blood.

CONTINUED

Calcium Channel Blockers

C

Drugs that reduce blood pressure either directly or indirectly, such as monoamine oxidase (MAO) inhibitors or opioid analgesics: calcium channel blockers may increase the hypotensive action of these drugs, possibly leading to dangerously low blood pressure. Your doctor may have to adjust your dosage of all medicines.

Estrogens: may elevate blood pressure and thus increase the need for calcium channel blockers.

Grapefruit juice: recent tests indicate that drinking grapefruit juice can increase blood levels of certain calcium channel blockers, including nifedipine and verapamil.

Lithium: nausea, vomiting, diarrhea, or tremors; increased or decreased blood lithium levels (verapamil).

Rifampin: reduced effect of calcium channel blockers.

TARGET AILMENTS
Angina
Heart-rhythm problems (especially diltiazem or verapamil)
High blood pressure
Raynaud's syndrome (nifedipine)
Control of cluster headaches and panic attacks (verapamil)

SIDE EFFECTS

NOT SERIOUS

- Muscle cramps
- Drowsiness; fatigue
- Lightheadedness
- Headache
- Weakness
- Flushing
- Gastrointestinal upset (rare)

CALL YOUR DOCTOR IF THESE EFFECTS BECOME TROUBLESOME.

SERIOUS

- Heart problems, such as congestive heart failure, heart-rhythm irregularities, or increased angina (heart pain)
- Low blood pressure
- Swelling of the lower extremities
- Allergic reactions, such as skin rash
- Swelling of the gums

CONTACT YOUR DOCTOR IMMEDIATELY.

Calcium Polycarbophil

C

Vital Statistics

DRUG CLASS
Laxatives

BRAND NAME
FiberCon

OTHER DRUGS IN THIS CLASS
methylcellulose, psyllium hydrophilic mucilloid

GENERAL DESCRIPTION
Calcium polycarbophil is a bulk-forming laxative used for the temporary relief of both constipation and diarrhea, and to prevent straining during bowel movements. Bulk-forming laxatives, considered the safest and therefore the first choice in treating constipation, work by absorbing water and expanding, thus increasing the moisture content of the stool to make passage easier. They may also be especially beneficial to people on low-fiber diets and to those with irritable bowel syndrome (spastic colon), diverticulitis, or hemorrhoids. See Laxatives for more information, including possible drug interactions.

Precautions

SPECIAL INFORMATION
- When taking this laxative, be sure to drink plenty of water or other fluid to avoid obstruction of the throat and esophagus. Taking this medication without enough liquid may cause choking.
- You may not experience the effects of this laxative for 12 to 72 hours after taking it.
- Bulk-forming laxatives are best for geriatric patients with poorly functioning colons.
- If you have difficulty swallowing, do not take bulk-forming laxatives, which can cause an esophageal obstruction.
- Call your doctor if this drug fails to have the desired effect after one week of use.

POSSIBLE INTERACTIONS
Laxatives that may contain danthron, mineral oil, or phenolphthalein: increased absorption of these substances, increasing the possibility of toxic effects.

Oral anticoagulants, digitalis, salicylate, tetracycline: these drugs may be less effective when taken concurrently with bulk-forming laxatives. After taking any of these drugs, wait two hours before taking a laxative.

TARGET AILMENTS
Constipation
Diarrhea
Irritable bowel syndrome (spastic colon)
Straining during bowel movements following rectal surgery or heart attacks, or when hemorrhoids are present

SIDE EFFECTS

NOT SERIOUS
- Harmless urine discoloration
- Skin rash

Calendula

LATIN NAME
Calendula officinalis

Vital Statistics

GENERAL DESCRIPTION

The therapeutic use of calendula originated in ancient Egypt and spread to Europe. Many varieties of the plant exist, one of which is the common marigold. Calendula's medicinally active parts are its flowers. A natural antiseptic and anti-inflammatory agent, calendula is one of the best herbs for treating wounds, skin abrasions, and infections. Taken internally, it also helps alleviate the symptoms of indigestion and other gastrointestinal disorders. Calendula's healing power appears to come from components known as terpenes. One of these, calenduloside B, is known as a sedative and for its healing effect on ulcers. For visual characteristics, see the Color Guide to Prescription Drugs and Herbs.

PREPARATIONS

Over the counter:

Available for both internal and external use in the form of lotions, ointments, oils, tinctures, and fresh or dried leaves and florets.

At home:

Lotions, ointments, and oils: Rub on injuries, rashes, and infections as needed.

Poultice: Mash up the leaves, then apply directly to minor burns or scalds.

Infusion: Steep covered 1 oz dried herb in 1 pt boiling water. For acute internal symptoms, drink two to four times a day until symptoms lessen.

Combinations: A mixture of marsh mallow root, American cranesbill, and calendula may help digestive problems. Calendula is often combined with slippery elm and applied to soothe skin inflammations and wounds. A mixture of goldenseal, calendula, and myrrh makes an antiseptic lotion.

Consult a qualified practitioner for the dosage appropriate for you and the specific condition being treated.

Precautions

SPECIAL INFORMATION

Do not apply calendula salve or ointment (any oil-based preparation) to a fresh burn or deep wound.

POSSIBLE INTERACTIONS

Combining calendula with other herbs may necessitate a lower dosage.

TARGET AILMENTS
Take internally for:
Indigestion
Gastric and duodenal ulcers
Gallbladder problems
Irregular or painful menstruation
Apply externally for:
Cuts
Burns
Skin rashes

SIDE EFFECTS

None expected

CAMPHOR

LATIN NAME
Cinnamomum camphora

VITAL STATISTICS

GENERAL DESCRIPTION

Camphor is native to China, Taiwan, and Japan, although it is also grown in California and Sri Lanka. This aromatic evergreen, a relative of the cinnamon and cassia trees, grows to a great age, and its trunk is sometimes of an enormous size. Its white flowers are followed by red berries. The older the tree, the more oil it contains.

The pale yellow oil is steam-distilled from the clippings, wood, and roots of the camphor tree. The oil is then vacuum-rectified and filter-pressed to produce three fractions; the white fraction (white camphor) is used medicinally. It has anti-inflammatory, antiseptic, antiviral, and bactericidal properties. White camphor can also be used as a stimulating agent, a diuretic, and an expectorant. The other fractions are highly toxic and have industrial uses. Camphor has a sharp, pungent scent.

PREPARATIONS

Camphor oil can be used on the skin if the oil is diluted first. Mix 2 to 4 drops in 2 tsp vegetable or nut oil or aloe gel. Apply to appropriate areas for each ailment. Use only 2 drops for sensitive areas, such as the face.

For an aromatic bath, add 5 to 10 drops of camphor oil to the bathwater.

For colds, the flu, and other respiratory ailments, sprinkle a few drops of camphor oil on a cloth or tissue and inhale, or use the oil in a room diffuser.

PRECAUTIONS

☠ *WARNING*

Camphor is a very powerful oil. It can be harmful to people who suffer from epilepsy, asthma, or allergies.

SPECIAL INFORMATION

- Avoid using camphor if you are pregnant.
- Do not use camphor with homeopathic treatment; the oil counters many homeopathic remedies.

TARGET AILMENTS
Acne and oily skin conditions
Arthritis
Muscle and joint pains
Rheumatism
Sprains
Bronchitis
Colds and flu
Fever

SIDE EFFECTS

WHITE CAMPHOR IS RELATIVELY NONIRRITATING, BUT SEE WARNING ABOVE.

CAMPHOR

C

VITAL STATISTICS

BRAND NAME
Vicks VapoRub

GENERAL DESCRIPTION
A resin from a type of cinnamon tree, camphor has been used for centuries as an insect repellent and as a medication for minor skin irritations. By itself or in combination with menthol, phenol, or methyl salicylate, camphor is found in many over-the-counter products, ranging from pain-relieving liniments to decongestants and cough suppressants.

Camphor is absorbed rapidly through the skin and by inhalation. Exposure to high concentrations of the substance can result in serious, even toxic side effects. Because deaths have occurred from camphor poisonings, the FDA has banned all products with a camphor concentration greater than 11 percent, including camphorated oil.

PRECAUTIONS

WARNING
In rare cases, overdose or poisoning can cause respiratory failure or extreme convulsions; death may result. See Serious Side Effects *(right)* for symptoms of overdose or poisoning.

SPECIAL INFORMATION
- Because it can affect the developing fetus or pass to an infant through breast milk, camphor is not considered safe for pregnant or nursing women.
- Do not apply camphor to deep or serious wounds, since this may allow the drug to enter the bloodstream.

TARGET AILMENTS

Cough

Nasal congestion

Pain from arthritis and minor skin irritations

Minor cuts and scrapes (as an antiseptic)

SIDE EFFECTS

NOT SERIOUS

- Minor irritation when applied to skin

CALL YOUR DOCTOR IF THE IRRITATION IS TROUBLESOME.

SERIOUS

- Headache
- Dizziness
- Delirium
- Hallucinations
- Restlessness
- Confusion
- Tremors
- Jerky motions
- Convulsions
- Drowsiness
- Shallow breathing
- Coma

THESE SYMPTOMS INDICATE OVERDOSE OR POISONING. IF ANY OF THESE SYMPTOMS OCCUR, CALL YOUR DOCTOR OR A POISON CONTROL CENTER IMMEDIATELY.

CANNABIS

C

VITAL STATISTICS

GENERAL DESCRIPTION

Cannabis, better known as marijuana, is a so-called recreational drug believed by a growing number of physicians to have therapeutic value. There is evidence that smoking cannabis increases appetite, reduces nausea, and reduces spasticity in people with multiple sclerosis. Evidence of cannabis's ability to provide pain relief in safe dosages is mixed.

The drug dronabinol, a synthetic form of an active ingredient of marijuana, tetrahydrocannabinol (THC), exhibited benefits similar to those of cannabis in clinical trials. The relative benefits of the two forms remain controversial.

Two states, California and Arizona, have passed voter initiatives to allow the medicinal use of marijuana.

PRECAUTIONS

SPECIAL INFORMATION

- Cannabis causes sleepiness and alters perception and mood. Avoid driving and other hazardous activities during and after use.
- Use with caution if you have a cardiac disorder. Cannabis may affect heart rate and blood pressure.
- Although marijuana is not physically addictive, long-term use may result in psychological addiction and abuse. Use with caution if you have a history of substance abuse.
- Anxiety and panic are possible, especially during the first use. Use this drug with caution if you have a history of a psychiatric disorder such as mania, depression, or schizophrenia. Obtain instruction in its use from a physician experienced with medicinal marijuana, and make sure someone is with you when you take it for the first time.
- The therapeutic effect of cannabis in reducing intraocular pressure in patients with glaucoma is not long lasting, necessitating frequent use in these patients.
- Do not use this drug if you are pregnant or nursing a baby.

POSSIBLE INTERACTIONS

Alcohol, sedatives, sleeping pills: increased drowsiness.

Anticholinergics and antihistamines: increased heart rate and drowsiness.

Antidepressants: increased drowsiness, heart rate, and blood pressure.

Theophylline: decreased effectiveness of theophylline.

SIDE EFFECTS

NOT SERIOUS

- Congestion of the conjunctiva (red eyes)
- Sleepiness; weakness
- Sore throat
- Slightly increased heart rate
- Nausea; vomiting
- Intoxication with possible altered perception, mood changes, anxiety, or hallucinations (rare)

CALL YOUR DOCTOR IF THESE EFFECTS PERSIST.

TARGET AILMENTS

AIDS wasting syndrome; glaucoma; nausea from cancer chemotherapy and AIDS treatment; movement disorders such as multiple sclerosis

CANTHARIS

LATIN NAME
Cantharis vesicatoria

C

VITAL STATISTICS

GENERAL DESCRIPTION

Popularly known as Spanish fly, cantharis is actually a beetle found in southern France and Spain. It produces an irritant so caustic that the skin will blister if exposed to it.

Cantharis has had a long career in medicine. It has been used for all manner of disorders from baldness to rheumatism, and even as an aphrodisiac. In high concentrations the irritant can be toxic, prompting abdominal cramps and burning pains in the throat and stomach, vomiting of blood, diarrhea, kidney damage, convulsions, coma, and death. Homeopaths prescribe *Cantharis* for patients whose ailments are coupled with symptoms like those of cantharis poisoning.

According to homeopathic tradition, the beetles are collected at daybreak, when they are still sluggish from the cool of the night, and heated in the steam of boiling vinegar until dead. The beetles are then crushed and mixed with successively greater amounts of milk sugar, undergoing a pharmaceutical process called trituration. The resulting powder is highly dilute.

Like most homeopathic prescriptions, *Cantharis* was developed as a remedy by observation of the reactions of healthy individuals to doses of various strengths. The mental, emotional, and physical changes induced by *Cantharis* were then cataloged. When a patient exhibits a set of symptoms that matches the cataloged symptoms brought on by *Cantharis,* the homeopathic practitioner then prescribes it in an extremely dilute form. It is presumed that in this highly dilute dosage, *Cantharis* can counter the symptoms that are similar to the ones it induces when it is at full strength. For more information on homeopathic medicine, see page 14.

PREPARATIONS

Cantharis is available in various potencies, in liquid and tablet form, at selected stores and pharmacies. Consult your homeopathic practitioner for more precise information.

PRECAUTIONS

SPECIAL INFORMATION

- When a remedy is administered, no one but the patient should touch the pills. If tablets are spilled, throw them away.
- The mouth should be clear of flavors 15 minutes before and after taking a remedy, and strong flavors and aromas, such as coffee, camphor, and heavily scented perfumes, should be avoided for the duration of treatment.

TARGET AILMENTS
Bladder infections or cystitis, with a constant desire to urinate accompanied by blood and pain during urination
Sunburns
Scalds
Blistering second-degree burns

SIDE EFFECTS

NONE EXPECTED

CAPTOPRIL

C

VITAL STATISTICS

DRUG CLASS
Angiotensin-Converting Enzyme (ACE) Inhibitors

BRAND NAME
Capoten

OTHER DRUGS IN THIS CLASS
benazepril, enalapril, fosinopril, lisinopril, quinapril, ramipril

GENERAL DESCRIPTION
Introduced in 1979, the ACE inhibitor captopril is prescribed for the control of high blood pressure (hypertension) and congestive heart failure. The drug works by blocking a body enzyme essential for the production of a substance that causes blood vessels to constrict. This action relaxes arterial walls, lowering blood pressure and decreasing the work load of the heart. For increased effectiveness in lowering blood pressure, captopril may be combined with hydrochlorothiazide, a diuretic that reduces water retention. For visual characteristics of Capoten, a brand of captopril, see the Color Guide to Prescription Drugs and Herbs. For further information, see Angiotensin-Converting Enzyme (ACE) Inhibitors.

PRECAUTIONS

WARNING
Get medical attention immediately if you notice swelling of your face, tongue, or vocal cords or have difficulty swallowing or breathing; this reaction can be life threatening.

This drug should not be taken during pregnancy; it has been associated with death of the fetus and newborn.

SPECIAL INFORMATION
- Captopril causes an increase in blood levels of potassium. Do not use potassium-rich products, including salt substitutes and low-salt milk, without first consulting your doctor. The potassium in your blood could rise to dangerous levels, leading to heart-rhythm problems.
- Do not abruptly stop taking this drug. Your doctor may tell you to reduce the dosage gradually.

TARGET AILMENTS

High blood pressure

Sometimes congestive heart failure (in conjunction with digitalis preparations and diuretics)

SIDE EFFECTS

SEE ANGIOTENSIN-CONVERTING ENZYME (ACE) INHIBITORS.

CARBACEPHEMS

C

VITAL STATISTICS

GENERIC NAME
loracarbef

GENERAL DESCRIPTION
Carbacephem drugs, a subclass of antibiotics, work in much the same way as penicillins and cephalosporins to kill growing bacteria.

PRECAUTIONS

SPECIAL INFORMATION

- Tell your doctor if you are allergic to penicillins or cephalosporins; if so, you are likely to be allergic to carbacephems as well. Allergic reactions to these drugs can be life threatening.
- Tell your doctor if your kidneys are impaired; you may require a smaller dose of a carbacephem drug or you may need a different drug altogether.
- Take carbacephems one hour before or two hours after a meal.
- If carbacephems cause severe diarrhea, consult your doctor before taking any antidiarrheal medicine. For mild diarrhea, use only antidiarrheal preparations containing kaolin or attapulgite.
- To prevent reinfection, take the full course of your prescription, even if you feel better before you've taken all the medicine.
- Carbacephems kill not only harmful bacteria but also "good" intestinal bacteria that keep harmful fungi and intestinal bacteria in check. Eating yogurt containing *Lactobacillus acidophilus* culture or taking acidophilus tablets may help restore the body's normal bacteria.
- Prolonged use of any antibiotic can lead to fungal infections, including candidiasis, or to bacterial infections such as pseudomembranous colitis.
- Unless they are clearly needed, avoid taking carbacephem drugs if you are pregnant or breast-feeding.

POSSIBLE INTERACTIONS
Carbacephems are a relatively new antibiotic subclass, and research into their interactions is still in progress. See the entries for two similar antibiotic subclasses, Penicillins and Cephalosporins, for other possible drug interactions.

Probenecid: decreases the kidneys' ability to excrete carbacephems. Possible carbacephem toxicity.

TARGET AILMENTS

Bacterial infections, such as bronchitis, otitis media, strep throat, some pneumonias, sinusitis, infections of the skin and soft tissue, and urinary tract infections

SIDE EFFECTS

NOT SERIOUS

- Nausea; abdominal pain; mild diarrhea; loss of appetite

CONSULT YOUR DOCTOR IF THESE SYMPTOMS CONTINUE FOR MORE THAN TWO DAYS OR ARE BOTHERSOME.

SERIOUS

SEE LORACARBEF.

CARBAMAZEPINE

VITAL STATISTICS

DRUG CLASS
Anticonvulsant Drugs

BRAND NAME
Tegretol

OTHER DRUGS IN THIS CLASS
phenytoin, valproic acid

GENERAL DESCRIPTION
When first introduced in 1962, carbamazepine was approved as a pain reliever for rare forms of neuralgia. It is now used primarily in the control of several types of epileptic seizures, including tonic-clonic (grand mal) seizures, partial seizures, and mixed seizure patterns. Carbamazepine is considered a first-choice anticonvulsant drug because of its low toxicity and the rarity of serious adverse effects. Although this drug is a pain reliever, carbamazepine should never be used to relieve ordinary aches and pains.

Anticonvulsants are not curatives, but they can reduce the possibility of seizure-related brain damage. They are usually prescribed, either alone or in combination, to control specific types of epileptic seizures. Since every case of epilepsy is unique and all anticonvulsants have toxic effects when taken in large dosages, a period of trial and error is usually needed to determine the appropriate drug and dosage. For visual characteristics of carbamazepine and the brand Tegretol, see the Color Guide to Prescription Drugs and Herbs. For more information, see Anticonvulsant Drugs.

PRECAUTIONS

WARNING
Do not abruptly discontinue the drug or switch to another anticonvulsant drug unless advised to do so by your physician. Sudden withdrawal can cause a series of uninterrupted seizures.

SPECIAL INFORMATION
- Do not use carbamazepine if you have had an allergic reaction to it or to any tricyclic antidepressant drug in the past; are nursing or are in the first three months of pregnancy; have a blood cell disorder, a bone marrow disorder, or an active liver disease.
- Tell your doctor if you are taking any other drugs (prescription or over-the-counter); consume more than two alcoholic drinks a day; have a history of kidney or liver disease, thrombophlebitis, or a severe mental depression or disorder; are planning any medical or dental surgery requiring a general anesthesia.
- If you are over the age of 60, this drug may aggravate glaucoma, angina, and prostate problems.
- Carbamazepine should be taken with food to lessen stomach upset and improve absorbency.
- Routine testing for early indications of bone marrow or blood cell toxicity is essential.
- Carbamazepine may affect blood cell counts, liver function tests, urine pregnancy tests, and various blood tests.

CONTINUED

CARBAMAZEPINE

C

POSSIBLE INTERACTIONS

Anticoagulants, doxycycline, oral contraceptives with estrogen, and valproic acid: carbamazepine can decrease the effect of these drugs.

Monoamine oxidase (MAO) inhibitors and lithium: may cause severe toxic reactions when taken with carbamazepine.

Tranquilizers, narcotics, alcohol, and sedatives and hypnotics: increased sedative effects.

TARGET AILMENTS

Certain types of epileptic seizures

Relief of pain in trigeminal (tic douloureux) and glossopharyngeal neuralgia

SIDE EFFECTS

NOT SERIOUS

- Constipation
- Impaired urination
- Dry throat and mouth
- Water retention
- Mild nausea and vomiting
- Loss of appetite
- Drowsiness
- Fatigue
- Increased sensitivity to sunlight (sunburn, rash, itching, redness)
- Headache
- Dizziness
- Unsteadiness
- Confusion

CONSULT YOUR DOCTOR IF THESE OR OTHER EFFECTS PERSIST OR ARE BOTHERSOME.

SERIOUS

- Blurred or double vision
- Severe dermatitis
- Bone marrow depression (weakness, fever, abnormal bleeding or bruising)
- Liver damage (jaundice)
- Behavioral changes (agitation, hostility)
- Mental depression

CALL YOUR DOCTOR AT ONCE.

CARBO VEGETABILIS

LATIN NAME
Carbo vegetabilis

VITAL STATISTICS

GENERAL DESCRIPTION
Carbo vegetabilis is better known as wood charcoal. It is made from beech, birch, or poplar wood. Charcoal is a form of carbon, an element found in all living matter. *Carbo vegetabilis* is known as a purifier and in earlier times was used to absorb gases and check fermentation.

Homeopathic practitioners now use *Carbo vegetabilis* as another form of purification: to treat a variety of digestive complaints, including sour stomach, heartburn, indigestion, regurgitation of food, and flatulence. People recovering from an infection or an accident, or who are sluggish and lack mental energy, can also benefit from this remedy. In such patients symptoms are worse during warm, wet weather, in the evening, and when the patient is lying down.

The homeopathic preparation is usually made with beechwood, which is stripped of bark, cut into small pieces, and heated to scalding. It is then immediately smothered in a tightly fitted container. For more information on homeopathic medicine, see page 14.

PREPARATIONS
Carbo vegetabilis is available in various potencies at selected stores and pharmacies or from your homeopathic practitioner. Consult your practitioner for more precise dosage information.

PRECAUTIONS

SPECIAL INFORMATION
- When a remedy is administered, no one but the patient should touch the pills. If tablets are spilled, throw them away.
- The mouth should be clear of flavors 15 minutes before and after taking a remedy, and strong flavors and aromas, such as coffee and heavy perfume, should be avoided for the duration of treatment.

TARGET AILMENTS
Coughing, in fits, accompanied by wheezing
Bronchitis
Common cold, with hoarseness and itching throat
Exhaustion
Flatulence
Food poisoning
Gas
Headache, especially after overeating
Heartburn
Indigestion
Sluggishness
Stomach bloating

SIDE EFFECTS
NONE EXPECTED

Rx CARDIZEM

C

VITAL STATISTICS

DRUG CLASS
Calcium Channel Blockers

GENERIC NAME
diltiazem

OTHER DRUGS IN THIS CLASS
amlodipine, isradipine, nifedipine, verapamil

GENERAL DESCRIPTION
Cardizem is a brand name for the generic drug diltiazem. This calcium-channel-blocking drug has been used since 1977 to treat heart-rhythm problems, hypertension, and angina. Like other drugs in its class, Cardizem works to inhibit the passage of calcium into body cells. This relaxes the muscles that surround the arteries, dilating them. Cardizem slows the contraction of the heart, which, together with the relaxation of the arteries, decreases the work load on the heart, lowering blood pressure and preventing some spasms of the coronary arteries. Cardizem is used alone or in carefully selected combinations with other heart and blood pressure medications. For visual characteristics of Cardizem, see the Color Guide to Prescription Drugs and Herbs. For information on possible drug interactions, see Calcium Channel Blockers.

PRECAUTIONS

SPECIAL INFORMATION
- Recent findings have prompted warnings from some healthcare professionals about the safety of calcium channel blockers. Before using Cardizem, be sure to discuss this matter thoroughly with your doctor. If you are already taking this drug, do not stop the medication without first consulting your doctor.
- Pregnant and nursing women should use Cardizem only if clearly needed.
- Let your doctor know if you are suffering from low blood pressure (hypotension), heart or kidney disease, heart arrhythmias, or a recent heart attack with pulmonary congestion.

TARGET AILMENTS

Angina

Heart-rhythm problems

High blood pressure

SIDE EFFECTS

NOT SERIOUS
- Constipation; diarrhea; nausea; vomiting
- Edema
- Headache
- Dizziness; weakness
- Flushing; rash
- Cough
- Flulike symptoms

CALL YOUR DOCTOR IF THESE EFFECTS BECOME TROUBLESOME.

SERIOUS
- Low blood pressure (hypotension)
- Slow heartbeat (bradycardia)
- Angina, congestive heart failure, heart palpitations (rare)

CONTACT YOUR DOCTOR IMMEDIATELY.

Rx CARISOPRODOL

C

VITAL STATISTICS

DRUG CLASS
Muscle Relaxants

BRAND NAMES
Rela, Sodol, Soma, Soprodol

OTHER DRUGS IN THIS CLASS
cyclobenzaprine

GENERAL DESCRIPTION
Carisoprodol is used, along with rest and therapeutic exercise, to relieve painful muscle spasms and strains. This drug does not relax skeletal muscles directly; rather, its sedative effects promote relaxation. For visual characteristics of carisoprodol and of Soma, a brand of carisoprodol, see the Color Guide to Prescription Drugs and Herbs. For more information, see Muscle Relaxants.

PRECAUTIONS

WARNING
Severe allergic reactions, including anaphylactic shock, may occur after the first to fourth dose. Symptoms include itching, rash, or hives; breathing problems; swelling. Seek immediate emergency treatment.

On rare occasions, the first dose of carisoprodol will cause the following: agitation or disorientation, vision problems, extreme weakness, euphoria, speech problems, or temporary paralysis of arms and legs. Call your doctor immediately.

An overdose of carisoprodol may result in breathing problems, stupor, or even coma. Contact a poison control center or seek emergency care if you've taken more than the prescribed amount.

SPECIAL INFORMATION
- Do not use carisoprodol if you have acute intermittent porphyria (a blood disorder).
- Before using carisoprodol, inform your doctor if you are allergic to it or to any other carbamate derivative, if you have a history of drug dependency, or if you have any kidney or liver dysfunction. If you are allergic to tartrazine, don't use Rela tablets.
- Carisoprodol is not recommended for pregnant or nursing women, or for children.
- Do not drive or operate machinery while taking carisoprodol; this drug may impair your judgment and coordination.

POSSIBLE INTERACTIONS
Alcohol and other central nervous system depressants: increased effects of central nervous system depressants; do not take these drugs while taking carisoprodol.
Monoamine oxidase (MAO) inhibitors or tricyclic antidepressants: may increase respiratory depression and hypotensive effects.

TARGET AILMENTS
Muscle spasms and strains

SIDE EFFECTS

SERIOUS

SEE WARNING.

CATNIP

LATIN NAME
Nepeta cataria

C

VITAL STATISTICS

GENERAL DESCRIPTION

Herbalists have used the flowers and leaves of catnip, an aromatic member of the mint family, for more than 2,000 years. Today it is prescribed for easing digestion, calming nerves, alleviating the discomforts of respiratory illnesses, and relieving muscle spasms, including menstrual cramps. Cats are strongly attracted to catnip and may become intoxicated by eating it; the herb has no such effect on humans.

PREPARATIONS

Over the counter:

Available in dried bulk flowers and leaves, tincture, and tea bags.

At home:

Leaves: Press crushed catnip leaves into minor cuts and scrapes before washing and bandaging them.

Infusion: Pour 1 cup boiling water onto 2 tsp dried leaves and steep for 10 to 15 minutes. Drink three times a day.

Combinations: Mix with boneset, elder, yarrow, or cayenne for colds.

Consult a qualified practitioner for the dosage appropriate for you and the specific condition being treated.

SIDE EFFECTS

NOT SERIOUS

- Upset stomach

DISCONTINUE USE AND CALL YOUR DOCTOR.

PRECAUTIONS

SPECIAL INFORMATION

- During pregnancy, avoid catnip or use only under a healthcare professional's supervision.
- Weak, cool infusions can be given to infants with colic. For older children and people over 65, start with weak preparations and increase the strength as necessary.

POSSIBLE INTERACTIONS

Combining catnip with other herbs may necessitate a lower dosage.

TARGET AILMENTS

Take internally for:

Indigestion

Gas

Tension, muscle spasms

Difficulty in sleeping

Colds

Flu

Bronchial congestion

Fever

Colic in infants

Diarrhea in children

Apply externally for:

Cuts and scrapes

CAT'S-CLAW

LATIN NAME
Uncaria tomentosa

VITAL STATISTICS

GENERAL DESCRIPTION
Cat's-claw, or *uña de gato* in Spanish, is a woody vine that grows up to 100 feet on trees in the Peruvian rain forest; it gets its name from the thorns on its stem. Native Ashanica Indians long harvested the root and used it to treat a variety of ailments. Research and anecdotal evidence indicate the herb possesses anti-inflammatory and antiviral properties and can stimulate the immune system, enhancing the power of tumor-fighting white blood cells. Acclaimed for its ability to cleanse the intestinal tract and correct bowel disorders, it may also stimulate blood circulation, inhibiting atherosclerosis and reducing the risk of heart disease. In addition, it helps relieve stress and depression, is considered a uterine stimulant, and has been used traditionally to help relieve PMS symptoms.

Modern research on cat's-claw began in the 1950s in France, and the plant continues to receive attention in European, South American, and U.S. laboratories. Because of its immune-stimulating properties, it may be incorporated into tests for AIDS treatments.

Concerned the plant would be cultivated out of existence, the government of Peru has outlawed use of the root; the bark is now sold in its place, but because harvesting may pose a threat to the rain forest, some herbalists choose not to recommend it.

PREPARATIONS
Over the counter:
Available as a capsule, tablet, tea, liquid, or extract. Cat's-claw may also be combined with aloe to help cleanse the intestinal tract.

Consult a qualified practitioner for the dosage appropriate for you and the specific condition being treated.

PRECAUTIONS

WARNING
Cat's-claw might cause the immune system to reject foreign cells; those with organ or tissue transplants should avoid the herb.

Do not use cat's-claw during pregnancy. Do not give to children under two; older children and people over 65 should begin with mild doses and increase the strength gradually, if needed. Use of this herb by children for more than seven to 10 days should be done in conjunction with a healthcare practitioner.

POSSIBLE INTERACTIONS
Combining cat's-claw with other herbs may necessitate a lower dosage.

TARGET AILMENTS

Take internally for:

Arthritis; gastritis; bowel problems; Crohn's disease; diverticulitis; ulcers; urinary infections; asthma; diabetes; cancer; menstrual disorders; emotional disorders; debility; viral diseases

Apply externally for:

Hemorrhoids; acne; wounds; fungus

SIDE EFFECTS

NOT SERIOUS
- Diarrhea

DISCONTINUE OR DECREASE DOSE.

CAUSTICUM

LATIN NAME
Causticum

C

VITAL STATISTICS

GENERAL DESCRIPTION

Causticum, also called potassium hydrate, is a mixture of slaked lime (calcium hydroxide) and potassium bisulfate. It was first developed by Samuel Hahnemann, the founding father of homeopathy.

Causticum has a burning, astringent taste on the tongue, qualities that provide a clue to its homeopathic uses. *Causticum* is said to be particularly effective for serious, third-degree burns, and any conditions involving burning sensations, blisters, soreness, or rawness. Hoarseness, a raw, scraped feeling in the throat, and loss of voice also may be alleviated with *Causticum.* It is said to benefit people who tend to be anxious, emotional, irritable, and full of foreboding, as well as those grieving the loss of a loved one. It may also help children who wet the bed shortly after falling asleep or who have bladder-control problems when they cough during the day.

Like most homeopathic prescriptions, *Causticum* was developed as a remedy by observation of the reactions of healthy individuals to doses of various strengths. The mental, emotional, and physical changes induced by *Causticum* were then cataloged. When a patient exhibits a set of symptoms that matches the cataloged symptoms brought on by *Causticum,* the homeopathic practitioner then prescribes it in an extremely dilute form. For more information on homeopathic medicine, see page 14.

PREPARATIONS

Over the counter:

Causticum is available in various potencies at selected stores and pharmacies.

Consult your homeopathic practitioner for more precise information.

PRECAUTIONS

SPECIAL INFORMATION

- When a remedy is administered, no one but the patient should touch the pills. If tablets are spilled, throw them away.
- The mouth should be clear of flavors 15 minutes before and after taking a remedy, and strong flavors and aromas, such as coffee, camphor, and heavily scented perfumes, should be avoided for the duration of treatment.

TARGET AILMENTS
Bedwetting
Blisters
Constipation
Hoarse voice
Indigestion
Joint pain
Burning, dry, raw throat
Scalds
Third-degree burns

SIDE EFFECTS

NONE EXPECTED

CAYENNE

LATIN NAME
Capsicum frutescens

VITAL STATISTICS

GENERAL DESCRIPTION

Herbalists regard cayenne as a powerful tonic. The fruit stimulates the heart and promotes circulation, improves digestion, and boosts energy. Like other species of hot garden pepper, cayenne contains the stimulant known as capsaicin. For visual characteristics, see the Color Guide to Prescription Drugs and Herbs.

PREPARATIONS

Over the counter:
Available as powder, capsules, tincture, or oil.

At home:

OIL: Rub oil on sprains, swelling, sore muscles, and joints to ease pain.

INFUSION: Pour 1 cup boiling water onto 1/2 to 1 tsp cayenne powder and steep for 10 minutes. Mix 1 tbsp of the infusion with hot water and drink as needed.

GARGLE: Combine cayenne with myrrh to treat laryngitis and to use as an antiseptic wash.

Consult a practitioner for the dosage appropriate for you and the specific ailment.

PRECAUTIONS

WARNING

Use with caution during pregnancy. Patients with ulcers, gastritis, or bowel diseases should avoid cayenne or use only under the supervision of a healthcare practitioner.

SPECIAL INFORMATION

Because it is hot and spicy when used in the form of an infusion or a tincture, cayenne can cause mild nausea when first taken. It's best to start with a small amount and increase gradually to the recommended dosage.

POSSIBLE INTERACTIONS

Combining cayenne with other herbs may necessitate a lower dosage.

TARGET AILMENTS
Take internally for:
Poor circulation
Gas, indigestion
Physical or mental exhaustion
Reversing lowered energy or vitality, particularly in the elderly
Apply externally for:
Pain, including that of arthritis and diabetes
Strains, sore muscles and joints
Poor blood circulation
Bleeding

SIDE EFFECTS

NOT SERIOUS

- Vomiting
- Stomach pain
- Intoxication

LARGE DOSES CAN CAUSE THESE SIDE EFFECTS. DO NOT EXCEED PRESCRIBED DOSAGES.

CEPHALOSPORINS

C

VITAL STATISTICS

GENERIC NAMES

cefaclor, cefadroxil, cefixime, cefprozil, ceftibuten, cefuroxime, cephalexin, cephalexin hydrochloride

BRAND NAMES

Ceclor (cefaclor); Cedax (ceftibuten); Ceftin (cefuroxime); Cefzil (cefprozil); Duricef (cefadroxil); Keflex (cephalexin); Keftab (cephalexin hydrochloride); Suprax (cefixime)

GENERAL DESCRIPTION

Cephalosporins, a subclass of antibiotics related to penicillins, act by destroying growing bacteria. They do not kill fungi or viruses, such as those responsible for colds and the flu. Your doctor may prescribe these drugs if you have an infection caused by bacteria resistant to penicillins. Cephalosporins are available in forms that can be taken orally or injected. Oral forms may be taken on a full or an empty stomach.

See the Color Guide to Prescription Drugs and Herbs for the visual characteristics of the generic drugs cefaclor and cephalexin, and for the brand-name drugs Ceclor, Cedax, Ceftin, Cefzil, Keflex, Keftab, and Suprax.

PRECAUTIONS

SPECIAL INFORMATION

- Let your doctor know if you have ever had an allergic reaction to a cephalosporin drug or to penicillins, penicillamine, or a penicillin derivative. Your doctor may decide to prescribe a different drug. About 10 percent of people with allergies to penicillin are also allergic to cephalosporins. Reactions range from mild rashes and fever to life-threatening anaphylaxis.
- People with the congenital disorder phenylketonuria should avoid cefprozil in oral suspension, which contains phenylalanine.
- Tell your doctor if you have kidney or liver impairment, phenylketonuria, or a history of bleeding disorders or gastrointestinal disease; cephalosporins can exacerbate these conditions.
- Take the full course of your prescription, even if you feel better before finishing the medication; otherwise, the infection may return.
- These drugs may cause false-positive results for the Clinitest urine glucose test. (They do not affect results of Clinistix or Tes-Tape.) Cefuroxime causes false-negative results in some blood glucose tests.
- Although most of these drugs are absorbed more quickly on an empty stomach, cefuroxime is better absorbed when taken with food.
- If possible, avoid taking these drugs if you are pregnant or breast-feeding.

- Cephalosporins also kill "good" intestinal bacteria that keep harmful fungi and intestinal bacteria in check. Eating yogurt containing *Lactobacillus acidophilus* culture or taking acidophilus tablets may help restore the body's normal bacteria.
- Prolonged use of any antibiotic drug can lead to fungal infections, including candidiasis, or to bacterial infections such as pseudomembranous colitis.

POSSIBLE INTERACTIONS

Aminoglycosides (amikacin, gentamicin, kanamycin, neomycin, netilmicin, streptomycin, tobramycin): risk of kidney failure.

Bacteriostatic drugs (tetracycline, erythromycin, chloramphenicol, sulfonamides): may impair cephalosporins' bacteria-killing action.

Loop diuretics: risk of kidney failure.

Nephrotoxic drugs (vancomycin, colistin, polymyxin B): risk of kidney failure.

Probenecid: decreases the kidneys' ability to excrete cephalosporins. Possible cephalosporin toxicity. However, this combination is sometimes prescribed to treat serious infections that require high, prolonged serum levels of cephalosporins.

TARGET AILMENTS

Otitis media

Infections of the respiratory tract, genitourinary tract, skin, or soft tissue

Serious infections of the blood, bones, joints, abdomen, lungs, or heart

SIDE EFFECTS

NOT SERIOUS

- Mild nausea or diarrhea
- Yeast infections of the mouth (sore mouth or tongue)
- Vaginal yeast infections (vaginal itching or discharge)

TELL YOUR DOCTOR WHEN CONVENIENT.

SERIOUS

- Dizziness
- Serum sickness (fever accompanied by joint pains and rash)
- Severe diarrhea
- Severe allergic reaction
- Unusual bruising or bleeding
- Severe stomach cramps

CALL YOUR DOCTOR IMMEDIATELY.

Cetirizine

C

Vital Statistics

DRUG CLASS
Antihistamines

BRAND NAME
Zyrtec

OTHER DRUGS IN THIS CLASS
astemizole, brompheniramine, chlorpheniramine, clemastine, dexbrompheniramine, diphenhydramine, doxylamine, loratadine, promethazine, terfenadine, triprolidine

GENERAL DESCRIPTION
Cetirizine is an antihistamine that relieves the symptoms of seasonal allergies—stuffy and runny nose, itching eyes, scratchy throat—and other allergic symptoms, such as rash, itching, or hives. It is also prescribed for allergy-induced asthma. Cetirizine causes less drowsiness than other antihistamines and is less likely to interact with other drugs. For visual characteristics of the brand-name drug Zyrtec, see the Color Guide to Prescription Drugs and Herbs.

Precautions

SPECIAL INFORMATION
- Cetirizine is considered safe and effective for adults and children six and older but is not recommended for pregnant and nursing women or newborn or premature babies.
- People with kidney disease should receive a reduced dosage of this drug.

POSSIBLE INTERACTIONS
Cetirizine should be taken on an empty stomach, but in the event of gastrointestinal upsets, it may be taken with food or milk.

Although cetirizine is less sedating than most other antihistamines, drowsiness may still occur, and the drug should not be mixed with alcohol or other CNS depressants.

Do not mix cetirizine with MAO inhibitors. See Monoamine Oxidase (MAO) Inhibitors for additional information.

TARGET AILMENTS

Nasal and respiratory allergies (seasonal and nonseasonal)

Allergy-induced asthma

Allergic skin reactions, including poison ivy, insect bites, and hives

SIDE EFFECTS

NOT SERIOUS
- Unusual fatigue or weakness not present before use
- Sore throat and fever
- Dry mouth, nose, or throat
- Excessive drowsiness, especially when dose is exceeded
- Dizziness or slower movement or reaction time
- Unusual bleeding or bruising
- Nervousness, restlessness, or insomnia
- Gastrointestinal upsets
- Weight gain

SERIOUS
- Severe episodes of the above side effects (rare)
- Irregular heartbeat

CHAMOMILE

LATIN NAME
Matricaria recutita

VITAL STATISTICS

GENERAL DESCRIPTION

Native to Europe and Asia, this widely cultivated aromatic herb (commonly known as German chamomile) has feathery leaves and white flowers that bloom from May through August. The dried flowers produce an inky blue, strong-scented oil. German chamomile has anti-inflammatory, sedative, and pain-killing properties. It also is used as an anti-allergenic and antiseptic.

PREPARATIONS

Aromatherapy treatments employ both the flowers themselves and the oil produced from the flowers. The dried flowers are used in tisanes and inhalations.

For relief of headache from sinusitis, mix 4 drops German chamomile oil with 1 tsp soy oil and rub the mixture around the sinus area and eyes, from nose to temple. To apply to a larger area or to use as a body massage oil, mix 10 to 12 drops in 2 tbsp vegetable or nut oil or aloe gel.

For baths, add no more than 2 drops to the water. For inhalation, scent the air with a diffuser or sniff drops placed on a tissue.

German chamomile is one of the gentlest essential oils. It is ideal for use with children and makes an effective teething remedy. Mix 1 drop German chamomile oil with 2 tsp grape-seed oil. Put a small amount on your index finger and rub the infant's inflamed gum.

PRECAUTIONS

SPECIAL INFORMATION

The oil should be blue in color. If it is brown, the oil is too old.

TARGET AILMENTS

- Digestive upsets
- Menstrual and menopausal symptoms
- Inflamed skin, burns, and sunburn
- Acne and boils
- Eczema and other skin problems
- Headache
- Anxiety and stress
- Arthritis
- Low back pain
- Muscular pain
- Hay fever
- Bronchitis

SIDE EFFECTS

NOT SERIOUS

- Dermatitis

Chamomile

LATIN NAME
Matricaria recutita

C

Vital Statistics

GENERAL DESCRIPTION

Of the three types of chamomile plant, the most popular and thoroughly studied is German chamomile, used medicinally around the world for thousands of years. Modern herbalists have identified elements in the oil of the chamomile flower that appear to calm the central nervous system, relax the digestive tract, and speed the healing process.

For visual characteristics, see the Color Guide to Prescription Drugs and Herbs.

PREPARATIONS

Over the counter:
Available as prepared tea, tincture, essential oil, and dried or fresh flowers.

At home:

Tea: Pour 8 oz boiling water over 2 tsp chamomile flowers and steep for 10 minutes. Drink 1 cup three or four times daily, or dilute and use as an eye compress.

Eye compress: Strain the tea through a coffee filter and dilute with an equal amount of water. Always use fresh tea (less than 24 hours old) and refrigerate unused portions. (Bring the dilute tea to room temperature before using it.) To make the compress, pour the liquid on a cloth and apply to the closed eye. Discontinue if your eye becomes irritated.

Fomentation: Apply three or four times daily to sore muscles; sore, swollen joints; varicose veins; and burns and skin wounds.

Herbal bath: Run bathwater over 2 or 3 oz chamomile flowers tied in cloth, or add no more than 2 drops essential oil of chamomile to bathwater.

Consult a practitioner for the dosage appropriate for you and the specific ailment.

Precautions

SPECIAL INFORMATION

Allergies to chamomile are rare. However, anyone allergic to other plants in the daisy family (chrysanthemum, ragweed, and aster, for example) should be alert to possible allergic reactions to chamomile, ranging from contact dermatitis to life-threatening anaphylaxis (itching, rash, and difficulty in breathing).

POSSIBLE INTERACTIONS

Combining chamomile with other herbs may necessitate a lower dosage.

TARGET AILMENTS

Take internally for:

Stomach cramps, gas, nervous stomach, indigestion, ulcers, colic; menstrual cramps; insomnia; anxiety

Apply externally for:

Joint swelling and pain; skin inflammation; sunburn; cuts and scrapes; teething pain; varicose veins; hemorrhoids; sore or inflamed eyes

Use as a gargle for:

Gingivitis; sore throat

SIDE EFFECTS

None expected

CHAMOMILLA

LATIN NAME
Chamomilla

VITAL STATISTICS

GENERAL DESCRIPTION

Chamomilla is made from the flowering German chamomile plant common in Europe. The whole plant is crushed, and its juices are mixed with equal parts of alcohol, then succussed. In homeopathy, *Chamomilla* is considered to work best for people who are extremely sensitive to pain, irritable, impatient, and implacable. *Chamomilla* patients sweat easily and are sensitive to wind and chills. *Chamomilla* is most often given to children who work themselves into violent temper tantrums.

Like most homeopathic prescriptions, *Chamomilla* was developed as a remedy by observation of the reactions of healthy individuals to doses of various strengths. The mental, emotional, and physical changes induced by *Chamomilla* were then cataloged. When a patient exhibits a set of symptoms that matches the cataloged symptoms brought on by *Chamomilla,* the homeopathic practitioner then prescribes it in an extremely dilute form. It is presumed that in this highly dilute dosage, *Chamomilla* can counter symptoms similar to the ones that it induces when it is at full strength. For more information on homeopathic medicine, see page 14.

PREPARATIONS

Chamomilla is available over the counter or from your homeopathic practitioner. Consult your practitioner for dosage information.

PRECAUTIONS

SPECIAL INFORMATION

- When a remedy is administered, no one but the patient should touch the pills. If tablets are spilled, throw them away.
- The mouth should be clear of flavors 15 minutes before and after taking a remedy, and strong flavors and aromas, such as coffee, camphor, and heavily scented perfumes, should be avoided for the duration of treatment.

TARGET AILMENTS
Irritability
Toothaches aggravated by cold air and warm food
Painful menstrual periods with severe cramping and a feeling of anger or restlessness
Extremely painful earaches
Teething pain, especially if the child is irritable
Difficulty getting to sleep

SIDE EFFECTS

NONE EXPECTED

CHARCOAL, ACTIVATED

C

VITAL STATISTICS

BRAND NAMES
Charcocaps, Actidose-Aqua, Charcodote, Liquid-Antidose, Charcosalanti Dote

DAILY DOSAGE
For diarrhea or gas pain, 2 capsules three or four times a day
For gout, 1 tsp three times a day

GENERAL DESCRIPTION
Activated charcoal, a type of chemically treated carbon used in medicine, has little in common with the charcoal used on the grill. Activated charcoal takes the form of tiny particles suspended in water and is often used by doctors to cleanse the intestinal tract of toxic substances. It is sometimes given as an antidote for poisoning or for overdose of such medications as aspirin and acetaminophen.

Introduced into the body, activated charcoal attracts and collects toxins, then carries them out through the stool. Because it does not enter the bloodstream, charcoal is generally considered safe, and overdose is unlikely.

PREPARATIONS
Available in capsules, powder, or suspension.

PRECAUTIONS

WARNING
Charcoal can interfere with the body's absorption of other drugs, particularly heart medications. Take activated charcoal at least two hours before or after taking other medications or vitamin supplements.

SPECIAL INFORMATION
- Contact a doctor in the case of poisoning. Do not try to treat the condition yourself.
- Heat and moisture can inhibit the action of charcoal. Store in a cool, dry place away from children.
- Women who are pregnant or breast-feeding should consult a doctor before using activated charcoal supplements.
- Although overdose is unlikely, if extreme amounts of charcoal are ingested, you should notify a doctor, emergency room, or poison control center right away.

TARGET AILMENTS

Diarrhea

Gout

Gas and gas pains

Poisoning and drug overdose

Hangover

Hiccups

SIDE EFFECTS

NOT SERIOUS
- Blackened stool; constipation; diarrhea; vomiting (if taken in large doses)

Chaste Tree

LATIN NAME
Vitex agnus-castus

C

Vital Statistics

GENERAL DESCRIPTION

Chaste tree's natural compounds seem to aid in regulating the menstrual cycle by bringing into balance the female sex hormones estrogen and progesterone. Besides treating menstrual irregularities, chaste tree is prescribed for relieving premenstrual syndrome and to counter symptoms of menopause. It also aids in readjusting the body after withdrawal from long-term use of birth-control pills, in preventing miscarriage in the first three months of pregnancy, and in promoting lactation. In past eras, the herb was used to dampen the sexual longings of Roman women whose husbands were abroad on military expeditions and to curb the sex drives of medieval monks. Paradoxically, chaste tree has also had a reputation as an aphrodisiac. For visual characteristics, see the Color Guide to Prescription Drugs and Herbs.

PREPARATIONS

Over the counter:
Available as berries, powder, dried herb, capsules, and tincture.

At home:
Tea: Pour 1 cup boiling water onto 1 tsp ripe berries and let them infuse, covered, for 10 to 15 minutes. Drink three times a day.
Consult a qualified practitioner for the dosage appropriate for you and the specific condition being treated.

SIDE EFFECTS
None expected

Precautions

SPECIAL INFORMATION

- Chaste tree seems to regulate hormonal imbalances within 10 days and to relieve premenstrual syndrome by the second menstrual cycle, but for optimal benefit it should be taken for six months or longer.
- To avoid premature production of milk, discontinue after the third month of pregnancy.

POSSIBLE INTERACTIONS

Combining chaste tree with other herbs may necessitate a lower dosage.

TARGET AILMENTS
Premenstrual syndrome
Menstrual irregularities
Symptoms of menopause
Prevention of miscarriage (in first three months of pregnancy only)
Promotion of lactation
Endometriosis (disorder of the uterine lining)
Fibroid cysts in smooth muscle tissue
Acne in both male and female teenagers (Note: Chaste tree should not be used with children unless prescribed by a healthcare practitioner knowledgeable about herbs.)

CHICKWEED

LATIN NAME
Stellaria media

C

VITAL STATISTICS

GENERAL DESCRIPTION

Rubbed on the body, this common weed is a good herb for relieving the discomfort of insect bites and other itchy skin conditions. The components of chickweed known as saponin glycosides exert a soothing effect on the skin. Taken internally, chickweed has a similar soothing and moistening effect on the lungs and stomach. Chickweed is high in vitamin C, and the fresh herb can be eaten raw in a salad or cooked as a green, as you would spinach. Juice squeezed from the leaves with a mortar and pestle is particularly effective in healing scalp problems when applied externally. Because it contains vitamin C, chickweed has been used as a remedy for scurvy.

PREPARATIONS

Over the counter:

Available in dried bulk, oil, ointment, and tincture.

At home:

TEA: Pour 1 cup boiling water onto 2 tsp dried herb; steep covered 5 minutes. Apply three times a day to reduce itching.

BATH: Pour fresh herbs or a strong infusion into bathwater to relieve itching.

COOL DRINK: Combine a handful of fresh herbs with pineapple juice, process in a blender, and strain. This drink may relieve skin irritation and rheumatism.

OINTMENT: Add marsh mallow root to the fresh herbs and juice, blend with petroleum jelly.

POULTICE: Grind up fresh leaves and apply to leg ulcers.

Consult a qualified practitioner for the dosage appropriate for you and the specific condition being treated.

PRECAUTIONS

POSSIBLE INTERACTIONS

Combining chickweed with other herbs may necessitate a lower dosage.

TARGET AILMENTS
Take internally for:
Rheumatism
Take internally as a tonic for:
Constipation
Fatigue; debility
Apply externally for:
Cuts
Wounds
Insect bites
Eczema, psoriasis, and other itchy skin irritations
Boils; abscesses; skin ulcers
Itchy scalp conditions

SIDE EFFECTS

NONE EXPECTED

CHICORY

LATIN NAME
Cichorium intybus

VITAL STATISTICS

GENERAL DESCRIPTION

Chicory flourishes both in gardens and in the wild, and it has been known to doctors at least as far back as the first century AD. Despite its many medicinal uses, chicory is often used as a food additive. The plant's leaves, like other green leafy vegetables, can be added to a salad or served by themselves, and the roasted and ground chicory root is a common addition to coffee in Europe as well as in the United States. Chicory added to coffee complements the popular drink, for experiments have shown that lactucin and lactucopicrin (two of the substances in chicory that make it taste somewhat bitter) may counteract the effects of caffeine by their sedative action on the central nervous system. Chicory is believed to be a laxative and is also said to increase the flow of bile. It may in addition be suitable for treating gout and rheumatism because it acts as a mild diuretic. Chicory leaves have also been used in compresses to treat skin inflammations and swellings.

PREPARATIONS

Over the counter:
Available as green leaves and dried roots.

At home:

TEA: Pour 1/2 cup boiling water over 1 tsp rootstock or dried herb; steep covered 10 minutes and strain. Drink 8 to 12 oz a day for jaundice and mild constipation.

NUTRITION AND DIET: Put chicory stem through a juicer; add 1 tbsp juice to milk or water and take three times a day. Use the fresh greens in a salad, or sauté them.

Consult a qualified practitioner for the dosage appropriate for you and the specific condition being treated.

PRECAUTIONS

SPECIAL INFORMATION

Chicory is best taken with a meal or at the end of a meal.

POSSIBLE INTERACTIONS

Combining chicory with other herbs may necessitate a lower dosage.

TARGET AILMENTS

Take internally for:

- Caffeine-induced rapid heartbeat
- Jaundice
- Mild constipation
- Rheumatism
- Gout

Apply externally for:

- Skin inflammations

SIDE EFFECTS

NOT SERIOUS

- Red, swollen, or irritated skin after handling chicory

COVER HANDS WITH GLOVES AND TREAT THE IRRITATED AREA AS NEEDED.

Chien Chin Chih Tai Wan

C

Vital Statistics

ENGLISH NAME
Thousand Gold Pieces Stop Vaginal Discharge Pills

PINYIN NAME
Qian Jin Zhi Dai Wan

GENERAL DESCRIPTION
Chien Chin Chih Tai Wan is a remedy commonly used to treat a number of gynecological conditions. It is basically for a woman whose body tends to be damp, as determined by a practitioner of Chinese medicine. Signs of dampness may include vaginal discharge, abdominal bloating, and a white tongue coating. Because the combined herbs help to smooth and regulate the menstrual cycle, this formula is often used to treat irregular or painful menstrual periods.

Chinese medicine takes a holistic approach to healthcare, fashioning remedies to treat the entire being as well as the specific parts or areas. Precise combinations of herbs are used to prevent and combat disease, which is thought to arise from disturbances in the flow of a bodily energy called chi (pronounced "chee") and blood, or from a lack of balance in the complementary states of yin and yang. Crucial to a practitioner's diagnosis is a careful examination of the tongue, considered a good barometer of the disharmonies in the body. A patent formula, *Chien Chin Chih Tai Wan* is made by using a standardized combination of herbs and method of preparation.

INGREDIENTS
dang gui, white atractylodes, fennel seed, corydalis, aucklandia, dipsacus, codonopsis, baked oyster shell, indigo

PREPARATIONS
This formula is available in pill form at many Chinese pharmacies and Oriental grocery stores.

TARGET AILMENTS

- White vaginal discharge
- Painful menstrual periods
- Irregular menstrual periods
- Amenorrhea (lack of menstruation)

SIDE EFFECTS
None expected

CHINA

LATIN NAME
China officinalis

VITAL STATISTICS

GENERAL DESCRIPTION
China, or Peruvian bark, comes from the dried bark of an evergreen tree found in South America. Beginning around the 17th century in Europe, *China* was used in extracts, infusions, and powders to treat various ailments, particularly malaria and fevers. In the early 1800s, pure quinine was extracted from the bark. Excessive use of quinine can have serious consequences. It can cause contractions of the uterus, bronchi, and spleen; nausea, headache, and ear and eye ailments; loss of protein through urine; and fever and sweating. These qualities make the homeopathic version of *China* useful in treating those with debilitating illness or an excessive loss of body fluids. People who suffer from diarrhea, vomiting, excessive sweating, or anemia can benefit from *China,* because the substance can accelerate their recovery time. *China* can also restore appetite in those who have none and relieve the exhaustion stemming from a prolonged illness.

For the homeopathic remedy, the bark is collected between May and November. It is first dried and ground into a powder, then mixed with alcohol and left to stand for eight days. After that, it is strained and filtered. When a patient exhibits a set of symptoms that matches the cataloged symptoms brought on by *China,* the homeopathic practitioner then prescribes it in an extremely dilute form. For more information on homeopathic medicine, see page 14.

PREPARATIONS
China is available in various potencies at selected stores and pharmacies. Consult your homeopathic practitioner for more precise information.

PRECAUTIONS

SPECIAL INFORMATION
- When a remedy is administered, no one but the patient should touch the pills. If tablets are spilled, throw them away.
- The mouth should be clear of flavors 15 minutes before and after taking a remedy, and strong flavors and aromas, such as coffee, camphor, and heavily scented perfumes, should be avoided for the duration of treatment.

TARGET AILMENTS

- Anemia
- Diarrhea
- Exhaustion associated with a long illness
- Flatulence
- Headache
- Hepatitis
- Indigestion
- Malaria
- Stomach bloating
- Vomiting

SIDE EFFECTS
NONE EXPECTED

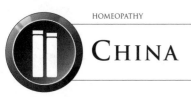

CHINESE FOXGLOVE ROOT

LATIN NAME
Rehmannia glutinosa

C

VITAL STATISTICS

GENERAL DESCRIPTION

Chinese foxglove root is commonly cooked in wine and used as a tonic for treating disorders associated with aging or dying. The herb is classified as cold and sweet when raw; cooked, it is characterized as warm and sweet.

Chinese medicine takes a holistic approach to healthcare, fashioning remedies to treat the entire being as well as the specific parts or areas. Single herbs may be used alone or in combination with other herbs to prevent and combat disease, which is thought to arise from disturbances in the flow of a bodily energy called chi (pronounced "chee") and blood, or from a lack of balance in the complementary states of yin and yang.

PREPARATIONS

Both raw and prepared Chinese foxglove root are available at Chinese pharmacies, Asian markets, and some Western health food stores.

COMBINATIONS: A mixture with gelatin is prescribed for coughing and vomiting blood, nosebleeds, and bleeding from the uterus. Practitioners also use combinations of the cooked root with cornus and Chinese yam, or with freshwater turtle shell, to treat lightheadedness, insomnia, forgetfulness, and related symptoms. See a practitioner for information on dosages and further herbal combinations.

PRECAUTIONS

WARNING

People with digestive problems or a tendency to develop gas or abdominal bloating should use this herb carefully; the cooked herb can distend the abdomen and cause loose stools.

SPECIAL INFORMATION

Grains-of-paradise fruit is often added to Chinese foxglove root to prevent side effects such as diarrhea, nausea, and abdominal pain.

TARGET AILMENTS

Take internally for:

Lightheadedness; palpitations; low back pain and weak knees; weak, stiff joints; premature graying of hair

Blurred vision or "floaters" in vision; hearing loss or tinnitus (ringing in the ears)

Insomnia or the inability to be still and restful; chronic low-grade fever; night sweats; hot flashes

Constipation with dry, hard stools; irregular menstruation or uterine bleeding, especially after childbirth

SIDE EFFECTS

NOT SERIOUS

- Diarrhea
- Nausea
- Abdominal pain

CALL YOUR DOCTOR IF THESE SYMPTOMS PERSIST OR BECOME TROUBLESOME.

Chinese Motherwort

LATIN NAME
Leonurus heterophyllus

Vital Statistics

GENERAL DESCRIPTION

In a literal translation of the Chinese name, *yì mu cao,* motherwort means "benefit mother herb." Indeed, the leaves of Chinese motherwort are popular among Chinese women as a treatment for menstrual difficulties. In traditional Chinese medicine, this herb is classified as acrid, bitter, and slightly cold.

Chinese medicine takes a holistic approach to healthcare, fashioning remedies to treat the entire being as well as the specific parts or areas. Single herbs may be used alone or in combination with other herbs to prevent and combat disease, which is thought to arise from disturbances in the flow of a bodily energy called chi (pronounced "chee") and blood, or from a lack of balance in the complementary states of yin and yang.

PREPARATIONS

Chinese motherwort is available as leaves or powder at Chinese pharmacies, Asian food markets, and some Western health food stores. When seeking the best variety, look for thin stems and pure green coloring.

COMBINATIONS: Chinese motherwort is often mixed with red peony root, dong quai, and aucklandia to regulate the appropriate timing of the menstrual cycle and alleviate the pain and discomfort of menstruation. Herbalists prescribe a combination with imperata to treat edema associated with the kidney disease nephritis. A mixture containing Chinese motherwort, polygonati, pyrrosia leaves, and musk mallow seeds is used to treat kidney stones and bloody urine. Check with a practitioner of Chinese medicine for information on dosages and additional herbal combinations.

Precautions

WARNING

Do not use Chinese motherwort if you are pregnant. In laboratory trials this herb has caused rabbits to miscarry.

TARGET AILMENTS

Take internally for:

- Irregular menstruation or light menstrual flow
- Premenstrual abdominal pain
- Uterine fibroids
- Postpartum abdominal pain
- Infertility
- Difficulty in urinating; edema (swelling), particularly if accompanied by blood in the urine

SIDE EFFECTS

NONE EXPECTED

C

CHINESE YAM

LATIN NAME
Dioscorea opposita

C

VITAL STATISTICS

GENERAL DESCRIPTION

Chinese yam, a thick, firm root with a white cross section, is used by practitioners of Chinese medicine as a tonic for treating a variety of conditions and ailments. Classified as neutral and sweet, the herb is harvested in the winter in the mountains of Hunan and in many other Chinese provinces.

Chinese medicine takes a holistic approach to healthcare, fashioning remedies to treat the entire being as well as the specific parts or areas. Single herbs may be used alone or in combination with other herbs to prevent and combat disease, which is thought to arise from disturbances in the flow of a bodily energy called chi (pronounced "chee") and blood, or from a lack of balance in the complementary states of yin and yang.

PREPARATIONS

Chinese yam is available as a fresh or dried vegetable in Chinese pharmacies, Asian food markets, and some Western health food stores. For symptoms of diabetes, drink a tea made by steeping slices of the fresh root in hot water.

COMBINATIONS: A mixture of Chinese yam, poria, and atractylodes (white) may be prescribed for loose, watery stools. A preparation of Chinese yam and codonopsis root is used to treat fatigue, general weakness, and reduced appetite. Consult a practitioner of Chinese medicine for information on dosages and other herbal combinations.

PRECAUTIONS

SPECIAL INFORMATION

If symptoms include abdominal swelling and pain, do not use Chinese yam.

POSSIBLE INTERACTIONS

Some practitioners warn against taking Chinese yam with kan-sui root.

TARGET AILMENTS

Take internally for:

- Weak digestion with diarrhea and fatigue
- Reduced appetite
- Frequent urination
- Excessive vaginal discharge
- Chronic coughing and wheezing
- Symptoms that accompany diabetes (such as weight loss, excessive urination)

SIDE EFFECTS

NONE EXPECTED

Ching Wan Hung

Vital Statistics

ENGLISH NAME
Capital Myriad Red

GENERAL DESCRIPTION
Ching Wan Hung is a topical ointment prescribed by practitioners of Chinese medicine to relieve pain, reduce inflammation, and promote regeneration of burned tissue. The formula is used to treat all kinds of burns, including sunburn and those caused by steam, hot water, flame, chemicals, and radiation therapy. The ointment is also used in the treatment of hemorrhoids.

Chinese medicine takes a holistic approach to healthcare, fashioning remedies to treat the entire being as well as the specific parts or areas. Precise combinations of herbs are used to prevent and combat disease, which is thought to arise from disturbances in the flow of a bodily energy called chi (pronounced "chee") and blood, or from a lack of balance in the complementary states of yin and yang. A patent formula, *Ching Wan Hung* is made by using a standardized combination of herbs and method of preparation.

INGREDIENTS
Chinese quince, burnet-bloodwort root, frankincense, Chinese lobelia, myrrh, safflower flower, dang gui, borneol camphor

PREPARATIONS
Ching Wan Hung ointment is sold by the tube or by the jar at many Chinese pharmacies and Oriental grocery stores.

Precautions

SPECIAL INFORMATION
- This formula should be used only for first- or second-degree burns with no infection.
- If the ointment is used with gauze dressing, the dressing should be changed daily.

TARGET AILMENTS

Sunburn and burns from steam, hot water, flame, hot oil, chemicals, and radiation therapy

Hemorrhoids

SIDE EFFECTS

None expected

Chin So Ku Ching

C

Vital Statistics

ENGLISH NAME
Metal Lock Pills to Stabilize the Essence

ALSO SOLD AS
Jin Suo Gu Jing Wan

GENERAL DESCRIPTION
Chin So Ku Ching is used in certain conditions to treat urinary incontinence, nocturnal emissions of semen, and impotence. According to practitioners of Chinese medicine, the formula stabilizes the lower abdomen by helping to prevent inappropriate loss of body fluids. The remedy is said to strengthen kidney function, which in Chinese medicine also involves the ears and hearing. For this reason, the formula is used to treat some kinds of tinnitus, or ringing in the ears.

Chinese medicine takes a holistic approach to healthcare, fashioning remedies to treat the entire being as well as the specific parts or areas. Precise combinations of herbs are used to prevent and combat disease, which is thought to arise from disturbances in the flow of a bodily energy called chi (pronounced "chee") and blood, or from a lack of balance in the complementary states of yin and yang. A patent formula, *Chin So Ku Ching* is made by using a standardized combination of herbs and method of preparation.

INGREDIENTS
astragalus seeds, euryale seeds, lotus stamen, cooked fossilized bones, cooked oyster shell, lotus seeds

PREPARATIONS
This formula is sold in pill form at many Chinese pharmacies and Oriental grocery stores.

Precautions

WARNING
This remedy should be used only for a person who has been diagnosed as cool and weak with a pale tongue. It should not be used if the tongue is red, or if the person has a urinary tract infection or conditions characterized as hot.

TARGET AILMENTS
Urinary incontinence
Nocturnal emissions of semen
Impotence
Tinnitus (ringing in the ears)
Weakness of the lower back

SIDE EFFECTS
None expected

CHITOSAN

VITAL STATISTICS

OTHER NAME
marine fiber

GENERAL DESCRIPTION
Chitosan is a fiber product made from the shells of oysters, crustaceans, and the exoskeletons of some insects. The substance effectively soaks up grease and other toxins in liquid. In fact, long before it gained recognition as a nutritional supplement, chitosan was used to remove impurities from drinking water. In the body, chitosan can add bulk to the stool for better digestive function, and it may help lower blood cholesterol levels, thereby reducing the risk of heart disease.

Chitosan has been hailed by some nutritionists and diet experts as a weight-loss wonder drug, surpassing plant fiber in its ability to collect and dispose of fatty deposits in the intestinal tract. Some proponents say that the substance also promotes blood clotting and, when used topically, fights staph infection in wounds. Other claims include its effectiveness in treating ulcers, fighting acne, and preventing tooth decay. However, chitosan's actual therapeutic benefits remain highly speculative.

NATURAL SOURCES
oysters, crabs, lobsters, shrimp, insects

PREPARATIONS
Available as capsules in select health food stores.

PRECAUTIONS

WARNING
Do not use chitosan if you are allergic to shellfish or if you are pregnant or breast-feeding.

SPECIAL INFORMATION
- Consult your doctor before using chitosan, since its benefits are still speculative.
- Do not give supplements to children under age two except upon a doctor's advice.
- Drink at least eight glasses of water a day when taking fiber supplements.

POSSIBLE INTERACTIONS
Chitosan works best for weight loss when taken just before a meal.

Taking any fiber supplement may interfere with the action of prescription and nonprescription drugs, other supplements, or herbal therapies. Consult your doctor for guidance.

TARGET AILMENTS
High cholesterol
Constipation
Obesity
High blood pressure

SIDE EFFECTS
NONE EXPECTED

Rx CHLORHEXIDINE

C

VITAL STATISTICS

DRUG CLASS
Antibiotics [Topical Antibiotics]

BRAND NAME
Peridex

OTHER DRUGS IN THIS SUBCLASS
Rx: mupirocin (for skin); combination of neomycin, polymyxin B, and hydrocortisone (antibiotic-corticosteroid for ears)
OTC: bacitracin, neomycin, polymyxin B

GENERAL DESCRIPTION
Chlorhexidine is used as an oral rinse in the treatment of gingivitis. By reducing the amount of bacteria in the mouth, the drug helps reduce inflammation (redness and swelling) and bleeding in the gums.

Topical antibiotics are used to prevent or clear up bacterial infections of the skin, ears, or gums. They should never be used interchangeably; drugs for the skin, for example, should not be applied to the ears or mouth. Each drug is effective against a specific group of bacteria. For more information, see Topical Antibiotics.

PRECAUTIONS

SPECIAL INFORMATION
- Check with your doctor if you notice no improvement after using this medication for two or three days.
- Prolonged use of a prescription topical antibiotic may result in fungal superinfection.
- The use of topical antibiotics increases the risk of kidney damage or hearing loss in people with impaired kidney function who are already taking nephrotoxic medicines.
- If you are pregnant or nursing, check with your doctor before using this drug.

TARGET AILMENTS
Gingivitis

SIDE EFFECTS

NOT SERIOUS
- Stained teeth
- Increased tartar
- Irritation on the inside of the mouth
- Temporary changes in your sense of taste

CALL YOUR DOCTOR IF THESE SYMPTOMS BECOME BOTHERSOME.

SERIOUS
- Anaphylactic reaction (nasal congestion, difficulty in breathing, rash, hives, facial swelling)

SEEK MEDICAL HELP IMMEDIATELY.

CHLORIDE

VITAL STATISTICS

GENERAL DESCRIPTION

A natural salt of the mineral chlorine, chloride works with sodium and potassium to help maintain the proper distribution and pH of all body fluids and encourage healthy nerve and muscle function. Independently, chloride contributes to digestion and to waste elimination. It is a key component of hydrochloric acid, one of the gastric juices that digest food.

Chloride deficiency is extremely rare and is usually due to illness.

EMDR

Adults: 750 mg

NATURAL SOURCES

A diet of unprocessed natural foods provides more than enough chloride for human health. Just a pinch of table salt contains about 250 mg, one-third of the RDA.

PRECAUTIONS

SPECIAL INFORMATION

- Excessive vomiting can reduce the stomach's chloride level, upsetting its pH balance and causing sweating, diarrhea, loss of appetite, slow and shallow breathing, listlessness, and muscle cramps.
- Although toxic in large amounts, excess chloride is excreted in urine, preventing potentially dangerous accumulation.

TARGET AILMENTS

Hypochlorhydria (low stomach acid) (given as a supplement)

Dehydration

SIDE EFFECTS

NONE EXPECTED

CHOLESTEROL-REDUCING DRUGS

C

VITAL STATISTICS

GENERIC NAMES

cholestyramine, colestipol, fluvastatin, gemfibrozil, lovastatin, niacin, pravastatin, simvastatin

GENERAL DESCRIPTION

As their name suggests, cholesterol-reducing drugs are used to alter levels of cholesterol and other fats in the blood. These fats combine with proteins to form lipoproteins. It has been shown that high levels of low-density lipoprotein (LDL) cholesterol increase the risk of heart disease, whereas high levels of high-density lipoprotein (HDL) seem to protect against it. These drugs help both to reduce the "bad" LDL cholesterol and to raise the "good" HDL cholesterol.

Cholesterol-reducing drugs are usually prescribed only after diet modification has failed to lower blood cholesterol levels. The medicines serve as a supplement to a proper diet and exercise program. They will not cure cholesterol disorders, but they do help to control them. No one drug is appropriate for treating all cholesterol disorders.

There are four major groups of cholesterol-reducing drugs: antihyperlipidemic (gemfibrozil); HMG-CoA reductase inhibitors (fluvastatin, lovastatin, pravastatin, simvastatin); bile-acid-binding resins (cholestyramine, colestipol); and niacin.

The drugs work alone or in carefully prescribed combinations to normalize blood lipid levels. Some work by inhibiting the synthesis of cholesterol and lipoproteins. Others accelerate the clearance of lipoproteins in the bloodstream or hasten their breakdown and elimination. For more information, see the entries for the generic drugs listed above.

PRECAUTIONS

SPECIAL INFORMATION

- If you are pregnant or nursing, check with your doctor before using any of these drugs. Fluvastatin, lovastatin, pravastatin, and simvastatin are not recommended if you are nursing, pregnant, or planning to become pregnant.
- Do not use any of these drugs if you have had an allergic reaction to them in the past.
- Do not use these drugs without telling your physician if you have or have had impaired liver or kidney function, gallstones or gallbladder disease, peptic ulcers, bleeding disorders, allergies, alcohol abuse, convulsions, organ transplants, cataracts or visual problems, chronic muscular disorder, gout or diabetes, low blood pressure, constipation, major surgery (or plan surgery soon), or any other medical problem.
- Carefully follow the special diet your doctor has recommended: This is essential if the medication is to work effectively.
- See your doctor regularly to have your progress measured and monitored.

- Do not stop taking the medication without first checking with your doctor; your blood cholesterol levels may increase again.
- Cholesterol-reducing drugs may affect the results of laboratory tests. Be sure to inform the healthcare practitioner performing the test if you are taking any of these drugs.
- Before undergoing emergency treatment or medical or dental surgery, be sure to tell your healthcare practitioner if you are taking any of these drugs.

POSSIBLE INTERACTIONS

Anticoagulants (such as warfarin): increased or decreased blood-thinning effects.

Oral medications: cholestyramine and colestipol interfere with the absorption of nearly every other drug, as well as with vitamins A, D, E, and K. Be sure to take your other medications at different times of the day.

TARGET AILMENTS

The major types of cholesterol disorders, particularly those in which high levels of blood fats (cholesterol and triglycerides) have been linked to an increased risk of heart disease

SIDE EFFECTS

NOT SERIOUS

- Mild stomach pain
- Diarrhea
- Heartburn
- Nausea and vomiting
- Dizziness
- Headache

CALL YOUR DOCTOR IF THESE EFFECTS BECOME BOTHERSOME.

SERIOUS

- Severe stomach pain with nausea and vomiting
- Unusual fatigue or weakness

CALL YOUR DOCTOR RIGHT AWAY.

Cholestyramine

C

Vital Statistics

DRUG CLASS
Cholesterol-Reducing Drugs

BRAND NAME
Questran

OTHER DRUGS IN THIS CLASS
colestipol, fluvastatin, gemfibrozil, lovastatin, niacin, pravastatin, simvastatin

GENERAL DESCRIPTION
Introduced in 1959, cholestyramine is in the group of medicines known as bile-acid-binding resins. These drugs lower blood levels of cholesterol by binding to the bile acids from which cholesterol is made and removing them from the body. For more information, see Cholesterol-Reducing Drugs.

Precautions

SPECIAL INFORMATION
- Never take cholestyramine in dry form, as it may cause you to choke. Mix powder as directed with water or fruit juice.
- Do not use this drug if you have had an allergic reaction to it in the past.
- Cholestyramine may interfere with your body's ability to absorb certain nutrients. While on this medication, you may need to take supplements of vitamins A, D, E, and K; folic acid; and calcium. Consult your doctor.

POSSIBLE INTERACTIONS
Other medications should be taken two hours before or four to six hours after taking cholestyramine.

Target Ailments

The major types of cholesterol disorders

Side Effects

Not Serious
- Belching
- Bloating
- Mild stomach pain
- Diarrhea
- Heartburn
- Nausea and vomiting

Call your doctor if these effects persist or become bothersome.

Serious
- Constipation
- Weight loss
- Black, tarry stools

Call your doctor.

Chondroitin Sulfate

Vital Statistics

GENERAL DESCRIPTION
Chondroitin sulfate is a complex carbohydrate that is produced naturally in the bodies of all mammals, including humans, and in parts of oysters and mussels. Most people have no need for additional amounts of the substance. But some, including individuals with weak bones or joints, heart problems, or arthritis, may benefit from supplements because chondroitin sulfate is thought to be an effective blood thinner and cell rejuvenator. A number of researchers think chondroitin sulfate can reduce the risk of blood clots and may help strengthen artery walls, bones, and joints. Some evidence suggests that chondroitin sulfate has antiviral properties as well.

A variety of claims have been made about chondroitin sulfate; it has been hailed as an effective antiaging drug, for example, and even as a mild aphrodisiac. So far, however, there is little scientific evidence that the substance has any real therapeutic effect.

NATURAL SOURCES
mussels, oysters, meat from mammals

PREPARATIONS
Chondroitin sulfate is available in capsule form at many health food stores.

Precautions

WARNING
Do not take chondroitin sulfate if you are pregnant, planning a pregnancy, or breastfeeding.

If you are taking anticoagulant drugs or have a blood-clotting disorder, consult your doctor before taking chondroitin sulfate.

Do not give this supplement to children under two years of age except upon the advice of a doctor.

SPECIAL INFORMATION
No standard recommended dosage has been determined for chondroitin sulfate. Consult your doctor for dosages.

POSSIBLE INTERACTIONS
Taking chondroitin sulfate may interfere with the action of prescription and nonprescription drugs, other supplements, or herbal therapies. Consult your doctor for guidance.

TARGET AILMENTS
Joint problems; weak cartilage; headache
Respiratory ailments; allergies
Arthritis; bursitis

SIDE EFFECTS

None expected

Chromium

C

Vital Statistics

GENERAL DESCRIPTION
As a component of a natural substance called glucose tolerance factor, chromium works with insulin to regulate the body's use of sugar and is essential to fatty-acid metabolism. Its contribution to metabolism makes chromium a helpful supplement in weight-loss programs.

Supplemental chromium may be used to treat some cases of adult-onset diabetes, to reduce insulin requirements of some diabetic children, and to relieve symptoms of hypoglycemia.

Inadequate chromium can result in alcohol intolerance, cause variable, inconsistent blood sugar levels, and possibly induce diabetes-like symptoms such as tingling in the extremities and reduced muscle coordination, or hypoglycemic symptoms such as fatigue and dizziness.

In addition, because chromium lowers cholesterol and triglyceride levels in both diabetic and nondiabetic subjects, deficiencies may result in an increased risk of atherosclerosis or cardiovascular disease.

EMDR
Adults: 50 mcg to 200 mcg

NATURAL SOURCES
Trace amounts of chromium are found in many foods, including brewer's yeast, liver, lean meats, poultry, molasses, whole grains, eggs, and cheese.

Precautions

WARNING
Taken regularly in supplements greater than 1,000 mcg, chromium inhibits insulin's activity and can be toxic to the liver and kidneys.

SPECIAL INFORMATION
Chromium is not absorbed well, so the body uses only a small portion of what is taken in through diet. Most people do not get enough dietary chromium, and some may benefit from a multinutrient supplement, such as chromium citrate or chromium picolinate. Nevertheless, care should be taken to avoid supplementing beyond the EMDR.

TARGET AILMENTS
Diabetes
Heart disease
Hypoglycemia
Alcoholism

SIDE EFFECTS

NONE EXPECTED

Chrysanthemum Flower

LATIN NAME
Chrysanthemum indicum

Vital Statistics

GENERAL DESCRIPTION

The wild chrysanthemum, found throughout China, is valued for its anti-inflammatory and antibiotic effects. The best flowers for medicinal purposes are yellow and fragrant and have an acrid, bitter taste. In traditional Chinese medicine, this herb is characterized as acrid, bitter, and slightly cold. It is harvested in the fall, when the flowers bloom.

Chinese medicine takes a holistic approach to healthcare, fashioning remedies to treat the entire being as well as the specific parts or areas. Single herbs may be used alone or in combination with other herbs to prevent and combat disease, which is thought to arise from disturbances in the flow of a bodily energy called chi (pronounced "chee") and blood, or from a lack of balance in the complementary states of yin and yang.

PREPARATIONS

Dried flowers are available in bulk at Chinese pharmacies, Asian food markets, and some Western health food stores.

COMBINATIONS: Chrysanthemum flower mixed with honeysuckle flowers and other herbs is a formula for colds and flu. This herb combined with prunella and white mulberry leaf is prescribed for painful, red, swollen eyes. A mixture of chrysanthemum flower and honeysuckle is taken for red, swollen, and painful sores. Modern practitioners use a blend containing chrysanthemum, honeysuckle, and dandelion to treat high blood pressure. Check with a practitioner of Chinese medicine for details about dosages and additional herbal combinations.

Precautions

SPECIAL INFORMATION

Use chrysanthemum flower cautiously if you have diarrhea; in some cases the herb can make the problem worse.

TARGET AILMENTS
Take internally for:
Headache
Dizziness
Hearing problems
Hypertension (high blood pressure)
Apply externally as a compress or wash for:
Conjunctivitis
Red or dry eyes
Blurred vision; spots in front of the eyes

SIDE EFFECTS

NONE EXPECTED

Chuan Qiong Cha Tiao Wan

Vital Statistics

ENGLISH NAME
Ligusticum Chuanxiong Pills to Be Taken with Green Tea

ALSO SOLD AS
Chuan Xiong Cha Tiao Wan

GENERAL DESCRIPTION
The Chinese patent formula *Chuan Qiong Cha Tiao Wan* is strictly used for headaches that are brought about by weather changes, for headaches with sinus congestion, or for headaches accompanied by chills, fever, and a stuffy nose. *Chuan Qiong Cha Tiao Wan* is traditionally taken with green tea, though it can be taken alone or with water.

Chinese medicine takes a holistic approach to healthcare, fashioning remedies to treat the entire being as well as the specific parts or areas. Precise combinations of herbs are used to prevent and combat disease, which is thought to arise from disturbances in the flow of a bodily energy called chi (pronounced "chee") and blood, or from a lack of balance in the complementary states of yin and yang. *Chuan Qiong Cha Tiao Wan* is made by using a standardized combination of herbs and method of preparation.

INGREDIENTS
mint, ligusticum, schizonepeta, ledebouriella, notopterygium, angelica, licorice, Chinese wild ginger

PREPARATIONS
This formula may be found in Chinese pharmacies and Asian food markets.

Precautions

WARNING
Do not use for any kinds of headaches other than those listed below.

TARGET AILMENTS

- Headache with weather changes
- Headache with sinusitis
- Headache with chills, fever, and stuffy nose

SIDE EFFECTS
None expected

CICADA

LATIN NAME
Cryptotympana atrata

C

VITAL STATISTICS

GENERAL DESCRIPTION
A winged insect with a large head, the cicada is recognized by its characteristic chirping sound. The molted skin of the creature is used as a treatment for skin rashes, sore throats, and other ailments. In traditional Chinese medicine cicada is characterized as sweet and slightly cold.

Chinese medicine takes a holistic approach to healthcare, fashioning remedies to treat the entire being as well as the specific parts or areas. Single herbs may be used alone or in combination with other herbs to prevent and combat disease, which is thought to arise from disturbances in the flow of a bodily energy called chi (pronounced "chee") and blood, or from a lack of balance in the complementary states of yin and yang.

PREPARATIONS
Dried cicada can be obtained at Chinese pharmacies. Look for yellow, lightweight skins.

COMBINATIONS: A blend with field mint is prescribed to ease itchy, red eyes and also to bring the rash out in the early stage of measles, to help shorten the duration of the illness. Herbalists may add chrysanthemum flowers *(Chrysanthemum morifolium)* and white mulberry leaves to strengthen the mixture's fever-reducing qualities. Another treatment for the early stage of measles is a blend of cicada skins with kudzu root and great burdock fruit. A preparation containing cicada skins and sterculia seeds may be prescribed for hoarseness. Check with a Chinese medicine practitioner for details of dosages and other herbal combinations.

PRECAUTIONS

WARNING
Be careful about using cicada if you are pregnant, because it might induce a miscarriage. Check with a Chinese herbalist before using.

TARGET AILMENTS
Take internally for:
Swollen, sore throat with loss of voice
Skin rashes, particularly during the early stage of measles or chickenpox
Red, painful, swollen eyes and blurred vision
High fever in childhood illnesses such as measles, which can cause convulsions, spasms, delirium, and terrifying nightmares in children

SIDE EFFECTS
NONE EXPECTED

Rx CIMETIDINE

C

VITAL STATISTICS

DRUG CLASS
Antiulcer Drugs [Histamine H_2 Blockers]

BRAND NAMES
Rx: Tagamet
OTC: Tagamet HB

OTHER DRUGS IN THIS CLASS
lansoprazole, omeprazole, sucralfate
Histamine H_2 blockers: famotidine, nizatidine, ranitidine

GENERAL DESCRIPTION
Cimetidine is used both to treat and to prevent ulcers of the stomach and duodenum (upper intestine). It is also prescribed for other conditions characterized by an overproduction of stomach acid, such as Zollinger-Ellison syndrome and gastroesophageal reflux (in which stomach acid flows backward into the esophagus). In some cases, cimetidine is used to help stop upper gastrointestinal bleeding.

In the over-the-counter form, cimetidine is used not for ulcers but to relieve acid indigestion and heartburn. Although the OTC version is a lower dose of cimetidine than the prescription form, essentially the same interactions apply, though the side effects are milder.

Like other histamine H_2 blockers, cimetidine works by blocking the stomach's response to the chemical compound histamine, thereby reducing the secretion of the digestive juice hydrochloric acid. For more information on side effects and possible drug interactions, see Antiulcer Drugs. For visual characteristics of cimetidine and the brand-name drug Tagamet, see the Color Guide to Prescription Drugs and Herbs.

PRECAUTIONS

SPECIAL INFORMATION
- Inform your doctor if you have a history of arthritis, kidney or liver disease, organic brain syndrome, asthma, or low sperm count.
- Avoid this drug if you are pregnant or nursing.
- Cimetidine may affect the results of some medical tests, including blood cholesterol levels, liver function tests, and sperm counts. Inform the person giving you the test that you are taking this medication.
- This drug may inhibit your body's ability to absorb vitamin B_{12}. Talk to your doctor about B_{12} supplements.

TARGET AILMENTS
Duodenal ulcer
Gastric ulcer
Upper gastrointestinal bleeding associated with gastric ulcer or duodenal ulcer, or with gastritis
Zollinger-Ellison syndrome
Multiple endocrine neoplasia
Other conditions characterized by an overproduction of stomach acid
Gastroesophageal reflux
Acid indigestion and heartburn (OTC)

CIMETIDINE

POSSIBLE INTERACTIONS

This drug interacts with many prescription and over-the-counter medications, some of which are listed here. Make sure you inform your doctor of any other drugs you may be taking.

Alcohol: cimetidine may interfere with the elimination of alcohol from the body, prolonging alcohol's intoxicating effects.

Antacids: blocked absorption of cimetidine; space dosages of cimetidine and antacids at least an hour apart.

Anticoagulants (such as warfarin), oral antidiabetic drugs, benzodiazepines, calcium channel blockers (such as amlodipine and diltiazem), carbamazepine, cyclosporine, lidocaine, metoprolol, pentoxifylline, phenytoin, procainamide, propranolol, quinidine, theophylline, triamterene, tricyclic antidepressants: increased effects of these drugs, possibly leading to toxicity.

Carmustine: increased risk of blood disorders.

Enteric-coated tablets: changes in stomach acidity may cause these drugs to dissolve prematurely in the stomach; avoid taking enteric-coated medications with cimetidine.

Itraconazole, ketoconazole, tetracycline: decreased absorption of these drugs into the body.

Sucralfate: decreased absorption of cimetidine.

Tobacco (smoking): may block the beneficial effects of cimetidine.

SIDE EFFECTS

NOT SERIOUS

- Mild diarrhea
- Mild skin rash or hives
- Dizziness
- Headache
- Blurred vision
- Fatigue
- Muscle and joint pain

CONTACT YOUR DOCTOR IF THESE SYMPTOMS CONTINUE OR BECOME BOTHERSOME.

SERIOUS

- Confusion
- Nervousness
- Delirium and hallucinations
- Slowed or irregular heartbeat
- Abnormal bleeding or bruising
- Combined weakness, fever, and sore throat (signs of bone marrow depression)
- Hair loss
- Rash
- Enlarged or painful breasts (in women or men)
- Male impotence
- Jaundice

CALL YOUR DOCTOR IMMEDIATELY.

CIMICIFUGA

LATIN NAME
Cimicifuga foetida (or Cimicifuga dahurica)

C

VITAL STATISTICS

GENERAL DESCRIPTION

Commonly known as bugbane, cimicifuga has medicinal properties in the root, which should have a black skin without rootlets. The Chinese name of this herb literally translated means "ascending hemp," an allusion to its alleged ability to lift the patient's energy level. Depending on the species of cimicifuga, the cross section of the root is white, light green, or gray. Chinese herbalists, following traditional medical practice, characterize cimicifuga as acrid, sweet, and cool.

Chinese medicine takes a holistic approach to healthcare, fashioning remedies to treat the entire being as well as the specific parts or areas. Single herbs may be used alone or in combination with other herbs to prevent and combat disease, which is thought to arise from disturbances in the flow of a bodily energy called chi (pronounced "chee") and blood, or from a lack of balance in the complementary states of yin and yang.

PREPARATIONS

Cimicifuga is available in dried form at Chinese pharmacies, Asian food markets, and some Western health food stores.

COMBINATIONS: When it is combined with great burdock fruit and indigo, the blend brings out skin rashes, such as those that accompany measles. This action helps the disease run its course faster. A mixture with coptis is prescribed for swollen gums, toothache, and ulcers of the mouth and tongue. It is taken internally and also rubbed on the affected areas. Together with bupleurum it is used to treat prolapses of internal organs, and also diarrhea. A Chinese medicine practitioner can provide details of dosages and additional herbal combinations.

PRECAUTIONS

☠ *WARNING*

Although cimicifuga effectively brings out the skin rash caused by measles in its early stage, the herb should not be used when the disease is fully developed.

This herb should not be taken by patients with breathing difficulties.

SPECIAL INFORMATION

Beware of taking too much cimicifuga; it may cause headaches, vomiting, tremors, and gastroenteritis. If you develop these symptoms, discontinue use and call your doctor or Chinese herbalist.

TARGET AILMENTS

Take internally for:

- Skin rashes, including those of measles
- Headache accompanying measles
- Sore teeth and gums, canker sores, and sore throats
- Prolapse (dropping) of the uterus, rectum, or bladder

SIDE EFFECTS

NONE EXPECTED

CINNAMON BARK

LATIN NAME
Cinnamomum cassia

VITAL STATISTICS

GENERAL DESCRIPTION

A popular stimulant in Chinese medicine, cinnamon is harvested from trees usually after they have reached seven years of age. Its outer bark is the common spice; the inner bark contains more oil and has stronger medicinal effects. Cinnamon bark is used to treat abdominal disorders, menstrual pain, infertility, and some forms of asthma. In a clinical trial, an alcohol-based preparation of the bark, injected at an acupuncture point associated with the lung, seemed to have a beneficial effect on bronchial asthma. Cinnamaldehyde, a major constituent of cinnamon bark, has shown tranquilizing and pain-relieving effects in mice. Characterized as hot, acrid, and sweet according to traditional Chinese medicine, the best quality has a thick skin and is oily and fragrant.

Chinese medicine takes a holistic approach to healthcare, fashioning remedies to treat the entire being as well as the specific parts or areas. Single herbs may be used alone or in combination with other herbs to prevent and combat disease, which is thought to arise from disturbances in the flow of a bodily energy called chi (pronounced "chee") and blood, or from a lack of balance in the complementary states of yin and yang.

PREPARATIONS

Cinnamon bark is available at Chinese pharmacies, Asian food markets, and some Western health food stores. It is normally taken in the form of powder, pill, or tincture, in which the crushed bark is mixed with alcohol.

COMBINATIONS: Chinese herbalists prescribe cinnamon bark together with the roots of Asian ginseng and Chinese foxglove cooked in wine to treat palpitations of the heart and shortness of breath. A Chinese medicine practitioner can advise you on dosages and additional herbal combinations.

PRECAUTIONS

SPECIAL INFORMATION

- Large doses of cinnamon bark can cause changes in breathing, dilation of blood vessels, and convulsions. If you develop these symptoms, discontinue use and call your doctor.
- Use this herb cautiously if you are pregnant.
- Do not use the herb if you have a fever or an inflammation or are hemorrhaging.

TARGET AILMENTS

- Poor digestion; diarrhea with undigested food; lack of appetite
- Abdominal spasms; excessive urination
- Impotence; lack of sexual desire
- Menstrual pain; lack of menstruation
- Infertility
- Wheezing from asthma caused by exposure to cold

SIDE EFFECTS

NONE EXPECTED

CINNAMON TWIG

LATIN NAME
Cinnamomum cassia

C

VITAL STATISTICS

GENERAL DESCRIPTION

Cinnamon twigs, sometimes called cassia twigs, are prescribed for colds, influenza, arthritis, and minor gynecological problems. Preparations of cinnamon twig have shown a possible antibiotic effect against organisms such as staphylococcus and salmonella. The herb is considered a diuretic.

Cinnamon twigs of good quality can be discerned by their strong fragrance and brownish red color. While this herb has many properties in common with cinnamon bark, Chinese herbalists use each part of the plant to treat a different set of ailments. Cinnamon twigs are characterized in traditional Chinese medicine as warm, acrid, and sweet.

Chinese medicine takes a holistic approach to healthcare, fashioning remedies to treat the entire being as well as the specific parts or areas. Single herbs may be used alone or in combination with other herbs to prevent and combat disease, which is thought to arise from disturbances in the flow of a bodily energy called chi (pronounced "chee") and blood, or from a lack of balance in the complementary states of yin and yang.

PREPARATIONS

Cinnamon twigs can be purchased in Chinese pharmacies, Asian markets, and some Western health food stores.

COMBINATIONS: A preparation containing cinnamon twigs and licorice that has been fried with honey is recommended by Chinese herbalists for palpitations and shortness of breath. When mixed with evodia fruit, the herb is prescribed for abdominal pain and menstrual disorders. Consult a Chinese medicine practitioner about dosages and additional herbal combinations.

PRECAUTIONS

WARNING

Do not use the herb to treat cases of influenza with high fever.

SPECIAL INFORMATION

Be careful about using cinnamon twigs if you are pregnant or if you menstruate heavily, because they may cause more bleeding or difficulties with the pregnancy.

TARGET AILMENTS
Take internally for:
Colds, influenza, and low-grade fever accompanied by chills
Arthritis
Rheumatism
Gynecological problems, such as painful menstruation or uterine fibroids

SIDE EFFECTS

NONE EXPECTED

CIPRO

VITAL STATISTICS

DRUG CLASS
Antibiotics [Fluoroquinolones]

GENERIC NAME
ciprofloxacin

GENERAL DESCRIPTION
Cipro is a brand name for the generic drug ciprofloxacin. Introduced in 1984, ciprofloxacin is a synthetic fluoroquinolone that is used to treat a number of infections, including bone and joint infections, and genital ulcers caused by *Hemophilus ducreyi*. For visual characteristics of Cipro, see the Color Guide to Prescription Drugs and Herbs. For more information, see Fluoroquinolones.

TARGET AILMENTS
Diarrhea
Infectious diarrhea
Pneumonia
Infections of the skin, soft tissues, or bone
Urinary tract infections

SIDE EFFECTS
SEE FLUOROQUINOLONES.

PRECAUTIONS

SPECIAL INFORMATION
Cipro may be taken with meals (to prevent stomach upset); food does not affect overall absorption of the drug.

POSSIBLE INTERACTIONS
Alkalizers (urinary), such as sodium bicarbonate, and citrates: these drugs reduce the solubility of Cipro in urine and can, in rare instances, lead to crystalluria (crystals in urine) or kidney toxicity.
Antacids, didanosine (antiviral), ferrous sulfate, laxatives containing magnesium, sucralfate (antiulcer), zinc: reduced fluoroquinolone effect. Take Cipro at least two hours before or six hours after taking any of these medications.
Cyclosporine (immunosuppressant): increased blood levels of cyclosporine. Your doctor may have to adjust your dose of cyclosporine.
Phenytoin (anticonvulsant): reduced phenytoin levels and effectiveness.
Theophyllines (asthma drugs): Cipro may inhibit metabolism of these drugs, increasing the risk of adverse effects and theophylline toxicity.

CISAPRIDE

C

VITAL STATISTICS

DRUG CLASS
Antigastroesophageal Reflux Drugs

BRAND NAME
Propulsid

GENERAL DESCRIPTION
Cisapride is used to treat gastroesophageal reflux disease, a digestive disorder in which the contents of the stomach flow back up into the esophagus. The drug stimulates release of the neurotransmitter acetylcholine in the gastrointestinal tract, resulting in a strengthening of the lower esophageal sphincter and thus inhibiting backflow. Cisapride also accelerates the emptying of food from the stomach into the intestines. For visual characteristics of Propulsid, a brand name for the generic drug cisapride, see the Color Guide to Prescription Drugs and Herbs. For more information, including possible drug interactions and additional side effects, see Antigastroesophageal Reflux Drugs.

PRECAUTIONS

SPECIAL INFORMATION
- Do not take this drug if you have intestinal or stomach bleeding, obstruction of the bowel, or any other gastrointestinal problem.
- Do not take this drug if you have epilepsy or a history of seizures.
- Weigh the benefit-to-risk ratio with your doctor if you are pregnant or are considering pregnancy. If you are nursing, discuss use of this drug with your doctor, since low levels of cisapride pass into breast milk.
- Inform your doctor if you have a history of liver, kidney, or heart problems.
- Do not take cisapride if you are taking ketoconazole, troleandomycin, or itraconazole.
- Take this medication at least 15 minutes before meals and at bedtime.

POSSIBLE INTERACTIONS
Alcohol and benzodiazepines: increased absorption of these drugs, causing increased sedation.

TARGET AILMENTS

Heartburn and acid indigestion caused by gastroesophageal reflux disease

SIDE EFFECTS

NOT SERIOUS
- Diarrhea or constipation
- Abdominal discomfort
- Runny nose (rhinitis)
- Nausea
- Fatigue; drowsiness
- Headache; dizziness
- Dry mouth; sore throat
- Muscle or joint pain
- Nervousness
- Frequent urination

CONSULT YOUR DOCTOR IF THESE SYMPTOMS PERSIST.

SERIOUS
- Tremors; heart palpitations
- Visual changes; severe stomach pain
- Hepatitis; migraines
- Swelling of the legs or feet

CALL YOUR DOCTOR PROMPTLY.

Clarithromycin

Vital Statistics

DRUG CLASS
Antibiotics [Erythromycins]

BRAND NAME
Biaxin

OTHER DRUGS IN THIS SUBCLASS
azithromycin, erythromycin

GENERAL DESCRIPTION
Clarithromycin is a type of erythromycin but has fewer side effects than other drugs in that class. Clarithromycin's action varies with the type of bacteria it is used to fight; it kills some and stops the growth and reproduction of others. This drug may be used to treat respiratory tract infections, including sinusitis, pharyngitis due to strep, tonsillitis, bronchitis, and some types of pneumonia as well as skin infections and AIDS-related infections due to *Mycobacterium avium* or *Mycobacterium intracellulare.*

Precautions

SPECIAL INFORMATION
- Some infections may require 14 days of treatment. Take the full course to prevent bacteria from becoming resistant to the medicine.
- Tell your doctor if your kidneys or liver is impaired. You may need to have your dose adjusted.
- Let your doctor know if you are allergic to erythromycin, azithromycin, or troleandomycin, because you may also be allergic to this drug.
- Do not use clarithromycin during pregnancy unless clearly needed. Avoid using this drug while nursing.

POSSIBLE INTERACTIONS
See Erythromycin for other possible interactions.
Astemizole: WARNING: risk of life-threatening heart problems. Do not take with clarithromycin.
Rifabutin: decreased clarithromycin effect.
Terfenadine: WARNING: risk of life-threatening heart problems. Do not take with clarithromycin.
Zidovudine: decreased zidovudine effect.

TARGET AILMENTS

Respiratory tract infections

Infections of the skin and soft tissue

SIDE EFFECTS

NOT SERIOUS
- An unusual taste in the mouth
- Abdominal pain; headache
- Mild diarrhea; nausea
- Yeast infections

CONSULT YOUR DOCTOR IF SYMPTOMS ARE PROLONGED OR BOTHERSOME.

SERIOUS
- Unusual bleeding or bruising
- Rash; vomiting
- Diarrhea that lasts more than 24 hours, cramps, fever (inflammation of the colon)

DISCONTINUE USE AND CALL YOUR DOCTOR IMMEDIATELY.

C

Rx CLARITIN

C

VITAL STATISTICS

DRUG CLASS
Antihistamines

GENERIC NAME
loratadine

OTHER DRUGS IN THIS CLASS
Rx: astemizole, cetirizine, diphenhydramine, fexofenadine, promethazine, terfenadine
OTC: brompheniramine, chlorpheniramine, clemastine, dexbrompheniramine, diphenhydramine, doxylamine, triprolidine

GENERAL DESCRIPTION
Claritin is the brand name for loratadine, a newer, relatively nonsedating antihistamine commonly prescribed for seasonal allergies. It generally doesn't cause the drowsiness, jitters, or dry mouth associated with other drugs of its kind. See Antihistamines for additional precautions, side effects, and interaction information. For visual characteristics, see the Color Guide to Prescription Drugs and Herbs.

PRECAUTIONS

SPECIAL INFORMATION
- If your liver is impaired, this medication can build up in your body and provoke serious heart problems. Depending on the severity of your liver condition, your doctor may prescribe a different antihistamine.
- Check with your doctor before using Claritin if you have asthma, liver disease, or kidney disease; loratadine may exacerbate these conditions.
- Let your doctor know if you are pregnant or breast-feeding. Your doctor may advise you to stop using Claritin or to stop breast-feeding while you're using the drug.
- Claritin may be prescribed for children over six years of age.

POSSIBLE INTERACTIONS
Azithromycin, cimetidine, clarithromycin, erythromycin, itraconazole, ketoconazole, ranitidine, theophylline, and troleandomycin: may interfere with the body's metabolism of loratadine, possibly causing life-threatening cardiac effects.

TARGET AILMENTS

Nasal and respiratory allergies, including hay fever

SIDE EFFECTS

NOT SERIOUS
- Sedation
- Insomnia
- Dry nose, mouth, or throat

CALL YOUR DOCTOR IF THESE SYMPTOMS CONTINUE.

SERIOUS
- Fainting
- Heart palpitations or change in heartbeat

CALL YOUR DOCTOR RIGHT AWAY. THESE EFFECTS ARE RARE BUT MAY OCCUR IF PROPER DOSAGE IS EXCEEDED OR IF YOU HAVE LIVER DAMAGE.

CLARITIN-D

VITAL STATISTICS

DRUG CLASS
Antihistamines; Decongestants

GENERIC NAME
loratadine and pseudoephedrine (combination)

BRAND NAMES
Claritin-D 12 Hour, Claritin-D 24 Hour

OTHER DRUGS IN THIS CLASS
Rx: astemizole, cetirizine, diphenhydramine, fexofenadine, promethazine, terfenadine
OTC: brompheniramine, chlorpheniramine, clemastine, dexbrompheniramine, diphenhydramine, doxylamine, triprolidine

GENERAL DESCRIPTION
The brand-name drugs Claritin-D 12 Hour and Claritin-D 24 Hour are formulas that combine an antihistamine and a decongestant. They are prescribed to relieve the symptoms of seasonal allergies, including sneezing, runny nose, nasal congestion, itching, and watery eyes. The antihistamine ingredient is loratadine, a new and relatively nonsedating medication; and the decongestant in Claritin-D is pseudoephedrine. Claritin-D generally doesn't cause the drowsiness, jitters, or dry mouth associated with antihistamines. For visual characteristics of Claritin-D 12 Hour, see the Color Guide to Prescription Drugs and Herbs.

PRECAUTIONS

SPECIAL INFORMATION

- If your liver is impaired, loratadine can build up in your body and provoke serious heart problems. Depending on the severity of your liver condition, your doctor may prescribe a different antihistamine.
- Check with your doctor before taking Claritin-D if you have asthma, liver disease, kidney disease, cardiovascular disease (including angina, coronary artery disease, and hypertension), hyperthyroidism (overactive thyroid), prostate enlargement, diabetes, or glaucoma; this drug may exacerbate these conditions.
- Let your doctor know if you are pregnant or breast-feeding. Your doctor may advise you to stop using Claritin-D or to stop breast-feeding while you're using this drug.
- This medication may cause palpitations, fainting, cardiac arrest, or other serious disorders if taken in dosages that are even slightly higher than those recommended. Follow the dosage instructions carefully.
- Do not use Claritin-D with other over-the-counter decongestants or antihistamines.
- Do not take Claritin-D within 14 days of taking a monoamine oxidase (MAO) inhibitor. The combination may lead to hypertensive crisis and heart problems.

TARGET AILMENTS

Nasal and respiratory allergies, including hay fever

CONTINUED

Claritin-D

POSSIBLE INTERACTIONS

Azithromycin, cimetidine, clarithromycin, erythromycin, itraconazole, ketoconazole, ranitidine, theophylline, and troleandomycin: may interfere with the body's metabolism of loratadine, possibly causing life-threatening cardiac effects. WARNING: Do not combine these drugs with Claritin-D.

Beta blockers: the pseudoephedrine in Claritin-D can lessen the effectiveness of beta blockers, causing hypertension.

Digoxin: possible heart-rhythm problems.

High blood pressure drugs: decreased antihypertensive effect.

Levodopa (anti-Parkinsonism drug): increased risk of heart-rhythm problems.

Monoamine oxidase (MAO) inhibitors: possible heart problems or hypertensive crisis. Do not take Claritin-D concurrently with MAO inhibitors; do not take Claritin-D within 14 days of taking an MAO inhibitor.

Rauwolfia: decreased effectiveness of pseudoephedrine.

Stimulants (such as other decongestants, amphetamines, caffeine): increased stimulant effects, leading to excessive nervousness, insomnia, irregular heart rhythm, or seizures.

Thyroid hormones: increased effects of both combined drugs. Your doctor may have to adjust the dosage of both medications.

SIDE EFFECTS

NOT SERIOUS

- Sedation
- Mild insomnia
- Dry nose, mouth, or throat
- Lightheadedness
- Headache
- Nausea
- Mild nervousness

CALL YOUR DOCTOR IF THESE SYMPTOMS CONTINUE.

SERIOUS

- Fainting
- Heart palpitations or change in heartbeat
- Tremors
- Dizziness
- Severe headache
- Nervousness
- Trouble breathing
- High blood pressure
- Cardiac arrest

CALL YOUR DOCTOR RIGHT AWAY. THESE EFFECTS ARE RARE BUT MAY OCCUR IF PROPER DOSAGE IS EXCEEDED OR IF YOU HAVE LIVER DAMAGE.

Clary Sage

LATIN NAME
Salvia sclarea

Vital Statistics

GENERAL DESCRIPTION

The southern European plant clary sage has small blue or white flowers and large, hairy leaves. Even though it is closely related to common sage, clary sage yields an entirely different essential oil. Clary sage oil is a powerful, quick-acting relaxant with several uses: It can help treat high blood pressure. It has warming effects and eases inflammation. It may also be used as an anticonvulsive and as an antiseptic. Clary sage oil is nontoxic, nonirritating, and nonsensitizing. It is colorless or pale yellow-green. The oil is used extensively in foods and drinks.

PREPARATIONS

The essential oil is distilled from the flowering tops and leaves of the clary sage plant. It can be used as an inhalant, in vaporizers and baths, or as a body massage oil.

For baths, add 5 to 10 drops to the water. For inhalation, either scent the air with a diffuser or sniff a few drops placed on a cloth.

To apply to your skin or to use as a body massage oil, mix 10 to 15 drops in 2 tbsp vegetable oil, nut oil, or aloe gel.

Precautions

WARNING

Do not use clary sage oil if you are pregnant.

SPECIAL INFORMATION

- Do not drink alcohol while using clary sage.
- Use for short periods only, preferably at the end of the day.

Target Ailments

- Anxiety and stress
- Depression
- Menstrual and menopausal symptoms
- Digestive cramps
- Burns
- Eczema and other skin problems
- Asthma
- Sore throat
- Excessive sweating

Side Effects

NOT SERIOUS

- Inhalation may cause sleepiness

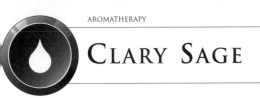

Clean Air Pills

C

Vital Statistics

PINYIN NAME
Qing Qi Hua Tan Wan

ALSO SOLD AS
Pinellia Expectorant Pills

GENERAL DESCRIPTION
Clean Air Pills are a classic Chinese formula used to treat sticky phlegm in the chest and the sinuses, often indicated by a thick yellow coating on the tongue. Clean Air Pills help treat strong coughs, including those that induce vomiting, as well as a sense of heavy fullness in the chest or sinuses.

Chinese medicine takes a holistic approach to healthcare, fashioning remedies to treat the entire being as well as the specific parts or areas. Precise combinations of herbs are used to prevent and combat disease, which is thought to arise from disturbances in the flow of a bodily energy called chi (pronounced "chee") and blood, or from a lack of balance in the complementary states of yin and yang. A patent formula, Clean Air Pills are made by using a standardized combination of herbs and method of preparation.

INGREDIENTS
treated jack-in-the-pulpit, pinellia, trichosanthes seed, scutellaria, dried mandarin orange peel, bitter almond, immature citrus, poria

PREPARATIONS
This formula is sold in pill form at many Chinese pharmacies and Oriental grocery stores.

Precautions

WARNING
This formula should not be used in the early stages of a cold or if you have a dry cough.

TARGET AILMENTS
Cough with thick sputum
Pneumonia
Bronchitis
Thick sinus congestion
Heavy fullness in the chest

SIDE EFFECTS
NONE EXPECTED

CLEAVERS

LATIN NAME
Galium aparine

VITAL STATISTICS

GENERAL DESCRIPTION

Cleavers, an herb with varied applications, is considered especially beneficial for cleansing and stimulating the immune system. In a tea it acts as a diuretic to help wash toxins from the body, and it has traditionally been used to treat urinary infections. Cleavers can also be applied externally for wounds or for skin disorders such as eczema and psoriasis. Taken internally or applied externally, cleavers can help reduce inflammation in such areas as the lymph nodes, tonsils, and adenoids, and it is used by some to help reduce cancerous growths, especially those associated with lymphatic cancer. Cleavers can be cooked and eaten like a vegetable, and it also has traditional cosmetic uses as a tea for improving the complexion, as a shampoo, and as a deodorant.

PREPARATIONS

Over the counter:
Available in dried bulk and as tincture.

At home:

TEA: Pour 1 cup boiling water over 2 to 3 tsp dried herb; steep covered 10 to 15 minutes. Drink up to 3 cups a day.

TINCTURE: Take ¼ to ½ tsp three times a day.

INFUSION: Can be applied to the face to help relieve sunburn or reduce freckles.

POULTICE: May be applied to help reduce inflammation. Chop or crush fresh leaves and apply to the inflamed area.

COMBINATIONS: To help cleanse the lymphatic system, combine cleavers with pokeweed or echinacea; use up to two weeks only. For psoriasis, mix tinctures of burdock, skullcap, yellow dock, and cleavers in equal parts; take 1 to 2 tsp a day. Or steep covered 1 tbsp fresh nettles and fresh cleavers in 1 cup boiling water for 10 minutes, strain, and drink 2 to 3 cups a day. Mix with buchu or bearberry for a diuretic.

Consult a qualified practitioner for the dosage appropriate for you and your specific condition.

PRECAUTIONS

SPECIAL INFORMATION

Cleavers can be used to treat a child with tonsillitis or swollen glands; dosage depends on weight and is significantly less than for adults. Consult a doctor or qualified practitioner for correct dosage.

POSSIBLE INTERACTIONS

Combining cleavers with other herbs may necessitate a lower dosage.

TARGET AILMENTS

Take internally for:

- Urinary infections
- Viral infections
- Swollen glands; tonsillitis (in children)

Apply externally for:

- Skin diseases
- Inflammation

SIDE EFFECTS

NONE EXPECTED

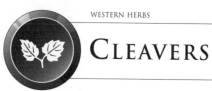

Clindamycin

C

Vital Statistics

DRUG CLASS

Antibiotics

BRAND NAME

Cleocin T

GENERAL DESCRIPTION

Introduced in 1973, clindamycin is a semisynthetic antibiotic derived from *Streptomyces lincolnensis* bacteria. Available in a variety of forms—including gels, lotions, creams, vaginal creams, and pills—clindamycin is most frequently used as a topical preparation for treating skin infections and irritations. The drug works by inhibiting protein synthesis in certain bacteria, thereby killing or disabling them. Clindamycin also decreases the concentration of fatty acids in skin secretions and may have other effects.

Precautions

SPECIAL INFORMATION

- In some cases, clindamycin applied topically can be absorbed in quantities sufficient to produce systemic side effects.
- Women who are pregnant or nursing should exercise caution when using this medication.
- Antibiotics kill not only harmful bacteria but also "good" bacteria that keep unwanted fungi and intestinal organisms in check. Eating yogurt containing *Lactobacillus acidophilus* culture or taking acidophilus tablets may help restore the body's normal bacteria.
- Prolonged use of any antibiotic drug can lead to fungal infections, including candidiasis, or to bacterial infections such as pseudomembranous colitis.
- The safety of clindamycin for children under age 12 has not been established because no studies have been performed on this age group.
- Use of topical clindamycin may cause increased skin sensitivity to this medication (either topical or systemic) during subsequent use.
- Side effects are more likely if you have a history of allergic skin reactions to medications.
- Adverse gastrointestinal reactions are more likely if you have had such responses to other antibiotics in the past.

CLINDAMYCIN

POSSIBLE INTERACTIONS

Peeling agents (including resorcinol, salicylic acid, sulfur): concurrent use with topical clindamycin can increase irritation of skin.

Shaving creams, lotions, aftershave products, medicated cosmetics, or cover-ups: may cause excessive irritation when used with topical clindamycin.

Soaps, cleansers, or astringents with drying action or that contain abrasives, medications, or alcohol: using topical clindamycin with these products may produce additional irritation or dryness.

TARGET AILMENTS

Moderate acne vulgaris, with inflammatory lesions (topical forms only)

Minor bacterial skin infections, such as rosacea (topical forms only)

Skin ulcers (topical forms only)

SIDE EFFECTS

NOT SERIOUS

- Peeling skin
- Scaliness
- Dry skin
- Burning or stinging of the skin
- Excess oiliness (topical forms only)
- Mild gastrointestinal problems (less frequent)

CALL YOUR DOCTOR IF THESE SYMPTOMS BECOME TROUBLESOME.

SERIOUS

- Allergic or hypersensitive reactions, such as skin rash, swelling, or any other irritation not apparent before drug use
- Severe diarrhea
- Other gastrointestinal problems

CALL YOUR DOCTOR IF YOU EXPERIENCE THESE SYMPTOMS.

Rx CLONAZEPAM

C

VITAL STATISTICS

DRUG CLASS
Antianxiety Drugs [Benzodiazepines]

BRAND NAME
Klonopin

OTHER DRUGS IN THIS SUBCLASS
alprazolam, diazepam, lorazepam, temazepam, triazolam

GENERAL DESCRIPTION
Introduced in 1977, clonazepam is a benzodiazepine that is prescribed alone or in combination with other drugs to control epileptic absence (petit mal) seizures as well as myoclonic and akinetic seizures. The effects of this drug start after the first dose. See Benzodiazepines for information on side effects and possible drug interactions.

PRECAUTIONS

WARNING
Never combine alcohol with clonazepam; the combination can cause dangerous central nervous system and respiratory depression.

Do not abruptly stop taking clonazepam. Sudden cessation can provoke withdrawal symptoms, including seizures; irritability; insomnia; confusion; mental depression; hypersensitivity to pain, noise, or light; and feelings of suspicion and distrust. Slowly reduce the dosage under your doctor's guidance.

SPECIAL INFORMATION
- Do not confuse clonazepam's brand name Klonopin with the generic name clonidine. Clonidine is used to treat high blood pressure.
- Clonazepam can impair your alertness, judgment, and coordination. Avoid driving and performing hazardous activities until you know how the drug affects you.
- Let your doctor know if you have narrow-angle glaucoma, a liver or kidney impairment, chronic respiratory disease, myasthenia gravis, depression, sleep apnea, or a history of drug abuse or addiction. Clonazepam may exacerbate these conditions.
- This drug can cause sleep apnea in people with chronic respiratory disease, such as emphysema.
- Clonazepam can cause physical and psychological dependence, sometimes after only one or two weeks, but usually after prolonged use.
- People with a history of drug or alcohol abuse are at a greater risk of psychological dependence on clonazepam.
- Tolerance may increase with prolonged use; as your body adjusts to clonazepam, the drug becomes less effective. Never increase the dose without consulting your doctor, because the risk of clonazepam dependence increases with higher doses.
- Do not take clonazepam if you are pregnant or breast-feeding.

TARGET AILMENTS
Convulsions or seizures

SIDE EFFECTS
SEE BENZODIAZEPINES.

Clonidine

Vital Statistics

DRUG CLASS
Antihypertensive Drugs

BRAND NAME
Catapres

OTHER DRUGS IN THIS CLASS
guanfacine

GENERAL DESCRIPTION
Clonidine relaxes the walls of blood vessels and is used to treat mild to moderate high blood pressure. For visual characteristics of clonidine and the brand-name drug Catapres, see the Color Guide to Prescription Drugs and Herbs.

Precautions

WARNING
Overdoses of clonidine may cause slow heartbeat, diminished reflexes, shortness of breath, fatigue, vomiting, dizziness, fainting, stupor, and coma. Seek emergency treatment.

SPECIAL INFORMATION
- Do not take clonidine if you are allergic to any $alpha_1$-adrenergic blocker.
- Tell your doctor if you are planning to have surgery or if you have heart disease, angina, slow heart rate, kidney or liver disease, diabetes, a peripheral circulation disorder, or a history of depression.
- Do not stop taking this drug without consulting your doctor. Abrupt cessation can cause serious symptoms.
- Do not take clonidine if you are pregnant. Consult your doctor if you are nursing.
- Do not give to children under age 12.
- Contact your doctor before taking any over-the-counter cold medicines.

POSSIBLE INTERACTIONS
Clonidine may react with other prescription and over-the-counter drugs. Tell your doctor about any other medications you are taking.
Beta-adrenergic blocking agents: precipitous change in blood pressure.
Central nervous system depressants (including alcohol): increased effects of these drugs and excessive drop in blood pressure.
Tricyclic antidepressants: decreased clonidine effect.

TARGET AILMENTS

High blood pressure; congestive heart failure; menstrual problems; vascular headache

SIDE EFFECTS

NOT SERIOUS
- Dizziness, drowsiness; dry mouth and nose
- Weight gain; fatigue, insomnia, nervousness; constipation; loss of appetite
- Decreased libido; impotence

CALL YOUR DOCTOR IF THESE EFFECTS PERSIST.

SERIOUS
- Abnormal heart rhythm
- Depression; fever
- Headache; nausea; vomiting
- Dry, burning eyes; edema

CALL YOUR DOCTOR IMMEDIATELY.

Rx CLOTRIMAZOLE

C

VITAL STATISTICS

DRUG CLASS
Antifungal Drugs

BRAND NAMES
Rx: Lotrisone
OTC: Lotrimin AF

OTHER DRUGS IN THIS CLASS
Rx: ketoconazole, fluconazole, miconazole, terconazole
OTC: miconazole, tolnaftate, undecylenate

GENERAL DESCRIPTION
Clotrimazole, available in topical or vaginal preparations, is used to treat a variety of yeast and ringworm infections of the mouth, throat, skin, and vaginal tract. See Antifungal Drugs for more information. Also see Vaginal Antifungal Drugs for information about other medications commonly used to treat vaginal yeast infections.

PRECAUTIONS

SPECIAL INFORMATION
Lotrisone, a combination of clotrimazole and betamethasone, is an antifungal-corticosteroid medication. Its purpose is to destroy fungi and relieve any accompanying skin inflammation. See also Betamethasone.

TARGET AILMENTS

Yeast infections (candidiasis) of the vulva and vagina, mouth, throat, and skin

Ringworm (tinea) of the body, scalp, nails, hands, feet (athlete's foot), and groin (jock itch)

Tinea versicolor, a ringworm infection that produces white-brown patches on the skin

SIDE EFFECTS

NOT SERIOUS

- Mild skin irritation in the infected area
- Headache
- Drowsiness
- Dizziness
- Nausea or vomiting
- Stomach pain
- Constipation or diarrhea

CALL YOUR DOCTOR IF THESE SYMPTOMS PERSIST.

SERIOUS

- Allergic skin reactions such as a rash or hives (topical preparations)
- Redness, burning, or itching of the genitals; abdominal cramps or menstrual irregularities; itching and burning of a sexual partner's penis (vaginal preparations)

CALL YOUR DOCTOR RIGHT AWAY.

CNIDIUM SEEDS

LATIN NAME
Cnidium monnieri

C

VITAL STATISTICS

GENERAL DESCRIPTION

Cnidium seeds grow throughout China and are prescribed typically for skin complaints. A good specimen is round, dusky yellow, and fragrant. Practitioners of Chinese medicine categorize cnidium seeds as acrid, bitter, and warm.

Chinese medicine takes a holistic approach to healthcare, fashioning remedies to treat the entire being as well as the specific parts or areas. Single herbs may be used alone or in combination with other herbs to prevent and combat disease, which is thought to arise from disturbances in the flow of a bodily energy called chi (pronounced "chee") and blood, or from a lack of balance in the complementary states of yin and yang.

PREPARATIONS

Over the counter:

Cnidium seeds are available in bulk at Chinese pharmacies, Asian markets, and some Western health food stores. They can occasionally be found in pill and powder form in herbal combinations.

At home:

TREATMENT OF ECZEMA AND OTHER SKIN DISORDERS: Soak the skin with a cnidium-seed solution; use as a douche for vaginal problems.

COMBINATIONS: Cnidium seeds mixed with the roots of the herbs sophora and stemona are prescribed for itchy, weeping skin lesions. A preparation containing cnidium seeds and calomel is applied to skin lesions associated with acute flareups of eczema, genital eczema, and scabies. Chinese herbalists recommend an oral preparation of cnidium seeds mixed with cuscuta and schisandra for impotence or infertility. Consult a practitioner for information about dosages.

PRECAUTIONS

WARNING

Do not use cnidium seeds for hot, sore skin that is excessively dry.

POSSIBLE INTERACTIONS

Chinese herbalists caution against using cnidium seeds (externally as well as internally) if you are also using bark of the tree peony root, croton seed, or fritillaria.

TARGET AILMENTS

Apply externally for:

- Itching skin
- Eczema
- Scabies, ringworm, or itchy, weeping skin lesions, especially in the genital area
- Vaginal discharge (use as a douche)

Take internally for:

- Male impotence
- Female infertility

SIDE EFFECTS

NONE EXPECTED WITH RECOMMENDED DOSAGE.

COBALT

C

VITAL STATISTICS

GENERAL INFORMATION

The mineral cobalt, a constituent of cobalamin (vitamin B_{12}), helps in the formation of red blood cells and in the maintenance of nerve tissue.

Inorganic cobalt has no nutritional value but is sometimes added to beer as an antifoaming agent.

RDA/EMDR

Not established.

NATURAL SOURCES

To be biologically useful, cobalt must be obtained from foods such as liver, kidneys, milk, oysters, clams, or sea vegetables, or from vitamin B_{12} supplements.

PRECAUTIONS

WARNING

Consuming large amounts of inorganic cobalt stimulates growth of the thyroid gland and may lead to the overproduction of red blood cells, a disorder known as polycythemia.

TARGET AILMENTS

Anemia

SIDE EFFECTS

NONE EXPECTED

COCCULUS

LATIN NAME
Cocculus indicus

VITAL STATISTICS

GENERAL DESCRIPTION

East India and neighboring countries are the habitat of this climbing plant, also called India berry and fishberry, whose fruit contains a poison that stimulates the central nervous system and can cause convulsions. *Cocculus* has an inglorious history that includes the adulteration of beer and use by thieves to make victims groggy. It has had few medicinal uses apart from the external treatment of lice, scabies, and ringworm. The poison, however, called picrotoxin, has been used to treat depression that results from overdose of barbiturates.

The homeopathic preparation, used to treat motion sickness and exhaustion, is prepared from the powdered seeds, which are mixed with alcohol, heated slowly, and strained.

Like most homeopathic prescriptions, *Cocculus* was developed as a remedy by observation of the reactions of healthy individuals to doses of various strengths. The mental, emotional, and physical changes induced by *Cocculus* were then cataloged. When a patient exhibits a set of symptoms that matches the cataloged symptoms brought on by *Cocculus,* the homeopathic practitioner then prescribes it in an extremely dilute form. It is presumed that in this highly dilute dosage, *Cocculus* can counter symptoms that are similar to the ones it induces when it is at full strength. For more information on homeopathic medicine, see page 14.

PREPARATIONS

Cocculus is available over the counter in various potencies, in both liquid and tablet form, at selected stores and pharmacies. Consult your homeopathic physician for further information.

PRECAUTIONS

SPECIAL INFORMATION

- When a remedy is administered, no one but the patient should touch the pills. If tablets are spilled, throw them away.
- The mouth should be clear of flavors 15 minutes before and after taking a remedy; strong flavors and aromas, such as coffee, camphor, and heavy perfumes, should be avoided for the duration of treatment.

TARGET AILMENTS

Severe nausea, worsened by looking out the window of a moving vehicle; dizziness caused by motion, improved by lying down, and worsened by noise, rising, and the sight or smell of food

Hot flashes

Exhaustion from overwork and lack of sleep, worsened by fresh air and especially when combined with worry about a loved one's health

Feeling of numbness and pins and needles

SIDE EFFECTS

NONE EXPECTED

C

Rx Codeine

Vital Statistics

DRUG CLASS
Analgesics [Opioid Analgesics]

BRAND NAME
Tylenol with Codeine

OTHER DRUGS IN THIS SUBCLASS
hydrocodone, oxycodone, propoxyphene, tramadol

GENERAL DESCRIPTION
Codeine is a narcotic analgesic, acting on the central nervous system (the spinal cord and brain) to alter the perception of pain. It is often combined with nonnarcotic analgesics such as aspirin and acetaminophen, which act at the site of the pain. Prescribed for decades for moderate pain relief, codeine also helps control coughing. For more information, see Opioid Analgesics.

Precautions

SPECIAL INFORMATION

- Although codeine is less habit forming than most other opioid analgesics, it should be used with caution; it can lead to addiction, both physical and psychological.
- Seek emergency medical care if you overdose on codeine. Symptoms include pinpoint pupils; slow, shallow, or troubled breathing, and slow heartbeat; dizziness or weakness; confusion; convulsions.
- Do not drink alcoholic beverages while you are taking this drug.
- Because some codeine-containing drugs also contain a nonnarcotic analgesic, read the label carefully before taking any other medication to avoid accidental overdose.

Target Ailments

Mild-to-severe pain, especially from acute trauma or surgery

Moderate-to-severe tension headaches

Nonproductive cough in bronchial disorders

Side Effects

Not Serious

- Dizziness or drowsiness
- Dry mouth
- Headache
- Nervousness
- Difficulty in urination
- Frequent urge to urinate
- Mild nausea, constipation

CONSULT YOUR DOCTOR IF THESE SYMPTOMS CONTINUE.

Serious

- Slow or shallow breathing
- Somnolence
- Skin rash, hives or itching, or facial swelling
- Decrease in blood pressure or heart rate
- Fast heartbeat with increased sweating and shortness of breath
- Severe constipation, nausea, stomach pain, or vomiting

DISCONTINUE USE AND CALL YOUR DOCTOR IF YOU NOTICE THESE SYMPTOMS.

Codonopsis Root

LATIN NAME
Codonopsis pilosula

Vital Statistics

GENERAL DESCRIPTION

Codonopsis root, found throughout northeastern China, is the basis of a tonic for treating lethargy and related symptoms. In laboratory tests, oral and intravenous doses of codonopsis increased red blood cell counts and blood hemoglobin levels of rabbits. The herb also appeared to improve the physical stamina of mice. Classified as sweet and neutral in traditional Chinese medicine, codonopsis root is considered milder and safer than Asian ginseng, and it is often used as a substitute for the stronger herb. Ideally, the root should be thick, moist, and tight skinned.

Chinese medicine takes a holistic approach to healthcare, fashioning remedies to treat the entire being as well as the specific parts or areas. Single herbs may be used alone or in combination with other herbs to prevent and combat disease, which is thought to arise from disturbances in the flow of a bodily energy called chi or qi (pronounced "chee") and blood, or from a lack of balance in the complementary states of yin and yang.

PREPARATIONS

Codonopsis is available in bulk form at Chinese pharmacies, Asian markets, and some Western health food stores. It is also included in several preparations designed as tonics.

Combinations: A mixture of codonopsis and white atractylodes is prescribed for reduced appetite, diarrhea, and vomiting. Codonopsis combined with astragalus is recommended in cases where shortness of breath is added to these symptoms. A preparation containing the roots of codonopsis and dong quai combined with Chinese foxglove root cooked in wine is given to patients who are suffering from dizziness, weakness, and lassitude.

See a Chinese medicine practitioner for information on dosages and appropriate herbal combinations.

Precautions

POSSIBLE INTERACTIONS

Some Chinese herbalists believe that codonopsis is incompatible with veratrum.

TARGET AILMENTS

Take internally for:

- Diabetes
- Chronic cough and shortness of breath
- Prolapsed (fallen) uterus, stomach, or rectum
- Lack of appetite, fatigue, and tired limbs
- Diarrhea and vomiting
- Excessive thirst

SIDE EFFECTS

None expected

Coenzyme Q10

C

Vital Statistics

OTHER NAME
ubiquinone

DAILY DOSAGE
Usually 50 mg to 150 mg, though higher doses are sometimes used. Check with your doctor for the dosage that is appropriate for you.

GENERAL DESCRIPTION
An antioxidant involved in the production of energy in cells, coenzyme Q10 (CoQ10) is sometimes called ubiquinone, from the word ubiquitous, because it is found in cells throughout the body. Levels of CoQ10 decrease as a person ages, a fact that leads some nutritionists to speculate that supplementation might slow down the aging process. In Japan, CoQ10 is used extensively to reduce the risk of heart attack, lower blood pressure, treat congestive heart failure, and boost the immune system. Some research suggests that supplements are useful in treating angina and may help prevent heart damage after surgery.

PREPARATIONS
CoQ10 is sold in the United States as a dietary supplement in the form of capsules, tablets, and soft gelatin capsules.

Keep CoQ10 cool and dry and away from light, and don't allow it to freeze.

SIDE EFFECTS
None expected

Precautions

WARNING
Do not take CoQ10 supplements if you are pregnant or breast-feeding.

SPECIAL INFORMATION
- Check labels carefully; not all products offer CoQ10 in its purest form.
- If you have heart disease, consult your doctor before taking supplements.

TARGET AILMENTS
Allergies; asthma
Alzheimer's disease
Cancer
Candidiasis
Cardiovascular disease; congestive heart failure; cardiomyopathy; angina pectoris
Diabetes mellitus
Hypertension
Muscular dystrophy
Obesity
Periodontal disease
Respiratory disease
Schizophrenia

COFFEA CRUDA

LATIN NAME
Coffea arabica

C

VITAL STATISTICS

GENERAL DESCRIPTION

Like the widely used drink, this remedy comes from the coffee plant, an evergreen shrub found in tropical regions worldwide. Historically coffee has been used most often as a social drink, first in the Arab world and then in Europe, but it has also been used medicinally as a diuretic, to relieve headache, to prevent sleepiness, and as an antidote to poisoning from morphine and some snake venoms. The effect of coffee on wakefulness is believed to have been discovered by an Ethiopian goatherd, who first noticed its effect on his goats.

The homeopathic form is said to have a relaxing effect on people who are overexcited, oversensitive, wired up, or unable to sleep after receiving either good or bad news. The stimulating effect of sudden strong emotions has in fact been compared to the effect of drinking coffee. A homeopathic dose of *Coffea* can help counteract the wakeful effect of coffee drunk during the day.

The berries of the plant are sun-dried to produce the coffee "bean." The beans are ground to a powder to make the homeopathic preparation—they are not roasted as in the preparation of coffee—and left to sit for eight days in an alcohol mixture. The sediment is then reduced by boiling, and the resulting remedy is, as with other homeopathic remedies, prescribed in an extremely dilute form. For more information on homeopathic medicine, see page 14.

PREPARATIONS

Coffea cruda is available over the counter in various potencies, in both liquid and tablet form, at selected stores and pharmacies. Consult your homeopathic physician for further information.

PRECAUTIONS

SPECIAL INFORMATION

- Only the patient should touch the pills. If tablets are spilled, throw them away.
- The mouth should be clear of flavors 15 minutes before and after taking a remedy, and strong flavors and aromas, such as coffee, camphor, and heavy perfume, should be avoided for the duration of treatment.

POSSIBLE INTERACTIONS

Like the coffee drink, the remedy *Coffea* can counteract the effects of some homeopathic remedies. Practitioners often advise patients to avoid this remedy when taking other homeopathic remedies.

TARGET AILMENTS
Excitability; oversensitivity
Overexcitement after receiving good or bad news
Headache with one-sided pain that worsens with noise
Insomnia from an overactive mind
Toothache, especially shooting, spasmodic pain that is made worse by heat and warm drinks and is relieved by cold water in the mouth

SIDE EFFECTS

NONE EXPECTED

Coix

LATIN NAME
Coix lachryma jobi

C

Vital Statistics

GENERAL DESCRIPTION

The seeds are the functional parts of the coix plant, which is also known as Job's-tears. The full, round, white fruit is used as a food, and its seeds can be ingested over a long period of time without producing side effects other than a feeling of dryness. In traditional Chinese medicine the seeds are categorized as sweet, bland, and slightly cold. The fruit is grown throughout China and harvested at the end of fall when the seeds have ripened.

Chinese medicine takes a holistic approach to healthcare, fashioning remedies to treat the entire being as well as the specific parts or areas. Single herbs may be used alone or in combination with other herbs to prevent and combat disease, which is thought to arise from disturbances in the flow of a bodily energy called chi (pronounced "chee") and blood, or from a lack of balance in the complementary states of yin and yang.

PREPARATIONS

Coix seeds are available in bulk at Chinese pharmacies, Asian food markets, and some Western health food stores. The herb can also be obtained in tablet form from some Chinese pharmacies.

Combinations: A preparation of coix mixed with poria mushrooms, kudzu root, and white atractylodes is often prescribed for traveler's diarrhea, weak digestion, nausea, vomiting, diarrhea, constipation, morning sickness, bloating, and cramps. Combine with winter melon seed, adzuki beans, and akebia caulis for inadequate urination. Other combinations are prescribed for diarrhea and internal abscesses. Consult a Chinese medicine practitioner for information on herbal preparations and dosages.

Precautions

SPECIAL INFORMATION

Practitioners urge pregnant women to use the seeds with caution because of the herb's drying effect on body tissues.

Clinical trials have indicated an effect of the oil from coix seeds on breathing: Low doses of the oil appear to stimulate breathing, while high doses seem to inhibit it.

TARGET AILMENTS

Take internally for:

- Urinary difficulty, marked by edema (retention of body fluids)
- Carbuncles
- Lung or intestinal abscesses
- Diarrhea
- Coated tongue (symptomatic of digestive problems)
- Arthritic pains from weather changes
- Fever accompanied by inadequate urination
- Plantar warts

SIDE EFFECTS

NOT SERIOUS

- Feeling of dryness

Rx COLCHICINE

VITAL STATISTICS

DRUG CLASS
Antigout Drugs

BRAND NAME
ColBenemid

OTHER DRUGS IN THIS CLASS
allopurinol

GENERAL DESCRIPTION
Colchicine, a medication taken from the cro-cuslike *Colchicum* plant, has been used for centuries as the treatment of choice for many physicians treating acute or chronic gout attacks. It is indicated for the treatment of chronic gouty arthritis when the patient also experiences frequent, recurring acute attacks of gout with acute pain in the joints.

Gout is a reaction of the immune system to deposits of uric acid in the joints. An anti-inflammatory agent, colchicine decreases the acidity of joint tissues and prevents deposits of uric acid crystals. Its exact mechanism in combating gout is unknown: It is neither a uricosuric agent (an aid in increasing the excretion of uric acid) nor an analgesic—yet it relieves pain in acute gout attacks. This is most likely due to its ability to reduce the acid level in joint tissues, which decreases deposits of uric acid, and to its ability to inhibit the function of immune system cells.

The antigout combination drug ColBenemid has the dual action of probenecid, a uricosuric agent, and colchicine. Together, these two drugs are effective in the long-term management of gout. For visual characteristics of colchicine, see the Color Guide to Prescription Drugs and Herbs.

PRECAUTIONS

WARNING
Overdosage amounts vary and can occur one to three days before symptoms begin. Exact dosing, and using the smallest dose that works, are important rules to observe when using colchicine. Overdose symptoms include nausea, vomiting, stomach pain, diarrhea, and burning sensations in the throat, stomach, or skin. Discontinue use and call your doctor immediately.

SPECIAL INFORMATION
- Colchicine (and colchicine with probenecid) should not be taken if you have a serious liver or kidney disorder or if you have any of the following: a previous allergic reaction to colchicine, active stomach or duodenal ulcers or ulcerative colitis, a serious heart condition, or a history of blood cell disorders.

TARGET AILMENTS
Gout; gouty arthritis
Mediterranean fever
Amyloidosis
Bençet's syndrome
Calcium pyrophosphate deposits
Pericarditis
Hepatic cirrhosis; primary biliary cirrhosis

CONTINUED

COLCHICINE

C

- Prolonged use of colchicine may lead to bone marrow depression and disorders of the blood.
- Use colchicine with caution if you are pregnant or breast-feeding. Discuss possible adverse effects on the fetus or infant with your doctor.
- Colchicine may adversely affect sperm production, impairing fertility. It has caused birth defects in animals.
- Those with compromised immune systems, including the elderly and the sick, should use this drug with caution.
- A low-purine diet (e.g., one that eliminates such foods as organ meats, shellfish, fatty fish, dried beans, spinach) should be observed while taking this medicine.
- Since colchicine may cause false-positive laboratory test results, be sure to remind your doctor that you are taking this drug.

POSSIBLE INTERACTIONS

Alcohol: increased sensitivity to alcohol and increased uric acid blood levels, resulting in interference with gout treatment.

Anticancer drugs, anticoagulants, bone marrow depressants, NSAIDs, aspirin, methotrexate, and zidovudine, among other drugs that affect the blood: increased sensitivity to the side effects of these drugs.

Cyanocobalamin (vitamin B_{12}): decreased cyanocobalamin absorption.

Cyclosporine: may result in cyclosporine toxicity.

Erythromycins: may result in colchicine toxicity.

Penicillin and beta-lactams: increased occurrence of adverse reactions to these antibiotics when used with colchicine-probenecid combination drugs (the interaction is with probenecid).

Phenylbutazone and other NSAIDs: increased side effects of these drugs and colchicine.

Sulfinpyrazone: may lead to leukemia in some patients.

Tranquilizers: increased sensitivity to tranquilizers when taking colchicine-probenecid combination drugs (the interaction is with probenecid).

SIDE EFFECTS

NOT SERIOUS

- Lowered body temperature
- Loss of appetite
- Muscular weakness
- Loss of hair (long-term use)

CALL YOUR DOCTOR IF THESE EFFECTS PERSIST.

SERIOUS

- Nausea; vomiting; diarrhea
- Abdominal pain
- Skin rash or hives, swelling of the face or lips, indicating an allergic reaction (anaphylaxis)
- Fever; sore throat; unusual bruising; severe weakness; blood in urine (long-term use) (bone marrow depression with blood disorders such as anemia)

DISCONTINUE USE AND CALL YOUR DOCTOR IMMEDIATELY. IN THE CASE OF A SEVERE ALLERGIC REACTION, SEEK EMERGENCY TREATMENT.

COLESTIPOL

VITAL STATISTICS

DRUG CLASS
Cholesterol-Reducing Drugs

BRAND NAME
Colestid

OTHER DRUGS IN THIS CLASS
cholestyramine, fluvastatin, gemfibrozil, lovastatin, niacin, pravastatin, simvastatin

GENERAL DESCRIPTION
Introduced in 1974, colestipol is in the group of medicines known as bile-acid-binding resins. These drugs lower blood levels of cholesterol by binding to the bile acids from which cholesterol is made and removing them from the body. For more information, see Cholesterol-Reducing Drugs.

SIDE EFFECTS

NOT SERIOUS
- Belching; bloating

CALL YOUR DOCTOR IF THESE SYMPTOMS PERSIST OR BECOME BOTHERSOME.

SERIOUS
- Constipation
- Loss of weight
- Black, tarry stools

CALL YOUR DOCTOR; YOU MAY NEED TO DECREASE YOUR DOSAGE OR DISCONTINUE USE.

PRECAUTIONS

SPECIAL INFORMATION
- Never take this drug in dry form, as it may cause you to choke. Mix powder as directed with water or fruit juice.
- Colestipol may interfere with your body's ability to absorb certain nutrients. While on this medication, you may need to take supplements of vitamins A, D, E, and K; folic acid; and calcium. Consult your doctor.
- If you are pregnant or nursing, check with your doctor before using this drug.
- Do not use colestipol if you have had an allergic reaction to it in the past.
- Do not stop taking the medication without first checking with your doctor; your blood cholesterol levels may increase again.
- Before undergoing emergency treatment or medical or dental surgery, be sure to tell your healthcare practitioner if you are taking this drug.

POSSIBLE INTERACTIONS
Other medications should be taken two hours before or four to six hours after taking colestipol.

TARGET AILMENTS

The major types of cholesterol disorders, particularly those in which high levels of blood fats (cholesterol and triglycerides) have been linked to an increased risk of heart disease

COLOCYNTHIS

LATIN NAME
Citrullus colocynthis

C

VITAL STATISTICS

GENERAL DESCRIPTION

The remedy *Colocynthis* comes from a vine with a hairy stem and yellow flowers that grows in the sand in hot, dry climates. It is probably because the stem resembles a cucumber that the plant has been nicknamed bitter cucumber. The remedy is made from the pulp of the fruit, which is yellow and as large as an orange. Although the seeds are believed to be highly nutritious, the pulp of the fruit contains a strong poison that acts on the bowels, causing extreme pain and straining during passage of stools. Historically, the fruit has been noted for its intense purgative effects and has been used to treat symptoms such as lethargy and "mania."

Today the homeopathic form is prescribed commonly to relieve anger, irritability, and severe abdominal pain, including infant colic and menstrual cramps. In preparing the homeopathic remedy, the dried fruit is made into a powder and steeped in alcohol. It is shaken twice a day for one week, strained, and then put through the standard shaking procedure. For more information on homeopathic medicine, see page 14.

PREPARATIONS

Colocynthis is available over the counter in various potencies, in both liquid and tablet form, at selected stores and pharmacies. Consult your homeopathic practitioner for further information.

SIDE EFFECTS

NONE EXPECTED

PRECAUTIONS

SPECIAL INFORMATION

- Only the patient should touch the pills. If tablets are spilled, throw them away.
- The mouth should be clear of flavors 15 minutes before and after taking a remedy, and strong flavors and aromas should be avoided for the duration of treatment.

TARGET AILMENTS
Anger and indignation
Irritability worsened by questioning
Humiliation or embarrassment over offensive remarks
Menstrual cramps relieved by doubling up, pressure, or warmth
Severe abdominal pain with nausea and vomiting, relieved by pressure, lying on the abdomen, or passing of stool
Diarrhea that is worse after eating, especially fruit
Headache on left side of face spreading to the ear
Sciatica, especially right-sided, better from lying on the pain
Gout or rheumatism, relieved by heat or pressure, aggravated by anger

COLTSFOOT

LATIN NAME
Tussilago farfara

C

VITAL STATISTICS

GENERAL DESCRIPTION

As many as 2,000 years ago, Asians and Europeans used coltsfoot as a cough suppressant for respiratory ailments, and both the dried flowers and the leaves are still used as an expectorant and a cough suppressant. They contain a substance called mucilage, which may have a soothing effect on the respiratory tract. For visual characteristics, see the Color Guide to Prescription Drugs and Herbs.

PREPARATIONS

Over the counter:
Available in tincture, capsules, and in bulk.

At home:

TEA: Pour 1 cup boiling water onto 1 to 2 tsp dried flowers or leaves; steep covered 10 minutes. Drink hot three times a day.

COMPRESS: Soak a pad in a coltsfoot infusion for several minutes, wring out, then apply to the affected area.

COMBINATIONS: For a cough, coltsfoot is often combined with horehound and mullein.

Consult a qualified practitioner for the dosage appropriate for your specific condition.

TARGET AILMENTS

Take internally for:

Lung-related coughs, such as those caused by asthma, bronchitis, and emphysema; whooping cough

Apply externally for:

Skin ulcers; abscesses; boils

PRECAUTIONS

WARNING

Do not give coltsfoot to children under two years old, pregnant or nursing women, alcoholics, or anyone with liver disease. Use of this herb by children for more than seven to 10 days should be done in conjunction with a healthcare practitioner.

Use coltsfoot only under a practitioner's supervision for short periods of time.

SPECIAL INFORMATION

- Today coltsfoot is banned in Canada, and the U.S. Food and Drug Administration (FDA) classifies it as an herb with "undefined safety." Coltsfoot contains an alkaloid that can seriously damage the liver, and a Japanese study concluded that the flower buds may be carcinogenic. Many practitioners in Europe and the U.S., however, still use coltsfoot on a short-term basis to treat coughs and other respiratory ailments.
- Coltsfoot is best taken on an empty stomach.

POSSIBLE INTERACTIONS

Combining coltsfoot with other herbs may necessitate a lower dosage.

SIDE EFFECTS

SERIOUS

- Fever
- Nausea, vomiting, loss of appetite, or diarrhea
- Jaundice or pain in the upper-right abdomen

DISCONTINUE USE AND CALL YOUR DOCTOR IMMEDIATELY.

COMFREY

LATIN NAME
Symphytum officinale

C

VITAL STATISTICS

GENERAL DESCRIPTION
Praised for centuries by herbalists throughout the world, who still use it to treat disorders ranging from cuts to cancer, comfrey nevertheless is rejected by many practitioners in the United States as too dangerous for any type of internal use. Comfrey contains pyrrolizidine alkaloids, which can cause liver damage when consumed in large amounts. The active agent in comfrey is allantoin, which fosters the growth of new cells. Although the dried roots and leaves are used for medicinal purposes, the comfrey root contains up to twice as much allantoin as the other parts. While its internal use remains questionable, comfrey can be used safely on external injuries such as cuts and other wounds. For visual characteristics, see the Color Guide to Prescription Drugs and Herbs.

PREPARATIONS
Over the counter:
Available in dry bulk.

At home:
POULTICE: Sprinkle a powder made from dry comfrey over cuts, bruises, insect bites, or wounds, and cover with a clean cloth. Or chop up fresh root and then apply. This poultice is good for sprains, strains, and joint injuries.

SIDE EFFECTS

NOT SERIOUS
- Rash

THIS SYMPTOM MAY OCCUR WHEN COMFREY IS APPLIED EXTERNALLY. DISCONTINUE USE.

PRECAUTIONS

WARNING
The American Herb Products Association has placed comfrey on its restricted list and suggests that this herb be used for external ailments only.

Do not use comfrey for deep wounds. Superficial tissue may heal faster than deep tissue, allowing abscesses to form.

This herb should not be used with children unless it is specifically prescribed by a healthcare practitioner who is knowledgeable about herbs.

POSSIBLE INTERACTIONS
Combining comfrey with other herbs may necessitate a lower dosage.

TARGET AILMENTS
Apply externally for:
Sprains; strains
Joint pain, especially rheumatism
Cuts; superficial wounds
Insect bites
Bruises
Ulcers
Inflammations

COPPER

C

VITAL STATISTICS

GENERAL DESCRIPTION

Copper is indispensable to human health. Its many functions include the following: helping to form hemoglobin in the blood; facilitating the absorption and use of iron so red blood cells can transport oxygen to tissues; assisting in the regulation of blood pressure and heart rate; strengthening blood vessels, bones, tendons, and nerves; promoting fertility; and ensuring normal skin and hair pigmentation. Some evidence suggests that copper helps prevent cardiovascular problems such as high blood pressure and heart arrhythmias and that it may help treat arthritis and scoliosis. Copper may also protect tissue from damage by free radicals, support the body's immune function, and contribute to preventing cancer.

Excess calcium and zinc will interfere with copper absorption, but a true copper deficiency is rare and tends to be limited to people either with certain inherited diseases that inhibit copper absorption, such as albinism, or with acquired malabsorption ailments, such as Crohn's disease and celiac disease. The deficiency may also occur in infants who are not breast-fed and in some premature babies. Symptoms of copper deficiency include brittle, discolored hair; skeletal defects; anemia; high blood pressure; heart arrhythmias; and infertility.

Some research suggests that high levels of copper and iron may play a role in hyperactivity and autism.

Common supplemental forms are copper aspartate, copper citrate, and copper picolinate.

EMDR

Adults: 1.5 mg to 3 mg

NATURAL SOURCES

Most adults get enough copper from a normal, varied diet. Seafood and organ meats are the richest sources; blackstrap molasses, nuts, seeds, green vegetables, black pepper, cocoa, and water passed through copper pipes also contain significant quantities.

TARGET AILMENTS

Cancer

Heart disease

Immune problems

SIDE EFFECTS

NONE EXPECTED

PRECAUTIONS

WARNING

Supplemental copper should be taken only on a doctor's advice.

SPECIAL INFORMATION

- Taking more than 10 mg of copper daily can bring on nausea, vomiting, muscle pain, and stomachaches.
- Women who are pregnant or are taking birth-control pills are susceptible to excess blood levels of copper.

COPTIS

LATIN NAME
Coptis chinensis
(or Coptis deltoidea)

C

VITAL STATISTICS

GENERAL DESCRIPTION

The rhizome of the coptis plant, sometimes called Chinese goldthread, is an antibiotic and fever-reducing herb frequently prescribed by Chinese medicine practitioners. It contains the antimicrobial substance berberine, which seems to inhibit many of the bacteria that cause dysentery. Look for a reddish yellow cross section in *Coptis chinensis,* the form most often available commercially, or for a pure yellow cross section in *Coptis deltoidea.* Chinese herbalists characterize the herb as cold and bitter. For more information on Chinese medicine, see page 12.

PREPARATIONS

You can obtain coptis in bulk or tablet form at Chinese pharmacies, Asian food stores, and some Western health food stores. Use powder or ointment on eye or mouth problems.

COMBINATIONS: With skullcap and gardenia, coptis is used to treat conditions marked by high fever, irritability, dry mouth and throat, and dark urine. With Chinese foxglove root, coptis is prescribed for insomnia and delirium and for serious illnesses with high fever. Coptis and aucklandia are mixed to treat dysentery. A combination of coptis and Chinese wild ginger, usually with gypsum, is used for toothaches, swollen gums, and ulcers of the tongue and mouth. Consult a Chinese medicine practitioner for dosages and other combinations.

PRECAUTIONS

POSSIBLE INTERACTIONS

Some herbalists believe that coptis should not be taken with pork. They also advise patients to avoid the herb in combination with chrysanthemum flowers *(Chrysanthemum morifolium),* scrophularia, dictamnus root bark, and silkworm. Coptis is also believed to counteract the beneficial effects of coltsfoot flower and achyranthes root.

TARGET AILMENTS

Take internally for:

High fever with irritability, disorientation, or delirium

Dysentery with hot, burning diarrhea

Nosebleeds or bright red blood in the urine, stool, or vomit

Bad breath or belching with bad odor

Apply externally for:

Toothache; swollen gums; ulcers of the tongue and mouth; red, painful eyes

SIDE EFFECTS

SERIOUS

- Digestive problems

LONG-TERM USE MAY CAUSE THIS EFFECT; DISCONTINUE USE AND CALL YOUR DOCTOR.

CORNUS

LATIN NAME
Cornus officinalis

C

VITAL STATISTICS

GENERAL DESCRIPTION

Chinese practitioners use cornus berries in several medicinal tonics. Known also as Asiatic cornelian cherry fruit and Asiatic dogwood, it is prescribed for kidney and bladder disorders and for menstrual irregularity. Laboratory tests indicate that cornus may have an antibiotic effect on staphylococcus bacteria; in tests with animals, cornus increased urination and reduced blood pressure. Grown in several parts of China, it is harvested in October and November, when the fruit becomes purplish red. The best variety is fat, thick, soft, and seedless. Traditional Chinese medicine attributes sour and slightly warm characteristics to cornus.

Chinese medicine takes a holistic approach to healthcare, fashioning remedies to treat the entire being as well as the specific parts or areas. Single herbs may be used alone or in combination with other herbs to prevent and combat disease, which is thought to arise from disturbances in the flow of a bodily energy called chi (pronounced "chee") and blood, or from a lack of balance in the complementary states of yin and yang.

PREPARATIONS

The berries are available at Chinese pharmacies, Asian food markets, and some Western health food stores.

COMBINATIONS: A preparation designed to overcome urinary frequency, tinnitus (ringing in the ears), and low-back pain contains cornus berries as well as Chinese foxglove root, Chinese yam, and other minor ingredients. A blend of cornus and Cherokee rose hip is prescribed for urinary incontinence. Check with a Chinese herbalist for recommended doses and additional combinations.

PRECAUTIONS

SPECIAL INFORMATION

While cornus is believed to have low toxicity, herbalists warn against prescribing it for some forms of painful, difficult urination involving infection or cystitis.

POSSIBLE INTERACTIONS

Some Chinese herbalists advise against using cornus in combination with the herbs platycodon, siler, and stephania.

TARGET AILMENTS

Take internally for:

- Excessive urination
- Incontinence
- Impotence, and other symptoms related to kidney and bladder problems
- Excessive sweating
- Lightheadedness with weakness of the back and knees
- Excessive menstrual bleeding or prolonged menstruation

SIDE EFFECTS

NONE EXPECTED

CORTICOSTEROIDS

C

VITAL STATISTICS

GENERIC NAMES

Rx: beclomethasone, betamethasone, fluticasone, methylprednisolone, mometasone furoate, prednisone, triamcinolone
OTC: hydrocortisone

GENERAL DESCRIPTION

The term *corticosteroids* refers both to natural hormones produced by the adrenal glands and to synthetic versions of these hormones. Corticosteroids are powerful drugs, prescribed for a variety of conditions ranging in severity from skin rash to multiple sclerosis. Because they affect almost all parts of the body, these drugs must be used with caution.

Corticosteroid medications are available in topical creams, nasal inhalers and sprays, lung inhalers and sprays, and oral forms (tablets, syrup, and solutions). For more information, see individual entries for each of the generic drugs listed above.

PRECAUTIONS

SPECIAL INFORMATION

- Corticosteroid topical creams, as well as nasal and oral sprays or inhalers, may be absorbed into your system after prolonged use. Tell your doctor if you are taking any other medication, and watch for any significant side effects or drug interactions.
- Ask your doctor about the risks and benefits of corticosteroid treatment if you have or have had any of the following conditions: HIV infection or AIDS, heart disease, hypertension, ulcerative colitis, diabetes, diverticulitis, gastritis or peptic ulcers, recent chickenpox or measles, candidiasis or other fungal infections, glaucoma, herpes simplex, liver or kidney disease, myasthenia gravis, osteoporosis, anastomoses, lupus, tuberculosis, recent intestinal problems, or any infection, such as a cold or flu.
- Prolonged use of corticosteroids can cause birth defects. Pregnant and nursing women should avoid these drugs.
- Prolonged use of corticosteroids increases the risk of osteoporosis, cataracts, glaucoma, Cushing's syndrome (moon face), and diabetes. It can also reactivate tuberculosis.
- Check with your doctor before you stop using these drugs. It may be necessary to reduce the dosage gradually to avoid serious consequences.

POSSIBLE INTERACTIONS

Aminoglutethimide, antacids, barbiturates, phenytoin, and rifampin: decreased effectiveness of corticosteroids.

Diuretics: decreased effectiveness of both combined drugs.

Growth hormones, isoniazid, potassium supplements, and salicylates: corticosteroids may decrease the effectiveness of these drugs.

Oral anticoagulants: corticosteroids may increase or decrease the effectiveness of oral anticoagulants.

Vaccines (live virus, other immunizations): corticosteroids may make you more susceptible to the injected virus.

CORTICOSTEROIDS

C

TARGET AILMENTS

Skin disorders, for symptomatic relief of rash, inflammation, itching; treatment of psoriasis, eczema, sunburn, and other skin diseases (hydrocortisone and mometasone furoate)

Nasal inflammations, including hay fever (allergic rhinitis) and nonallergic inflammation of the nasal passages (beclomethasone and triamcinolone)

Respiratory ailments such as severe asthma (beclomethasone and triamcinolone)

Rheumatic disorders (arthritis, bursitis, tendinitis); ulcerative colitis; Crohn's disease (prednisone)

Itchiness and inflammation associated with fungal infections such as athlete's foot, jock itch, and yeast infections (betamethasone, in combination with the antifungal drug clotrimazole)

SIDE EFFECTS

NOT SERIOUS

- Mild and transient skin rash, burning, irritation, dryness, redness, itchiness, or scaling (topical corticosteroids)
- Stomach upset; increased or decreased appetite; restlessness; dizziness; sleeplessness; change in skin color; unusual hair growth on face or body (other corticosteroids)

SERIOUS

- Eye pain
- Vision loss or blurred vision
- Stomach pain or burning sensation in the stomach
- Black, tarry stools
- Severe and lasting skin rash, hives, or burning, itching, or painful skin
- Blisters, acne, or other skin problems
- Nausea or vomiting
- High blood pressure
- Foot or leg swelling
- Rapid weight gain
- Fluid retention (edema)
- Unusual bruising
- Menstrual irregularities
- Prolonged sore throat, fever, cold, or other sign of infection

CONTACT YOUR DOCTOR IMMEDIATELY.

CORYDALIS

LATIN NAME
Corydalis yanhusuo

C

VITAL STATISTICS

GENERAL DESCRIPTION

Grown in China's Zhejiang, Hubei, Hunan, and Jiangsu provinces, corydalis is considered among the most effective painkillers in traditional Chinese medicine. Herbalists use the root alone or in combination with other herbs to treat almost any kind of pain. The best roots are large, hard, and bright yellow on the inside. According to the tenets of traditional Chinese medicine, corydalis is classified as acrid, bitter, and warm.

Chinese medicine takes a holistic approach to healthcare, fashioning remedies to treat the entire being as well as the specific parts or areas. Single herbs may be used alone or in combination with other herbs to prevent and combat disease, which is thought to arise from disturbances in the flow of a bodily energy called chi or qi (pronounced "chee") and blood, or from a lack of balance in the complementary states of yin and yang.

PREPARATIONS

Corydalis is available in Chinese pharmacies, Asian markets, and some Western health food stores. Toasting or frying in vinegar enhances its effects in cases of menstrual pain and pain caused by trauma. Powdered corydalis root is considered an especially potent painkiller.

COMBINATIONS: A mixture of corydalis and cnidium root *(Ligusticum chuanxiong)* is prescribed for body aches and headaches. Corydalis combined with fennel is used for abdominal pain and hernial disorders. Herbalists prescribe a preparation containing corydalis and cinnamon bark for painful menstruation. Consult a practitioner of Chinese medicine for information on appropriate dosages and additional combinations.

PRECAUTIONS

☠ *WARNING*

Do not use this herb if you are pregnant.

SPECIAL INFORMATION

In clinical tests, corydalis has shown a slight hypnotic effect on many animal species, causing a lack of alertness.

TARGET AILMENTS

Take internally for:

- Abdominal pain
- Chest pain
- Pain resulting from traumatic injuries
- Menstrual pain
- Rheumatism pain
- Arthritis pain

SIDE EFFECTS

NONE EXPECTED

Cough Suppressants

C

Vital Statistics

GENERIC NAME
dextromethorphan

GENERAL DESCRIPTION
Cough suppressants (antitussives) are used to reduce the intensity and frequency of the dry, nonproductive type of cough associated with allergies, colds, and the flu. The drugs should not be used with a productive (phlegm- or mucus-producing) cough unless the cough is extremely bothersome or disrupts sleep.

Some cough suppressants work in the brain to suppress the cough reflex; others act on the throat and bronchial passages to soothe irritation and relax the muscles. For more information on a potent, nonnarcotic drug found in many over-the-counter products, see Dextromethorphan. For information about other drugs that help suppress the cough reflex, see Codeine, Hydrocodone, and Opioid Analgesics.

TARGET AILMENTS

Dry, nonproductive, and temporary coughing

SIDE EFFECTS

NOT SERIOUS

- Mild drowsiness
- Mild dizziness
- Stomach pain
- Nausea or vomiting

CALL YOUR DOCTOR IF THESE SYMPTOMS PERSIST.

Precautions

SPECIAL INFORMATION

- Symptoms of dextromethorphan overdose include confusion, hyperactivity, feeling of intoxication, lack of coordination, hallucinations, irritability, and severe nausea and vomiting. Seek immediate medical help.
- Do not take dextromethorphan if you have had an allergic reaction to any medications containing this drug.
- Before taking dextromethorphan, consult your doctor if you have asthma or impaired liver function, or if your cough is producing mucus or phlegm.
- Use dextromethorphan only as instructed by your doctor or the label directions. Take it only as long as needed; some reports suggest that this drug may be habit forming if you use too much for too long.
- Check with your doctor if your cough persists for more than seven to 10 days or if it is accompanied by a skin rash, high fever, or continuing headache. These symptoms may indicate the presence of other medical problems.

POSSIBLE INTERACTIONS

Central nervous system depressants (alcohol, anesthetics, antidepressants, antihistamines, anti-insomnia drugs, barbiturates, benzodiazepines, muscle relaxants, narcotics or prescription pain medicines, tranquilizers): increased sedative and depressant effects when these substances are taken with dextromethorphan.

MAO inhibitors: combining these drugs with dextromethorphan can cause disorientation, psychotic behavior, and coma.

COUMADIN

C

VITAL STATISTICS

DRUG CLASS
Anticoagulant and Antiplatelet Drugs

GENERIC NAME
warfarin

OTHER DRUGS IN THIS CLASS
aspirin, dalteparin, dipyridamole, heparin

GENERAL DESCRIPTION
This powerful anticoagulant inhibits blood clotting by blocking the action of vitamin K, a central ingredient in the production of four blood-clotting factors. It is administered orally and can be extremely dangerous if not used properly. You must have periodic blood tests to monitor clotting time. See Anticoagulant and Antiplatelet Drugs for important information on serious side effects and drug interactions. For visual characteristics, see the Color Guide to Prescription Drugs and Herbs.

TARGET AILMENTS

Prevention and treatment of blood clots

To reduce the risk of recurrent myocardial infarction and blood clot formation after myocardial infarction

SIDE EFFECTS

NOT SERIOUS
- Minor bleeding; skin rash

PRECAUTIONS

WARNING
Do not use without telling your physician if you have had a heart attack, uncontrolled high blood pressure, ulcers, or a stroke.

Do not take if you are pregnant; Coumadin can cause serious birth defects.

SPECIAL INFORMATION
- Nursing women should check with a physician before taking Coumadin.
- Tell your doctor if you have or have had low blood pressure, an impaired kidney or liver, a bleeding disease or disorder, chest pains, allergies, asthma, colitis, diabetes, active tuberculosis, a recent childbirth, medical or dental surgery, spinal anesthesia, x-rays, a bad fall, heavy bleeding or menstrual periods, diarrhea, or any other medical problem. Also, tell your doctor if you are using an intrauterine device (IUD) for birth control or a catheter.
- Tell your pharmacist, dentist, and physician that you are taking the medicine. You may be advised to carry a medication identification card.
- Avoid dangerous activities that might cause injuries. Be sure to report all falls and blows to your doctor. Internal bleeding may occur without symptoms.

POSSIBLE INTERACTIONS
A number of drugs can increase or decrease Coumadin's effects. Tell your doctor about all prescription and over-the-counter drugs you are taking.

Vitamin K: counteracts Coumadin. Avoid eating large quantities of foods rich in vitamin K, including leafy green vegetables, dairy products, bacon, beef liver, cabbage, cauliflower, and fish.

Cramp Bark

LATIN NAME
Viburnum opulus

Vital Statistics

GENERAL DESCRIPTION

Cramp bark is known traditionally for its effectiveness in relieving muscular cramps and spasms. The herb is especially recommended to help ease cramps associated with menstruation and pregnancy and to help with related problems such as an excessive menstrual flow during menopause. The herb, which is a stimulant as well as a relaxant, helps strengthen the uterus and is credited with the ability to guard against miscarriage. Its effectiveness as a muscle relaxant also leads to its use in treating arthritis, anxiety, and severe headaches.

PREPARATIONS

Over the counter:
Available as extract, capsules, or bulk herb.

At home:

Decoction: Add 2 tsp cramp bark to 1 cup water and bring to boil; simmer covered 10 to 15 minutes. Drink hot three times a day.

Tincture: Take 1/4 to 1/2 tsp every 4 hours as needed for cramps.

Combinations: For menstrual cramps, use with prickly ash and wild yam or with dong quai. To help prevent miscarriage during pregnancy, mix with black haw or mix with equal parts button snakeroot. Migraines brought on by stress may benefit from a combination of equal parts hawthorn, linden, wood betony, skullcap, and cramp bark, taken three times a day as a tea or tincture. Cramp bark is also used with linden blossoms to help relieve anxiety associated with high blood pressure. A tincture of cramp bark and lobelia can help relieve arthritis or bursitis.

Consult a qualified practitioner for the dosage appropriate for you and the specific condition being treated.

Precautions

WARNING

Fresh cramp bark berries are poisonous.

This herb should not be used with children unless it is specifically prescribed by a healthcare practitioner who is knowledgeable about herbs.

POSSIBLE INTERACTIONS

Combining cramp bark with other herbs may necessitate a lower dosage.

TARGET AILMENTS
Muscular cramps
Menstrual cramps
Menopausal problems

SIDE EFFECTS

None expected

Cromolyn

C

Vital Statistics

DRUG CLASS
Asthma Therapy

BRAND NAME
Intal

GENERAL DESCRIPTION
Cromolyn is an antiasthmatic and antiallergenic drug used to prevent bronchial asthma episodes and bronchospasm caused by allergens, dry air, airborne pollutants, or other triggering factors. The drug, available as a pill, powder, oral inhalant, and nasal spray, can also be used immediately before exercise to control exercise-induced bronchial problems. Because cromolyn is not fast acting, it should not be used for relief during acute asthma attacks.

See Asthma Therapy, Bronchodilators, and Corticosteroids for more information on asthma medications.

Precautions

SPECIAL INFORMATION
- Women who are pregnant or nursing should consult a doctor before using this drug.
- Let your doctor know if you have a history of heart arrhythmias or coronary artery disease; cromolyn inhalants may affect your condition.

POSSIBLE INTERACTIONS
- **Cortisone drugs:** increased cortisone effect.
- **Ipratropium (asthma inhalant):** increased cromolyn effect.

TARGET AILMENTS

- Bronchial asthma attacks
- Bronchospasm
- Respiratory allergies
- Allergic rhinitis (nasal spray)

SIDE EFFECTS

NOT SERIOUS
- Cough, hoarseness; an unpleasant taste in the mouth
- Dryness of the mouth or throat; sneezing; nasal congestion; watery eyes; throat irritation

CALL YOUR DOCTOR IF THESE EFFECTS BECOME TROUBLESOME.

SERIOUS
- Swelling of the face, lips, eyelids, hands, feet, or inside of mouth; increased bronchospasm (wheezing, chest tightness, trouble breathing); difficult, painful, or frequent urination; joint pain or swelling; severe or continuous headache; nausea, skin rash or itching; difficulty swallowing; pneumonia

THESE EFFECTS ARE UNCOMMON. CALL YOUR DOCTOR RIGHT AWAY IF YOU EXPERIENCE ANY OF THEM.

CUSCUTA

LATIN NAME
Cuscuta chinensis

C

VITAL STATISTICS

GENERAL DESCRIPTION

A common parasitic growth on plants, cuscuta yields grayish yellow seeds, sometimes called Chinese dodder seeds, that are said to have medicinal effects. Among its many uses, cuscuta is prescribed to prevent miscarriages. Practitioners of Chinese medicine characterize this herb as sweet, acrid, and neutral.

Chinese medicine takes a holistic approach to healthcare, fashioning remedies to treat the entire being as well as the specific parts or areas. Single herbs may be used alone or in combination with other herbs to prevent and combat disease, which is thought to arise from disturbances in the flow of a bodily energy called chi or qi (pronounced "chee") and blood, or from a lack of balance in the complementary states of yin and yang.

PREPARATIONS

Cuscuta seeds are available in bulk from Chinese pharmacies, Asian markets, and some Western health food stores.

COMBINATIONS: Practitioners recommend a mix of cuscuta seeds, psoralea fruit, and eucommia bark for premature ejaculation. A preparation of cuscuta and astragalus seeds *(Astragalus complanatus)* may help in the treatment of blurred vision, dizziness, and tinnitus. A mixture of cuscuta, Japanese teasel root, mulberry mistletoe stems, and eucommia bark is often prescribed to prevent miscarriages. Check with a practitioner of Chinese medicine for further combinations and doses.

PRECAUTIONS

SPECIAL INFORMATION

The herb is not recommended for patients with constipation and scanty, dark urine.

TARGET AILMENTS

Take internally for:

- Impotence
- Nocturnal emissions; premature ejaculation
- Prostate problems
- Frequent urination
- Incontinence
- Diarrhea with lack of appetite
- Habitual or threatened miscarriage
- Backache from muscular weakness
- Dizziness
- Tinnitus (ringing in the ears)
- Blurred vision

SIDE EFFECTS

NONE EXPECTED

CYCLOBENZAPRINE

C

VITAL STATISTICS

DRUG CLASS
Muscle Relaxants

GENERAL DESCRIPTION
Cyclobenzaprine is used along with other medications to relieve acute pain associated with muscle spasms. Although not actually a sedative, the drug acts to reduce muscle hyperactivity, thereby producing a sedative effect. For more information, see Muscle Relaxants. For visual characteristics, see the Color Guide to Prescription Drugs and Herbs.

PRECAUTIONS

SPECIAL INFORMATION
- Since cyclobenzaprine may reduce saliva production, you should maintain good dental hygiene to avoid problems such as caries and periodontal disease.
- Before taking this drug, tell your doctor if you are pregnant or nursing, or have glaucoma, urinary retention, congestive heart failure, hypertension, or arrhythmia.

POSSIBLE INTERACTIONS
Since cyclobenzaprine is closely related to tricyclic antidepressants, drug interactions specific to those drugs may also apply to cyclobenzaprine. See Tricyclic Antidepressants for more interaction information.

Any central nervous system depressant (including sedatives, antihistamines, MAO inhibitors, and alcohol): may boost effects of the combined drugs while also increasing risks associated with side effects.

TARGET AILMENTS

Acute, painful muscle spasms

SIDE EFFECTS

NOT SERIOUS

- Dryness of the mouth; blurred vision; drowsiness

CALL YOUR DOCTOR IF THESE SYMPTOMS PERSIST.

- Headache; confusion or nervousness; numbness, tingling, pain, or weakness in limbs; muscle twitching or weakness; insomnia; gastrointestinal problems; pounding heartbeat; change in the sense of taste

THESE EFFECTS ARE RARE. CALL YOUR DOCTOR IF THEY PERSIST OR BECOME TROUBLESOME.

SERIOUS

- Allergic reactions, including swelling of the face, lips, or tongue
- Skin rash, hives, or itching
- Mania, unusual dreaming, or clumsiness
- Fainting or disorientation
- Depression
- Ringing in the ears
- Yellow skin
- Heart-rhythm problems or low blood pressure
- Breathing difficulties

CALL YOUR DOCTOR IF YOU EXPERIENCE THESE SIDE EFFECTS.

CYPERUS

LATIN NAME
Cyperus rotundus

VITAL STATISTICS

GENERAL DESCRIPTION

The large, reddish brown root of a plant found in marshy areas and river bottoms throughout China, cyperus is considered one of the best menstrual regulators known to traditional Chinese medicine. Practitioners also prescribe this fragrant herb, sometimes called nut-grass rhizome, for digestive problems. Injections of cyperus under the skin have increased the pain thresholds of mice in laboratory experiments. In traditional Chinese medicine, cyperus is classified as acrid, slightly bitter, and neutral.

Chinese medicine takes a holistic approach to healthcare, fashioning remedies to treat the entire being as well as the specific parts or areas. Single herbs may be used alone or in combination with other herbs to prevent and combat disease, which is thought to arise from disturbances in the flow of a bodily energy called chi or qi (pronounced "chee") and blood, or from a lack of balance in the complementary states of yin and yang.

PREPARATIONS

Cyperus root is available in bulk from Chinese pharmacies, Asian markets, and some Western health food stores. To increase its pain-reducing effects, practitioners suggest frying the root in vinegar; to speed its action, they recommend cooking it in wine.

COMBINATIONS: A preparation of cyperus, bupleurum, and white peony root is prescribed for pain and bloating in the chest, sides, and breasts. Combined with aucklandia and finger citron fruit, cyperus is used to treat pain in the upper abdomen, indigestion, vomiting, and diarrhea. A preparation of cyperus, dong quai, and cnidium root *(Ligusticum chuanxiong)* is often prescribed for irregular menstruation. A mixture of cyperus, bupleurum, and trichosanthes fruit is recommended for breast swelling during menstruation.

For information on specific dosages and other herbal combinations, consult a qualified practitioner of Chinese medicine.

TARGET AILMENTS

Take internally for:

- Irregular menstruation
- Menstrual cramps
- Digestive problems, such as gas and bloating
- Depression
- Moodiness and instability

SIDE EFFECTS

NONE EXPECTED

CYPRESS

LATIN NAME
Cupressus sempervirens

C

VITAL STATISTICS

GENERAL DESCRIPTION

Cypress has a long history as a medicinal agent. Used by the ancient Chinese, Greeks, and Egyptians, the oil was considered especially helpful to treat bleeding problems. The Egyptians used the wood to build sarcophagi for their mummies; the Greeks dedicated the tree to the god of the underworld. Cypress trees today are often found in cemeteries.

Aromatherapists use cypress oil to help stanch blood loss, to support the vascular and urinary systems, and to counter the excessive loss of fluids that accompanies diarrhea, menstruation, and heavy perspiration. The oil can be applied externally to reduce swelling of varicose veins, hemorrhoids, and other types of painful swelling.

Cypress is native to southern Europe, although it is now cultivated throughout Europe and in North America. Also known as the Mediterranean or Italian cedar, the tall, conical evergreen bears small flowers and round brownish gray cones. Cypress oil ranges in color from colorless to pale yellow and has a rich woody-balsamic scent.

PREPARATIONS

Cypress aromatherapy treatments employ the oil that comes from the needles, twigs, and cones of the cypress tree.

FOR TOPICAL APPLICATIONS, such as for relief from varicose veins or arthritis, mix 15 drops of cypress oil with 2 oz grape-seed oil and 3 drops of wheat-germ oil or aloe gel. Apply to the skin daily.

FOR INHALATIONS, either place a few drops of cypress oil on a pillow to inhale while sleeping or scent the air with a diffuser.

FOR BATHS, add 5 to 10 drops of cypress oil to the water.

PRECAUTIONS

SPECIAL INFORMATION

Avoid using cypress if you have high blood pressure or are pregnant.

TARGET AILMENTS
Insomnia
Varicose veins
Coughs; bronchitis; asthma
Menstrual pain
Menopause problems
Rheumatism and arthritis
Diarrhea
Excessive sweating

SIDE EFFECTS

NONE EXPECTED. CYPRESS IS A NONIRRITATING, NONTOXIC OIL.

DALTEPARIN

VITAL STATISTICS

DRUG CLASS
Anticoagulant and Antiplatelet Drugs

BRAND NAME
Fragmin

OTHER DRUGS IN THIS CLASS
aspirin, dipyridamole, heparin, warfarin

GENERAL DESCRIPTION
Dalteparin is an injectable anticoagulant used to prevent thrombosis (formation of blood clots) in patients having abdominal surgery who are at high risk of this complication, to prevent blood clots in patients with renal failure who are treated with extracorporeal blood circulation (hemodialysis), and to treat established deep vein thrombosis. Deep vein thrombosis, common after surgery, can lead to pulmonary embolism, a potentially fatal complication in which a blood clot travels to the lungs. Dalteparin acts by inhibiting factors that contribute to coagulation, reducing the formation of new clots and the propagation of existing ones. See Anticoagulant and Antiplatelet Drugs for more information, including possible interactions and additional special information.

PRECAUTIONS

WARNING
An overdose can cause serious problems such as bleeding and shortness of breath. Seek emergency treatment if you think you have taken too much, or if you notice any bleeding.

Tell your doctor if you have a bleeding or platelet disorder, liver or kidney disease, retinal disease, or severe hypertension, or have had recent surgery or gastrointestinal bleeding.

If you are sensitive to heparin or pork products, you might also be sensitive to dalteparin.

SPECIAL INFORMATION
- Maintain regular contact with your doctor while taking dalteparin; monitoring may be necessary.
- There is no evidence that dalteparin will harm a fetus, but this drug should be avoided during pregnancy. Dalteparin should be avoided if you are breast-feeding.
- The safety and effectiveness of dalteparin for children under 18 has not been established.

TARGET AILMENTS
Treatment or prevention of blood clots

SIDE EFFECTS

NOT SERIOUS
- Pain at injection site

SERIOUS
- Itching, hives, or rash; fever
- Difficulty swallowing; trouble breathing; swelling in face
- Dizziness or fainting
- Blood under the skin at injection site; hemorrhage
- Bleeding, bruising, or petechiae (showers of tiny red spots on the skin) (low platelet count)

CALL YOUR DOCTOR IMMEDIATELY.

DAMIANA

LATIN NAME
Turnera diffusa

VITAL STATISTICS

GENERAL DESCRIPTION

Since 1874, when damiana became commercially available in the United States, its effectiveness as an aphrodisiac has been touted by some even as it was being dismissed by herbalists and the public. It has been used as a food additive in sweets, in baked goods, and in liqueurs, and a few of its believers have smoked the leaves and reported a high lasting about 90 minutes. Although some contemporary herbalists think damiana has no medicinal value, others recommend it to support the nervous and endocrine systems. How damiana renders this support has not been proved, but anecdotal evidence suggests that the herb is useful in testosterone production and may stimulate the central nervous system, aiding in the alleviation of depression. It is prescribed to reduce anxiety, depression, or mood disorders of a sexual origin. Damiana may also promote digestion and serve as a laxative. The FDA has approved damiana as a food additive.

PREPARATIONS

Over the counter:
Damiana is available in dry bulk, tinctures, and capsules.

At home:

TEA: Pour 1 cup boiling water over 1 tsp dried leaves, steep covered for 10 to 15 minutes. Drink three times daily.

COMBINATIONS: For nervous anxiety or depression, damiana can be combined with any or all of the following: oats, skullcap, or kola.

Consult a qualified practitioner for the dosage appropriate for you and the specific condition being treated.

PRECAUTIONS

WARNING

This herb should not be used with children unless it is specifically prescribed by a healthcare practitioner who is knowledgeable about herbs.

POSSIBLE INTERACTIONS

Combining damiana with other herbs may necessitate a lower dosage.

TARGET AILMENTS

Take internally for:

Anxiety-induced stomach indigestion

Hormone-based disorders such as impotence, testosterone deficiency

Depression, anxiety, or listlessness

SIDE EFFECTS

NOT SERIOUS

- Insomnia
- Headache

LARGE DOSES OF DAMIANA MAY CAUSE THESE SYMPTOMS. DISCONTINUE USE.

SERIOUS

NONE EXPECTED

DANDELION

LATIN NAME
Taraxacum mongolicum

VITAL STATISTICS

GENERAL DESCRIPTION

While the Chinese dandelion differs slightly from the Western variety, both have roots with similar medicinal properties. Chinese medical practitioners use dandelion frequently for hepatitis, stomach disorders, and fluid retention. Test-tube studies suggest that the herb may kill staph and other bacteria that resist other antimicrobial treatments. Dandelion root, according to traditional Chinese medicine, is characterized as bitter, sweet, and cold.

Chinese medicine takes a holistic approach to healthcare, fashioning remedies to treat the entire being as well as the specific parts or areas. Single herbs may be used alone or in combination with other herbs to prevent and combat disease, which is thought to arise from disturbances in the flow of a bodily energy called chi (pronounced "chee") and blood, or from a lack of balance in the complementary states of yin and yang.

PREPARATIONS

Dandelion is available in bulk form from Chinese pharmacies, Asian markets, and some Western health food stores. It is also possible to obtain it in tablet form.

COMBINATIONS: Mixed with trichosanthes fruit, fritillaria, and myrrh, dandelion root is applied to breast abscesses, carbuncles, and furuncles. Dandelion blended with chrysanthemum flower *(Chrysanthemum morifolium)* and skullcap is used to treat red, swollen eyes. A preparation that contains dandelion and honeysuckle flower is prescribed for painful, deep-rooted boils. Adding forsythia fruit and chrysanthemum flower strengthens the effect. Consult your herbalist for information on additional combinations and doses.

PRECAUTIONS

WARNING

Overdoses of the herb can cause mild diarrhea; some preparations using Chinese dandelion root may cause heartburn.

D

TARGET AILMENTS
Take internally for:
Hepatitis
Jaundice and other liver conditions
Poor lactation in nursing mothers
Painful and difficult urination
Red, painful, swollen eyes
Use both internally and topically for:
Abscesses
Boils, carbuncles, and sores, particularly on the breast

SIDE EFFECTS

NONE EXPECTED

DANDELION

LATIN NAME
Taraxacum officinale

D

VITAL STATISTICS

GENERAL DESCRIPTION

Dandelion acts as a natural diuretic while also supplying potassium, a nutrient often lost through diuretic use. The plant is rich in vitamins A and C—antioxidants that are believed to help prevent cancer. The young leaves can be eaten fresh or used in herbal preparations. For visual characteristics, see the Color Guide to Prescription Drugs and Herbs.

PREPARATIONS

Over the counter:

Available in tinctures, prepared tea, capsules, and dried or fresh leaves or roots.

At home:

TEA: Steep covered 1 tbsp dried or 2 tbsp fresh leaves per cup of boiling water for 10 minutes. Drink as many as 4 cups a day.

DECOCTION: Simmer covered 1 tbsp fresh or dried root per cup of water for 15 minutes. Drink as many as 4 cups a day.

NUTRITION AND DIET: Add fresh leaves to a salad, or blend in a juicer with other green vegetables. Use with barberry for liver and gallbladder problems. Use with yarrow for water retention.

Consult a qualified practitioner for the dosage appropriate for your specific condition.

TARGET AILMENTS

Poor digestion; gallbladder problems; inflammation of the liver

Water retention accompanying congestive heart failure, high blood pressure, menstrual problems, and general joint pain

PRECAUTIONS

SPECIAL INFORMATION

- If any of these conditions apply, use dandelion only in consultation with a professional herbalist or naturopath: pregnancy, heart condition, or inflamed stomach or colon. Consult a herbalist if you plan to use the herb longer than two or three months.
- Use low-strength preparations for adults over 65 and children between two and 12. Do not give to children younger than two.

POSSIBLE INTERACTIONS

Combining dandelion with other herbs may necessitate a lower dosage.

For those taking either lithium or potassium, dandelion may increase the concentrations of these substances in the blood.

Check with your doctor before combining this herb with prescription diuretics.

SIDE EFFECTS

NOT SERIOUS

- Allergic dermatitis
- Stomach upset and diarrhea
- Flulike symptoms
- Liver pain

DISCONTINUE USE AND CALL YOUR DOCTOR WHEN CONVENIENT.

DECONGESTANTS

VITAL STATISTICS

GENERIC NAMES

Rx: phenylpropanolamine
OTC: oxymetazoline, phenylephrine, phenylpropanolamine, pseudoephedrine

GENERAL DESCRIPTION

Available as sprays or pills in over-the-counter and prescription forms, decongestants relieve nasal and sinus congestion and headaches by constricting blood vessels in the nose and other parts of the respiratory system. Because the drugs affect certain receptors in the nervous system, high doses (doses above recommended amounts) may produce central nervous system side effects. Some of those medications used orally are chemically related to amphetamines and are banned for athletic use.

Decongestants come in both pill and spray forms; the form selected depends on the purpose to be achieved. Nasal sprays give the fastest results and are used for short-term treatment of nasal congestion. Use of these sprays for extended periods of time or at higher-than-recommended doses may result in nasal irritation or rebound congestion (nasal stuffiness, swelling, and redness without underlying illness).

In pill form, decongestants are used alone or in combination with other drugs to relieve the symptoms of colds, allergies, and other respiratory problems. Decongestant pills do not usually produce rebound congestion and therefore are useful for long-term treatment of nasal congestion. Decongestant pills can also be used to treat problems caused by pressure changes during air travel. For more information, see individual entries for the generic drugs listed above.

PRECAUTIONS

SPECIAL INFORMATION

- In rare cases, phenylpropanolamine has been associated with serious cardiovascular side effects, including severe high blood pressure and heart-rhythm problems, as well as psychotic problems, such as hallucinations and seizures. These effects are associated with high doses of phenylpropanolamine and may be more likely in individuals with similar preexisting problems, such as high blood pressure or neurological or psychiatric disease.
- Check with your doctor before taking any decongestants if you have cardiovascular disease (including angina, coronary artery disease, and hypertension), hyperthyroidism (overactive thyroid), diabetes, or glaucoma. Decongestants may exacerbate these conditions.

TARGET AILMENTS

Congestion of the nose and sinuses caused by allergy or upper respiratory infection

Congestion of Eustachian tubes, which join the ear with the nose and throat (pseudoephedrine)

Bronchial asthma (phenylpropanolamine)

Obesity (phenylpropanolamine, used as an appetite suppressant)

Urinary incontinence (phenylpropanolamine)

D

CONTINUED

DECONGESTANTS

D

POSSIBLE INTERACTIONS

Anticoagulant (blood-thinning) drugs: decreased anticoagulant effect.

Beta blockers: oral decongestants can lessen the effectiveness of beta blockers, causing hypertension.

Digitalis preparations: taking these drugs with oral decongestants may result in heart-rhythm problems.

High blood pressure drugs containing rauwolfia: decreased effectiveness of oral decongestants.

MAO inhibitors: increased stimulant action of oral decongestants, causing effects such as hypertension and heart-rhythm problems.

Stimulants (such as other decongestants, amphetamines, caffeine): increased stimulant effects, leading to excessive nervousness, insomnia, irregular heart rhythm, or seizures.

Tricyclic antidepressants (such as amitriptyline): increased action of oxymetazoline and phenylpropanolamine, making serious central nervous system side effects more likely.

SIDE EFFECTS

NOT SERIOUS

- Mild nervousness
- Mild restlessness
- Mild insomnia
- Dizziness
- Lightheadedness
- Nausea
- Dryness of mouth or nose
- Rebound congestion
- Sneezing; burning, stinging, or dryness of nose (spray and topical forms)

CALL YOUR DOCTOR IF THESE SYMPTOMS CONTINUE OR BECOME TROUBLESOME.

SERIOUS

- Severe headache
- Nervousness
- Restlessness
- Insomnia
- Pounding or irregular heartbeat
- High blood pressure

CONTACT YOUR DOCTOR IMMEDIATELY.

DEVIL'S CLAW

LATIN NAME
Harpagophytum procumbens

D

VITAL STATISTICS

GENERAL INFORMATION

An extremely bitter herb, devil's claw grows in arid regions in southern and eastern Africa, where the root is collected at the end of the rainy season. Traditionally, the dried root was made into a tea used to treat indigestion, fevers, and blood disorders, whereas the fresh root was used for an ointment to put on boils and skin lesions.

Since the herb's active ingredient, harpagoside, is believed to reduce pain and inflammation, devil's claw is sometimes recommended for arthritis; this use, however, was not validated when the herb was clinically tested. Herbalists do recommend trying devil's claw for arthritis on a case-by-case basis, especially if the arthritis is accompanied by severe pain and swelling.

Some herbalists believe that devil's claw is helpful in the treatment of liver and lymphatic disorders, and that it also may lower blood sugar levels. It is also used to stimulate the appetite and aid digestion. Since it must be imported from Africa, devil's claw is very expensive.

PREPARATIONS

Over the counter:

Devil's claw is available in bulk and in tinctures and capsules.

At home:

DECOCTION: Put ½ to 1 tsp devil's claw ground to a powder in 1 cup boiling water; simmer covered for 15 minutes and strain; drink three times a day for at least one month.

COMPRESS: Soak a pad in an infusion of devil's claw for several minutes; wring out and apply to the affected area.

COMBINATIONS: Devil's claw can be used with bogbean, celery seed, and meadowsweet for arthritis.

Consult a qualified practitioner for the dosage appropriate for you and the specific condition being treated.

PRECAUTIONS

WARNING

Avoid devil's claw during pregnancy.

Use of this herb by children for more than seven to 10 days should be done in conjunction with a healthcare practitioner.

POSSIBLE INTERACTIONS

Combining devil's claw with other herbs may necessitate a lower dosage.

TARGET AILMENTS

Take internally for:

Arthritis; gout

Liver dysfunctions

Gallbladder disorders

Digestive problems

Diabetes

Apply externally for:

Skin lesions and boils

SIDE EFFECTS

NONE EXPECTED

DEXTROMETHORPHAN

VITAL STATISTICS

DRUG CLASS
Cough Suppressants

BRAND NAMES
Some types of Comtrex, Contac, and Thera-Flu; Benylin Adult Formula Cough Suppressant, Benylin DM Cough Syrup, Benylin Pediatric Cough Suppressant, Buckley's Mixture, Dextromethorphan Hydrobromide Cough Syrup, Dimetapp DM Elixir, DM Syrup, Drixoral Cough Liquid Caps, Hold DM 4 Hour Cough Relief, Iodrol, NyQuil, PediaCare (various forms), Pertussin CS, Robitussin Cough Calmers, Robitussin Pediatric Cough Suppressant, Robitussin Maximum Strength Cough Suppressant, Robitussin-CF, Robitussin-DM, St. Joseph Cough Suppressant for Children, Sucrets 4 Hour Cough Suppressant, Triaminic Nite Light, Triaminic Sore Throat Formula, Triaminic DM Syrup, Triaminicol Multi-Symptom Relief, Trocal, Tylenol Cold (adults and children), Vicks DayQuil Liquid or LiquiCaps, Vicks Pediatric Formula 44 Cough Medicine, Vicks Formula 44 Maximum Strength Cough Suppressant

GENERAL DESCRIPTION
Dextromethorphan is the main ingredient in a large number of widely available over-the-counter cough suppressants (antitussives) and common cold medications. The drug is used for the temporary relief of dry coughs caused by the common cold or flu. It should not be used for chronic coughs or for coughs that produce secretions.

Some cough suppressants act on the throat and bronchial passages to soothe irritation and relax the muscles. Others, including dextromethorphan, work in the brain to suppress the cough reflex. Like codeine, from which it is derived, dextromethorphan inhibits the cough reflex by acting directly on the cough center, located in the medulla of the brain. Unlike codeine, however, dextromethorphan is not a narcotic. When taken at the recommended dosages, it lacks analgesic and addictive properties and does not depress respiration. For more information, see Codeine, Cough Suppressants, and Opioid Analgesics.

DEXTROMETHORPHAN

PRECAUTIONS

☠ ***WARNING***

Overdose symptoms include confusion, hyperactivity, feeling of intoxication, lack of coordination, hallucinations, irritability, and severe nausea and vomiting. Seek immediate medical help.

SPECIAL INFORMATION

- Do not take dextromethorphan if you have had an allergic reaction to any medications containing this drug.
- Before taking dextromethorphan, consult your doctor if you have asthma or impaired liver function, or if your cough is producing mucus or phlegm.
- Use dextromethorphan only as instructed by your doctor or the directions on the label. Take it only as long as needed; some reports suggest that this drug may be habit forming if you use too much for too long.
- Check with your doctor if your cough persists for more than seven to 10 days or if it is accompanied by a skin rash, high fever, or continuing headache. These symptoms may indicate the presence of other medical problems.

POSSIBLE INTERACTIONS

Central nervous system depressants (anesthetics, antidepressants, antihistamines, anti-insomnia drugs, barbiturates, benzodiazepines, muscle relaxants, narcotics or prescription pain medicines, tranquilizers): increased sedative and depressant effects.

Monoamine oxidase (MAO) inhibitors: disorientation, psychotic behavior, coma.

TARGET AILMENTS

Dry, nonproductive, and temporary coughing

SIDE EFFECTS

NOT SERIOUS

- Mild drowsiness
- Mild dizziness
- Stomach pain
- Nausea
- Vomiting

CALL YOUR DOCTOR IF THESE SYMPTOMS PERSIST OR BECOME BOTHERSOME.

SERIOUS

ADVERSE EFFECTS AT THE RECOMMENDED NONPRESCRIPTION DOSAGES ARE MILD AND RARE. FOR OVERDOSE SYMPTOMS, SEE WARNING ABOVE, LEFT.

D

DGL

D

VITAL STATISTICS

OTHER NAME
deglycyrrhizinated licorice

DAILY DOSAGE
As directed.

GENERAL DESCRIPTION
When the substance glycyrrhizin is removed from the herb licorice root, a derivative known as deglycyrrhizinated licorice, or DGL, is formed. Glycyrrhizin, regarded as one of licorice root's most active ingredients, possesses many therapeutic properties for which licorice root is famous, such as anti-inflammatory, antiviral, and antidepressant properties. However, glycyrrhizin is also responsible for the harmful side effects associated with licorice, including high blood pressure, fluid retention, weakness, and irregular heart rate.

The derivative DGL causes none of the side effects associated with licorice root yet still offers healing benefits, especially in the treatment of peptic ulcers resulting from the overuse of aspirin, ibuprofen, caffeine, or alcohol. DGL helps increase mucous secretion, which helps protect the gastric lining, inhibiting the development of ulcers. DGL may be effective not only in treating existing ulcers but also in helping prevent injury to the stomach lining during long-term therapeutic use of aspirin or nonsteroidal anti-inflammatory drugs, or other medications that may tend to promote gastric ulcers.

PREPARATIONS
Available as a chewable tablet, liquid, or extract.

PRECAUTIONS

SPECIAL INFORMATION
- Since some ulcers need to be treated with antibiotics or other medications, consult your doctor if you think you have an ulcer.
- Do not give DGL supplements to children under two years of age except upon the advice of a doctor.
- If you have an existing medical condition or if you are pregnant, planning a pregnancy, or breast-feeding, consult your doctor before taking DGL supplements.

POSSIBLE INTERACTIONS
If you are taking any other supplements, prescription or nonprescription medications, or herbal therapies, consult your doctor before taking DGL supplements.

TARGET AILMENTS

Peptic ulcers

Mouth sores

SIDE EFFECTS
NONE EXPECTED

DHEA

D

VITAL STATISTICS

OTHER NAME
dehydroepiandrosterone

DAILY DOSAGE
5 mg to 50 mg

GENERAL DESCRIPTION
DHEA is a hormone produced by the adrenal glands. Since levels of this hormone are highest in puberty and young adulthood, DHEA supplements have acquired a reputation as an anti-aging drug. DHEA's purported benefits include the ability to strengthen the immune system, increase energy, enhance sex drive, reduce memory loss, reduce stress, and treat diseases such as cancer, diabetes, Alzheimer's disease, and Parkinson's disease, though none of these claims has been proved. Used cautiously and in low doses, DHEA may provide some benefits as a hormone replacement therapy.

DHEA is widely available as a nutritional supplement in health food stores for the public to purchase and use, perhaps indiscriminately. In large doses DHEA is known to cause harmful side effects, and its other long-term effects and possible drug interactions are unknown. While many experts are hopeful about DHEA's health benefits, a doctor's supervision is strongly advised when taking this supplement.

PREPARATIONS
Available in capsules and sublingual capsules.

TARGET AILMENTS

Depression; mood swings; heart disease; obesity; memory loss; weak bones; autoimmune disorders

PRECAUTIONS

WARNING
Use only under a doctor's supervision.
Do not take if you are pregnant or breast-feeding. Large doses may complicate prostate or ovarian cancer.

SPECIAL INFORMATION
- Most healthy people under the age of 40 have no reason to use this supplement because the body produces it naturally. Also, DHEA supplements can inhibit the body's natural production of the hormone.
- Consult a knowledgeable doctor about which brand of DHEA supplements to buy.
- Synthetic DHEA is created in a laboratory using a constituent of Mexican wild yam. The plant itself will not provide the health benefits; any commercial claims to the contrary should be ignored.

POSSIBLE INTERACTIONS
Since DHEA may interact with prescription or over-the-counter drugs, herbal therapies, or other supplements, tell your doctor if you are taking any drugs or natural medicines.

Estrogen therapy: your dosage may need to be altered if you begin taking DHEA.

SIDE EFFECTS

NOT SERIOUS

Acne; unwanted hair growth in women; enlarged breasts in men; mood swings; fatigue; insomnia

CALL YOUR DOCTOR IF THESE EFFECTS PERSIST.

DIAZEPAM

D

VITAL STATISTICS

DRUG CLASS
Antianxiety Drugs [Benzodiazepines]

BRAND NAME
Valium

OTHER DRUGS IN THIS CLASS
alprazolam, clonazepam, lorazepam, temazepam, triazolam

GENERAL DESCRIPTION
Since 1963, diazepam has been used to reduce anxiety and nervous tension. Despite its history of being overprescribed, particularly in the years immediately following its introduction, diazepam is effective in up to 80 percent of anxiety patients and is now considered one of the drugs of choice for treating mild to moderate anxiety. However, diazepam should not be used for the stress and anxiety of everyday living.

Like other benzodiazepines, the drug is potentially habit forming, especially when used for extended periods of time or at high dosages. Diazepam may also be used to treat acute alcohol withdrawal and presurgery anxiety, and as an adjunct treatment for skeletal muscle spasms and seizure disorders. For visual characteristics of diazepam and the brand Valium, see the Color Guide to Prescription Drugs and Herbs.

TARGET AILMENTS
Anxiety and panic disorders
Alcohol withdrawal
Convulsions or seizures; skeletal muscle pain and spasticity; presurgery anxiety (as an adjunct)

PRECAUTIONS

WARNING
Never combine alcohol with diazepam; the combination can cause dangerous central nervous system and respiratory depression.

Do not abruptly stop taking diazepam. Sudden cessation can provoke withdrawal symptoms, including seizures; irritability; insomnia; confusion; mental depression; hypersensitivity to pain, noise, or light; and feelings of suspicion and distrust. Slowly reduce the dosage under your doctor's guidance.

Rarely, diazepam may cause the following serious side effects: rash or itching, indicating an allergic reaction; jaundice; low blood pressure; anemia; unusual bruising or bleeding, indicating low platelet count. Call your doctor immediately.

SPECIAL INFORMATION
- Diazepam can impair your alertness, judgment, and coordination. Avoid driving and performing hazardous activities until you know how the drug affects you.
- Let your doctor know if you have narrow-angle glaucoma, a liver or kidney impairment, chronic respiratory disease, myasthenia gravis, depression, sleep apnea, or a history of drug abuse or addiction. Diazepam may exacerbate these conditions.
- This drug can cause sleep apnea in people with chronic respiratory disease, such as emphysema.
- Diazepam can cause physical and psychological dependence, sometimes after only one or two weeks, but usually after prolonged use.
- People with a history of drug or alcohol abuse are at a greater risk of psychological dependence on diazepam.

DIAZEPAM

- Tolerance may increase with prolonged use; as your body adjusts to diazepam, the drug becomes less effective. Never increase the dose without consulting your doctor, because the risk of diazepam dependence increases with higher doses.
- Do not take diazepam if you are pregnant or breast-feeding.

POSSIBLE INTERACTIONS

Alcohol, anticonvulsants, antihistamines that cause drowsiness (clemastine, diphenhydramine), barbiturates, MAO inhibitors, opioids, tricyclic antidepressants: increased sedative effects, such as excessive mental (central nervous system) depression, sleepiness, and slow or shallow breathing. It is very important that you avoid taking diazepam in combination with any of these drugs.

Antacids: may slow the absorption of diazepam. Separate from diazepam dose by an hour.

Beta blockers, cimetidine, disulfiram, erythromycin, ketoconazole, omeprazole, oral contraceptives, probenecid: may prolong the amount of time diazepam remains in your body, leading to increased diazepam effects and possible toxicity.

Tobacco (smoking): decreased diazepam effects.

Clozapine: risk of profound hypotension (low blood pressure), slow or shallow breathing, cessation of breathing, and cardiac arrest leading to death.

Isoniazid: increased diazepam effect and possible toxicity.

Levodopa: decreased levodopa effect.

Phenytoin: possible phenytoin toxicity.

Rifampin: decreased diazepam effect.

Valproic acid: increased diazepam effects, including mental depression.

Zidovudine: risk of zidovudine toxicity.

SIDE EFFECTS

NOT SERIOUS

- Clumsiness or unsteadiness
- Lethargy
- Dry mouth
- Nausea
- Change in bowel habits
- Temporary amnesia (especially "traveler's amnesia" when taken to treat insomnia associated with jet lag)

TELL YOUR DOCTOR IF THESE SYMPTOMS PERSIST OR BECOME BOTHERSOME. CONTACT YOUR DOCTOR IF YOU ARE HAVING DIFFICULTY WITH YOUR MEMORY.

SERIOUS

- Drowsiness
- Dizziness or blurred vision
- Persistent or severe headache
- Confusion
- Depression
- Changes in behavior (outbursts of anger, difficulty concentrating)
- Hallucinations
- Uncontrolled movement of body or eyes
- Muscle weakness
- Chills or fever
- Sore throat

TELL YOUR DOCTOR ABOUT THESE SYMPTOMS RIGHT AWAY.

Rx DICLOFENAC

D

VITAL STATISTICS

DRUG CLASS
Analgesics [Nonsteroidal Anti-Inflammatory Drugs (NSAIDs)]

BRAND NAMES
Cataflam (immediate release); Voltaren (delayed release)

OTHER DRUGS IN THIS SUBCLASS
etodolac, flurbiprofen, ibuprofen, ketoprofen, ketorolac, nabumetone, naproxen, oxaprozin

GENERAL DESCRIPTION
Diclofenac is a type of pain reliever acting at the site of the pain. It may be used by people who cannot tolerate aspirin, or when aspirin or acetaminophen is not effective. It comes in timed-release form for treating symptoms of rheumatoid arthritis, osteoarthritis, and arthritis of the spine. In addition to reducing inflammation, diclofenac is also used for relief of menstrual discomfort and pain in general. For further information, including additional possible interactions, see Nonsteroidal Anti-Inflammatory Drugs (NSAIDs). For visual characteristics of diclofenac and the brand Voltaren, see the Color Guide to Prescription Drugs and Herbs.

TARGET AILMENTS

Inflammation, especially related to osteoarthritis and rheumatoid arthritis

Pain, especially from inflammation, dental and other surgeries, menstruation, or migraines

PRECAUTIONS

POSSIBLE INTERACTIONS
Antidiabetic drugs and insulin: diclofenac may either increase or decrease the hypoglycemic effect of antidiabetic drugs.

SIDE EFFECTS

NOT SERIOUS
- Dizziness, drowsiness; headache; abdominal pain or cramps
- Constipation; diarrhea; indigestion; nausea

CONSULT YOUR DOCTOR IF THESE SYMPTOMS PERSIST.

SERIOUS
- Hives, rash, intense itching, and trouble breathing (anaphylactic reaction)

SEEK EMERGENCY HELP.

- Chest pain or irregular heartbeat; diminished hearing or ringing in the ears
- Trouble breathing; fluid retention; blood in urine
- Black or tarry stools (gastrointestinal bleeding; ulceration of stomach
- Photosensitivity
- Bleeding, bruising, fatigue, tenderness in upper abdomen, and yellow eyes or skin (jaundice)

DISCONTINUE USE AND CALL YOUR DOCTOR IMMEDIATELY.

DICYCLOMINE

VITAL STATISTICS

DRUG CLASS
Antispasmodic Drugs

BRAND NAME
Bentyl

GENERAL DESCRIPTION
Introduced in 1954, dicyclomine is an antispasmodic drug used to reduce muscle spasms in the gastrointestinal tract. The drug acts directly on the smooth muscles of the gastrointestinal tract. Dicyclomine also has an anticholinergic effect, meaning that it inhibits the action of a body chemical called acetylcholine. This prevents muscles in the GI tract from contracting, thereby eliminating spasms.

Antispasmodic drugs are used to treat a number of disorders, including asthma, urinary incontinence, motion sickness, irritable bowel syndrome, infant colic, and peptic ulcers. Besides preventing involuntary muscle contractions, these medications also inhibit glandular secretions such as saliva, bronchial mucus, and stomach acids. For visual characteristics of dicyclomine and the brand-name drug Bentyl, see the Color Guide to Prescription Drugs and Herbs.

PRECAUTIONS

SPECIAL INFORMATION

- Do not give this drug to infants under the age of six months.
- Do not use dicyclomine if you have ulcerative colitis, paralytic ileus (obstruction of the bowel), urinary retention, myasthenia gravis (muscle weakness), gastroesophageal reflux, esophagitis, or an allergic reaction to anticholinergic drugs.
- Before taking this medication, inform your doctor if you have glaucoma, hypertension, angina, coronary artery disease, congestive heart failure, tachycardia, asthma or bronchitis, an enlarged prostate, a peptic ulcer, or kidney, liver, or thyroid disease. You should also tell your doctor if you plan to have surgery within two months that will require anesthesia.
- If you are pregnant, consult your doctor and weigh the benefit-to-risk ratio of taking this drug.
- Dicyclomine passes into breast milk and lessens the flow; avoid the drug if you are nursing.
- Take this medication 30 minutes before meals and at bedtime.
- Prolonged use of dicyclomine can result in chronic constipation and possible fecal impaction.
- Dicyclomine may cause drowsiness or blurred vision; use caution when driving or operating machinery.

CONTINUED

DICYCLOMINE

D

POSSIBLE INTERACTIONS

Antacids and some antidiarrheal drugs: decreased dicyclomine effect.

Ketoconazole: decreased ketoconazole effect.

Other anticholinergics, amantadine, antihistamines, certain antiviral drugs, benzodiazepines, buclizine, MAO inhibitors, meperidine, methylphenidate, orphenadrine, phenothiazines, quinidine, tricyclic antidepressants: increased dicyclomine effect.

Potassium chloride: risk of intestinal ulcers.

TARGET AILMENTS

Irritable bowel syndrome (spastic colon)

Infant colic

SIDE EFFECTS

NOT SERIOUS

- Altered sense of taste
- Decreased perspiration
- Nasal congestion
- Insomnia
- Dizziness
- Drowsiness
- Constipation
- Dry mouth, ears, and throat

CALL YOUR DOCTOR IF THESE EFFECTS BECOME BOTHERSOME.

SERIOUS

- Hives or skin rash
- Intense itching
- Headaches
- Difficulty urinating
- Nausea and vomiting
- Confusion or delirium
- Agitation
- Heart palpitations
- Blurred vision
- Dilated pupils
- Eye pain
- Difficulty swallowing and breathing
- Muscle weakness
- Lightheadedness

DISCONTINUE USE AND CONTACT YOUR DOCTOR IMMEDIATELY.

DIGOXIN

VITAL STATISTICS

DRUG CLASS
Digitalis Preparations

BRAND NAMES
Lanoxin, Lanoxicaps

GENERAL DESCRIPTION
Digoxin is a digitalis preparation that has been used since 1934 to strengthen the heart and to treat heart arrhythmias. Digitalis preparations are effective, but toxicity is a major concern with their use, since the effective dose is often only slightly smaller than a toxic dose. Additionally, digoxin interacts with many over-the-counter and prescription drugs.

PRECAUTIONS

SPECIAL INFORMATION
- Do not discontinue this medication without your doctor's knowledge; to do so might cause heart problems.
- Check your pulse if directed by your doctor; be sure to report any low pulse rate (less than 60 beats per minute) to your doctor immediately.
- Digoxin can cross the placenta and affect the fetus, and it can pass to infants through breast milk. Pregnant and nursing women should therefore use caution when taking this medication. The dosage often must be reduced for women who have given birth recently (within six weeks).
- Avoid all over-the-counter antacids as well as cough, cold, allergy, and diet drugs, except when advised otherwise by your doctor.
- Foods high in fiber may interfere with the absorption of digoxin.
- Heart failure may cause potassium levels in your body to drop. Talk with your doctor about adding potassium-rich foods, such as bananas and oranges, to your diet, since digoxin toxicity is increased if serum potassium is low.
- Patients with kidney failure require lower doses of digoxin.

POSSIBLE INTERACTIONS
Following is a partial list of the drugs and other substances that can interact with digoxin. To compensate for these interactions, your doctor may have to adjust the dosages of digoxin and any other drugs you may be taking.

Amiodarone (an antiarrhythmia drug): increased amounts of digoxin circulating in the blood, which can lead to heart-rhythm problems.

Other antiarrhythmia drugs, calcium supplements, rauwolfia (an antihypertensive drug): increased heart arrhythmias.

Antacids, antidiarrheal drugs (such as kaolin and pectin), antiulcer drugs (including sulfasalazine), dietary fiber, laxatives: inhibited absorption of digoxin, reducing its effectiveness.

TARGET AILMENTS

Congestive heart failure (all degrees)

Prevention and treatment of heart arrhythmias (atrial fibrillation and flutter, atrioventricular tachycardia, and paroxysmal nodal tachycardia)

CONTINUED

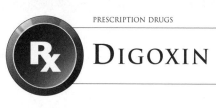

DIGOXIN

D

Calcium channel blockers: increased amounts of digoxin circulating in the blood, possibly leading to heart-rhythm problems.

Diuretics: may increase or decrease the effects of digoxin.

Erythromycin: increased absorption of digoxin into the body, thereby increasing its actions and side effects.

Fluoxetine: increased digoxin effects.

Indomethacin, a nonsteroidal anti-inflammatory drug (NSAID): increased amounts of digoxin circulating in the blood.

Potassium supplements (salts): increased risk of excess potassium, possibly leading to heart-rhythm problems; do not take potassium supplements with digoxin.

Quinidine or quinine: increased blood concentration of digoxin.

Stimulant drugs, such as amphetamines or over-the-counter decongestants: increased risk of heart-rhythm problems.

SIDE EFFECTS

NOT SERIOUS

NONE EXPECTED; ALL SIDE EFFECTS ARE POTENTIALLY SERIOUS.

SERIOUS

- Slow or irregular heartbeat; in children, fast heartbeat
- Visual disturbances, such as blurred vision or halos around objects
- Drowsiness, confusion, or depression
- Headache
- Fainting
- Digestive problems, such as pain in the lower stomach, diarrhea, nausea, vomiting, or loss of appetite
- Unusual fatigue or weakness
- Allergic reactions (rare), such as skin rash or hives

CALL YOUR DOCTOR IMMEDIATELY IF YOU EXPERIENCE ANY OF THESE EFFECTS.

DILANTIN

VITAL STATISTICS

DRUG CLASS
Anticonvulsant Drugs

GENERIC NAME
phenytoin

OTHER DRUGS IN THIS CLASS
carbamazepine, valproic acid

GENERAL DESCRIPTION
Dilantin is a brand name for the generic drug phenytoin. Introduced in 1938, this drug is one of several hydantoin anticonvulsant drugs used primarily in the suppression and control of epileptic seizures. Although the exact mechanisms by which these drugs work are unknown, anticonvulsants appear to inhibit the sudden spread of excessive or abnormal electrical impulses in the brain, thereby limiting or preventing epileptic convulsions. Dilantin is used to treat all types of epilepsy except absence (petit mal) seizures. It may be used alone or in combination with other anticonvulsants. For visual characteristics, see the Color Guide to Prescription Drugs and Herbs. For more information, see Anticonvulsant Drugs.

TARGET AILMENTS
Epileptic seizures, except absence (petit mal) type
Prevention and treatment of seizures during and following neurosurgery
Relief of pain in trigeminal neuralgia (tic douloureux). May be used alone or with carbamazepine.

PRECAUTIONS

WARNING
Seek immediate medical help for overdose. Overdose signs include double or blurred vision; jerky or rolling eye movements; slurred speech or stuttering; severe clumsiness, unsteadiness, confusion, and trembling; and staggering walk.

SPECIAL INFORMATION
- Do not use Dilantin if you have had an allergic reaction to this drug or to any of the hydantoin drugs in the past.
- Tell your doctor if you are taking any other drugs (prescription or over-the-counter); have diabetes, heart disease, or low blood pressure; have a history of impaired liver function or liver disease; or may soon have surgery under general anesthesia.
- Using Dilantin during pregnancy increases the risk of birth defects (fetal hydantoin syndrome). Be sure to tell your doctor if you are pregnant or planning to become pregnant soon.
- Since Dilantin may cause folic acid deficiency, talk with your doctor about taking a daily multivitamin supplement.
- Since Dilantin can cause gum problems (bleeding, tenderness, abnormal growth), good oral hygiene is essential: Be sure to brush and floss your teeth and massage your gums regularly and carefully. You should also see your dentist every three months to have your teeth cleaned.
- Dilantin may affect complete blood cell counts; blood cholesterol, calcium, glucose, thyroid hormone and other hormone levels; and liver function tests.
- Do not abruptly discontinue this drug or switch to another brand or generic unless so advised by your physician.

CONTINUED

DILANTIN

D

POSSIBLE INTERACTIONS

Dilantin interacts with a vast number of drugs, only a few of which are described here. Be sure to check with your physician before taking any other medication.

Alcohol, antacids, antidepressants (tricyclic), antihistamines, central nervous system depressants, diazoxide, and rifampin: decreased effectiveness of Dilantin in controlling epileptic seizures.

Anticoagulants, caffeine, corticosteroids, cyclosporine, doxycycline, drugs for high blood pressure, oral contraceptives, propranolol and other beta-adrenergic blockers, and sedatives: Dilantin may increase or decrease the effects of these drugs.

Cimetidine, sulfonamides, and valproic acid: increased effects of Dilantin and increased risk of severe side effects.

SIDE EFFECTS

NOT SERIOUS

- Mild sluggishness and fatigue; diarrhea
- Excessive growth of facial and body hair; enlargement of jaw; widening of nose tip; thickening of lips
- Swollen breasts (in males)
- Muscle twitching
- Nausea and vomiting
- Headache; dizziness
- Insomnia

CONSULT YOUR DOCTOR IF THESE EFFECTS PERSIST OR ARE BOTHERSOME.

SERIOUS

- Gum overgrowth
- Bleeding or tender gums
- Fever
- Enlarged glands in underarms or neck
- Mood changes
- Increase in seizures
- Muscle pain or weakness
- Excitability or nervousness
- Severe skin rash
- Joint pain and swelling
- Blurred or double vision
- Elevated blood sugar
- Sore throat, weakness, fever, or abnormal bruising or bleeding (bone marrow depression)
- Discolored urine; drug-induced hepatitis or nephritis

CONTACT YOUR DOCTOR IMMEDIATELY.

DILTIAZEM

VITAL STATISTICS

DRUG CLASS
Calcium Channel Blockers

BRAND NAMES
Cardizem, Dilacor XR

OTHER DRUGS IN THIS CLASS
amlodipine, isradipine, nifedipine, verapamil

GENERAL DESCRIPTION
The calcium channel blocker diltiazem has been used since 1977 to treat heart-rhythm problems, hypertension, and angina. Like other drugs in its class, diltiazem works to inhibit the passage of calcium into body cells. This relaxes the muscles that surround the arteries, dilating them. Diltiazem slows the contraction of the heart, which, together with the relaxation of the arteries, decreases the work load on the heart, lowering blood pressure and preventing some spasms of the coronary arteries. Diltiazem is used alone or in carefully selected combinations with other heart and blood pressure medications. For visual characteristics of the brand Dilacor XR, see the Color Guide to Prescription Drugs and Herbs. For information on possible drug interactions, see Calcium Channel Blockers.

PRECAUTIONS

SPECIAL INFORMATION
- Recent findings have prompted warnings from some healthcare professionals about the safety of calcium channel blockers. Before using diltiazem, be sure to discuss this matter thoroughly with your doctor. If you are already taking this drug, do not stop the medication without first consulting your doctor.
- Pregnant and nursing women should use diltiazem only if clearly needed.
- Let your doctor know if you are suffering from low blood pressure (hypotension), heart or kidney disease, heart arrhythmias, or a recent heart attack with pulmonary congestion.

D

TARGET AILMENTS

Angina

Heart-rhythm problems

High blood pressure

SIDE EFFECTS

NOT SERIOUS
- Constipation; diarrhea; nausea; vomiting
- Edema
- Headache
- Dizziness; weakness
- Flushing; rash
- Cough
- Flulike symptoms

CALL YOUR DOCTOR IF THESE EFFECTS BECOME TROUBLESOME.

SERIOUS
- Low blood pressure (hypotension)
- Slow heartbeat (bradycardia)
- Angina; congestive heart failure; heart palpitations (rare)

CONTACT YOUR DOCTOR IMMEDIATELY.

Rx

DIPHENHYDRAMINE

D

VITAL STATISTICS

DRUG CLASS
Antihistamines

BRAND NAMES
Rx: Benadryl
OTC: Benadryl, Excedrin PM, Tylenol Cold Night Time Medication Liquid, Tylenol PM, Unisom

OTHER DRUGS IN THIS CLASS
Rx: astemizole, cetirizine, fexofenadine, loratadine, promethazine, terfenadine
OTC: brompheniramine, chlorpheniramine, clemastine, dexbrompheniramine, doxylamine, triprolidine

GENERAL DESCRIPTION
Introduced in 1946, diphenhydramine was one of the first antihistamines. Its sedating and drying effects are more pronounced than those of the newer antihistamines. Diphenhydramine is used to treat symptoms of allergies, insomnia, chronic cough, vertigo, and mild Parkinson's disease. One form of diphenhydramine, a drug called dimenhydrinate, is used to treat motion sickness. See Antihistamines for additional information, including side effects.

PRECAUTIONS

SPECIAL INFORMATION
- Diphenhydramine causes drowsiness in varying degrees; avoid driving or operating machinery until you know how the drug affects you.
- Check with your doctor before using diphenhydramine if you have asthma, glaucoma, hyperthyroidism, high blood pressure, an enlarged prostate, a stomach ulcer, a bladder obstruction, or heart disease; this drug may exacerbate these conditions.
- Diphenhydramine is not recommended for pregnant and breast-feeding women. Consult your doctor and use only if clearly needed.

POSSIBLE INTERACTIONS
Alcohol: likely to increase the sedative effects of dipenhydramine; do not drink when you take these drugs.
Antianxiety drugs; barbiturates or other sedatives: do not take with antihistamines, as the combination may result in excessive sedation.
MAO inhibitors: can cause hypotension and dryness of the respiratory passages when taken with antihistamines. Do not combine these with antihistamines.

TARGET AILMENTS

Nasal and respiratory allergies (seasonal and nonseasonal), including hay fever

Common cold (used in combination with other drugs)

Insomnia

Motion sickness

Vertigo

SIDE EFFECTS
SEE ANTIHISTAMINES.

Rx DIPYRIDAMOLE

VITAL STATISTICS

DRUG CLASS
Anticoagulant and Antiplatelet Drugs

OTHER DRUGS IN THIS CLASS
aspirin, dalteparin, heparin, warfarin

GENERAL DESCRIPTION
Introduced in 1959, dipyridamole is used to prevent the formation and migration of blood clots (thromboembolism) following heart valve surgery and in other heart and blood conditions. It may be used alone or in combination with aspirin or one of the anticoagulants. Dipyridamole seems to inhibit the action of certain enzymes, thus preventing the aggregation of blood platelets (the smallest type of blood cell) and reducing the chance of blood clot formation. For additional information on side effects, special information, and drug interactions, see Anticoagulant and Antiplatelet Drugs.

PRECAUTIONS

WARNING
Before you use dipyridamole, be sure to tell your physician if you have or have had uncontrolled high blood pressure, ulcers, a heart attack, or a stroke.

SPECIAL INFORMATION
- Pregnant women and women who are nursing should check with a physician before taking dipyridamole.
- Avoid dangerous activities that might cause injuries. Be sure to report all falls and blows to your doctor. Internal bleeding may occur without symptoms.

POSSIBLE INTERACTIONS
Aspirin: taken concurrently, aspirin may make it possible to reduce the dosage of dipyridamole; it may also lessen the drug's side effects. Do not take aspirin for this purpose without first consulting your doctor.

TARGET AILMENTS

To reduce the risk of:

Formation and migration of blood clots (thromboembolism)

SIDE EFFECTS

NOT SERIOUS
- Dizziness; lightheadedness
- Flushing (infrequent)
- Weakness (infrequent)
- Stomach irritation

CALL YOUR DOCTOR IF THESE EFFECTS PERSIST OR ARE BOTHERSOME.

SERIOUS
- Chest pains
- Severe headaches
- Low or high blood pressure
- Rash
- Breathing problems
- Wheezing
- Runny nose
- Chest tightness

CALL YOUR DOCTOR IMMEDIATELY.

Rx DIURETICS

D

VITAL STATISTICS

GENERIC NAMES

amiloride, bumetanide, furosemide, hydrochlorothiazide, indapamide, potassium chloride (adjunct therapy), spironolactone, triamterene

GENERAL DESCRIPTION

Diuretics, sometimes referred to as water pills, work by increasing the elimination of fluids from the body through urination. This action lowers blood volume (and blood pressure), helps reduce swelling, and decreases excess fluid in body tissues. During the excretion of fluid, minerals such as sodium, potassium, magnesium, and calcium are also eliminated, a side effect that can cause problems with the heart, muscles, and other organs.

The heart, in particular, can be affected by either too much or too little potassium. For this reason, doctors often prescribe the newer, so-called potassium-sparing diuretics, designed to lessen the excretion of potassium. In some cases, supplements of potassium chloride are prescribed to restore supplies of that mineral lost through use of diuretics. For more information, see the entries for each of the generic drugs listed above.

PRECAUTIONS

SPECIAL INFORMATION

- Taking diuretics in hot weather or while engaged in heavy exertion can cause a dangerous loss of fluids or minerals. Watch for signs of dehydration (fatigue, dizziness, headache, nausea).
- If you are not taking a potassium-sparing diuretic, you may be given a potassium supplement (such as potassium chloride). If you are currently taking a potassium-sparing diuretic, you should avoid potassium supplements, salt substitutes (which are high in potassium), and potassium-rich foods such as bananas.
- When triamterene is suddenly discontinued after prolonged use, a rebound effect may occur, causing a rapid and potentially dangerous buildup of potassium in the body. Gradual discontinuation of this drug is important to prevent potassium toxicity.
- Because diuretics can affect glucose (blood sugar) levels, people with diabetes or who have been diagnosed with borderline diabetes should have their blood sugar levels monitored closely.

TARGET AILMENTS

General edema (swelling caused by water retention)

Edema associated with various medical conditions, including congestive heart failure and cirrhosis of the liver

High blood pressure (hypertension)

DIURETICS

POSSIBLE INTERACTIONS

Alcohol: increased action of diuretics.

Amiodarone: low blood potassium levels and subsequent heart arrhythmias.

Anticoagulants (such as coumarin derivatives or heparin): thiazide diuretics and furosemide may decrease the action of these drugs.

Antigout medications (including probenecid): thiazide diuretics may increase blood uric acid levels. Your doctor may need to adjust your dosage of the antigout medicine.

Digitalis and other heart drugs: though thiazide diuretics and furosemide are sometimes taken with heart medications, such combinations can increase the risk of potassium loss and additional heart-rhythm problems. Your doctor will closely monitor your progress.

Foods high in potassium (such as bananas and low-salt milk), salt substitutes, potassium supplements: may lead to potassium toxicity if ingested in sufficient amounts while taking a potassium-sparing diuretic.

Lithium: thiazide diuretics and furosemide may increase the risk of lithium toxicity.

Nonsteroidal anti-inflammatory drugs (NSAIDs), especially indomethacin: reduced effectiveness of diuretics.

Oral antidiabetic drugs, insulin: in rare cases, diuretics may interfere with these medicines or raise blood glucose levels.

Other blood pressure drugs, including angiotensin-converting enzyme (ACE) inhibitors: although diuretics are frequently taken with medications to lower blood pressure, caution should be exercised to ensure that blood pressure does not go too low.

SIDE EFFECTS

NOT SERIOUS

- Headache
- Blurred vision
- Diarrhea
- Dizziness or lightheadedness when getting up (orthostatic hypotension)
- Increased risk of sunburn

LET YOUR DOCTOR KNOW IF THESE SYMPTOMS CONTINUE OR BECOME TROUBLESOME.

SERIOUS

- Nausea or vomiting
- Fatigue or weakness
- Irregular or weak pulse
- Increased thirst
- Dry mouth
- Muscle pain or cramps
- Mood changes
- Mental confusion
- Blood in urine or stools
- Unusual bruising
- Skin rash

TELL YOUR DOCTOR IMMEDIATELY IF YOU EXPERIENCE ANY OF THESE SYMPTOMS. YOU MAY BE ADVISED TO LOWER YOUR DOSAGE AND INCREASE YOUR INTAKE OF FLUIDS AND MINERALS.

DMSO

D

Vital Statistics

GENERAL DESCRIPTION

The chemical dimethyl sulfoxide, or DMSO, was developed in the 1940s as an industrial solvent and is still used for that purpose today. Its popularity as a topical medicine for sprains, strains, and arthritis flourished in the 1960s, but the U.S. Food and Drug Administration (FDA) eventually rejected DMSO as a topical treatment after serious side effects were discovered. One danger of this potent solvent is that it can immediately penetrate the skin and enter the bloodstream, carrying with it germs from the skin's surface as well as harmful contaminants in the solvent preparation itself.

After extensive testing, the FDA approved DMSO as a therapy for interstitial cystitis, a disease that causes damage to the bladder walls and occurs primarily in women. Although most doctors discourage the use of DMSO because of its potentially harmful effects, some doctors still prescribe it.

DMSO is currently being researched for possible safe applications in the treatment of cancer, stroke, autoimmune disorders, injuries to the brain and spine, and skin problems.

PREPARATIONS

Available as a topical gel and as a liquid for bladder instillations.

TARGET AILMENTS

Interstitial cystitis

Precautions

WARNING

Use only under a doctor's supervision.

DMSO is a potent solvent. Upon contact with the skin it will be immediately absorbed into the bloodstream, carrying with it germs or chemicals from the skin's surface as well as contaminants present in the DMSO preparation itself.

DMSO sold over the counter is not as pure as that developed for prescription use and may contain harmful contaminants.

SPECIAL INFORMATION

- DMSO is no longer commonly recommended because of serious side effects. Each patient's reaction should be monitored closely.
- DMSO has an unpleasant smell that exudes from the body within minutes of application.

SIDE EFFECTS

NOT SERIOUS

- Rash
- Itching
- Body odor

CALL YOUR DOCTOR IF THESE EFFECTS PERSIST OR BECOME BOTHERSOME.

SERIOUS

- Blurred vision
- Cataracts
- Blood poisoning (sepsis)

DISCONTINUE USE AND CALL YOUR DOCTOR.

DOCUSATE

VITAL STATISTICS

DRUG CLASS
Laxatives

BRAND NAMES
Correctol, Colace, some types of Ex-Lax

OTHER DRUGS IN THIS CLASS
calcium polycarbophil, methylcellulose, psyllium hydrophilic mucilloid, phenolphthalein, sennosides

GENERAL DESCRIPTION
Docusate, a stool-softening type of laxative, is used to relieve constipation. Stool softeners add to the bowels' liquid content, softening the stool. They are often taken as a prophylactic to prevent straining during bowel movements after heart attacks, childbirth, or rectal surgery, or when hemorrhoids are present. See Laxatives for more information about side effects and possible drug interactions.

SIDE EFFECTS
NONE EXPECTED

TARGET AILMENTS

Constipation

Straining during bowel movements following rectal surgery, heart attacks, or childbirth, or when hemorrhoids are present

PRECAUTIONS

WARNING
In rare cases, side effects ranging from skin rashes and kidney problems to breathing difficulty and cardiac arrest have occurred when docusate is combined with the laxative phenolphthalein.

SPECIAL INFORMATION
- This type of laxative should never be taken with mineral oil; stool softeners increase the toxicity of mineral oil.
- Laxatives can be habit forming. Use them infrequently, at the lowest effective dosage, and for no longer than one week. Long-term use can cause physical dependence, resulting in loss of normal bowel function and chronic constipation.
- Call your doctor if the laxative fails to have the desired effect after one week of use.
- For more information, see Laxatives.

POSSIBLE INTERACTIONS
Laxatives that may contain danthron, mineral oil, or phenolphthalein: increased absorption of these substances, increasing the possibility of toxic effects.

DONG QUAI

LATIN NAME
Angelica sinensis

D

VITAL STATISTICS

GENERAL DESCRIPTION

Also known as Chinese angelica root, dong quai is used by Chinese herbalists as a treatment for several gynecological complaints. Modern acupuncturists sometimes also inject the herb into acupuncture points to treat pain, especially that from neuralgia and arthritis. Look for a long, moist, oily plant as the source of the root, which has brown bark and a white cross section. This fragrant herb is characterized as sweet, acrid, bitter, and warm, according to traditional Chinese medicine.

Chinese medicine takes a holistic approach to healthcare, fashioning remedies to treat the entire being as well as the specific parts or areas. Single herbs may be used alone or in combination with other herbs to prevent and combat disease, which is thought to arise from disturbances in the flow of a bodily energy called chi (pronounced "chee") and blood, or from a lack of balance in the complementary states of yin and yang.

PREPARATIONS

This root is widely available in bulk and in tablet form at Chinese pharmacies, Asian markets, and Western health food stores. You should avoid the herb if it is dry or has a greenish brown cross section. Frying the herb in vinegar or wine improves its tonic effect on blood circulation. Toasting it to ash increases its ability to stop bleeding.

COMBINATIONS: Mixed with astragalus, dong quai provides a tonic for treating fatigue and other symptoms associated with loss of blood. A blend of dong quai, white peony root, Chinese foxglove root cooked in wine, and cnidium root *(Ligusticum chuanxiong)* is prescribed for menstrual irregularity and similar conditions. Dong quai is also combined with honeysuckle flowers and red peony root to form a preparation that reduces the swelling and alleviates the pain of abscesses and sores.

Consult a Chinese medicine practitioner for further information on mixtures and doses.

PRECAUTIONS

SPECIAL INFORMATION

- You should not take dong quai during the early stages of pregnancy.
- Check on the use of this herb with your Chinese medicine practitioner if you have diarrhea or abdominal bloating; it is not recommended in some cases.

TARGET AILMENTS

Take internally for:

Menstrual irregularity; lack of menstruation; painful or insubstantial menstruation; stabbing pain; pain caused by traumatic injury; poor blood circulation; pale complexion; possible anemia; carbuncles that, according to traditional Chinese medicine, arise from stagnant blood; abscesses; sores; lightheadedness; blurred vision; heart palpitations

SIDE EFFECTS

NONE EXPECTED IF USED AS DIRECTED.

Rx DORZOLAMIDE

VITAL STATISTICS

DRUG CLASS
Carbonic Anhydrase Inhibitors

BRAND NAME
Trusopt

GENERAL DESCRIPTION
A type of eye drop, dorzolamide reduces the amount of fluid in the eye, thereby restoring normal eye pressure. Eye drops of various kinds are often the initial treatment for open-angle (chronic) glaucoma and have proved effective in controlling this condition in a majority of patients. Dorzolamide eye drops may be especially beneficial to glaucoma patients who are unable to use eye drops containing beta-adrenergic blockers, such as timolol. Dorzolamide may also be effective in treating ocular hypertension.

Since this medication is relatively new, no long-term studies about its ultimate effectiveness and possible long-term side effects have been completed.

TARGET AILMENTS
Open-angle (chronic) glaucoma
Ocular hypertension

PRECAUTIONS

SPECIAL INFORMATION
- Do not take dorzolamide if you are also taking an oral carbonic anhydrase inhibitor, including acetazolamide, dichlorphenamide, and methazolamide.
- Dorzolamide may be absorbed into the bloodstream and circulate throughout the body, causing the side effects associated with oral carbonic anhydrase inhibitors. These effects include increased urinary frequency, tingling in fingers and toes, poor appetite, diarrhea, and fatigue.
- Before taking dorzolamide, tell your doctor if you are using any other eye drops, have a kidney or liver disease, or have a history of sensitivity to carbonic anhydrase inhibitors or to sulfa drugs, including oral antidiabetic agents.
- If you are sensitive to other carbonic anhydrase inhibitors, you may experience similar effects while taking dorzolamide.
- Normal dosage is one drop three times daily. If dorzolamide is being used in conjunction with other eye drops, the patient should wait at least 10 minutes in between dosages of these two medicines. As with all eye drops, keep the tip of the dispensing container from touching your eye.
- Dorzolamide should not be used while wearing soft contact lenses, because the drug may damage them.
- Dorzolamide has not been proved safe for use during pregnancy. Consult your doctor before using the drug.
- Dorzolamide is not recommended for use by breast-feeding mothers, and its safety and efficacy for children has not been established.
- If you develop increased sensitivity to sunlight while taking dorzolamide, avoid bright

CONTINUED

DORZOLAMIDE

light or wear sunglasses.

- Do not drive or operate machinery until you know how dorzolamide might affect your eyesight.
- Regular checkups with your doctor while taking this medication are recommended.

POSSIBLE INTERACTIONS

Amphetamines, mecamylamine, or quinidine: possible decreased elimination of these drugs and increased risk of side effects.

Aspirin therapy (high dose): may increase toxicity of dorzolamide.

Ophthalmic silver preparations, such as silver nitrate: also in eye-drop form, these are incompatible with dorzolamide. Do not take these eye drops together.

SIDE EFFECTS

NOT SERIOUS

- Fatigue; unusual fatigue or weakness
- Headache; nausea
- Feeling of something in eye (superficial punctate keratitis); dry or watery eyes
- Burning or stinging sensation in eyes; discomfort; blurred vision
- Photophobia; sensitivity to light
- Bitter taste

CALL YOUR DOCTOR IF THESE SYMPTOMS PERSIST OR BECOME TROUBLESOME.

SERIOUS

- Persistent allergic reaction in eye; itching; redness; swelling
- Persistent eye pain; persistent tearing; blurred vision
- Conjunctivitis
- Skin rash
- Blood in urine; nausea; pain in side, back, or abdomen (indicating kidney stones)

DISCONTINUE USE AND CALL YOUR DOCTOR.

Rx DOXAZOSIN

VITAL STATISTICS

DRUG CLASS
Alpha$_1$-Adrenergic Blockers

BRAND NAME
Cardura

OTHER DRUGS IN THIS CLASS
terazosin

GENERAL DESCRIPTION
Introduced in 1986, doxazosin is one of several alpha$_1$-adrenergic blocking agents used in the treatment of high blood pressure. Doxazosin works by selectively blocking nerve endings called alpha receptors; the blockage allows the blood vessels to relax and expand, which enables blood to pass through more easily and lowers blood pressure.

Doxazosin can be used alone or in conjunction with other drugs, such as beta-adrenergic blockers or diuretics, depending on the degree of hypertension. This drug does not cure high blood pressure, but it can help control it. Doxazosin is also used to relax the muscles in the prostate gland and increase urine flow. This drug will not, however, shrink an enlarged prostate. For visual characteristics of the brand-name drug Cardura, see the Color Guide to Prescription Drugs and Herbs. See Alpha$_1$-Adrenergic Blockers for possible drug interactions and side effects.

TARGET AILMENTS

High blood pressure

Benign prostatic hyperplasia (benign enlargement of the prostate)

PRECAUTIONS

SPECIAL INFORMATION
- Avoid driving and hazardous tasks for 24 hours after the first dose, after a dosage increase, or after resumption of treatment.
- The effects of doxazosin on pregnant women, nursing mothers, and children under 12 years of age are not yet known. Use only if directed by your physician.
- Before taking doxazosin, tell your doctor if you have previously experienced an unusual or allergic reaction to doxazosin, prazosin, or terazosin or have encountered dizziness, faintness, or lightheadedness with other drugs.
- Inform your doctor if you have a history of mental depression, stroke, or impaired circulation to the brain; coronary artery disease; impaired liver function or active liver disease; impaired kidney function; or any plans to undergo surgery in the near future.
- To minimize dizziness, take the first doxazosin dose at bedtime. Dosages must be adjusted on an individual basis.
- Doxazosin may affect some laboratory tests. Effects may include a mild decrease in white blood cell counts, certain cholesterol ratios, and blood sugar levels.
- The symptoms of prostate cancer are similar to those of benign prostate enlargement. Ask your doctor to test for prostate cancer before starting treatment with alpha$_1$-adrenergic blockers.

SIDE EFFECTS
SEE ALPHA$_1$-ADRENERGIC BLOCKERS.

Rx DOXEPIN

D

VITAL STATISTICS

DRUG CLASS
Antidepressants [Tricyclic Antidepressants (TCAs)]

OTHER DRUGS IN THIS SUBCLASS
amitriptyline, nortriptyline

GENERAL DESCRIPTION
Introduced in 1969, doxepin is among the group of drugs called tricyclic antidepressants, which are commonly prescribed in the treatment of depressive illnesses. Like other antidepressants, this drug works to restore serotonin and other brain chemicals to their normal levels. Doxepin is also used to treat some kinds of chronic pain, peptic ulcers, and urticaria (hives, skin ulcers). See Antidepressants for information about side effects and other possible drug interactions.

PRECAUTIONS

SPECIAL INFORMATION
- Before taking doxepin, tell your doctor if you suffer from glaucoma, urinary retention, epilepsy, hyperthyroidism, or heart disease.
- Doxepin may cause drowsiness. Use care while driving, operating machinery, or performing tasks that require mental alertness.
- Doxepin can trigger manic attacks in individuals with manic-depression. Be sure to tell your doctor if you have manic-depression.
- Doxepin can affect blood sugar (glucose tolerance) tests by causing fluctuation in blood sugar levels.
- The full effects of doxepin may not be felt for several weeks.
- Check with your doctor if you are pregnant, nursing, or planning a pregnancy.

POSSIBLE INTERACTIONS
Anticoagulant drugs (such as warfarin): doxepin may increase the anticlotting activity.
Barbiturates: decreased effectiveness of doxepin.
Cimetidine (antiulcer): increased doxepin effects.
Clonidine (blood pressure medication): may cause a dangerous increase in blood pressure.
Haloperidol (antipsychotic), oral contraceptives, phenothiazines (antipsychotic), levodopa (anti-Parkinsonism): increased levels of doxepin.
Thyroid medications: combining doxepin with thyroid drugs may increase the effects, including side effects, of both medications.
Tobacco (smoking): increased elimination of doxepin from the body, lessening its effectiveness.

TARGET AILMENTS
Major depressive disorders
Obsessive-compulsive disorders
Phobias
Eating disorders
Chronic pain
Peptic ulcers
Urticaria (hives, skin ulcers)

SIDE EFFECTS
SEE ANTIDEPRESSANTS.

Rx DOXYCYCLINE

D

VITAL STATISTICS

DRUG CLASS
Antibiotics [Tetracyclines]

BRAND NAME
Doryx

GENERAL DESCRIPTION
Introduced in 1967, doxycycline is a semisynthetic tetracycline antibiotic, used for the same ailments as other tetracyclines and for certain other conditions. These include use by short-term travelers to prevent malaria in areas where the disease is resistant to other preventives. Doxycycline also prevents and treats traveler's diarrhea in high-risk patients. For more information, see Tetracyclines.

For visual characteristics, see the Color Guide to Prescription Drugs and Herbs.

PRECAUTIONS

WARNING
Using tetracyclines during tooth development (from the last half of the mother's pregnancy to age eight) may cause permanent tooth discoloration.

SPECIAL INFORMATION
Unlike most other tetracyclines, doxycycline may be taken with food, milk and other dairy products, or carbonated beverages with no expected decrease in action.

POSSIBLE INTERACTIONS
Barbiturates and anticonvulsants (such as carbamazepine or phenytoin): decreased doxycycline effect, possibly requiring increased dosage of doxycycline or use of another tetracycline.

TARGET AILMENTS

Some sexually transmitted diseases, including syphilis, gonorrhea, and chlamydia; urinary tract infections; acne vulgaris

Malaria (preventive)

Tick-borne diseases, such as Rocky Mountain spotted fever and Lyme disease

Skin and soft-tissue infections

Chronic bronchitis; pneumonia

Sinusitis

Certain peptic ulcers

Traveler's diarrhea

SIDE EFFECTS

NOT SERIOUS

- Lightheadedness; dizziness; gastrointestinal upsets; photosensitivity
- Fungal infection of the mouth, genital, or rectal area; darkening or discoloration of the tongue

CALL YOUR DOCTOR IF THESE SYMPTOMS BECOME TROUBLESOME.

SERIOUS

- Serious photosensitivity; symptoms of diabetes

CALL YOUR DOCTOR IMMEDIATELY.

DROSERA

LATIN NAME
Drosera rotundifolia

VITAL STATISTICS

GENERAL DESCRIPTION
This remedy is derived from a perennial insect-trapping plant that grows on mossy wetlands in parts of Europe, Asia, and North America. Its flowers open only in the morning, and its leaves contain glands whose secretions attract insects and digest them. Because this fluid resembles a dewdrop, *Drosera* is often called the dew plant or sundew. Historically, the herb was given to treat toothache, was rubbed on the abdomen for relief during childbirth, was hung around the neck to cure madness, and was also used in an attempt to treat tuberculosis.

Today, the herbal form of *Drosera* is given for chest conditions, and the homeopathic remedy serves as a palliative for coughs, sore throats, and other chest complaints. The whole plant is used in making the homeopathic remedy. The plants are gathered in July, the usual time of blooming, and the juice is expressed and then prepared in the usual way. For more information on homeopathic medicine, see page 14.

PREPARATIONS
Drosera is available over the counter in various potencies, in both liquid and tablet form, at selected stores and pharmacies. Consult your homeopathic physician for further information.

PRECAUTIONS

SPECIAL INFORMATION
- When a remedy is administered, no one but the patient should touch the pills. If tablets are spilled, throw them away.
- The mouth should be clear of flavors 15 minutes before and after taking a remedy, and strong flavors and aromas, such as coffee, camphor, and heavily scented perfumes, should be avoided for the duration of treatment.

TARGET AILMENTS

Cough that is barking, deep, hacking, dry, spasmodic, or croupy

Cough that is worse after midnight, after eating or drinking, or on first lying down at night

Cough that is relieved by pressure on the chest

Cough with retching and vomiting, nosebleed, vomiting of mucus, pain in chest, labored rapid breathing

Whooping cough

Sore throat with sore, inflamed larynx and deep, husky voice, worse on swallowing

SIDE EFFECTS
NONE EXPECTED

Du Huo Ji Sheng Wan

Vital Statistics

ENGLISH NAME
Angelica Pubescens and Sangjisheng Pills

GENERAL DESCRIPTION
Du Huo Ji Sheng Wan is an herbal formula used for the treatment of joint stiffness, numbness, pain, and weakness especially in the lower body; it is said to be particularly effective in cases where the patient has a sore and weak lower back and knees. Practitioners of Chinese medicine recommend this remedy when the symptoms are made worse by coldness, and it may be particularly suited to people who find that their joints ache more when the weather is cold and damp. Another diagnostic sign pointing to the use of this formula is a pale tongue.

Chinese medicine takes a holistic approach to healthcare, fashioning remedies to treat the entire being as well as the specific parts or areas. Precise combinations of herbs are used to prevent and combat disease, which is thought to arise from disturbances in the flow of the bodily energy called chi (pronounced "chee") and blood, or from a lack of balance in the complementary states of yin and yang. A patent formula, *Du Huo Ji Sheng Wan* is made by using a standardized combination of herbs and method of preparation.

INGREDIENTS
angelica pubescens, Chinese wild ginger, ledebouriella, gentiana, loranthis, eucommia bark, achyranthes, cinnamon bark, dong quai, ligusticum, rehmannia, white peony root, ginseng, poria, honey-fried licorice

PREPARATIONS
This formula is sold in pill form at many Chinese pharmacies and Oriental grocery stores.

TARGET AILMENTS

Arthritis (rheumatoid arthritis and osteoarthritis)

Chronic low back pain

Chronic lower body pain, stiffness, or numbness

Joint pain that comes with cold, damp weather

SIDE EFFECTS

NONE EXPECTED

DULCAMARA

LATIN NAME
Solanum dulcamara

VITAL STATISTICS

GENERAL DESCRIPTION

A member of the nightshade family, this perennial plant, also called bittersweet, has poisonous berries that appear in the fall. Its stems contain a substance, solanine, that when taken in excess can cause nausea, vomiting, and convulsive muscular movements, as well as paralysis of the vagus nerve and increased heart rate. The juice of this plant was used historically in many different countries to treat cancers and warts. The plant also has been used for skin diseases such as psoriasis, for liver ailments, and for rheumatism.

The homeopathic remedy, which is used frequently by practitioners to treat coughs and colds, is made from the stems and leaves, gathered just before or at the start of blossoming. Juice is extracted from the plant parts and mixed with alcohol.

For more information on homeopathic medicine, see page 14.

PREPARATIONS

Dulcamara is available over the counter in various potencies, in both liquid and tablet form, at selected stores and pharmacies. Consult your homeopathic practitioner for further information.

PRECAUTIONS

SPECIAL INFORMATION

- Only the patient should touch the pills. Any spilled tablets should be thrown away.
- The mouth should be clear of flavors 15 minutes before and after taking a remedy, and strong flavors and aromas, such as coffee and heavy perfume, should be avoided for the duration of treatment.

TARGET AILMENTS

- Colds that occur after exposure to cold and wet weather, possibly accompanied by neck pain and stiffness
- Cough generating large amounts of phlegm, made worse by lying down
- Yellow or greenish diarrhea
- Cystitis with involuntary urination, brought on by cold and wet conditions
- Hives that are worse with warmth; itchy, bleeding, or encrusted eruptions on scalp or face
- Warts on face or back of hands, usually large, smooth, and flat
- Ringworm of the scalp
- Backache in lower back that improves with movement and worsens with wet weather
- Joint pain related to damp conditions that improves with movement
- Paralysis or weakness worsened by dampness and cold

SIDE EFFECTS

NONE EXPECTED

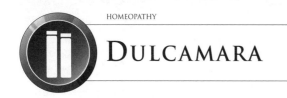

DYCLONINE

D

VITAL STATISTICS

DRUG CLASS
Anesthetics

BRAND NAME
Dyclone

OTHER DRUGS IN THIS CLASS
benzocaine, pramoxine

GENERAL DESCRIPTION
Dyclonine spray is used topically to temporarily relieve minor throat and mouth pain. It rapidly alleviates pain from canker sores, minor irritation or injury to the mouth and gums, minor dental procedures, dentures, or orthodontic appliances. It also suppresses the gag reflex, facilitating medical procedures in the oral cavity. It is also used to relieve pain associated with anogenital lesions. This drug works by blocking nerve impulses at sensory nerve endings in mucous membranes, impeding pain messages to the brain. As a rinse or gargle, dyclonine may provide relief for up to an hour. Drug interactions are unlikely. See Anesthetics for additional information.

PRECAUTIONS

SPECIAL INFORMATION
- Dyclonine is safe and effective for adults and children 12 and older but should be used by younger patients only on the advice of a physician or dentist. Geriatric patients may require lower doses.
- Consult your doctor before using this drug if you are pregnant or nursing.
- Consult your doctor if sore throat is severe, persists for more than two days, or is accompanied or followed by fever, headache, rash, nausea, or vomiting. If sore mouth symptoms do not improve in seven days, or if irritation, pain, or redness persists or worsens, see your physician or dentist.
- Use care not to inhale the drug, and avoid applying to the back of the throat or mouth unless so directed by a health professional.
- Do not eat or chew gum for one hour following use. Do not apply to traumatized or infected mucous membranes.

TARGET AILMENTS

Minor sore throat, sore mouth; canker sores; mouth or gum injury

Pain from dental procedures or appliances

Pain, burning, and itching from hemorrhoids

SIDE EFFECTS

SERIOUS
- Allergic skin reactions (e.g., hivelike swellings, burning, stinging, or tenderness)
- Nervousness, dizziness, blurred vision, tremors, seizures, or respiratory arrest (caused by overdose)
- Cardiovascular effects (e.g., fainting, irregular heart rhythm, hypotension, or cardiac arrest)

CALL YOUR DOCTOR IMMEDIATELY.

ECHINACEA

LATIN NAME
Echinacea spp.

E

VITAL STATISTICS

GENERAL DESCRIPTION

Herbalists value the dried root of echinacea for its broad-based action against many types of viral and bacterial illnesses such as colds, bronchitis, ear infections, influenza, and cystitis. Laboratory testing shows that it contains echinacoside, an ingredient that may have antibiotic effects. Another ingredient, echinacein, is believed to block some mechanisms that enable infectious viruses or bacteria to invade body tissue.

In the laboratory, echinacea seems to bolster white blood cells in their battle against foreign microorganisms; it may increase the production of T cells, which join other white blood cells in the fight against infectious agents. Echinacea can also be effective topically for eczema and other skin problems.

For visual characteristics, see the Color Guide to Prescription Drugs and Herbs.

PREPARATIONS

Over the counter:
Available in dried form in bulk, and in teas, capsules, and tinctures.

At home:
Tea: Boil 2 tsp dried root in 1 cup water and simmer covered for 15 minutes. Drink three times a day.
Combinations: Use echinacea with yarrow or uva ursi to treat cystitis.
Consult a practitioner for the dosage appropriate for you and the specific ailment.

SIDE EFFECTS
None expected

PRECAUTIONS

SPECIAL INFORMATION

- Do not use for more than a few weeks.
- Do not give to children younger than two at all or to older ones for more than seven to 10 days except in conjunction with a healthcare practitioner; start with minimal doses for older children and older adults.
- Check with your doctor before using echinacea if you are pregnant or nursing.

POSSIBLE INTERACTIONS

Combining echinacea with other herbs may necessitate a lower dosage.

TARGET AILMENTS

Take internally for:

Colds, the flu, and other respiratory illnesses; mononucleosis

Ear infections

Septicemia (blood poisoning)

Bladder infections

Apply externally for:

Cuts; burns; wounds

Abscesses; boils

Insect bites and stings

Hives; eczema

Herpes

EDTA

VITAL STATISTICS

GENERAL DESCRIPTION

EDTA, or ethylenediaminetetraacetic acid, is a synthetic amino acid used to cleanse the body of excess metals and calcium. Administered intravenously in a treatment known as chelation therapy, EDTA attracts metal or calcium deposits in the blood and carries them out of the body through the urine. The U.S. Food and Drug Administration (FDA) has approved chelation therapy for the treatment of lead poisoning.

EDTA has also been used to help rid the body of aluminum, a metal associated by some researchers with Alzheimer's disease. This application is controversial, as is the use of chelation therapy for cardiovascular problems. Many sufferers from angina, high blood pressure, and atherosclerosis seek chelation therapy because they believe it will clear the artery walls of life-threatening fatty deposits.

Advocates claim that chelation therapy is safer and less expensive than bypass surgery and other conventional treatments—and just as effective. Critics cite the lack of reliable scientific evidence and claim that chelation therapy is ineffective, can cost thousands of dollars, and is potentially dangerous (EDTA has been linked to kidney damage and osteoporosis). Supporters maintain that when administered properly in low doses, EDTA is unlikely to produce side effects, but until chelation therapy undergoes thorough scientific study, it remains a controversial treatment option.

PREPARATIONS

Available for intramuscular (IM) or intravenous (IV) injection.

PRECAUTIONS

WARNING

If you wish to try chelation therapy, seek a practitioner certified by one of the major American chelation societies. The treatment method is not universally accepted, could cause serious side effects, and is still being tested for safety and efficacy.

Do not use EDTA if you have a kidney disease or if you are pregnant or breast-feeding.

POSSIBLE INTERACTIONS

Chelation therapy may interfere with anticoagulant drugs.

TARGET AILMENTS
Lead poisoning
Atherosclerosis
Angina
High blood pressure
Circulatory problems
Alzheimer's disease

SIDE EFFECTS

EDTA CAN HAVE SERIOUS SIDE EFFECTS, INCLUDING KIDNEY DAMAGE, OSTEOPOROSIS, HYPOCALCEMIA, OR RECURRENCE OF TUBERCULOSIS. YOU SHOULD BE MONITORED BY YOUR HEALTHCARE PRACTITIONER.

ELDER

LATIN NAME
Sambucus nigra

E

VITAL STATISTICS

GENERAL DESCRIPTION

Often described in Europe as the "medicine chest of the country people," elder has been used for its many therapeutic and prophylactic qualities for centuries. Preparations made from the flowers have an expectorant effect and help treat conditions causing upper respiratory tract congestion. They also promote sweating, stimulate circulation, and act as a diuretic and mild laxative, as well as having anti-inflammatory properties. The berries have many of the same effects and are rich in vitamins A and C. Raw elderberries, however, are toxic and should not be eaten. The bark and leaves are considered toxic and should not be taken internally. Preparations made from the leaves, however, can be used for minor burns, bruises, sprains, chilblains, and wounds.

TARGET AILMENTS

Take internally for:

Colds and flu, coughs, rheumatic conditions, catarrhal conditions such as hay fever and sinusitis; neuralgia

Apply ointment externally for:

Skin irritations, including rashes, eczema, dry skin, and chilblains; bruises, sprains, and wounds; conjunctivitis

SIDE EFFECTS

SEE WARNING.

PREPARATIONS

Over the counter:

Available as dried blossoms, teas, salves, syrups, tinctures, and elixirs.

At home:

INFUSION: Pour 1 cup boiling water over 2 tsp dried or fresh flowers and steep covered for 10 minutes. May drink 3 cups a day.

JUICE: Fresh, ripe berries should be simmered in water for 2 to 3 minutes and the juice expressed. Drink 1 glass diluted with hot water once a day as a tonic or three times a day for 1 week or less for viral ailments. Juice may be preserved by bringing to a boil 10 parts juice to 1 part honey.

OINTMENT: Heat 3 parts fresh leaves with 6 parts melted petroleum jelly until the leaves are crisp. Strain and store.

TINCTURE: Take ⅛ to ½ tsp three times a day.

COMBINATIONS: Combine with peppermint, yarrow, or hyssop for colds and fevers; combine with goldenrod for catarrhal conditions.

Consult a practitioner for the dosage appropriate for you and the specific ailment.

PRECAUTIONS

WARNING

Raw elderberry seeds are toxic. Ripe berries should be eaten only after cooking.

The roots, stems, and leaves of this plant may cause cyanide poisoning. Do not take preparations made from them.

POSSIBLE INTERACTIONS

Combining elder with other herbs may necessitate a lower dosage.

ELECAMPANE

LATIN NAME
Inula helenium

VITAL STATISTICS

GENERAL DESCRIPTION

Traditionally elecampane has had a variety of applications. Once used to treat tuberculosis, it is today best known as a remedy for cough and other respiratory ailments. It may be especially helpful for treating bronchial infections in children. Like other herbs, elecampane contains both stimulating and relaxing agents, accounting for its usefulness as both an expectorant and a sedative. It was naturalized in the U.S. after arriving with the colonists and is cultivated widely in Europe and Asia; the flowers are popular in Chinese medicine.

PREPARATIONS

Over the counter:
Available as a tincture.

At home:

TEA: To clear the body of excess mucus, shred the root to yield 1 tsp and add a full cup of cold water; let stand covered for 10 hours, then strain and drink hot three times daily.

TINCTURE: Take anywhere from 1/8 to 1/2 tsp up to three times a day.

COMBINATIONS: Blend with horehound and bloodroot to relieve congestion. Also can be combined with coltsfoot, pleurisy root, and yarrow.

Consult a qualified practitioner for the dosage appropriate for your specific condition.

PRECAUTIONS

SPECIAL INFORMATION

- If your symptoms do not improve after two weeks of using the herb, or if you have any uncomfortable side effects, discontinue using the herb and consult your doctor.
- Do not use this herb during pregnancy.
- Do not give elecampane to children under the age of two. Older children and persons over the age of 65 should take mild preparations to begin with and increase the strength gradually, if necessary.
- Unconfirmed studies indicate elecampane may have an effect on blood sugar. People with diabetes should consult their doctor.

POSSIBLE INTERACTIONS

Combining elecampane with other herbs may necessitate a lower dosage.

TARGET AILMENTS
Cough and cold
Bronchitis
Asthma
Emphysema
Digestive problems
Intestinal parasites

SIDE EFFECTS

NOT SERIOUS

- Rash
- Stomach upset
- Diarrhea

DECREASE DOSAGE OR STOP USING THE HERB.

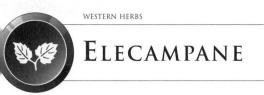

Enalapril

E

Vital Statistics

DRUG CLASS
Angiotensin-Converting Enzyme (ACE) Inhibitors

BRAND NAME
Vasotec

GENERAL DESCRIPTION
Like other ACE inhibitors, enalapril relaxes arterial walls, thereby lowering blood pressure and reducing the work load of the heart. For these reasons the drug, introduced in 1985, is used for high blood pressure (hypertension) and congestive heart failure. Enalapril is sometimes combined with hydrochlorothiazide, a diuretic that reduces water retention, for increased blood-pressure-lowering action. For further information, see Angiotensin-Converting Enzyme (ACE) Inhibitors. For visual characteristics of the brand-name drug Vasotec, see the Color Guide to Prescription Drugs and Herbs.

Precautions

WARNING
Get medical attention immediately if you notice swelling of your face, tongue, or vocal cords or have difficulty swallowing or breathing; this reaction can be life threatening.

Do not take enalapril during pregnancy; it has caused birth defects and death of the fetus and newborn.

SPECIAL INFORMATION
- Enalapril causes an increase in blood levels of potassium. Do not use potassium-rich products, including salt substitutes and low-salt milk, without first consulting your doctor. The potassium in your blood could rise to dangerous levels, leading to heart-rhythm problems.
- Do not abruptly stop taking this drug. The dosage must be reduced gradually.

TARGET AILMENTS

High blood pressure

Congestive heart failure (in conjunction with digitalis preparations and diuretics)

SIDE EFFECTS

NOT SERIOUS
- Dry, persistent cough
- Headache or fatigue
- Nausea or diarrhea
- Loss of sense of taste
- Temporary rash; itching
- Dizziness on suddenly rising or changing position

CALL YOUR DOCTOR IF THESE EFFECTS BECOME BOTHERSOME.

SERIOUS
- Fainting; drowsiness
- Persistent skin rash
- Joint pain
- Numbness and tingling
- Abdominal pain, vomiting, or diarrhea
- Fever and sore throat
- Chest pain; palpitations
- Jaundice

CALL YOUR DOCTOR RIGHT AWAY.

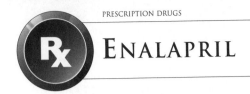

EPHEDRA

LATIN NAME
Ephedra sinica

VITAL STATISTICS

GENERAL DESCRIPTION
With its jointed, barkless branches that bear few leaves, the ephedra plant has been used by traditional Chinese healers for thousands of years. Its active ingredients are ephedrine, pseudoephedrine, and norpseudoephedrine, which are all central nervous system stimulants. Ephedrine affects the body by opening bronchial passages; this activates the heart, increasing blood pressure and speeding up metabolism. Excessive use of ephedra can lead to nervousness, insomnia, and high blood pressure. Known as *ma huang* in China, ephedra grows abundantly throughout the northern provinces of this country. It is described in traditional Chinese medicine as acrid, bitter, and warm.

PREPARATIONS
Over the counter:
Available as fluidextract, tablets, dried herb.

At home:
Prepare by combining 1 part honey, 4 parts dried herb, and a small amount of water in a wok. Allow to simmer over low heat until water has evaporated and herbs are light brown.
COMBINATIONS: For fever and chills, ephedra is mixed with cinnamon twig. Congestion is treated by ephedra combined with dried ginger.

PRECAUTIONS

WARNING
Do not take ephedra if you are pregnant or have heart disease, hypertension, diabetes, glaucoma, or hyperthyroidism.

Ephedra is an ingredient in several weight-loss aids. Its effectiveness in this regard, however, derives from its accelerating effect on the metabolism, considered an unwanted side effect; many healthcare professionals warn against using it for weight loss.

Use low-strength preparations for children or adults over 65. Do not administer to children under age two.

Because ephedra can cause a number of side effects—and in rare cases, death—consult a practitioner before using it.

If you are taking any medication, consult your physician before using this herb.

TARGET AILMENTS

Take internally for:

Fever and chills

Coughing; wheezing; nasal and chest congestion

Indigestion or stomachache

SIDE EFFECTS

NOT SERIOUS
- Insomnia; dry mouth
- Nervousness; irritability
- Headache; dizziness

CALL YOUR DOCTOR IF THESE EFFECTS PERSIST OR BECOME BOTHERSOME.

SERIOUS
- Increased blood pressure and heart rate; palpitations

STOP USING EPHEDRA. CONSULT YOUR PHYSICIAN IMMEDIATELY.

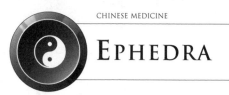

EPHEDRA

LATIN NAME
Ephedra sinica

VITAL STATISTICS

GENERAL DESCRIPTION
The roots and aboveground parts of this herb are used by Western practitioners as a bronchial decongestant and as a remedy for asthma, hay fever, and the common cold. One of its three active ingredients, ephedrine, opens the bronchial passages; this activates the heart, increasing blood pressure and speeding up metabolism. For this reason, herbalists warn that excessive use of ephedra can lead to nervousness, insomnia, and high blood pressure. In the United States, several states have set restrictions on the strength of over-the-counter products containing ephedra. For visual characteristics of ephedra, see the Color Guide to Prescription Drugs and Herbs.

PREPARATIONS
Over the counter:
Available as fluidextract, tablets, and dried bulk herb.

At home:
TEA: Simmer covered 1 to 2 tsp ephedra with 1 cup water for 10 to 15 minutes. Drink up to 2 cups a day.
Consult a qualified practitioner for the dosage appropriate for you and your specific condition.

PRECAUTIONS

WARNING
Do not take ephedra if you are pregnant or have heart disease, diabetes, glaucoma, high blood pressure, anxiety, or hyperthyroidism.

Several weight-loss aids contain ephedra. Its effectiveness derives from its accelerating effect on the metabolism, considered an unwanted side effect; thus, many healthcare professionals warn against using it to lose weight.

If you are taking any medication, consult your physician before using this herb.

This herb should not be used with children unless it is specifically prescribed by a healthcare practitioner who is knowledgeable about herbs. In any case, do not administer to children under age two. Use low-strength prescriptions for adults over 65.

Because ephedra can cause a number of side effects—and in rare cases, death—consult a practitioner before using it.

POSSIBLE INTERACTIONS
Combining ephedra with other herbs may necessitate a lower dosage.

TARGET AILMENTS

Colds; influenza; nasal and chest congestion

Asthma; hay fever

SIDE EFFECTS

NOT SERIOUS
- Insomnia
- Dry mouth
- Nervousness; irritability
- Headache; dizziness

DECREASE DOSE. CALL YOUR DOCTOR IF THESE EFFECTS PERSIST.

SERIOUS
- Increased blood pressure
- Increased heart rate
- Heart palpitations

STOP USING EPHEDRA IMMEDIATELY AND CONSULT YOUR DOCTOR.

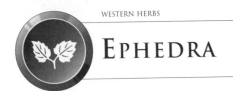

EPHEDRINE

VITAL STATISTICS

DRUG CLASS
Bronchodilators

BRAND NAMES
Primatene Dual Action Formula, Primatene Tablets

OTHER DRUGS IN THIS CLASS
Rx: albuterol, epinephrine, ipratropium, salmeterol, terbutaline, theophylline
OTC: epinephrine, theophylline

GENERAL DESCRIPTION
Ephedrine, a synthetically produced drug chemically similar to the herb ephedra, is a decongestant that also works as a bronchodilator. It is used to reduce the frequency and severity of recurrent asthma attacks. Ephedrine is available in both liquid and tablet form, sometimes in combination with aspirin or acetaminophen. For more information, see Bronchodilators. Also see warnings under Ephedra.

PRECAUTIONS

SPECIAL INFORMATION
- Bronchodilators (especially ephedrine and epinephrine) can cause adverse effects in individuals with high blood pressure, diabetes, heart disease, seizures, peptic ulcers, or thyroid or prostate problems. If you have any of these conditions do not use bronchodilators—even in their over-the-counter forms—without your doctor's permission.
- Women who are pregnant or breast-feeding should consult a doctor before using ephedrine.

POSSIBLE INTERACTIONS
Alpha and beta blockers: these drugs decrease the action of many bronchodilators, including ephedrine.
See also Bronchodilators.

TARGET AILMENTS
Bronchial asthma

SIDE EFFECTS

NOT SERIOUS
- Mild nausea
- Insomnia
- Nervousness
- Restlessness
- Dryness of nose and throat
- Rebound congestion

CALL YOUR DOCTOR IF THESE EFFECTS BECOME TROUBLESOME.

SERIOUS
- Change in blood pressure; change in heartbeat (irregular or pounding, for example)
- Trembling; weakness
- Breathing problems
- Unusual anxiety or nervousness
- Dizziness; lightheadedness
- Muscle cramps
- Nausea or vomiting
- Chest pain or discomfort (rare)

LET YOUR DOCTOR KNOW RIGHT AWAY IF YOU EXPERIENCE THESE SIDE EFFECTS.

Epinephrine

E

Vital Statistics

DRUG CLASS
Bronchodilators

BRAND NAMES
Rx: Adrenalin Chloride Solution, Ana-Kit, EpiPen, Sus-Phrine
OTC: Primatene Mist, Primatene Mist Suspension

OTHER DRUGS IN THIS CLASS
Rx: albuterol, ipratropium, salmeterol, terbutaline, theophylline
OTC: ephedrine, theophylline

GENERAL DESCRIPTION
Since 1900, epinephrine has been used to relieve the symptoms of bronchial asthma and allergic nasal congestion. In the form of eye drops, the drug is used to manage glaucoma. Other uses include the emergency treatment of heart problems and anaphylactic shock. For more information, see Bronchodilators.

Precautions

☠ ***WARNING***
Your body can build up tolerance to bronchodilator inhalants, causing them to become less effective. If this happens, discontinue the drug and tell your doctor. Do not increase the dose. Increasing the dose can lead to serious, perhaps fatal bronchial constriction.

SPECIAL INFORMATION
- Epinephrine can cause adverse effects in individuals with high blood pressure, diabetes, heart disease, seizures, peptic ulcers, or thyroid or prostate problems. If you have any of these conditions do not use epinephrine—even in over-the-counter forms—without your doctor's permission.
- If you are pregnant or breast-feeding, consult a doctor before using epinephrine.

POSSIBLE INTERACTIONS
See Bronchodilators.

TARGET AILMENTS
Anaphylactic shock from severe allergic reaction (injection)
Bronchial asthma
Heart-rhythm problems and cardiac arrest (intravenous infusion)
Nasal congestion from allergies
Glaucoma (eye drops)

SIDE EFFECTS

NOT SERIOUS
- Mild nausea, insomnia, nervousness, or restlessness

CALL YOUR DOCTOR IF THESE EFFECTS BECOME BOTHERSOME.

SERIOUS
- Change in blood pressure; change in heartbeat
- Breathing problems
- Trembling; dizziness
- Unusual anxiety
- Muscle cramps
- Severe nausea or vomiting

CALL YOUR DOCTOR RIGHT AWAY.

Er Chen Wan

Vital Statistics

ENGLISH NAME
Two-Cured Pills

GENERAL DESCRIPTION
Er Chen Wan is a versatile pill that is used for conditions that traditional Chinese medicine characterizes as "dampness" or "phlegm" in the body. The main symptom that *Er Chen Wan* addresses is coughing with a lot of white mucus. Other ailments said to be provoked by the presence of phlegm include congestion in the head with dizziness, a full, heavy feeling in the chest, nausea or vomiting, and even soft lumpy swellings like fatty tumors or goiter. According to Chinese medicine, the formula resolves the phlegm and also strengthens the functions of the body that keep dampness from accumulating.

Chinese medicine takes a holistic approach to healthcare, fashioning remedies to treat the entire being as well as the specific parts or areas. Precise combinations of herbs are used to prevent and combat disease, which is thought to arise from disturbances in the flow of a bodily energy called chi (pronounced "chee") and blood, or from a lack of balance in the complementary states of yin and yang. A patent formula, *Er Chen Wan* is made by using a standardized combination of herbs and method of preparation.

INGREDIENTS
pinellia, aged mandarin orange peel, poria, honey-fried licorice

PREPARATIONS
This formula is sold in pill form at many Chinese pharmacies and Oriental grocery stores.

Precautions

WARNING
Do not use with a dry cough.

TARGET AILMENTS
Upper respiratory tract infection
Chronic bronchitis
Ménière's disease
Chronic gastritis or ulcer
Goiter or lymph node swellings
Fatty tumors

SIDE EFFECTS

NOT SERIOUS
- Excessive thirst
- Dry throat

THESE SYMPTOMS MAY OCCUR IF *ER CHEN WAN* IS USED IMPROPERLY OR TOO LONG.

E

ERYTHROMYCIN

E

VITAL STATISTICS

DRUG CLASS

Antibiotics [Ophthalmic Antibiotics; Erythromycins (systemic)]

BRAND NAMES

Ophthalmic: Ilotycin
Systemic: E.E.S., E-Mycin, Ery-Tab, Erythromycin Base Filmtab, Erythrocin Stearate, PCE

OTHER DRUGS IN THESE SUBCLASSES

Erythromycins: azithromycin, clarithromycin
Ophthalmic antibiotics: tobramycin

GENERAL DESCRIPTION

Erythromycin, which was introduced in 1952, and other drugs in its class are used to treat many of the same infections for which penicillins are prescribed. Depending on its target and its concentration, erythromycin may kill bacteria outright (bactericidal action) or stop the growth and spread of bacteria (bacteriostatic action) by keeping the organisms from manufacturing protein. Once their growth has been halted, the bacteria can be eliminated by the body's defenses. Erythromycin is particularly useful for people who are allergic to penicillin or tetracycline.

When it is used for the eyes in the form of a solution or ointment, erythromycin has fewer side effects than it does when taken orally or by injection for systemic problems. The various systemic forms of this drug include erythromycin estolate, erythromycin stearate, erythromycin ethylsuccinate, and erythromycin base.

For visual characteristics of Ery-Tab and Erythrocin Stearate, see the Color Guide to Prescription Drugs and Herbs.

PRECAUTIONS

SPECIAL INFORMATION

- With long-term use, antibiotics can interfere with the action of "good" bacteria, which may cause diarrhea and fungal infections such as candidiasis. If you get a fungal infection while taking an antibiotic, continue the medication but call your doctor to find out how to treat these problems.
- Before starting erythromycin therapy, let your doctor know if you have ever had an allergic reaction to this drug or if you have ever used erythromycin estolate.
- Tell your doctor if you have hearing loss, cardiac arrhythmias, or an impaired liver, or if you are susceptible to allergies (asthma, eczema, or hives). The systemic forms of this drug may exacerbate these conditions.
- If you are pregnant, avoid erythromycin estolate, which can cause liver toxicity during pregnancy. If you're pregnant or nursing, be sure to tell your doctor before taking any form (systemic or ophthalmic) of this drug.

POSSIBLE INTERACTIONS (Systemic)

Acidic fruits or juices: decreased effect of erythromycin; do not consume within an hour of taking erythromycin.

Alcohol: possible liver damage.

Alfentanil, aminophylline, chloramphenicol, digoxin, midazolam, theophylline, triazolam: erythromycins increase the effects of these drugs; possible toxicity.

Anticoagulants: increased anticoagulant effect; risk of bleeding.

Astemizole, terfenadine: WARNING: may cause life-threatening heart problems. Do not take in combination with erythromycin.

Bactericidal antibiotics (penicillins, cephalosporins), lincomycin: erythromycins decrease the effectiveness of these drugs.

Carbamazepine, cyclosporine, phenytoin: possible toxicity of these drugs and of erythromycin; also risk of kidney damage with cyclosporine.

Ergotamine: possible ergotamine toxicity; impaired circulation, tingling, and burning pain in hands and feet.

Lovastatin: risk of rhabdomyolysis, a severe muscle disease.

TARGET AILMENTS

Ophthalmic:

Eye infections from strains of strep, staph, *Hemophilus influenzae,* and other bacteria (also used to prevent conjunctivitis in newborns exposed to chlamydia or gonorrhea)

Systemic:

Respiratory tract infections like pharyngitis and sinusitis caused by strep; otitis media; some types of pneumonia; whooping cough; legionnaire's disease

Amoebic dysentery

Skin and soft tissue infections

Nonspecific urethritis

Gonorrhea; syphilis; chlamydia

Rheumatic, congenital, or valvular heart disease (used in short-term therapy before dental or upper respiratory surgery to prevent endocarditis or in continuous therapy to prevent strep infections)

SIDE EFFECTS

NOT SERIOUS

- Systemic: mild nausea; oral candidiasis (sore mouth or tongue); vaginal candidiasis; unusual fatigue

CALL YOUR DOCTOR WHEN CONVENIENT.

SERIOUS

- Ophthalmic: eye irritation that develops and persists after you begin using this drug; also itching, redness, or swelling

THESE SYMPTOMS MAY INDICATE AN ALLERGY OR SUPERINFECTION. DISCONTINUE USE AND CALL YOUR DOCTOR RIGHT AWAY.

- Systemic: diarrhea, abdominal cramps, vomiting, and fever

CALL YOUR DOCTOR IF THESE SYMPTOMS ARE SEVERE OR PROLONGED.

- Hearing loss; jaundice (pale stools, dark urine, yellow eyes or skin); anaphylactic reaction (rash, redness, itching, and hives)

DISCONTINUE USE AND CALL YOUR DOCTOR RIGHT AWAY.

Rx ESTRACE

E

VITAL STATISTICS

DRUG CLASS
Estrogens and Progestins [Hormone Replacement]

GENERIC NAME
estradiol

OTHER DRUGS IN THIS SUBCLASS
Estrogens: conjugated estrogens, estropipate
Progestins: medroxyprogesterone

GENERAL DESCRIPTION
The brand-name drug Estrace replaces the body's estrogen at natural menopause or after surgical removal of the ovaries. This lessens symptoms of estrogen deficiency, such as hot flashes and vaginal dryness, and at the same time helps prevent osteoporosis and atherosclerosis. Estrace is also prescribed for young women whose ovaries do not produce enough estrogen. Estrace is available as oral tablets and vaginal cream, and as a skin patch that is prescribed under the brand name Estraderm. As a vaginal cream, Estrace is used short term to treat the degeneration of vaginal tissues and vulvar itching associated with estrogen deficiencies. See Estrogens and Progestins for more information about possible drug interactions. For visual characteristics of Estrace tablets, see the Color Guide to Prescription Drugs and Herbs.

PRECAUTIONS

WARNING
Do not use Estrace if you are pregnant or breast-feeding. If you suspect you are pregnant, discontinue use immediately to avoid severely harming the fetus.

Estrogens increase the risk of uterine cancer in menopausal and postmenopausal women. Abnormal vaginal bleeding is a possible symptom. If you experience unusual vaginal bleeding, call your doctor right away.

Get medical attention immediately if you experience any of the following: severe pain in leg, chest, or abdomen; sudden headaches; changes in speech, vision, or breathing; weakness or numbness in extremities. These symptoms may indicate blood clots.

TARGET AILMENTS
Hot flashes, vaginal dryness, and other symptoms occurring at natural menopause or after surgical removal of the ovaries
Other estrogen-deficiency conditions
Osteoporosis and heart disease in postmenopausal women (preventive treatment)
Degeneration of vulvar and vaginal tissues
Palliative treatment of advanced inoperable cancers: breast cancer in women and prostate cancer in men

SPECIAL INFORMATION

- Before taking Estrace, let your doctor know if you are a smoker or have liver disease, gallbladder disease, a history of breast cancer, fibrocystic breast changes, endometriosis, uterine fibroids, diabetes, asthma, epilepsy, heart disease, blood-clotting disorders, stroke or high blood pressure. Your doctor will use this information to determine whether or not you should use this drug and what your dosage should be.
- Long-term use of estrogens may increase your risk of blood clots and breast cancer. Women who use estrogen after menopause have a higher risk of gallbladder disease.
- Estrogens may increase blood glucose levels; if you are diabetic, your doctor may have to adjust your dosage of insulin or other antidiabetic drug.
- These hormones may cause fluid retention, which can aggravate asthma, epilepsy, migraines, and heart and kidney disease.
- Taking Estrace tablets with or after meals can help reduce nausea.

SIDE EFFECTS

NOT SERIOUS

- Acne
- Headache or migraine
- Mild nausea, diarrhea, vomiting, or abdominal pain
- Appetite or weight changes
- Fluid retention
- Breast tenderness
- Changes in sexual desire
- Blotchy spots on skin; increased body hair; loss of hair on scalp; photosensitivity; intolerance to contact lenses; mild dizziness (less common)

TELL YOUR DOCTOR WHEN CONVENIENT.

SERIOUS

- Lumps in the breasts or breast enlargement
- Spotting or changes in menstrual bleeding (may indicate uterine cancer)
- Painful or frequent urination
- Fainting
- Jaundice
- Gallbladder disease (painful right side of the abdomen)
- Increased blood pressure
- Skin rash not associated with skin patch; a new mole
- Cataracts
- Vaginitis (itching, irritation, or thick whitish discharge)

LET YOUR DOCTOR KNOW IF YOU EXPERIENCE THESE SYMPTOMS OR THE SYMPTOMS OF BLOOD CLOTS LISTED UNDER WARNING.

Estrogens and Progestins

E

Vital Statistics

GENERIC NAMES

Estrogens: conjugated estrogens, estradiol, estropipate, ethinyl estradiol, mestranol

Progestins: desogestrel, ethynodiol diacetate, levonorgestrel, medroxyprogesterone, norethindrone, norgestimate, norgestrel

BRAND NAMES

Abnormal uterine bleeding:

- *Provera,* Cycrin *(medroxyprogesterone)*

Estrogen replacement:

- Climara, Estrace, Estraderm, Estring (estradiol)
- Premarin (conjugated estrogens)
- Ogen (estropipate)
- Prempro (medroxyprogesterone and conjugated estrogens)

Oral contraceptives:

- *Ortho-Novum 1/35, Ortho-Novum 7/7/7, Genora 1/35,* Genora 0.5/35, *Loestrin,* Ovcon (norethindrone and ethinyl estradiol)
- *Levora,* Nordette, *Triphasil, Tri-Levlen* (levonorgestrel and ethinyl estradiol)
- *Demulen 1/35, Zovia 1/35* (ethynodiol diacetate and ethinyl estradiol)
- *Desogen, Ortho-Cept* (desogestrel and ethinyl estradiol)
- Genora 1/50, Ortho-Novum 1/50 (norethindrone and mestranol)
- *Lo/Ovral* (norgestrel and ethinyl estradiol)
- *Ortho Tri-Cyclen, Ortho-Cyclen* (norgestimate and ethinyl estradiol)

For visual characteristics of the medications listed in italics above, see the Color Guide to Prescription Drugs and Herbs.

GENERAL DESCRIPTION

Estrogens and progestins are natural and synthetic hormones or hormonelike substances that have strong effects on the reproductive organs. The drugs, used for birth control and a range of hormone-related medical conditions, also affect the heart, circulatory system, bones, and other organs. Estrogens and progestins come in different forms, depending on their target conditions: When used for contraception, they are usually taken as pills but may also be implanted or injected. When used for hormone replacement, estrogens and progestins are available as pills, skin patches, and vaginal creams or inserts.

Most oral contraceptives combine a progestin drug with an estrogen such as ethinyl estradiol or mestranol. There are also

TARGET AILMENTS

Estrogen- and progestin-deficiency conditions, such as hot flashes and vaginal dryness, occurring at natural menopause or after surgical removal of ovaries

Birth control

Osteoporosis and heart disease in postmenopausal women (preventive treatment)

Palliative treatment of advanced inoperable cancers: breast cancer in women and, occasionally, prostate cancer in men

Abnormal uterine bleeding or lack of menstruation due to hormonal imbalance (medroxyprogesterone)

Endometriosis (oral contraceptives)

estrogen-only and progestin-only contraceptives. Your doctor will select an oral contraceptive on the basis of the relative strength and proportion of each ingredient to best fit your menstrual cycle and medical history.

The drugs may be used for estrogen- and progestin-deficiency conditions. Estrogens, such as conjugated estrogens, estradiol, and estropipate, are prescribed to prevent hot flashes, vaginal dryness, and other symptoms occurring at natural menopause. They are also prescribed to prevent osteoporosis and atherosclerosis after surgical removal of the uterus or ovaries, and for young women whose ovaries do not produce enough estrogen. Many of the drugs used for estrogen replacement therapy contain estrogen only, but some combine estrogen and progestin. Estrogen is known to be cardioprotective; taken alone it offers some protection against heart disease. However, this benefit is lost when estrogen is combined with progestin. On the other hand, adding a small dose of progestin helps alleviate the side effects of estrogen and reduces the risk of endometrial hyperplasia (a precancerous uterine condition).

Progestin-deficiency conditions include both abnormal uterine bleeding (heavy or prolonged menstruation) and amenorrhea (absence of menstruation). Medroxyprogesterone is the progestin most often used to treat menstrual problems that are caused by hormonal imbalance. In certain doses, it induces uterine bleeding to allow the uterine lining to be shed. This drug also alleviates the side effects of estrogen in estrogen replacement therapy.

PRECAUTIONS

WARNING

Do not use estrogens and progestins if you are pregnant or breast-feeding. If you suspect you are pregnant, discontinue use immediately to avoid severely harming the fetus.

Estrogens increase the risk of uterine cancer in menopausal and postmenopausal women. Abnormal vaginal bleeding is a possible symptom. If you experience unusual vaginal bleeding, call your doctor right away.

Get medical attention immediately if you experience the following: severe pain in leg, chest, or abdomen; sudden headache; changes in speech, vision, or breathing; weakness or numbness in extremities. These symptoms may indicate blood clots.

SPECIAL INFORMATION

- Before taking estrogens and progestins, let your doctor know if you are a smoker or have liver disease, gallbladder disease, a history of breast cancer, fibrocystic breast changes, endometriosis, uterine fibroids, diabetes, asthma, epilepsy, heart disease, blood-clotting disorders, or high blood pressure. Your doctor will use this information to determine whether or not you should use these drugs and what your dosage should be.
- Long-term use of estrogens may increase your risk of blood clots. Do not use estrogens if you have a history of heart attack, stroke, thrombophlebitis, or embolism.
- Estrogens may increase blood glucose levels; if you are diabetic, your doctor may have to adjust the dosage of your antidiabetic drug.
- These hormones may cause fluid retention, which can aggravate asthma, epilepsy, migraines, and heart and kidney disease.
- Do not smoke if you are using oral contraceptives. The combination can increase the risk of heart-related side effects, including heart attack, stroke, and blood clots, especially in women over 35.

CONTINUED

Estrogens and Progestins

E

SIDE EFFECTS

NOT SERIOUS

- Acne
- Headache or migraine
- Mild nausea, diarrhea, vomiting, or abdominal pain
- Appetite or weight changes
- Fluid retention or swelling of ankles, feet, or breasts
- Changes in sexual desire
- Blotchy spots on skin; increased body hair; loss of hair on scalp; photosensitivity; intolerance to contact lenses
- Local skin irritation (with skin patch)

TELL YOUR DOCTOR IF THESE SYMPTOMS BECOME BOTHERSOME.

SERIOUS

- Lumps in the breasts or breast enlargement
- Spotting or changes in menstrual bleeding (may indicate uterine cancer)
- Painful or frequent urination
- Fainting; jaundice
- Pain in the right side of the abdomen (may indicate gallbladder disease)
- Increased blood pressure
- Skin rash not associated with skin patch; a new mole
- Cataracts; vaginitis

TELL YOUR DOCTOR IMMEDIATELY IF YOU EXPERIENCE THESE SYMPTOMS OR THE SYMPTOMS FOR BLOOD CLOTS LISTED UNDER WARNING.

- Progestin-only oral contraceptives have been associated with higher rates of ectopic (fallopian tube) pregnancy.
- Taking these drugs with or after meals can help reduce nausea.
- Taking them at night and avoiding prolonged exposure to ultraviolet light and sunlight will reduce the chance of chloasma (patches of brown skin, often on the face).
- Oral contraceptives cause thinning of the cervical mucus, which in turn increases susceptibility to vaginal infections.
- Medroxyprogesterone may cause mental depression.

POSSIBLE INTERACTIONS

Anticoagulants: estrogens and progestins may decrease the anticoagulant effect of these medicines.

Anti-infective drugs: may decrease the effectiveness of oral contraceptives by interfering with estrogen in the digestive system.

Barbiturates and rifampin: reduced effectiveness of estrogens and progestins.

Benzodiazepines and theophylline: oral contraceptives may alter the effectiveness of these drugs. Your doctor may have to adjust your dosage.

Beta blockers: birth-control pills may interfere with some beta blockers.

Calcium supplements: oral contraceptives may increase calcium absorption.

Hydrocortisone and related corticosteroid drugs: estrogens and progestins may increase the anti-inflammatory effects of these drugs. Your doctor may lower the dosage of corticosteroids.

Tamoxifen: estrogen may decrease the effects of tamoxifen.

Tricyclic antidepressants and maprotiline: estrogen may increase blood levels of these drugs.

Rx ETODOLAC

VITAL STATISTICS

DRUG CLASS
Analgesics [Nonsteroidal Anti-Inflammatory Drugs (NSAIDs)]

BRAND NAMES
Lodine, Lodine XL

OTHER DRUGS IN THIS SUBCLASS
diclofenac, flurbiprofen, ibuprofen, ketoprofen, ketorolac, nabumetone, naproxen, oxaprozin

GENERAL DESCRIPTION
Etodolac is prescribed for pain and for the acute symptoms and long-term management of osteoarthritis and rheumatoid arthritis. This drug may be used by people who cannot tolerate aspirin, or when aspirin or acetaminophen is not effective. For further information, see Nonsteroidal Anti-Inflammatory Drugs (NSAIDs). For visual characteristics of the brand-name drug Lodine, see the Color Guide to Prescription Drugs and Herbs.

PRECAUTIONS

SPECIAL INFORMATION
- Do not use etodolac if you are allergic to NSAIDs or to aspirin. It may cause bronchoconstriction or anaphylaxis in aspirin-sensitive asthmatics.
- Avoid this drug or consult your doctor before using it if you have asthma, peptic ulcer, enteritis (intestinal inflammation), high blood pressure, bleeding problems, or impaired liver or kidney function.
- Etodolac is not recommended during pregnancy or for nursing mothers.

TARGET AILMENTS

Inflammation, especially related to osteoarthritis and rheumatoid arthritis

Pain, especially from inflammation, dental and other surgeries, menstruation, and migraines

Fever

SIDE EFFECTS

NOT SERIOUS
- Dizziness or headache
- Mild abdominal pain; cramps; constipation or diarrhea; indigestion or nausea

CONSULT YOUR DOCTOR IF THESE SYMPTOMS PERSIST.

SERIOUS
- Anaphylactic reaction (hives, rash, intense itching, and trouble breathing)
- Gastrointestinal bleeding; ulceration; stomach perforation (black or tarry stools)
- Hypertension; irregular heartbeat; fluid retention
- Diminished hearing or ringing in the ears
- Jaundice; blood in urine

CALL YOUR DOCTOR IMMEDIATELY.

EUCALYPTUS

LATIN NAME
Eucalyptus globulus

E

VITAL STATISTICS

GENERAL DESCRIPTION

This native Australian evergreen is cultivated in several areas, including the state of California. The oil ranges in color from clear to yellow and has a penetrating smell.

Eucalyptus oil is distilled from the leaves and twigs. Eucalyptus has strong antiseptic, antiviral, and antibacterial properties. It also has stimulating, astringent, and analgesic actions. It is useful as a decongestant and as an insect repellent.

PREPARATIONS

For most of its target ailments, eucalyptus oil can be inhaled, used in baths, and rubbed on the skin.

INHALATION: Use a diffuser, or place a few drops of the oil on a handkerchief and hold it to the nose. For respiratory problems, add 6 drops oil to a bowl of steaming hot water and inhale the vapors for up to 5 minutes.

BATH: Add 10 drops to the bathwater.

SKIN APPLICATION: Apply a drop directly to minor cuts, sores, boils, and pimples. To cover larger areas of the body, mix 10 to 15 drops eucalyptus essential oil with a carrier oil such as almond oil or aloe gel. To ease nervousness and speed convalescence, apply the oil externally to the lower back, the tops of the hands, and the solar plexus.

PRECAUTIONS

☠ *WARNING*

Do not take the oil internally. If taken internally, even as little as a teaspoonful can be fatal.

Use recommended dilutions. Once absorbed by the bloodstream, eucalyptus can irritate the kidneys.

SPECIAL INFORMATION

Eucalyptus is not compatible with many homeopathic remedies; do not use if undergoing such treatment.

TARGET AILMENTS
Fevers
Colds and flu
Sinus problems
Coughing
Bronchitis
Boils and pimples
Cuts and sores
Joint and muscle pain

SIDE EFFECTS

WHEN USED EXTERNALLY AND IN RECOMMENDED DILUTIONS, EUCALYPTUS OIL HAS NO SIDE EFFECTS.

EUCALYPTUS

LATIN NAME
Eucalyptus globulus

VITAL STATISTICS

GENERAL DESCRIPTION

Native to Australia and a favorite meal for koalas, the eucalyptus tree is sometimes called the Australian fever tree or gum tree. The oil extracted from eucalyptus leaves is an important ingredient in over-the-counter mouthwashes and decongestants. Herbalists include small amounts of the oil in several preparations, including gargles for sore throat, topical antiseptics for skin injuries, rubs for arthritis, and inhalants for asthma, bronchitis, and other respiratory conditions.

PREPARATIONS

Over the counter:
Available in dry bulk, tinctures, and oils.

At home:

Inhalant: Put 1 to 3 drops of the oil in a bowl and add 1 pt boiling water; inhale steam until the vapors disappear.

Antiseptic: Dilute the oil with an equal amount of an alcohol-based topical antiseptic and apply to cuts and other open wounds after you have washed them with soap.

Rub: Mix 1 to 5 drops eucalyptus oil with 1 cup olive oil.

Consult a qualified practitioner for the dosage appropriate for your specific condition.

SIDE EFFECTS

NOT SERIOUS

- Skin rash

THIS SYMPTOM MAY OCCUR WITH EXTERNAL USE. IF IT DOES, DISCONTINUE USE.

PRECAUTIONS

WARNING

The oil of eucalyptus in concentrated form is poisonous if you ingest it. A teaspoonful can be fatal. Call your doctor immediately if you experience stomach upset or diarrhea with any dosage.

Do not administer internally to children under two years of age. For older children and older adults, start with minimal doses.

If you apply the oil to broken, irritated skin, use small amounts.

Close your eyes when inhaling eucalyptus in any form because the fumes are very powerful, and be especially careful to protect your eyes from any contact with the oils.

POSSIBLE INTERACTIONS

Combining eucalyptus with other herbs may necessitate a lower dosage.

TARGET AILMENTS

Apply externally for:

Arthritis; rheumatism

Minor cuts and scrapes

Use as an inhalant in an extremely dilute form for:

Asthma

Colds, flu, and other respiratory illnesses

Bronchitis

Whooping cough

E

EUCOMMIA BARK

LATIN NAME
Eucommia ulmoides

E

VITAL STATISTICS

GENERAL DESCRIPTION

Eucommia bark is used to strengthen the musculoskeletal system and to prevent miscarriages. In some clinical trials, eucommia bark reduced high blood pressure, with the fried herb having a stronger effect than the dried herb. Also, when tested in dogs, rats, and mice, the herb seemed to stimulate urination.

The bark is yellowish brown on the outside with a dark purple interior. When broken, the bark should produce thin white threads. According to traditional Chinese medicine, the herb has acrid, sweet, and warm characteristics. It is harvested in several provinces of China, from trees that are at least 15 years old.

PREPARATIONS

Eucommia bark is available in bulk or dried form at Chinese pharmacies, Asian markets, and some Western health food stores. It is sometimes possible to obtain it in pills or tablets. Herbalists recommend that you fry it in salt water when you use it as a tonic to strengthen the lower back and knees, and to treat fatigue and frequent urination.

COMBINATIONS: Eucommia bark is sometimes mixed with psoralea fruit, cornus, and cuscuta for impotence or urinary frequency and incontinence. It may be combined with Japanese teasel root, cuscuta, and mulberry mistletoe stems for low back pain and stabilizing pregnancy. A preparation containing eucommia bark, Japanese teasel root, and Chinese yam is prescribed for pregnant women who have suffered habitual miscarriages.

Consult a Chinese practitioner for advice about dosages and other herbal combinations.

PRECAUTIONS

POSSIBLE INTERACTIONS

Some herbalists suggest that eucommia bark should not be taken at the same time as scrophularia.

TARGET AILMENTS

Take internally for:

- Weak muscles and bones, especially in the back and knees, accompanied by poor circulation
- Low back pain and soreness, accompanied by frequent urination
- Mild abdominal pain or slight vaginal bleeding during pregnancy
- Prevention of miscarriage and stabilization of pregnancy
- Back pain in pregnant women
- Dizziness and lightheadedness caused by high blood pressure

SIDE EFFECTS

NOT SERIOUS

- Mild sedative effect

THIS EFFECT OCCURS WITH LARGE DOSES; CALL YOUR DOCTOR IF THE EFFECT PERSISTS OR BECOMES BOTHERSOME.

EUPHRASIA

LATIN NAME
Euphrasia officinalis

VITAL STATISTICS

GENERAL DESCRIPTION

The popular name of this plant, eyebright, suggests both its medicinal uses and its appearance. The red spots on white or purple flowers are said to resemble bloodshot eyes, and the dried stems, leaves, and flowers have long been used as a tonic for irritated or infected eyes. Its formal name, *Euphrasia,* is derived from the Greek word *euphrosyne,* meaning gladness, possibly because its effects on patients' eyes were so pleasing. The herb is still used for eye ailments, including conjunctivitis, and is taken as a tea to reduce nasal congestion and coughs that accompany hay fever, colds, and sinusitis.

Samuel Hahnemann, the founder of homeopathy, first demonstrated the effects of this substance, discovering that when taken full strength, orally, it irritated the eyes. Today, homeopathic practitioners prescribe *Euphrasia* for various eye conditions as well as for some kinds of headaches, colds, coughs, and hay fever. Preparation of the remedy involves expressing the juice of the whole, fresh plant and mixing it with an equal part of alcohol. For more information on homeopathic medicine, see page 14.

PREPARATIONS

Euphrasia is available over the counter in various potencies, in both liquid and tablet form, at selected stores and pharmacies. Consult your homeopathic physician for further information.

SIDE EFFECTS
None expected

PRECAUTIONS

SPECIAL INFORMATION

- Only the patient should touch the pills. If tablets are spilled, throw them away.
- The mouth should be clear of flavors 15 minutes before and after taking a remedy, and strong flavors and aromas, such as coffee and heavy perfume, should be avoided for the duration of treatment.

TARGET AILMENTS
Stinging, watery discharge from the eyes
Hot, red, swollen eyelids
Watering eyes
Conjunctivitis with copious burning tears and mucus discharge
Intolerance of bright light
Colds with watery discharge from nose and burning tears
Cough, worse during the day and relieved by eating and lying down
Hay fever with cold symptoms and eye inflammation
Measles, early stages
Short, painful menstrual periods
Prostatitis
Constipation

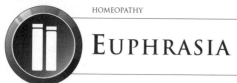

Evening Primrose Oil

LATIN NAME
Oenothera biennis

E

Vital Statistics

GENERAL INFORMATION

Herbalists recommend the oil from the seeds of the plant known as evening primrose for a wide range of ailments that includes arthritis and premenstrual syndrome. Evening primrose supplements may also benefit brittle hair and fingernails, and may help to keep dry eyes lubricated. Native Americans and early settlers in North America used the oil to treat asthma, gastrointestinal ills, and bruises.

The therapeutic component of evening primrose oil, known as gamma-linolenic acid (GLA), is an essential fatty acid that the Western diet often lacks. GLA supports the body's production of hormones known as prostaglandins, which affect the body's hormone balance. When the body's supply of essential fatty acids such as GLA is deficient, the effects of premenstrual syndrome, diabetes, and other disorders may become more pronounced.

Evening primrose oil may also, through its anti-inflammatory action, be useful in treating sore breasts in nursing mothers. In addition, recent studies suggest that evening primrose oil may have an anticlotting action. Some herbalists believe that this property may make the oil helpful in the treatment of coronary artery disease.

PREPARATIONS

Available in capsules and in liquid form. Consult a qualified practitioner for the dosage appropriate for you and the specific condition being treated.

Precautions

SPECIAL INFORMATION

- Evening primrose supplements must be taken regularly for at least a month before their beneficial effects can be noticed.
- Consult a practitioner before using evening primrose oil medicinally for children.

TARGET AILMENTS
Premenstrual syndrome
Arthritis
Dry eyes
Multiple sclerosis
High blood pressure
Eczema
Brittle hair and fingernails

SIDE EFFECTS

NOT SERIOUS

- Headache
- Skin rash
- Nausea

LOWER YOUR DOSAGE OR DISCONTINUE USE ALTOGETHER.

EVERLASTING

LATIN NAME
Helichrysum angustifolium

VITAL STATISTICS

GENERAL DESCRIPTION

This strongly scented herb is known by many names: helichrysum, everlasting, and immortelle. It has a multibranched stem and bright flowers and is native to the Mediterranean region. It also grows wild in the Pacific Northwest. The pale yellow to red oil is distilled from the flowers and flowering tops of the plant.

Everlasting is valued for its anti-inflammatory and painkilling properties. It can help prevent internal hemorrhaging and swelling after injury and assist in the healing of nearly all skin complaints.

PREPARATIONS

Everlasting oil can be applied undiluted to very small areas of the skin such as scars, stretch marks, and small bruises. For all other uses the oil should be diluted. To dilute, mix 10 to 15 drops of oil in 2 tbsp aloe gel or a carrier oil such as vegetable or nut oil. For scars, wrinkles, and stretch marks, rosa mosqueta oil (also known as rose hip oil) is a particularly effective carrier oil.

For a healing bath, add 10 drops everlasting oil to the bathwater.

TARGET AILMENTS

- Skin conditions such as scarring, stretch marks, sunburn, wounds
- Acne
- Dermatitis
- Bruises
- Wrinkles
- Liver or spleen congestion
- Bronchitis
- Colds and flu
- Tendinitis
- Arthritis pain
- Muscle aches
- Sprains and strains

SIDE EFFECTS

NONE EXPECTED

EVERLASTING IS NONTOXIC, NONIRRITATING, AND NONSENSITIZING.

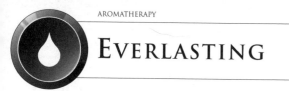

EVODIA FRUIT

LATIN NAME
Evodia rutaecarpa

VITAL STATISTICS

GENERAL DESCRIPTION

This extremely fragrant herb is prescribed for abdominal disorders and sometimes for its painkilling properties. In clinical tests, powdered evodia appeared to be helpful in treating eczema. Evodia fruit is grown in several Chinese provinces and is harvested between August and October, when it is brownish green in color and not fully ripe. Practitioners characterize the herb as hot, acrid, and bitter.

PREPARATIONS

Evodia fruit is available in bulk or powdered form at Chinese pharmacies, Asian markets, and some Western health food stores.

COMBINATIONS: Evodia fruit is often mixed with other herbs to treat vomiting. These preparations frequently include fresh or dried ginger, pinellia root, or coptis. In addition, practitioners recommend that powdered evodia be combined with vinegar to make a poultice. These pastes are then placed on the navel to relieve indigestion, or on the soles of the feet to treat high blood pressure and sores of the mouth and tongue.

PRECAUTIONS

WARNING

Herbalists consider evodia slightly toxic. They caution against long-term use and overdosage. They also believe it can dry out body tissues.

SPECIAL INFORMATION

- Practitioners often try to reduce side effects by giving patients a preparation of licorice before they take the evodia.
- An overdose of evodia fruit can cause the throat to become extremely dry.

POSSIBLE INTERACTIONS

Some herbalists believe that evodia should not be used in combination with sage root.

TARGET AILMENTS

Take internally or apply poultice externally for:

Diarrhea with undigested food, especially morning diarrhea

Headache with vomiting; nausea accompanied by lack of appreciation for the taste of food

Pain in the upper abdomen; hernia

Apply poultice externally for:

Indigestion; high blood pressure; sores of the mouth or tongue

SIDE EFFECTS

SERIOUS

- Visual disturbances
- Hallucinations

CAUSED BY LARGE DOSES. DISCONTINUE USE AND CALL YOUR DOCTOR IMMEDIATELY.

EXPECTORANTS

VITAL STATISTICS

GENERIC NAME
guaifenesin

GENERAL DESCRIPTION
Expectorants help people cough up and remove thick and excessive mucus (also known as phlegm or sputum) from the lungs and upper respiratory tract, thus providing symptomatic relief from persistent coughs that frequently accompany the common cold or flu. These drugs work by reducing the stickiness and adhesiveness of mucus, making it easier to cough up and expel. Expectorants are particularly useful with dry coughs that are producing little, if any, phlegm. Eventually, as the phlegm is expelled, the respiratory tract becomes less congested and the need to cough is reduced. For information about a specific generic expectorant drug, see Guaifenesin.

PRECAUTIONS

SPECIAL INFORMATION
- If you are using the extended-release tablet form of guaifenesin, swallow it whole; do not crush or chew the tablet before swallowing it.
- Guaifenesin is most effective when taken on an empty stomach.
- To help guaifenesin loosen mucus from the lungs, drink eight to 10 glasses of fluid each day, including a glass of water after each dose.
- If you are pregnant or nursing, check with your doctor before using guaifenesin.
- Do not give guaifenesin to a child under the age of two without first consulting the child's pediatrician.
- Do not take guaifenesin for persistent cough due to smoking, asthma, bronchitis, or emphysema.
- If your cough does not improve within seven days, see your doctor.

POSSIBLE INTERACTIONS
None expected when guaifenesin is taken as directed.

TARGET AILMENTS

Coughs due to cold, flu, or other minor upper respiratory conditions

SIDE EFFECTS

(GUAIFENESIN ONLY)

NOT SERIOUS
- Stomach pain
- Diarrhea
- Nausea
- Drowsiness
- Mild weakness

CALL YOUR DOCTOR IF THESE EFFECTS PERSIST OR BECOME BOTHERSOME.

SERIOUS
- Skin rash
- Persistent headache
- Vomiting
- High fever

CALL YOUR DOCTOR RIGHT AWAY.

E

EYEBRIGHT

LATIN NAME
Euphrasia officinalis

E

VITAL STATISTICS

GENERAL INFORMATION

Eyebright's name suggests both its action and appearance; its red-spotted white or purple flowers seem to resemble bloodshot eyes. In fact, its dried stems, leaves, and flowers have long been used as a tonic for irritated or infected eyes. Eyebright can be applied to eyes affected by hay fever, other allergies, or colds. Herbalists also recommend it to relieve conjunctivitis, and some suggest that drinking eyebright tea can help maintain good vision.

Eyebright teas are also used to diminish nasal congestion and the coughs that accompany hay fever, colds, and sinusitis. The herb, indigenous to heaths and pastures throughout Great Britain and other parts of Europe, by now has become naturalized in the United States. For visual characteristics, see the Color Guide to Prescription Drugs and Herbs.

TARGET AILMENTS

Apply externally for:

- Eye irritations including redness, itching, and tearing from hay fever
- Other allergies or colds
- Conjunctivitis

Take internally for:

- Nasal congestion
- Cough due to colds, sinusitis, or allergies

PREPARATIONS

Over the counter:
Available in bulk, capsules, and tinctures.

At home:

TEA: Pour 1 cup boiling water onto 2 tsp dried eyebright and steep covered for 10 minutes; drink three times a day.

COMPRESS: Boil 1 to 2 tbsp dried eyebright in 1 pt water for 10 minutes. When the water is lukewarm, strain the mixture to remove all parts of the herb, dip a sterile cloth in the liquid and wring it out, then put it over your eyes for 15 minutes several times daily.

COMBINATIONS TO BE TAKEN ORALLY: Combine with goldenrod, elder flowers, or goldenseal to treat respiratory and nasal congestion; combine with ephedra for hay fever that causes itchy or watery eyes.

Consult a qualified practitioner for the dosage appropriate for your specific condition.

PRECAUTIONS

WARNING
Consult a practitioner before using eyebright to treat children.

POSSIBLE INTERACTIONS

Combining eyebright with other herbs may necessitate a lower dosage.

SIDE EFFECTS

NOT SERIOUS

- Skin rash; nausea

REDUCE YOUR DOSAGE OR STOP TAKING COMPLETELY.

Famotidine

Vital Statistics

DRUG CLASS
Antiulcer Drugs [Histamine H_2 Blockers]

BRAND NAMES
Rx: Pepcid
OTC: Pepcid AC, Mylanta AR

OTHER DRUGS IN THIS CLASS
lansoprazole, omeprazole, sucralfate
Histamine H_2 Blockers: cimetidine, nizatidine, ranitidine

GENERAL DESCRIPTION
Famotidine is used mainly to treat ulcers of the stomach and duodenum. It is also prescribed for Zollinger-Ellison syndrome, gastroesophageal reflux (in which stomach acid flows back into the esophagus), and other conditions involving the overproduction of stomach acid. In some cases the drug is used to prevent upper gastrointestinal bleeding.

In the over-the-counter form, famotidine is used not for ulcers but to relieve acid indigestion and heartburn. The OTC form—a lower dose than the prescription version—has milder side effects. The same drug interactions may apply, although no interactions have been reported for the OTC drug.

Belonging to a subclass of antiulcer drugs known as histamine H_2 blockers, famotidine works by blocking the effects of the chemical histamine in the stomach, thereby reducing the secretion of the digestive juice hydrochloric acid. For more information on side effects and drug interactions, see Antiulcer Drugs. For visual characteristics of the brand-name drug Pepcid, see the Color Guide to Prescription Drugs and Herbs.

TARGET AILMENTS
Duodenal ulcer
Gastric ulcer
Upper gastrointestinal bleeding associated with gastric ulcer or duodenal ulcer, or with gastritis
Zollinger-Ellison syndrome
Multiple endocrine neoplasia
Other conditions characterized by an overproduction of stomach acid
Gastroesophageal reflux
Acid indigestion and heartburn (OTC)

CONTINUED

FAMOTIDINE

F

PRECAUTIONS

SPECIAL INFORMATION

- Avoid this drug while pregnant or nursing.
- Inform your doctor if you have a history of liver or kidney disease.
- This drug can interfere with skin allergy tests and cause false-negative results.
- You may need to avoid driving or other potentially hazardous activities while taking this drug.
- Antacids can be taken with famotidine.

POSSIBLE INTERACTIONS

Alcohol, tobacco: may cause decreased effectiveness of famotidine.

Enteric-coated tablets: changes in stomach acidity may cause these medications to dissolve prematurely in the stomach; avoid taking them with famotidine.

Itraconazole, ketoconazole: decreased absorption of these drugs into the body.

SIDE EFFECTS

NOT SERIOUS

- Headache
- Mild diarrhea or constipation
- Dizziness

CALL YOUR DOCTOR IF THESE EFFECTS PERSIST.

- Skin rash
- Dry mouth or skin
- Fatigue; insomnia
- Loss of appetite
- Nausea or stomach pains
- Swelling of the eyelids

THESE EFFECTS ARE RARE. CONTACT YOUR DOCTOR IF THEY CONTINUE OR BECOME BOTHERSOME.

SERIOUS

- Confusion, depression, or anxiety
- Hair loss
- Hallucinations
- Muscle or joint pain
- Ringing in the ears
- Shortness of breath
- Tingling in fingers or toes
- Unusual bleeding or bruising
- Jaundice (yellowing of skin and eyes)

IF YOU EXPERIENCE ANY OF THESE SYMPTOMS, CALL YOUR DOCTOR IMMEDIATELY.

Rx FENFLURAMINE

VITAL STATISTICS

DRUG CLASS
Appetite Suppressants

BRAND NAME
Pondimin

OTHER DRUGS IN THIS CLASS
phentermine

GENERAL DESCRIPTION
Fenfluramine is used for short-term treatment of obesity in patients in whom there is no physiological basis for the disorder; it is not intended for long-term or intermittent use. The drug is used to control appetite and is administered in conjunction with a low-calorie diet and behavior-modification techniques.

Fenfluramine is believed to work by stimulating the hypothalamus, the part of the brain thought to control appetite. Because it may improve glucose tolerance, this drug is especially useful in patients with non-insulin-dependent (Type 2) diabetes.

Fenfluramine is related chemically to the amphetamines, which can cause severe psychological dependence and produce harmful physical and mental effects. Although amphetamines and other appetite suppressant drugs stimulate the central nervous system and raise the blood pressure, fenfluramine is more likely to depress the central nervous system, and it may reduce blood pressure. It therefore can be useful for patients with anxiety or who need to avoid stimulation for any reason. For more information, see Appetite Suppressants, keeping in mind that fenfluramine differs in some ways from other drugs in its class. For visual characteristics of the brand-name drug Pondimin, see the Color Guide to Prescription Drugs and Herbs.

PRECAUTIONS

☠ ***WARNING***
Do not take fenfluramine if you have glaucoma, a history of drug abuse, severe hypertension, symptomatic cardiovascular disease, mental depression, or a history of psychotic illness.

Do not take this drug within 14 days of taking a monoamine oxidase (MAO) inhibitor. Combining these drugs poses the risk of a hypertensive crisis, causing symptoms such as severe headache and heart palpitations.

Avoid anesthesia, if possible, while taking fenfluramine. If surgery with anesthesia is unavoidable, intensive cardiac monitoring is required to avoid serious or even fatal cardiac arrhythmias.

Taking fenfluramine for longer than three months within a one-year period has been associated with an increased risk of the development of primary pulmonary hypertension, a serious, often fatal cardiopulmonary disease. Tell your doctor immediately if you notice reduced tolerance for exercise, including shortness of breath or chest pain; faintness; or swelling of your feet or ankles.

Overdoses of fenfluramine may produce a variety of symptoms, including drowsiness, confusion, flushing, tremor, fever, and sweating. Extreme overdoses can cause convulsions, coma, and even death. In case of overdose or ingestion by a child, seek emergency help immediately.

CONTINUED

FENFLURAMINE

F

SPECIAL INFORMATION

- Alcoholics and people with mental illness should check with a doctor before using this drug. Fenfluramine can increase the risk of paranoia, depression, delusions, or agitation in susceptible people. Severe depression may also result if fenfluramine is stopped abruptly.
- Avoid this drug if you are pregnant. It's also best to avoid fenfluramine when nursing a baby, although it is not known whether fenfluramine passes into human breast milk.
- The safety and efficacy of fenfluramine in children younger than 12 years is unknown.
- People with mild or moderate hypertension should have their blood pressure monitored when taking this drug.
- Avoid alcohol while taking fenfluramine.
- Refrain from driving or engaging in other potentially hazardous activities until you know how this drug will affect you.

POSSIBLE INTERACTIONS

Antihypertensive drugs (such as guanethidine, reserpine, methyldopa): increased effects of these drugs.

Central nervous system depressants: increased depressant effects.

Insulin: the combination may reduce the requirement for insulin. Glucose levels should be monitored.

Monoamine oxidase (MAO) inhibitors: may cause hypertensive crisis.

TARGET AILMENTS

Obesity without physiological basis

SIDE EFFECTS

NOT SERIOUS

- Drowsiness
- Diarrhea
- Dry mouth; bad taste in the mouth
- Sweating; fever; chills
- Dizziness
- Weakness; fatigue; insomnia
- Increased or decreased libido
- Constipation; abdominal pain; nausea
- Painful or frequent urination
- Muscle pain
- Rash
- Burning sensation

CALL YOUR DOCTOR IF THESE PROBLEMS PERSIST.

SERIOUS

- Blurred vision
- Palpitations
- Incoordination; confusion
- Elevated mood; depression; anxiety
- Nervousness; tension; agitation
- Difficulty articulating
- Eye irritation
- Chest pain
- Hives
- Shortness of breath
- Increased or decreased blood pressure

CONTACT YOUR DOCTOR IMMEDIATELY.

FENNEL

LATIN NAME
Foeniculum vulgare

VITAL STATISTICS

GENERAL DESCRIPTION

The tiny fruits (seeds) of fennel have been used since ancient times to treat colic and to increase lactation in nursing mothers. Fennel may help digestion by relaxing the stomach and other digestive organs; it may also relieve diarrhea. In addition, it is believed that fennel may have effects upon the body similar to those of estrogen. Because it acts as a mild diuretic, fennel has been used to aid in flushing kidney stones from the body. It can also be used as a soothing eyewash. Fennel oil is used to soothe the pain of inflamed joints.

PREPARATIONS

Over the counter:
Available in dry bulk, oil, and tinctures.

At home:
To help digestion, chew fresh fennel fruit.

TEA: Steep covered 2 tsp ground fennel in 1 cup boiling water for 10 minutes. Drink three times daily to aid digestion. For gas, drink a cup of the tea half an hour before eating. Use a weaker dosage when treating colic in children under age two.

Consult a qualified practitioner for the dosage appropriate for you and the specific condition being treated.

PRECAUTIONS

WARNING

Do not ingest the oil; it can cause nausea, vomiting, and seizures. Call your doctor if any of these symptoms develop.

SPECIAL INFORMATION

- Do not use fennel if you are pregnant or if you can't use birth-control pills or estrogen supplements.
- Do not take fennel if you have a history of alcoholism, hepatitis, liver disease, abnormal blood clotting, or estrogen-dependent breast tumors. Animal studies suggest that fennel may exacerbate liver damage.

POSSIBLE INTERACTIONS

Combining fennel with other herbs may necessitate a lower dosage.

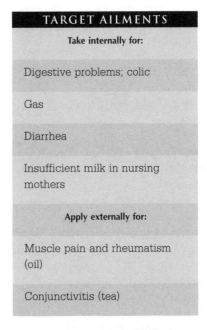

TARGET AILMENTS
Take internally for:
Digestive problems; colic
Gas
Diarrhea
Insufficient milk in nursing mothers
Apply externally for:
Muscle pain and rheumatism (oil)
Conjunctivitis (tea)

SIDE EFFECTS

NOT SERIOUS

- Rash

DISCONTINUE IF THIS OCCURS.

F

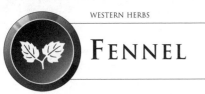

FENUGREEK

LATIN NAME
Trigonella foenum-graecum

VITAL STATISTICS

GENERAL DESCRIPTION

Members of a legume family that includes beans and peas, fenugreek seeds have been used for centuries for digestive problems, skin injuries, sore throats, fever, muscle aches, and impotence. The seeds contain a large amount of mucilage, which becomes gelatinous when mixed with water; in this form it was thought to soothe irritated tissue. Some recent studies suggest that fenugreek has a mild anti-inflammatory effect, which may be why herbalists find it useful in treating boils, rashes, and other skin wounds, as well as arthritis. It may also be taken internally for sore throats and coughs.

PREPARATIONS

Over the counter:

Available in bulk seeds, capsules, and tinctures.

At home:

Decoction: Bring to a boil 2 tsp ground fenugreek seeds in 1 cup water and simmer covered for 10 minutes; drink up to three times a day.

Gargle: Mix 1 tbsp ground seeds in 1 cup hot water; simmer covered for 10 minutes, then strain. Gargle three times daily, every 3 to 4 hours, for sore throat pain.

Poultice: Mix enough boiled seeds in 1 cup warm water to make a thick paste. Apply it directly to affected areas daily.

Consult a qualified practitioner for the dosage appropriate for you and the specific condition being treated.

PRECAUTIONS

SPECIAL INFORMATION

- Do not give to children under age two.
- For older children and elderly adults, start treatment with low-strength doses.
- Use with caution during pregnancy.

POSSIBLE INTERACTIONS

Combining fenugreek with other herbs may necessitate a lower dosage.

TARGET AILMENTS

Take internally for:

Digestive disorders

Sore throats and coughs

Lactation problems of nursing mothers

Apply externally for:

Skin injuries, such as boils, rashes, cuts, or other wounds

Pain caused by arthritis

SIDE EFFECTS

SERIOUS

- Uterine contractions

CALL YOUR DOCTOR RIGHT AWAY.

FERRUM PHOSPHORICUM

LATIN NAME
Ferrum phosphoricum

VITAL STATISTICS

GENERAL DESCRIPTION

Ferrum phosphoricum, also called *Ferrum phos* or iron phosphate, is a mineral compound of iron and phosphorus. Both elements are present in the body independently; phosphorus contributes to bone and muscle health, and iron aids the exchange of oxygen in the blood. *Ferrum phos* is derived from mixing solutions of iron sulfate, phosphate, and sodium acetate. The resulting iron phosphate is ground with large quantities of lactose (milk sugar) to render it nontoxic. Homeopathic practitioners consider *Ferrum phos* good for patients who suffer from conditions characterized by low energy and anemia. When a patient exhibits a set of symptoms that matches the cataloged symptoms brought on by *Ferrum phos,* the homeopathic practitioner then prescribes it in an extremely dilute form. For more information on homeopathic medicine, see page 14.

PREPARATIONS

Ferrum phos is available in various potencies, in both liquid and tablet form, at selected stores and pharmacies. Consult your practitioner for more information.

PRECAUTIONS

SPECIAL INFORMATION

- Only the patient should touch the pills. If tablets are spilled, throw them away.
- The mouth should be clear of flavors 15 minutes before and after taking a remedy, and strong flavors and aromas, such as coffee, camphor, and heavily scented perfumes, should be avoided for the duration of treatment.

TARGET AILMENTS

- Tickling, hacking coughs with chest pain
- Headache
- Fevers that begin slowly
- Ear infections
- Incontinence
- Rheumatic joints
- Early menstrual periods accompanied by headache
- Anemia
- Fatigue
- Nosebleeds
- Sore throat
- Vomiting
- Diarrhea
- Palpitations

SIDE EFFECTS

NONE EXPECTED

F

FEVERFEW

LATIN NAME
Tanacetum parthenium
(or Chrysanthemum parthenium)

F

VITAL STATISTICS

GENERAL DESCRIPTION

Feverfew is a perennial with small, daisylike blossoms and leaves that are medicinal. In the late 1970s, British researchers found feverfew leaves helpful in treating migraine headaches where other treatments had failed. They believe this relief is due to the chemical parthenolide, which blocks the release of inflammatory substances from the blood. The researchers consider these inflammatory elements, which affect the walls of the brain's blood vessels, to be key components in the onset of a migraine.

You may need to take feverfew daily for two to three months before it has any effect. For visual characteristics of feverfew, see the Color Guide to Prescription Drugs and Herbs.

PREPARATIONS

Over the counter:
Available in dry bulk, pills, capsules, and tinctures.

At home:
Chew two fresh or frozen leaves a day for migraines. If you find the leaves too bitter, substitute capsules or pills containing 85 mg of the leaf material, but fresh leaves are best for immediate results.

TEA: Steep covered 2 tsp dried herb in 1 cup boiling water for 5 to 10 minutes; drink 2 to 3 cups per day.

Consult a qualified practitioner for the dosage appropriate for you and the specific condition being treated.

PRECAUTIONS

SPECIAL INFORMATION

- Do not use feverfew if you are pregnant; it may stimulate uterine contractions.
- Feverfew may interfere with the blood's clotting ability; talk to your doctor before using if you have a clotting disorder or take anticoagulant medicine.
- Use of this herb by children for more than seven to 10 days should be done in conjunction with a healthcare practitioner.

POSSIBLE INTERACTIONS

Combining feverfew with other herbs may necessitate a lower dosage.

TARGET AILMENTS

Migraine headaches

SIDE EFFECTS

SERIOUS

- Internal mouth sores
- Abdominal pain

CHEWING FRESH OR DRIED FEVERFEW MAY CAUSE THESE SYMPTOMS. IF THEY DEVELOP, DISCONTINUE USE AND NOTIFY YOUR DOCTOR IMMEDIATELY.

FIBER, DIETARY

VITAL STATISTICS

DAILY DOSAGE
30 grams

GENERAL DESCRIPTION
Dietary fiber is the part of whole grains, fruits, and vegetables that remains undigested as it travels through the alimentary canal. Soluble fiber, such as that found in oat bran, beans, apples, and carrots, helps lower blood cholesterol. Insoluble fiber, such as that found in wheat bran, rice bran, and lentils, is especially helpful for adding bulk to improve digestion and prevent constipation. Most nutritionists favor food sources, but several over-the-counter supplements are available, such as psyllium seed for constipation.

NATURAL SOURCES
Good sources are fresh fruits and vegetables, nuts and seeds, and whole-grain foods.

PREPARATIONS
Available as psyllium seed, oat bran and rice bran, glucomannan, guar gum, or fennel seed.

Supplements are available as capsules, tablets, oral suspension, flakes, or wafers.

To help relieve constipation, mix bran with fruit juice or cereal. Start with 1 tbsp a day and gradually increase to 3 to 4 tbsp.

PRECAUTIONS

WARNING
Consult your doctor before taking fiber supplements if you have Crohn's disease.

SPECIAL INFORMATION
- Fiber intake should be increased gradually. Supplements may cause intestinal gas, but this effect will subside as the body adjusts.
- Increase water intake when increasing dietary fiber, because fiber absorbs water.

POSSIBLE INTERACTIONS
Digoxin: decreased effectiveness.
Minerals (calcium, iron, zinc, and copper): decreased absorption of these minerals.

TARGET AILMENTS
High cholesterol
Constipation; hemorrhoids
Diverticulitis
Obesity
Heart disease
Non-insulin-dependent diabetes
Cancers of the colon and breast

SIDE EFFECTS

NOT SERIOUS
- Flatulence or bloating

SERIOUS
- Blocked colon, indicated by pain, fever, lack of bowel movements, and distended abdomen

CALL YOUR DOCTOR IMMEDIATELY.

F

FIELD MINT

LATIN NAME
Mentha haplocalyx (or Mentha arvensis)

VITAL STATISTICS

GENERAL DESCRIPTION

Chinese herbalists believe that this fragrant mint speeds recovery in diseases such as measles by bringing rashes to the skin's surface. Field mint is also prescribed for a range of conditions that include gynecological problems and emotional disturbances. Characterized in Chinese medicine as an acrid, cool herb, field mint is cultivated throughout China.

Chinese medicine takes a holistic approach to healthcare, fashioning remedies to treat the entire being as well as the specific parts or areas. Single herbs may be used alone or in combination with other herbs to prevent and combat disease, which is thought to arise from disturbances in the flow of a bodily energy called chi (pronounced "chee") and blood, or from a lack of balance in the complementary states of yin and yang.

PREPARATIONS

You can buy field mint in its natural form at Chinese pharmacies, Asian and Western groceries, and health food stores. It is also available in tablet form.

COMBINATIONS: A mixture with prunella is prescribed for inflammation of the eyes and swelling of the lymph nodes. A preparation prescribed for a sore, swollen throat combines field mint with platycodon and silkworm. Mixed with chrysanthemum flower *(Chrysanthemum morifolium)*, field mint is used to relieve headaches and other pains, as well as redness and swelling of the eyes. Practitioners warn against overcooking when preparing medicinal solutions of the mint; it is usually added to combinations 5 minutes before the cooking is finished.

Consult your herbalist for further information on appropriate combinations and dosages.

PRECAUTIONS

SPECIAL INFORMATION

Nursing mothers should not use this herb, since it may cause insufficient production of milk.

TARGET AILMENTS

Take internally for:

- Rashes in the early stages
- Sore throat
- Red eyes
- Headache
- Emotional instability
- Gynecological problems
- Childhood convulsions

SIDE EFFECTS

NONE EXPECTED

Rx FIORINAL WITH CODEINE

VITAL STATISTICS

DRUG CLASS
Analgesics

GENERIC NAME
aspirin, butalbital, caffeine, and codeine (combination)

GENERAL DESCRIPTION
The brand-name drug Fiorinal with Codeine is a strong opiate pain reliever and muscle relaxant prescribed for the relief of tension headaches caused by stress and muscle contraction in the head, neck, and shoulder area. It combines butalbital (a sedative-barbiturate) with codeine (an opiate pain reliever and cough suppressant), aspirin (a pain-and-fever reliever), and caffeine (a stimulant).

Barbiturates like butalbital and opioid analgesics like codeine may be habit forming when taken in higher-than-recommended doses over long periods of time. For further information about side effects and interactions, see the entries for aspirin, caffeine, and codeine. For visual characteristics, see the Color Guide to Prescription Drugs and Herbs.

PRECAUTIONS

SPECIAL INFORMATION
- Fiorinal with Codeine should not be given to children under the age of 12 or to teenagers with chickenpox or the flu.
- Do not take this medication if you are sensitive to butalbital, codeine, aspirin, caffeine, or other pain relievers. Avoid Fiorinal with Codeine if you have a bleeding disorder, severe liver damage, nasal polyps, asthma due to aspirin or NSAIDs such as ibuprofen, edema, peptic ulcer, or porphyria.
- Do not take Fiorinal with Codeine if you must drive or operate dangerous machinery.
- Avoid taking this medication if you are pregnant or breast-feeding.

POSSIBLE INTERACTIONS
Alcohol: avoid alcohol while taking this medication.
Anticoagulants, antidiabetic drugs, insulin, mercaptopurine, methotrexate, NSAIDs: increased side effects of these drugs.
Antihistamines, opioid analgesics, sedatives and hypnotics, tranquilizers: increased sedative effects of these drugs.
Antigout drugs (probenecid, sulfinpyrazone): decreased effectiveness of these drugs.
MAO inhibitors: may cause drowsiness, dizziness, headache, or agitation.

TARGET AILMENTS
Tension headaches

SIDE EFFECTS

NOT SERIOUS
- Abdominal pain
- Dizziness; lightheadedness
- Drowsiness; nausea

CALL YOUR DOCTOR IF THESE EFFECTS PERSIST.

SERIOUS
- Confusion; coma
- Low blood pressure; shock
- Slow or labored breathing
- Gastric bleeding

CALL YOUR DOCTOR IMMEDIATLEY.

FLAXSEED

LATIN NAME
Linum usitatissimum

F

VITAL STATISTICS

GENERAL DESCRIPTION

Flaxseed, also known as linseed, is one of many herbs that contain mucilage, a substance composed mainly of sugar that builds up on the cell wall of the plant. When mixed with water, mucilage forms into a paste or gel, which can serve as a soothing emollient or poultice. This bulking agent also accounts for the herb's laxative effect. Although flaxseed is best known for its laxative benefits, it is also helpful for clearing mucus from the lungs, soothing sore throats and coughs, and cleansing the urinary tract, kidneys, and bladder. For a laxative, the seeds can be taken whole in water, hot cereal, or applesauce. A decoction is helpful for clearing mucus from bronchial tubes and may help relieve coughs and heal urinary infections.

PREPARATIONS

Over the counter:
Available in health food stores as seeds, in a liquid extract, or as an oil in soft gel capsules.

At home:

DECOCTION: Add 1 tbsp flaxseed to 1 qt water. Simmer partly covered until ½ qt remains. Strain; take in the morning or before bed for constipation.

POULTICE: For boils and other inflammations, make a paste by mixing the seeds, ground up or softened by cooking in hot water, with hot water.

COMBINATIONS: To treat burns, flaxseed can be combined with slippery elm powder in a poultice.

Consult a qualified practitioner for the dosage appropriate for you and the specific condition being treated.

PRECAUTIONS

☠ *WARNING*

The oil from flaxseed, called linseed oil, is often used in paint products. Be sure to use only oil that is prepared for human consumption.

Those with digestive complaints should consult a doctor before using flaxseed for medicinal purposes. Large quantities ingested at one time can cause poisoning. Immature seeds should be avoided.

POSSIBLE INTERACTIONS

Combining flaxseed with other herbs may necessitate a lower dosage.

TARGET AILMENTS

Take seeds internally for:

Constipation
Digestive disorders
Gallbladder problems

Take oil internally for:

Inflammation
Skin conditions
Arthritis

Apply externally for:

Burns
Boils

SIDE EFFECTS

NONE EXPECTED

Fluconazole

Vital Statistics

DRUG CLASS
Antifungal Drugs

BRAND NAME
Diflucan

GENERAL DESCRIPTION
Fluconazole is an orally administered antifungal drug that inhibits the growth of some types of fungal organisms and can even destroy them. It is used to treat yeast infections of the mouth, throat, esophagus, urinary tract, and vagina; systemic yeast infections; and cryptococcal meningitis. For more information, see Antifungal Drugs and Vaginal Antifungal Drugs. For visual characteristics of the brand-name drug Diflucan, see the Color Guide to Prescription Drugs and Herbs.

Precautions

WARNING
Dangerous adverse reactions to fluconazole include liver damage, anaphylaxis, and severe rash; seek emergency treatment.

Do not take fluconazole if you are allergic to it or have active liver disease.

SPECIAL INFORMATION
- Before you take fluconazole, tell your doctor if you have impaired kidneys or liver, allergies to any antifungal drugs, a history of alcoholism, or low blood potassium levels.
- It is important to take the full prescribed course of this drug. Do not stop taking it without talking to your doctor. If you are undergoing long-term treatment with this drug, be sure to contact your doctor for periodic evaluations and monitoring.
- Avoid this drug if you are pregnant or breast-feeding.

POSSIBLE INTERACTIONS
Antidiabetic drugs (oral), cyclosporine, phenytoin, theophylline, warfarin, zidovudine: increased effects of these drugs.
Astemizole, loratadine, terfenadine: potential for increased effects of these drugs.
Contraceptives, oral: decreased effectiveness of oral contraceptives in some people.
Hydrochlorothiazide: increased levels of fluconazole, loss of potassium.
See Ketoconazole for additional interactions.

TARGET AILMENTS
Yeast infections

SIDE EFFECTS

NOT SERIOUS
- Stomach pain, vomiting, diarrhea, or loss of appetite
- Headache or dizziness
- Mild itching or skin rash
- Hair loss (with high doses)

CALL YOUR DOCTOR IF THESE EFFECTS PERSIST.

SERIOUS
- Anaphylactic reaction (rash, difficulty breathing)
- Unusual bruising or bleeding
- Seizures (rare)
- Jaundice, dark urine, or abdominal pain
- Fever, chills, and sore throat

SEEK EMERGENCY TREATMENT.

FLUORIDE

VITAL STATISTICS

GENERAL DESCRIPTION

Fluoride, a natural form of the element fluorine, is required for healthy teeth and bones. It helps form the tough enamel that protects teeth from decay and cavities, and increases bone strength and stability. Since the 1950s, many U.S. cities have added fluoride to municipal drinking water at a ratio of about 1 part per million (ppm), or 1 mg per liter. Many believe that this practice is responsible for the 40 to 70 percent reduction in tooth decay that dentists have since observed. Fluoride's decay-reducing effects are strongest if children are exposed to the element while their teeth are forming. Fluoride toothpaste is helpful, but it is not nearly as effective as regularly ingested fluoride.

EMDR

Adults: 1.5 mg to 4 mg

NATURAL SOURCES

Fluoridated water provides most individuals with at least 1 mg of fluoride daily; other dietary sources are dried seaweed, seafood—especially sardines and salmon—cheese, meat, and tea.

PRECAUTIONS

SPECIAL INFORMATION

Nursing babies and children who do not regularly drink fluoridated water should be given supplements, but only as prescribed by a dentist or doctor, because excess fluoride can have adverse effects: At levels of 2 ppm to 8 ppm, the teeth may soften and discolor; at over 8 ppm, fluoride toxicity can depress growth, harden ligaments and tendons, make bones brittle, and induce degeneration of major body systems; 50 ppm may cause fatal poisoning. The low fluoride levels in fluoridated drinking water, however, pose no harmful effects to health.

TARGET AILMENTS
Osteoporosis
Tooth decay

SIDE EFFECTS

NONE EXPECTED

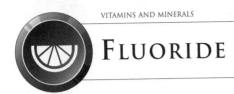

FLUOROQUINOLONES

VITAL STATISTICS

DRUG CLASS
Antibiotics

GENERIC NAMES
ciprofloxacin, ofloxacin

GENERAL DESCRIPTION
Introduced in the 1980s, fluoroquinolones are broad-spectrum antibiotics. The drugs, which belong to a group known as quinolones, work by inhibiting the ability of bacteria to make DNA, thereby preventing the organisms' growth and reproduction. Because they enter into many parts of the body and are effective against a wide range of organisms, fluoroquinolones have been used to treat many kinds of infections, including those of the bones, joints, skin, gastrointestinal tract, respiratory tract, and urinary tract, as well as infections that are sexually transmitted. For more information about specific fluoroquinolones, see the entries for Cipro, a brand of the generic drug ciprofloxacin, and for ofloxacin.

PRECAUTIONS

SPECIAL INFORMATION

- A rare condition known as pseudomembranous colitis may occur during or after the use of fluoroquinolones. Call your doctor at once if you experience abdominal or stomach cramps, severe pain and bloating, watery and severe diarrhea (may be bloody); fever, increased thirst; nausea or vomiting; fatigue or weakness; or unusual weight loss. These symptoms may occur at any time while you are using fluoroquinolones, or they may strike weeks after you have stopped taking the drug.
- Antibiotics kill not only harmful bacteria but also "good" bacteria that keep unwanted fungi and intestinal organisms in check. Eating yogurt containing *Lactobacillus acidophilus* culture or taking acidophilus tablets may help restore the body's normal bacteria.
- Prolonged use of any antibiotic drug can lead to fungal infections, including candidiasis, or to bacterial infections such as pseudomembranous colitis.
- Pregnant and nursing women should not take fluoroquinolones because these drugs can cause arthropathy (abnormal development of joints) in the fetus and infant.
- Except in very limited cases, children and adolescents under the age of 18 should not use fluoroquinolones because of the risk of arthropathy. Some researchers say these drugs may be safe for use by adolescents who have completed their skeletal growth.
- Fluoroquinolones may cause sensitivity to the sun or to sunlamps. Limit your exposure while on these medications.
- Take the full course of your prescription, even if you feel better before you've taken all the medication.

CONTINUED

FLUOROQUINOLONES

F

POSSIBLE INTERACTIONS

Antacids, didanosine (antiviral), ferrous sulfate, laxatives containing magnesium, sucralfate (antiulcer), zinc: reduced fluoroquinolone effect. (See Cipro and Ofloxacin for specific instructions on timing of these medications.)

Cimetidine (antiulcer) and probenecid (antigout): decreased elimination of fluoroquinolones, heightening risk of adverse effects and toxicity (especially with ofloxacin).

Warfarin (anticoagulant): increased anticoagulant effect.

TARGET AILMENTS
Bronchitis (bacterial exacerbations)
Gonorrhea
Pneumonia (bacterial)
Otitis media
Sinusitis
Prostatitis (bacterial)
Infections of the skin and soft tissue
Urinary tract infections; pelvic inflammatory disease (PID)
Traveler's diarrhea

SIDE EFFECTS

NOT SERIOUS

- Mild central nervous system effects, including dizziness, lightheadedness, drowsiness, headache, nervousness, and insomnia
- Minor gastrointestinal problems such as pain or discomfort, diarrhea, nausea, and vomiting
- Photosensitivity (rare)

CALL YOUR DOCTOR IF THESE SYMPTOMS PERSIST OR BECOME BOTHERSOME.

SERIOUS

- Central nervous system effects, including agitation, confusion, hallucinations, tremors, and psychosis
- Allergic reactions (skin rash, itching or redness; swelling of face or neck; shortness of breath)
- Fever or small ulcers on skin
- Bloody or cloudy urine
- Swelling of feet or legs
- Stevens-Johnson syndrome (fever, skin blisters, or blisters and open sores on mucous membranes and genitals; weakness; joint pain)

CALL YOUR DOCTOR IMMEDIATELY IF YOU HAVE THESE REACTIONS.

FLUOXETINE

VITAL STATISTICS

DRUG CLASS
Antidepressants [Selective Serotonin Reuptake Inhibitors (SSRIs)]

BRAND NAME
Prozac

OTHER DRUGS IN THIS SUBCLASS
paroxetine, sertraline

GENERAL DESCRIPTION
Fluoxetine, a well-known antidepressant drug, is prescribed for the control of a wide range of depressive illnesses. It is also used to treat alcohol dependence and obsessive-compulsive disorder.

Fluoxetine belongs to a subclass of antidepressants known as selective serotonin reuptake inhibitors (SSRIs). It works by enhancing the action of the neurotransmitter serotonin in the brain. See Antidepressants for information on side effects and possible drug interactions.

TARGET AILMENTS

Major depression

Obsessive-compulsive disorder

SIDE EFFECTS

SEE ANTIDEPRESSANTS.

PRECAUTIONS

SPECIAL INFORMATION
- Although fluoxetine benefits many of those who take it, a greater percentage of people experience side effects with this drug than with other antidepressants. If you have any questions about possible side effects, discuss them with your doctor.
- Rarely, fluoxetine can trigger manic attacks; this side effect may be more common in individuals with manic-depressive (bipolar) disorder. Be sure to tell your doctor if you have a history of manic-depression.
- Fluoxetine may exacerbate suicidal tendencies in some individuals. Be sure to tell your healthcare provider if you have ever had thoughts of suicide or believe you may be susceptible to such thoughts.
- This drug may cause drowsiness. When taking fluoxetine, use care while driving, operating machinery, or performing tasks that require mental alertness.
- Fluoxetine can affect blood sugar levels; dosage adjustment in oral antidiabetic medication or insulin may be required.
- If you are pregnant, nursing, or planning a pregnancy, check with your doctor before taking fluoxetine.
- The full effects of this drug may not occur for several weeks.
- The severity of any side effects may decrease with time (after two weeks) or with lowered dosages. If you have any questions about potential side effects, discuss them with your doctor.

Rx FLURBIPROFEN

VITAL STATISTICS

DRUG CLASS
Analgesics [Nonsteroidal Anti-Inflammatory Drugs (NSAIDs)]

BRAND NAME
Ansaid

OTHER DRUGS IN THIS SUBCLASS
diclofenac, etodolac, ibuprofen, ketoprofen, ketorolac, nabumetone, naproxen, oxaprozin

GENERAL DESCRIPTION
Flurbiprofen is an NSAID, a type of pain reliever that acts at the site of the pain. Because it reduces inflammation, this drug is useful for acute or long-term relief of the symptoms of rheumatoid arthritis and osteoarthritis. It may be used by people who cannot take aspirin, or when aspirin or acetaminophen is not effective. For further information, see Nonsteroidal Anti-Inflammatory Drugs (NSAIDs).

PRECAUTIONS

SPECIAL INFORMATION

- This drug may cause gastrointestinal bleeding and ulceration of the stomach, especially in the elderly.
- Do not use flurbiprofen if you are allergic to NSAIDs or to aspirin. It may cause bronchoconstriction or anaphylaxis in aspirin-sensitive asthmatics.
- Avoid this drug or consult your doctor before using it if you have asthma, peptic ulcer, enteritis (intestinal inflammation), high blood pressure, bleeding problems, or impaired liver or kidney function.
- Flurbiprofen is not recommended for use during pregnancy or by nursing mothers.

TARGET AILMENTS

Inflammation, especially related to osteoarthritis and rheumatoid arthritis

Pain, especially from inflammation, dental and other surgeries, menstruation, migraines

SIDE EFFECTS

NOT SERIOUS

- Dizziness
- Drowsiness
- Headache
- Abdominal pain or cramps
- Constipation or diarrhea
- Indigestion or nausea

CONSULT YOUR DOCTOR IF THESE SYMPTOMS PERSIST.

SERIOUS

- Anaphylactic reaction (hives, rash, intense itching, and trouble breathing)

SEEK EMERGENCY HELP.

- Vision changes or ringing in the ears
- Fluid retention
- Black or tarry stools
- Blood in urine
- Jaundice

DISCONTINUE USE AND CALL YOUR DOCTOR IMMEDIATELY.

FLUTICASONE

VITAL STATISTICS

DRUG CLASS
Corticosteroids

BRAND NAME
Flonase

OTHER DRUGS IN THIS CLASS
beclomethasone, betamethasone, hydrocortisone, methylprednisolone, mometasone furoate, prednisone, triamcinolone

GENERAL DESCRIPTION
Fluticasone is a corticosteroid drug—a synthetic version of a hormone produced by the adrenal glands. It is a relatively new and more potent type of corticosteroid. Although its mechanism of action is not completely known, the principal action of fluticasone is to reduce inflammation. The drug comes in the form of a nasal spray, an inhalant, and a topical cream or ointment, with different uses and different target ailments for each.

The nasal spray is used for inflammation of the nose (rhinitis) caused by either seasonal or perennial allergy. Many physicians consider it appropriate to use nasal corticosteroids such as fluticasone only when other treatments, primarily decongestants and antihistamines, have been unsuccessful or have produced serious side effects. The effect of this drug is not immediate but may take as long as 12 hours to appear after the initial treatment, and the maximal benefit may not be achieved for several days. It has not been shown to be effective in treating nonallergic rhinitis.

The topical form of fluticasone is helpful in treating various skin problems, including eczema, sunburn, and lupus. It is not used for skin conditions caused by fungi, for viruses such as herpes, or for tuberculosis.

The inhalant form is used in the treatment of chronic asthma, for which it reduces symptoms and improves lung function. Over time, its use may allow concomitant oral corticosteroid treatment to be decreased or eliminated. However, it is not intended to be used for the symptoms of acute asthma, for which quick bronchodilation is needed. For more information about this class of drugs, see Corticosteroids.

PRECAUTIONS

WARNING
Do not take fluticasone if you have ever had an allergic reaction to this drug in any form or to other steroid medications.

Tell your doctor if you are exposed to chickenpox or measles while taking this drug. Use of systemic corticosteroids can result in a serious or even fatal course of those illnesses, and nasal spray or topical fluticasone may reduce your body's ability to fight viruses. Try to avoid such exposure as much as possible.

TARGET AILMENTS
Allergic rhinitis (nasal spray)
Skin inflammations (topical form)
Asthma (inhalant form)

F

CONTINUED

FLUTICASONE

F

SPECIAL INFORMATION

- Use fluticasone nasal spray with caution if you have active or inactive tuberculosis, an untreated infection (fungal, bacterial, or viral), or ocular herpes simplex. Also discuss with your doctor the risks of using the drug if you have glaucoma.
- Do not use fluticasone nasal spray if you have had nasal septal ulcer or recent nasal surgery or trauma to the nose. Wait until the condition has healed.
- Tell your doctor if you take any other prescription or over-the-counter medications, particularly prednisone.
- Tell your doctor if you plan to become pregnant. Although specific information about the effect of this drug on the fetus is not available, it is known that systemic corticosteroids cross the placenta and have caused damage to the fetus.
- Although it is unknown whether this drug passes into breast milk, watch the infant closely and either stop taking the drug or stop nursing if you notice any effects.
- If you are taking fluticasone nasal spray on a long-term basis, consult your doctor for possible dosage adjustment. Your doctor may want to assess your adrenal gland function and examine your ears, nose, and throat periodically.
- Because fluticasone may cause dizziness, restrict driving and other hazardous activities until you know how it will affect you.
- Do not stop taking this drug abruptly; consult your doctor before discontinuing it.
- Intranasal fluticasone has not been established to be safe and effective for children under the age of 12. Use in children could cause suppression of the adrenal glands and retardation of growth.
- If you miss a dose of this medication, either take it as soon as you remember or, if it is almost time for the next one, skip it. Do not take a double dose.
- Be cautious about taking this drug if you are already taking a systemic corticosteroid.

POSSIBLE INTERACTIONS

Systemic steroids (for example, prednisone): increased risk of suppression of adrenal gland function.

SIDE EFFECTS

NOT SERIOUS

- Contact dermatitis
- Irritation of nasal membrane
- Dizziness; headache
- Nausea; vomiting; unpleasant taste in mouth
- Nosebleed; burning sensation in nose
- Cough; runny nose

THESE ARE POSSIBLE EFFECTS OF FLUTICASONE NASAL SPRAY. CALL YOUR DOCTOR IF THEY PERSIST.

SERIOUS

- Severe allergic reaction such as hives
- Cushing's syndrome
- Yeast infection in the nose
- Wheezing
- Nasal septum perforation
- Eye symptoms such as increased intraocular pressure (rare)

CALL YOUR DOCTOR NOW IF YOU NOTICE THESE EFFECTS WHILE USING FLUTICASONE NASAL SPRAY.

Rx FLUVASTATIN

VITAL STATISTICS

DRUG CLASS
Cholesterol-Reducing Drugs

BRAND NAME
Lescol

OTHER DRUGS IN THIS CLASS
cholestyramine, colestipol, gemfibrozil, lovastatin, niacin, pravastatin, simvastatin

GENERAL DESCRIPTION
Fluvastatin lowers blood cholesterol levels by inhibiting a liver enzyme that is essential to the body's production of cholesterol. The drug is used when a low-fat, low-cholesterol diet and weight loss have failed to reduce blood cholesterol sufficiently, and it is considered an adjunct to diet and exercise. Fluvastatin is also used to slow the advance of atherosclerosis. For visual characteristics, see the Color Guide to Prescription Drugs and Herbs.

PRECAUTIONS

SPECIAL INFORMATION
- Inform your doctor before you take fluvastatin if you are taking any drugs that suppress the immune system, if you are a heavy drinker, if you have low blood pressure, hormone abnormalities, liver or kidney disease, a seizure disorder, or an active infection, or if you have recently been in a major accident.
- Don't stop taking this drug without consulting your doctor. The dose may need to be reduced gradually, and dosages of other drugs you are taking may need to be adjusted.
- Do not take this drug if you are pregnant or nursing a baby.

POSSIBLE INTERACTIONS
Anticoagulants: increased risk of bleeding.
Cholestyramine, colestipol, rifampin: decreased effect of fluvastatin.
Cimetidine, ranitidine, omeprazole: increased fluvastatin effect.
Cyclosporine, erythromycins, gemfibrozil, immunosuppressants, niacin: increased risk of kidney and heart problems; increased risk of muscle inflammation.

F

TARGET AILMENTS
High cholesterol

Atherosclerosis

SIDE EFFECTS

NOT SERIOUS
- Constipation; nausea
- Headache; tiredness; weakness
- Dizziness
- Skin rash
- Impotence (rare)
- Insomnia (rare)

CALL YOUR DOCTOR IF THESE EFFECTS PERSIST.

SERIOUS
- Aching muscles
- Fever
- Blurred vision

CALL YOUR DOCTOR IMMEDIATELY.

Folic Acid (Vitamin B9)

F

Vital Statistics

OTHER NAMES

vitamin B9, folacin, folate

GENERAL DESCRIPTION

Healthy hair, skin, nails, nerves, mucous membranes, and blood all depend on folic acid—sometimes called vitamin B9, folacin, or folate. A critical component of RNA and DNA—the genetic material that controls the growth and repair of all cells—folic acid supports immune function and may help deter atherosclerosis as well as some cancers of the mucous membranes.

Extreme vitamin B9 deficiency may cause megaloblastic anemia, a disease characterized by red blood cells that are too few in number and malformed. Symptoms include headache; pallor; fatigue; loss of appetite; insomnia; diarrhea; and a red, inflamed tongue. Those who are most susceptible to folic acid deficiency include alcoholics, people with gastrointestinal diseases, adolescents who subsist mainly on junk food, women taking oral contraceptives, and pregnant women who are not taking supplements.

RDA

Men: 200 mcg
Women: 180 mcg
Women of childbearing age: 400 mcg

NATURAL SOURCES

Sources of folic acid include liver, kidneys, avocados, beans, beets, celery, eggs, fish, green leafy vegetables, nuts, seeds, peas, orange juice, and fortified breakfast cereals.

Precautions

WARNING

High doses of folic acid are not toxic but may mask the symptoms of vitamin B12 deficiency. Therefore, it's best to increase folic acid intake through diet or a multivitamin that contains low-dose folic acid, rather than through individual supplements, which have to be prescribed by a doctor.

SPECIAL INFORMATION

A healthy diet should provide adequate folic acid, but the need increases during pregnancy, with injury, with some diseases—especially cancer—and with long-term use of drugs such as aspirin and oral contraceptives. Supplements taken during pregnancy may help deter the birth defects spina bifida and cleft palate. For this reason, experts now recommend that all women of childbearing age consume 400 mcg daily.

TARGET AILMENTS
Cancer
Heart disease
Immune problems
Skin problems

SIDE EFFECTS

None expected

Fosinopril

Vital Statistics

DRUG CLASS
Angiotensin-Converting Enzyme (ACE) Inhibitors

BRAND NAME
Monopril

OTHER DRUGS IN THIS CLASS
benazepril, captopril, enalapril, lisinopril, quinapril, ramipril

GENERAL DESCRIPTION
Like other ACE inhibitors, fosinopril lowers blood pressure by apparently blocking an enzyme that is essential for the production of a substance that causes blood vessels to constrict. See Angiotensin-Converting Enzyme (ACE) Inhibitors for more information, including possible drug interactions. For visual characteristics, see the Color Guide to Prescription Drugs and Herbs.

Precautions

WARNING
Do not take this drug if you are pregnant or breast-feeding, are allergic to any ACE inhibitor, or have a high blood potassium level.

While taking fosinopril, do not use salt substitutes, which may contain potassium, without your doctor's approval.

SPECIAL INFORMATION
- Tell your doctor if you have any liver or kidney disease before taking this drug. You may need a lower-than-usual dose.
- Before taking this drug, tell your doctor if you have any form of heart disease, scleroderma or lupus, diabetes, a blood cell or bone marrow disorder, or cerebral artery disease; if you are planning a pregnancy or planning to have surgery under general anesthesia in the near future; or if you are taking any other antihypertensive drugs, diuretics, potassium supplements, or nitrates.

F

TARGET AILMENTS

High blood pressure

SIDE EFFECTS

NOT SERIOUS
- Drowsiness or fatigue; loss of taste; cough; indigestion; mood changes; sleep disturbances

SERIOUS
- Sore throat; nausea or diarrhea; unexpected weight gain; dizziness; fever; jaundice; reduced urine output or inability to urinate

TELL YOUR DOCTOR PROMPTLY IF YOU NOTICE THESE SYMPTOMS.

- Swelling of face, lips, tongue, or larynx
- Skin rash or itching
- Irregular heartbeat
- Chest pain
- Difficulty swallowing
- Difficulty breathing

DISCONTINUE USE AND SEEK EMERGENCY TREATMENT.

FRANKINCENSE

LATIN NAME
Boswellia carteri

F

VITAL STATISTICS

GENERAL DESCRIPTION

Frankincense, an aromatic oil distilled from tree resin, has been used in religious rituals since ancient times. Native to Africa and the Middle East, the trees that produce the resin have white or pink flowers and are related to the trees that produce the essential oil myrrh.

To collect the resin, the tree is gashed and allowed to exude its sap. The sap hardens and falls to the ground as teardrop-shaped balls. Essential oil of frankincense can be colorless to pale yellow, and it has a balsamic fragrance with lemon and camphor undertones.

Today, frankincense is valued as a cell regenerator and for its sedative and antiseptic properties. It also acts as an anti-inflammatory, astringent, digestive aid, and expectorant.

PREPARATIONS

Commercial frankincense is available as an essential oil and, for herbal use, as a powder or in solid blocks.

To relieve respiratory congestion, use as an inhalation or apply the oil as a lotion (see recipe below) to the area of the face over the sinuses, to the temples, to the chest, and to the ganglia behind the ears when sore.

Inhalation: Put 6 drops of oil in a bowl of hot water. Lean over the bowl and cover it and your head with a towel to capture the vapors. Breathe deeply for 7 to 10 minutes.

Lotion: Mix 6 drops of frankincense oil and 2 drops of wheat-germ oil with 2 tsp of soy oil. Apply a few times a day to the affected areas. For use in the bath, add 10 drops essential oil to the bathwater.

TARGET AILMENTS

- Asthma
- Bronchitis
- Coughing
- Anxiety and stress
- Colds and flu
- Cystitis
- Menstrual symptoms
- Gout
- Dermatitis; dry skin
- Stretch marks
- Scars and wrinkles

SIDE EFFECTS

NONE EXPECTED. FRANKINCENSE IS NONTOXIC, NONIRRITATING, AND NONSENSITIZING.

Fritillaria and Loquat Syrup

Vital Statistics

PINYIN NAME
Chuan Bei Pi Pa Gao

ALSO SOLD AS
Natural Herb Loquat Flavored Syrup
Similar mixtures: Fritillary and Loquat Leaf Mixture; *Chuan Bei Pi Pa Tang Jiang*

GENERAL DESCRIPTION
Fritillaria and Loquat Syrup, considered a good general cough syrup, is also used to treat a dry cough, smoker's cough, or coughing associated with asthma. The herbs in this mixture are said to help supress coughing and eliminate phlegm.

Chinese medicine takes a holistic approach to healthcare, fashioning remedies to treat the entire being as well as the specific parts or areas. Precise combinations of herbs are used to prevent and combat disease, which is thought to arise from disturbances in the flow of a bodily energy called chi or qi (pronounced "chee") and blood, or from a lack of balance in the complementary states of yin and yang. A patent formula, Fritillaria and Loquat Syrup is made by using a standardized combination of herbs and method of preparation.

INGREDIENTS
loquat leaf, fritillaria, adenophora, schisandra, dry mandarin orange peel, balloonflower, pinellia, mint, coltsfoot, bitter almond, honey

PREPARATIONS
This formula is sold in syrup form at many Chinese pharmacies and Oriental grocery stores.

TARGET AILMENTS

- Dry cough
- Cough associated with asthma
- Smoker's cough

SIDE EFFECTS
None expected

FUROSEMIDE

F

VITAL STATISTICS

DRUG CLASS
Diuretics

BRAND NAME
Lasix Oral

OTHER DRUGS IN THIS CLASS
amiloride, bumetanide, hydrochlorothiazide, indapamide, potassium chloride (adjunct therapy), spironolactone, triamterene

GENERAL DESCRIPTION
The fast-acting and powerful diuretic furosemide has been prescribed since 1964 to treat high blood pressure (hypertension) and excess fluid retention. The drug acts by increasing urine production, thereby removing water from the body and reducing swelling and blood volume. In the process, however, salts containing sodium, potassium, calcium, and other vital minerals are also eliminated, sometimes leading to muscle cramps and serious cardiovascular side effects. For more information, see Diuretics. For visual characteristics, see the Color Guide to Prescription Drugs and Herbs.

PRECAUTIONS

SPECIAL INFORMATION
- While taking this medicine you may become more photosensitive, meaning your skin will burn more readily when exposed to sunlight. To protect your skin, use a sunblocking lotion when outside and avoid prolonged exposure to the sun or sunlamps.
- Taking this drug in hot weather or while engaged in heavy exertion can cause a dangerous loss of fluids or minerals. Watch for signs of dehydration (fatigue, dizziness, headache, nausea).
- If you are taking furosemide, your doctor will closely monitor your potassium levels to prevent heart-rhythm problems. You may be given a potassium supplement (such as potassium chloride).

TARGET AILMENTS

General edema (swelling caused by water retention)

Edema associated with various medical conditions, including congestive heart failure and cirrhosis of the liver

High blood pressure (hypertension)

FUROSEMIDE

POSSIBLE INTERACTIONS

Alcohol: increased action of furosemide.

Aminoglycoside antibiotics, including streptomycin, kanamycin, neomycin, gentamicin: increased risk of ototoxicity, possibly resulting in hearing loss, ringing in the ears, and vertigo. Avoid combining these drugs except in emergency situations.

Digitalis and other heart drugs: although furosemide is sometimes taken with heart medications, such combinations can increase the risk of potassium loss and additional heart-rhythm problems. Your doctor will closely monitor your progress.

Lithium: furosemide may increase the risk of lithium toxicity.

Nonsteroidal anti-inflammatory drugs (NSAIDs), especially indomethacin: reduced effectiveness of furosemide.

Oral antidiabetic drugs, insulin: in rare cases, furosemide may interfere with these medicines or raise blood glucose levels.

Other blood pressure drugs, including angiotensin-converting enzyme (ACE) inhibitors: although diuretics are often taken with medications to lower blood pressure, caution should be exercised to ensure that blood pressure does not go too low.

SIDE EFFECTS

NOT SERIOUS

- Headache
- Blurred vision
- Diarrhea
- Dizziness or lightheadedness when getting up (orthostatic hypotension)
- Increased risk of sunburn

LET YOUR DOCTOR KNOW IF THESE SYMPTOMS CONTINUE OR BECOME TROUBLESOME.

SERIOUS

- Nausea or vomiting
- Fatigue or weakness
- Irregular or weak pulse
- Increased thirst
- Ringing in ears and hearing loss
- Dry mouth
- Muscle pain or cramps
- Mood changes
- Mental confusion
- Bleeding in urine or stools
- Unusual bruising
- Skin rash

TELL YOUR DOCTOR IMMEDIATELY IF YOU EXPERIENCE THESE SYMPTOMS. YOU MAY BE ADVISED TO LOWER YOUR DOSAGE AND INCREASE YOUR INTAKE OF FLUIDS AND MINERALS.

Gan Mao Ling

Vital Statistics

ENGLISH NAME
Common Cold Effective Remedy

ALSO SOLD AS
Su Xiao Ganmaoling

GENERAL DESCRIPTION
The Chinese patent formula *Gan Mao Ling* is used to treat the common cold or the flu if it is accompanied by any of the following symptoms: chills, high fever, swollen glands in the neck, sore throat, and stiff and achy upper back and neck. One of the actions of this formula is to help the body rid itself of the cold or influenza virus.

Chinese medicine takes a holistic approach to healthcare, fashioning remedies to treat the entire being as well as the specific parts or areas. Precise combinations of herbs are used to prevent and combat disease, which is thought to arise from disturbances in the flow of a bodily energy called chi (pronounced "chee") and blood, or from a lack of balance in the complementary states of yin and yang. *Gan Mao Ling* is made by using a standardized combination of herbs and method of preparation.

INGREDIENTS
ilex, evodia, dyer's woad root, chrysanthemum, vitex, honeysuckle flower, menthol crystal

PREPARATIONS
This formula is sold in pill form at many Chinese pharmacies and Oriental grocery stores.

TARGET AILMENTS

- Cold or flu
- Flu with body aches
- Swollen glands in throat (with flulike symptoms)
- High fever, with or without chills

SIDE EFFECTS
None expected

GANODERMA

LATIN NAME
Ganoderma lucidum

VITAL STATISTICS

GENERAL DESCRIPTION
A variety of mushroom also known as *ling zhi* in China and as *reishi* in the West, ganoderma grows in mountainous regions in China. It is a rare fungus that Chinese practitioners value highly for its multiple uses. Practitioners have traditionally used it to treat psychological disturbances as well as respiratory complaints and ulcers. In traditional Chinese medicine, where herbs are classified according to heating and cooling properties, ganoderma is categorized as neutral.

Ganoderma has also been prescribed to boost patients' immune systems. It appears to help the body to resist a wide range of physical, biological, and environmental stresses. This herb has also proved useful in conjunction with conventional medical treatment of AIDS and cancer. And in clinical studies, ganoderma seems to have reduced blood pressure in humans and animals.

Chinese medicine takes a holistic approach to healthcare, fashioning remedies to treat the entire being as well as the specific parts or areas. Single herbs may be used alone or in combination with other herbs to prevent and combat disease, which is thought to arise from disturbances in the flow of a bodily energy called chi (pronounced "chee") and blood, or from a lack of balance in the complementary states of yin and yang.

PREPARATIONS
Ganoderma can be found in bulk at Chinese pharmacies, Asian markets, and some Western health food stores (under the name *reishi*). It is also possible to obtain it in pill or tablet form, and in alcohol extracts. Consult a Chinese medicine practitioner for information on dosages. Unlike most other Chinese herbs, ganoderma is not traditionally combined with other substances.

TARGET AILMENTS

Take internally for:

- Nervousness
- Insomnia
- Dizziness
- Asthma
- Allergy-related chronic bronchitis
- Weakened immune system
- Tumors
- Ulcers
- Poor blood circulation
- Mushroom poisoning

SIDE EFFECTS

NOT SERIOUS
- Dizziness
- Sore bones
- Itchy skin
- Increased bowel movements
- Hardened feces and pimple-like eruptions

STOP USING THE HERB IMMEDIATELY AND SEE YOUR DOCTOR.

G

GARDENIA

LATIN NAME
Gardeniae jasminoides

G

VITAL STATISTICS

GENERAL DESCRIPTION

In traditional Chinese medicine gardenia is classified as a cold herb. As such, gardenia fruit are used to treat "hot" conditions such as burning urination, jaundice, sores on the face, irritability, restlessness, delirious speech, and sudden and bright red bleeding. Mixed with egg white or vinegar, gardenia can be used topically to treat bruises and swelling due to trauma. Decoctions of gardenia given orally or injected in some animals were found to have a long-lasting effect on lowering blood pressure. Good-quality gardenia fruit are thin skinned, round, and reddish yellow in color.

Chinese medicine takes a holistic approach to healthcare, fashioning remedies to treat the entire being as well as the specific parts or areas. Single herbs may be used alone or in combination with other herbs to prevent and combat disease, which is thought to arise from disturbances in the flow of a bodily energy called chi (pronounced "chee") and blood, or from a lack of balance in the complementary states of yin and yang.

PREPARATIONS

Over the counter:

Dried gardenia fruit are available in Chinese pharmacies.

At home:

DECOCTION: Gardenia fruit are usually mixed with other herbs and cooked at a low simmer for 20 minutes. If used to stop bleeding, char the fruit first. If gardenia causes nausea, some practitioners suggest frying it first.

COMBINATIONS: Gardenia may be mixed with prepared soybeans for insomnia and irritability due to weakness. Mixed with biota leaves and Chinese foxglove, gardenia is used to stop vomiting blood and nosebleeds. Check with your practitioner for further information on combinations and dosages.

PRECAUTIONS

WARNING

Do not use if you have loose stools or loss of appetite due to weakness.

TARGET AILMENTS

Irritability; restlessness; insomnia; delirious speech

Painful urination; sores of the nose, eyes, or mouth; jaundice (damp heat conditions)

Nosebleeds, vomiting blood, blood in the urine or stool

SIDE EFFECTS

NOT SERIOUS

- Diarrhea or loose stools

GARLIC

LATIN NAME
Allium sativum

VITAL STATISTICS

GENERAL DESCRIPTION

Worn or carried as a protective talisman throughout the ages and valued as a pungent culinary spice, the garlic bulb has gained recognition as a medicinal remedy in Chinese and Western cultures. To release its therapeutic effects, it can be eaten either raw or cooked.

In China this perennial herb is prescribed for colds and coughs, as well as for intestinal and digestive disorders. Chinese herbalists also believe that garlic can be used externally as an antibiotic to relieve skin infections. In traditional Chinese medicine, garlic is characterized as acrid, bitter, and warm.

Chinese medicine takes a holistic approach to healthcare, fashioning remedies to treat the entire being as well as the specific parts or areas. Single herbs may be used alone or in combination with other herbs to prevent and combat disease, which is thought to arise from disturbances in the flow of a bodily energy called chi (pronounced "chee") and blood, or from a lack of balance in the complementary states of yin and yang.

PREPARATIONS

Over the counter:

Garlic is available as cloves and in tablet form.

At home:

NOSE DROPS: Combine 1 part crushed root with 10 parts water.

EXTERNAL TREATMENT: Garlic is combined with sesame oil and applied externally to treat ringworm of the scalp, pinworm, carbuncles, swelling, athlete's foot, arthritis, and rheumatism.

COMBINATIONS: A mix of garlic and sugar water is sometimes prescribed for digestive disorders, diarrhea, colds, coughs, food poisoning from shellfish, and conditions that require an enema.

PRECAUTIONS

SPECIAL INFORMATION

- Consult your practitioner before using garlic if you are pregnant.
- Garlic has a blood-clot-preventing agent. If you have a blood-clotting disorder, consult a herbalist or a licensed healthcare professional.
- Garlic is thought to function as an adjunct treatment for cardiovascular disease. Consult your practitioner before using it in this capacity.

TARGET AILMENTS

Take internally for:

Digestive disorders; diarrhea; food poisoning from shellfish; conditions that require an enema; colds; coughs; rheumatoid arthritis

Apply externally for:

Hookworm; roundworm; ringworm of the scalp; carbuncles; swelling; pinworm; athlete's foot

SIDE EFFECTS

NOT SERIOUS

PEOPLE ALLERGIC TO GARLIC MAY DEVELOP A RASH FROM TOUCHING OR EATING THE HERB.

GARLIC

LATIN NAME
Allium sativum

VITAL STATISTICS

GENERAL DESCRIPTION

Worn or carried as a protective talisman throughout the ages and valued as a pungent culinary spice, the garlic bulb has gained recognition as a medicinal remedy in Chinese and Western cultures. To release its therapeutic effects, it can be eaten either raw or cooked, Garlic's active ingredient is allicin, an amino acid derivative that is also responsible for the herb's pungent smell.

Western herbalists prescribe garlic for many of the same ailments as do their Chinese counterparts. It is also thought to strengthen the cardiovascular system by reducing cholesterol and lowering blood pressure. Although no conclusive evidence has been found, a string of Western studies suggest that incorporating garlic into the daily diet may lower the risk of heart disease. For visual characteristics of garlic, see the Color Guide to Prescription Drugs and Herbs.

G

PREPARATIONS

Over the counter:
Available as cloves and in tablet form.

At home:
TINCTURE: Combine 1 cup crushed cloves with 1 qt brandy. Shake daily for two weeks. Take up to 3 tbsp a day.
Consult a qualified practitioner for the dosage appropriate for you and the specific condition being treated.

PRECAUTIONS

SPECIAL INFORMATION

- Consult your practitioner before using garlic if you are pregnant.
- Garlic contains a blood-clot-preventing agent. If you have a blood-clotting disorder, consult an herbalist or a licensed healthcare professional.
- Garlic is thought to function as an adjunct treatment for cardiovascular disease. Consult your practitioner before using it in this capacity.

TARGET AILMENTS
Take internally for:
Colds; coughs; flu
High cholesterol
High blood pressure
Atherosclerosis
Digestive disorders
Bladder infection
Liver and gallbladder problems
Apply externally for:
Athlete's foot; ringworm
Minor skin infections

SIDE EFFECTS

NOT SERIOUS

PEOPLE ALLERGIC TO GARLIC MAY DEVELOP A RASH FROM TOUCHING OR EATING THE HERB.

GASTRODIA

LATIN NAME
Gastrodia elata

VITAL STATISTICS

GENERAL DESCRIPTION

The root of this member of the orchid family is prescribed by Chinese medicine practitioners for conditions that they ascribe to disorders of the liver, where, in Chinese tradition, the soul resides. A literal English translation would be "heavenly hemp." Look for a fat, solid, translucent yellowish white root, probably imported from China's Sichuan, Yunnan, or Guizhou provinces. Gastrodia is categorized in traditional Chinese medicine as a sweet and neutral herb.

Chinese medicine takes a holistic approach to healthcare, fashioning remedies to treat the entire being as well as the specific parts or areas. Single herbs may be used alone or in combination with other herbs to prevent and combat disease, which is thought to arise from disturbances in the flow of a bodily energy called chi (pronounced "chee") and blood, or from a lack of balance in the complementary states of yin and yang.

PREPARATIONS

Gastrodia is found in bulk or in tablets at Chinese pharmacies, Asian markets, and some Western health food stores.

COMBINATIONS: Mixed with gambir, skullcap, and achyranthes root, it is used for dizziness. Adding scorpion to that mixture creates a preparation for treating seizures. Herbalists prescribe a mix containing gastrodia, Asian ginseng, atractylodes (white), and silkworm for chronic childhood convulsions.

Check with your practitioner for further information on combinations and dosages.

PRECAUTIONS

SPECIAL INFORMATION

Preparations of the herb have halted seizures and inhibited the development of epilepsy-like symptoms in rabbits. Gastrodia, however, proved not as effective for this purpose as phenobarbital.

TARGET AILMENTS

Take internally for:

Headaches, including migraines

Dizziness

Childhood convulsions

Epilepsy

SIDE EFFECTS

NONE EXPECTED

GELSEMIUM

LATIN NAME
Gelsemium sempervirens

G

VITAL STATISTICS

GENERAL DESCRIPTION

Sometimes called yellow jasmine, gelsemium is not really part of the jasmine family but is related to the plants *Ignatia* and *Nux vomica.* A climbing vine with trumpetlike yellow flowers, it is common in the woods and coastal shoreline of the southern United States. Taken in large doses, gelsemium causes paralysis of the motor nerves, impairing physical and mental functions like vision, balance, thought, and movement; ultimately, poisoning causes convulsions and death. Homeopathic physicians prescribe dilute solutions of gelsemium for ailments that are accompanied by symptoms like those of gelsemium poisoning. In its homeopathic form, *Gelsemium* is prepared from the fresh root, which is chopped, soaked in alcohol, strained, and diluted to the desired, highly dilute potencies.

Like most homeopathic prescriptions, *Gelsemium* was developed as a remedy by observation of the reactions of healthy individuals to doses of various strengths. The mental, emotional, and physical changes induced by *Gelsemium* were then cataloged. When a patient exhibits a set of symptoms that matches the cataloged symptoms brought on by *Gelsemium,* the homeopathic practitioner then prescribes it in an extremely dilute form. It is presumed that in this dilute dosage, *Gelsemium* can counter symptoms that are similar to the ones it induces when it is at full strength. For more information on homeopathic medicine, see page 14.

PREPARATIONS

Gelsemium is available in various potencies, in both liquid and tablet form, from selected stores and pharmacies. Consult your homeopathic practitioner for further information.

PRECAUTIONS

SPECIAL INFORMATION

- When a remedy is administered, no one but the patient should touch the pills. If tablets are spilled, throw them away.
- The mouth should be clear of flavors 15 minutes before and after taking a remedy, and strong flavors and aromas, such as coffee, camphor, and heavily scented perfumes, should be avoided for the duration of treatment.

TARGET AILMENTS

Anxiety

Flu with aches, chills, and exhaustion

Headache, beginning from the back of the head and moving forward

Measles

Sore throat

Fever with chills that move up and down the spine, although the patient may not feel cold

SIDE EFFECTS

NONE EXPECTED

GEMFIBROZIL

VITAL STATISTICS

DRUG CLASS
Cholesterol-Reducing Drugs

BRAND NAME
Lopid

OTHER DRUGS IN THIS CLASS
cholestyramine, colestipol, fluvastatin, lovastatin, niacin, pravastatin, simvastatin

GENERAL DESCRIPTION
Introduced in 1976, gemfibrozil is used to lower cholesterol and triglyceride levels in the blood, thus reducing the risk of coronary artery disease. The drug seems to work by inhibiting production of triglycerides in the liver and accelerating removal of cholesterol from the body. For visual characteristics of gemfibrozil and the brand Lopid, see the Color Guide to Prescription Drugs and Herbs. For more information, see Cholesterol-Reducing Drugs.

PRECAUTIONS

SPECIAL INFORMATION
This drug is usually taken twice a day, 30 minutes before the morning and evening meals.

POSSIBLE INTERACTIONS
Anticoagulants (such as warfarin): increased blood-thinning effect.
Chenodiol and ursodiol: these two medications, prescribed to treat gallstones, have decreased effectiveness when taken with gemfibrozil.
Lovastatin: may lead to kidney failure when it is taken concurrently with gemfibrozil.

TARGET AILMENTS

The major types of cholesterol disorders, particularly those in which high levels of blood fats (cholesterol and triglycerides) have been linked to an increased risk of heart disease

SIDE EFFECTS

NOT SERIOUS

- Moderate increase in blood sugar levels
- Reduced libido in men

CALL YOUR DOCTOR IF THESE EFFECTS PERSIST OR BECOME BOTHERSOME.

SERIOUS

- Fever
- Chills
- Sore throat
- Low back and side pain
- Difficult or painful urination
- Doubled risk of gallstone formation with long-term use

CALL YOUR DOCTOR IMMEDIATELY.

GENTIAN

LATIN NAME
Gentiana lutea

VITAL STATISTICS

GENERAL DESCRIPTION
Distinguished by oval leaves and orange blooms, gentian is believed to act as a general tonic, relieving exhaustion and helping the body rebuild its natural defenses against illness. The root of this herb has been used in different cultures for about 3,000 years to treat digestive disorders and to stimulate the appetite. It was introduced to Western herbalists by Native Americans, who used the plant to alleviate back pains. Today, gentian is prescribed in Western countries primarily as a digestive aid. Because of its bitter properties, it stimulates the secretion of stomach acid and produces saliva. For this reason, contemporary herbalists frequently recommend ingesting this herb before or with large meals. Its most common form is as an ingredient in liqueurs, vermouths, and a variety of other bitter-tasting cocktails.

PREPARATIONS
Over the counter:
Gentian is available in bulk as dried roots, and in tincture.

At home:
TEA: Simmer covered 1 oz gentian root with 1 cup water for 15 to 20 minutes. Drink 15 to 30 minutes before eating, to aid digestion.
COMBINATIONS: Use with ginger and cardamom for digestive disorders.
Consult a qualified practitioner for the dosage appropriate for you and the specific condition being treated.

PRECAUTIONS

☠ ***WARNING***
Use only under the direction of a herbalist or healthcare professional if you are pregnant or have high blood pressure (hypertension) or chronic gastrointestinal conditions.

Use of this herb by children for more than seven to 10 days should be done in conjunction with a healthcare practitioner. Use low-strength preparations for children and for adults over 65. Do not give gentian to children under two years of age.

POSSIBLE INTERACTIONS
Combining gentian with other herbs may necessitate a lower dosage.

TARGET AILMENTS
Digestive disorders
Loss of appetite
Arthritis
Constipation

SIDE EFFECTS

NOT SERIOUS
- Upset stomach
- Nausea
- Vomiting

G

GENTIANA

LATIN NAME
Gentiana scabra

VITAL STATISTICS

GENERAL DESCRIPTION

Several varieties of this herb grow throughout China. *Gentiana scabra,* the most widely used, is a long, thick yellow root, described as cold by Chinese herbalists. They prescribe the herb primarily for disorders of the liver and organs in the pelvic area. Gentiana is believed to have an antibiotic effect; it is also thought to be toxic to malarial parasites. Gentiana tastes so bitter that herbalists use it as a standard for judging bitterness in plants.

Chinese medicine takes a holistic approach to healthcare, fashioning remedies to treat the entire being as well as the specific parts or areas. Single herbs may be used alone or in combination with other herbs to prevent and combat disease, which is thought to arise from disturbances in the flow of a bodily energy called chi (pronounced "chee") and blood, or from a lack of balance in the complementary states of yin and yang.

PREPARATIONS

You can find gentiana in bulk at Chinese pharmacies, Asian markets, and some Western health food stores. While the Chinese variety is not available in pills or tablets, the European root can be obtained in that form.

COMBINATIONS: Chinese herbalists prescribe a preparation that contains gentiana, sophora root, and plantago seeds for genital itching and vaginal discharge. A combination of gentiana with cattle gallstone and gambir is given for convulsions, especially when the symptoms appear in children.

Check with your practitioner for advice on other combinations and dosages.

PRECAUTIONS

WARNING

Chinese herbalists advise against the use of this root when diarrhea is among the symptoms.

TARGET AILMENTS

Use internally for:

- Hepatitis
- Jaundice and other liver disorders
- Sexually transmitted diseases
- Vaginal discharge
- Inflammation of the pelvis
- Pain or swelling in the genital area
- Convulsions

SIDE EFFECTS

NONE EXPECTED

G

GERANIUM

LATIN NAME
Pelargonium graveolens

G

VITAL STATISTICS

GENERAL DESCRIPTION

Only a few of the hundreds of species of the geranium, a popular garden plant, are cultivated for essential oils. One of these species, rose-scented geranium *(Pelargonium graveolens),* originated in South Africa and was introduced to Europe in the late 17th century. Research indicates that the oil of this plant was first used in aromatherapy in the mid-19th century.

Applied externally, geranium is an all-purpose healing agent. Believed to balance hormones, it may help relieve premenstrual syndrome. Geranium oil can help ease fatigue when massaged into the temples. It can also be used as an insect repellent. The aromatic oil is also used in perfumes, often as a substitute for the more expensive rose oil.

PREPARATIONS

Geranium essential oil is distilled from the upper part of the plant, leaves, and flowers.

For skin applications: Mix 15 drops geranium oil with 2 tbsp vegetable oil, nut oil, or aloe gel.

For baths: Add 5 to 10 drops to the water. For inhalation, use a diffuser to scent the air or sniff drops placed on a cloth.

For hemorrhoids: Mix 1 drop geranium oil with 1 tsp wheat-germ oil, cold cream, or aloe gel. Apply with a gauze pad and leave in place. Repeat as needed.

For athlete's foot: Mix 10 drops geranium oil with 1 tbsp soy oil and 3 drops wheat-germ oil. Store in a dark bottle. Massage into feet morning and night. Before applying oil, soak feet in a footbath of warm water with sea salt and 5 drops geranium oil.

To make an insect repellent: Combine 16 drops geranium oil with 4 tsp soy oil. Massage into skin. To ease itching from insect bites, apply undiluted geranium oil directly to the bites.

PRECAUTIONS

SPECIAL INFORMATION

- Keep the oil away from the eyes.
- Do not use during pregnancy.
- Since the best-quality geranium oil is expensive, some brands may be adulterated with inferior oils. Buy geranium essential oil only from a reputable source.

TARGET AILMENTS
Small wounds and burns (apply undiluted)
Anxiety and stress
Menopausal and menstrual symptoms
Athlete's foot; eczema; shingles
Sore throat; mouth ulcers
Insect stings and bites (apply undiluted)
Headache
Hemorrhoids

SIDE EFFECTS

None expected

GINGER

LATIN NAME
Zingiber officinale

VITAL STATISTICS

GENERAL DESCRIPTION

Ginger is valued in many cultures as a remedy for a range of ailments as well as a culinary seasoning. Chinese herbalists believe it relieves motion sickness and dizziness, improves digestion, and alleviates menstrual cramps. In China, ginger may be applied to first- and second-degree burns. It is described in traditional Chinese medicine as acrid and warm.

Chinese medicine takes a holistic approach to healthcare, fashioning remedies to treat the entire being as well as the specific parts or areas. Single herbs may be used alone or in combination with other herbs to prevent and combat disease, which is thought to arise from disturbances in the flow of a bodily energy called chi (pronounced "chee") and blood, or from a lack of balance in the complementary states of yin and yang.

PREPARATIONS

Over the counter:

Ginger is available as fresh or dried root, liquid extract, tablets, capsules, or prepared tea.

At home:

TRADITIONAL PREPARATION: Wrap fresh gingerroot in five or six layers of rice paper. Bury under warm coals until the paper is blackened. Remove rice paper before using.

BLOT: Treat first- and second-degree burns by blotting fresh ginger juice, extracted from the root, on the wound.

COMBINATIONS: For vomiting, ginger is mixed with pinellia root; when there is also severe abdominal pain, the herb is combined with licorice or galangal. A preparation of ginger and chamomile is used to treat menstrual irregularity. For coughing and headaches, ginger is mixed with dried bamboo.

PRECAUTIONS

SPECIAL INFORMATION

If you are pregnant, consult a herbalist or a licensed healthcare professional before using.

TARGET AILMENTS

Take internally for:

Vomiting

Abdominal pain

Menstrual irregularity

Coughs

Apply externally for:

First- and second-degree burns

SIDE EFFECTS

NOT SERIOUS

- Heartburn

CALL YOUR DOCTOR WHEN CONVENIENT.

GINGER

LATIN NAME
Zingiber officinale

G

VITAL STATISTICS

GENERAL DESCRIPTION

Characterized by delicate yellow blooms rimmed with purple, ginger not only is a valued culinary seasoning but also is considered in many cultures to be a remedy for a range of ailments. Discovered by practitioners of traditional Ayurvedic (Hindu) medicine, gingerroot was originally thought of as a digestive aid. Today both Chinese and Western herbalists believe it relieves motion sickness and dizziness and improves digestion. Ginger is also believed to alleviate menstrual cramps. Its active constituents are gingerols, which soothe the abdomen and relieve excess gas. Some studies show that ginger may help prevent heart disease and strokes by reducing internal blood clotting and blood pressure.

For visual characteristics of ginger, see the Color Guide to Prescription Drugs and Herbs.

PREPARATIONS

Over the counter:

Ginger is available as fresh or dried root, liquid extract, tablets, capsules, or prepared tea.

At home:

COMBINATIONS: For vomiting, ginger is mixed with pinellia root; when there is also severe abdominal pain, the herb is combined with licorice or galanga. A preparation of ginger and chamomile is used to treat menstrual irregularity. For coughing and headaches, ginger is mixed with dried bamboo.

TEA: Simmer 1 to 2 tsp dried gingerroot in 1 cup water for 5 to 10 minutes.

Consult a qualified practitioner for the dosage appropriate for you and the specific condition being treated.

PRECAUTIONS

WARNING

If you are pregnant, consult a herbalist or a licensed healthcare professional before using.

POSSIBLE INTERACTIONS

Combining ginger with other herbs may necessitate a lower dosage.

TARGET AILMENTS
Motion sickness
Morning sickness
Digestive disorders
Menstrual cramps
Colds; flu
Arthritis
Elevated cholesterol level
High blood pressure

SIDE EFFECTS

NOT SERIOUS

- Heartburn

GINKGO

LATIN NAME
Ginkgo biloba

VITAL STATISTICS

GENERAL INFORMATION

Chinese herbalists have used the leaves of the ginkgo tree for thousands of years to treat asthma, chilblains, and swellings. Today, Western herbalists value ginkgo leaves for their action against vascular diseases that typically affect the elderly. One of ginkgo's most important benefits is its ability to increase vasodilation (expansion of blood vessels) and thereby improve blood flow in capillaries and arteries, especially in peripheral areas such as the lower legs and feet. It also appears to improve blood flow to the brain, decreasing symptoms such as dizziness and memory loss.

Ginkgo may also help reduce retinal damage from macular degeneration, a cause of blindness particularly threatening for diabetics. And it may help reverse deafness caused by reduced blood flow to the auditory nerves. For visual characteristics of ginkgo, see the Color Guide to Prescription Drugs and Herbs.

PREPARATIONS

Ginkgo leaves are available in dry bulk, capsules, or tincture. You can find a standardized product known as ginkgo biloba extract (GBE) in health food stores. Most herbalists recommend using only OTC ginkgo products.

PRECAUTIONS

SPECIAL INFORMATION

- Some people are unable to tolerate ginkgo, even in small doses.
- Do not use if you have a clotting disorder, or if you are pregnant or nursing.
- This herb should not be used with children unless specifically prescribed by a healthcare practitioner knowledgeable about herbs.
- Use in medicinal amounts only in consultation with a healthcare professional.

POSSIBLE INTERACTIONS

Combining ginkgo with other herbs may necessitate a lower dosage.

TARGET AILMENTS
Vertigo; tinnitus
Alzheimer's disease
Phlebitis; leg ulcers
Cerebral atherosclerosis
Diabetic vascular disease
Raynaud's syndrome
Headache; depression
In the elderly, lack of concentration or mental and emotional fatigue
Clotting disorders, including strokes and heart attacks

SIDE EFFECTS

SERIOUS

- Irritability; restlessness
- Diarrhea; nausea; vomiting

IF THESE SYMPTOMS DEVELOP, CHECK WITH YOUR PRACTITIONER TO SEE IF YOU SHOULD LOWER YOUR DOSAGE OR STOP TAKING GINKGO COMPLETELY.

G

GINSENG, AMERICAN

LATIN NAME
Panax quinquefolius

G

VITAL STATISTICS

GENERAL INFORMATION
Found in the Cumberland Gap region of the southern Appalachians, this native American plant is used by both American herbalists and Chinese medicine practitioners. Its active ingredients are panaxosides, thought to calm the stomach and the brain and act as a mild stimulant to vital organs. Ginseng is used to treat weakness and fatigue, particularly when these are the results of a long, fever-producing illness. It is also used to treat tuberculosis or other diseases characterized by a blood-producing cough, and is often used to treat AIDS.

American ginseng is considered an endangered species because of excessive harvesting.

PREPARATIONS
Over the counter:
Ginseng is available as fresh or dried root, root powder, capsules, tablets, prepared tea, freeze-dried root, and cured rock candy.

At home:
TEA: Simmer covered 1 tbsp fresh root with 1 cup water for 15 to 20 minutes. Drink up to 2 cups a day.
Consult a qualified practitioner for the dosage appropriate for your specific condition.

PRECAUTIONS

WARNING
This herb should not be used with children unless specifically prescribed by a healthcare practitioner knowledgeable about herbs.

POSSIBLE INTERACTIONS
Combining American ginseng with other herbs may necessitate a lower dosage.

TARGET AILMENTS

Take internally for (Western):

Depression; fatigue; stress

Colds

Inflammation

Damaged immune system

Take internally for (Chinese):

Weakness with fever, irritability, and thirst

Cough with blood in sputum, dry cough, or loss of voice with dryness

SIDE EFFECTS

NOT SERIOUS

- Headache
- Insomnia; anxiety
- Breast soreness
- Skin rashes
- Loose stools

CALL YOUR DOCTOR IF SYMPTOMS PERSIST.

SERIOUS

- Asthma attacks
- Increased blood pressure
- Heart palpitations
- Postmenopausal uterine bleeding

STOP USING GINSENG AND CONSULT YOUR DOCTOR.

GINSENG, ASIAN

LATIN NAME
Panax ginseng

VITAL STATISTICS

GENERAL DESCRIPTION

Asian ginseng, considered the most potent form of ginseng, strengthens the immune system and increases the body's ability to deal with fatigue and stress. Today herbalists prescribe Asian ginseng root for minor ailments such as fever, colds, coughs, and menstrual irregularities. For visual characteristics, see the Color Guide to Prescription Drugs and Herbs.

PRECAUTIONS

WARNING

If you have any of the following conditions, use ginseng only under the direction of a herbalist or a licensed healthcare professional: pregnancy, insomnia, hay fever, fibrocystic breasts, asthma, emphysema, high blood pressure, blood-clotting problems, heart disorders, diabetes. This herb should not be used with children unless specifically prescribed by a healthcare practitioner knowledgeable about herbs.

PREPARATIONS

Over the counter:

Ginseng is available as fresh or dried root, root powder, capsules, tablets, prepared tea, freeze-dried root, and cured rock candy.

At home:

CHINESE: Boil fresh roots, covered, in water for 3 to 7 minutes. Prick roots with needles. Dry roots in the sun and then soak in thick sugar 10 to 12 hours.

WESTERN: TEA: Boil covered 1 tbsp fresh root with 1 cup water for 15 to 20 minutes. Drink up to 2 cups a day.

Consult a qualified practitioner for the dosage appropriate for your specific condition.

TARGET AILMENTS

Take internally (Chinese) for:

Symptoms of shock
Profuse sweating
Ice-cold extremities
Shortness of breath
Fever; thirst
Irritability
Diarrhea, vomiting
Distention of the abdomen

Take internally (Western) for:

Depression
Fatigue; stress
Colds; influenza
Respiratory problems
Inflammation
Damaged immune system

SIDE EFFECTS

NOT SERIOUS

- Headache
- Insomnia or anxiety
- Breast soreness
- Skin rashes

CALL YOUR DOCTOR IF THESE EFFECTS PERSIST.

SERIOUS

- Asthma attacks
- Increased blood pressure
- Heart palpitations
- Postmenopausal bleeding

STOP USING GINSENG AND CONSULT YOUR DOCTOR.

GINSENG, SIBERIAN

LATIN NAME
Eleutherococcus senticosus

VITAL STATISTICS

GENERAL INFORMATION

Found in the Siberian regions of Russia and China, Siberian ginseng, also called eleuthero, affects the body in a manner similar to Asian and American ginseng, although these effects are subtler and result in less-pronounced reactions. The active elements of Siberian ginseng are eleutherosides, which stimulate the immune system, increasing the body's resistance to disease, stress, and fatigue. Siberian ginseng has gained popularity as a Western herb because it does not cause the insomnia and anxiety that sometimes result when Asian or American ginseng is used. Siberian ginseng gained popularity in Russia when an extract was mass-produced and used in a popular colalike drink called Bodust, meaning vigor.

PREPARATIONS

Over the counter:

Ginseng is available as fresh or dried root, root powder, capsules, tablets, prepared tea, freeze-dried root, and cured rock candy.

At home:

TEA: Simmer covered 1 tbsp fresh root with 1 cup water for 15 to 20 minutes. Drink up to 2 cups a day.

Consult a qualified practitioner for the dosage appropriate for you and the specific condition being treated.

PRECAUTIONS

WARNING

This herb should not be used with children unless it is specifically prescribed by a health-care practitioner who is knowledgeable about herbs.

POSSIBLE INTERACTIONS

Combining Siberian ginseng with other herbs may necessitate a lower dosage.

TARGET AILMENTS
Depression; fatigue; stress
Colds
Inflammation
Damaged immune system

SIDE EFFECTS

NOT SERIOUS

- Headaches
- Insomnia
- Anxiety
- Skin rashes

CALL YOUR DOCTOR IF THESE EFFECTS PERSIST.

SERIOUS

- Asthma attacks
- Increased blood pressure
- Heart palpitations

STOP USING GINSENG AND CONSULT YOUR DOCTOR.

GLANDULARS

VITAL STATISTICS

OTHER NAME
raw glandular concentrates

GENERAL DESCRIPTION
In ancient Rome, eating the glands of animals was considered an effective way to rejuvenate the body; ingesting the ground-up testicular gland of a donkey was not an uncommon way to attempt to revive lost or flagging sexual vigor. In recent years, ingesting glands has gained popularity. Today, the glands of animals, most often cows and pigs, are freeze-dried, pulverized, pressed into tablets, and sold as glandulars. Those on the market include adrenal, pituitary, testicular, ovarian, prostate, and thymus products.

The use of glandulars is controversial, and health benefits are unproved. Supporters cite studies suggesting that glandular supplements stimulate corresponding human glands, boosting hormone production. Health benefits may include fighting fatigue, strengthening the immune system, improving the sex drive, and increasing strength. Critics call glandulars mere snake oil, believing that they are inactivated by the digestive process and so are useless—and perhaps potentially harmful.

Fifty years ago, doctors sometimes used pulverized animal thyroid gland to treat thyroid disease. Today, synthetic versions of thyroid hormone are more commonly used instead, and many experts now recommend against using animal-derived thyroid gland.

PREPARATIONS
Glandulars are sold in the United States in tablet form as a dietary supplement.

PRECAUTIONS

WARNING
Do not take glandulars if you are pregnant or breast-feeding.

SPECIAL INFORMATION
- Using glandulars may inhibit normal hormone production. Consult with your doctor before taking glandular supplements.
- Glandulars may contain toxins the animals have been exposed to, including pesticides, fertilizers, antibiotics, and growth hormones.

TARGET AILMENTS

Problems involving the thyroid, pancreas, liver, thymus, spleen, testes, ovaries, pituitary gland, and adrenal cortex

SIDE EFFECTS

SERIOUS
- Intestinal upset, with nausea, vomiting, or diarrhea
- Numbness
- Tingling of feet and hands

CALL YOUR DOCTOR AT ONCE.

Rx GLIPIZIDE

G

VITAL STATISTICS

DRUG CLASS
Antidiabetic Drugs [Oral Hypoglycemics]

BRAND NAMES
Glucotrol, Glucotrol XL

OTHER DRUGS IN THIS CLASS
acarbose, glyburide, insulin, metformin, troglitazone

GENERAL DESCRIPTION
Glipizide, used to treat a form of non-insulin-dependent (Type 2) diabetes that cannot be controlled by diet and exercise alone, stimulates the release of existing insulin in people whose bodies are capable of producing it. See Oral Hypoglycemics for more information, including facts about side effects and possible drug interactions. For visual characteristics, see the Color Guide to Prescription Drugs and Herbs.

PRECAUTIONS

SPECIAL INFORMATION
- An overdose can result in hypoglycemia. Signs of hypoglycemia include excessive hunger, cold sweats, shakiness, nervousness or anxiety, rapid pulse, headache, drowsiness, confusion, nausea, and cool, pale skin. Keep hard candy, fruit juice, or glucose tablets handy to raise your blood sugar level and counteract hypoglycemia. Call your doctor.
- Tell your doctor if you are allergic to other sulfa drugs; you may also be allergic to oral hypoglycemics.
- People who are elderly, debilitated, or malnourished, as well as those with adrenal, thyroid, pituitary, kidney, or liver problems, have an increased susceptibility to the hypoglycemic action of antidiabetic drugs and should use them with caution.
- It is important to self-monitor your glucose level when taking these drugs.
- Strict adherence to your prescribed regimen of diet and exercise is required for these medications to be effective.

TARGET AILMENTS

Non-insulin-dependent (Type 2) diabetes

SIDE EFFECTS

NOT SERIOUS

- Constipation or diarrhea; nausea, vomiting, or stomach pain; dizziness; mild drowsiness; headache; heartburn; appetite change; skin allergies; weakness; tingling of hands and feet

CALL YOUR DOCTOR IF THESE SYMPTOMS CONTINUE OR BECOME BOTHERSOME.

SERIOUS

- Sore throat and unusual bleeding or bruising; water retention (edema); weight gain; yellowing of skin or eyes (jaundice); abnormally light-colored stools; low-grade fever, fatigue, chills

CONTACT YOUR DOCTOR IMMEDIATELY. ALSO SEE OVERDOSE SYMPTOMS LISTED IN SPECIAL INFORMATION.

GLUCOPHAGE

VITAL STATISTICS

DRUG CLASS
Antidiabetic Drugs [Oral Antihyperglycemics]

GENERIC NAME
metformin

OTHER DRUGS IN THIS CLASS
insulin; glipizide, glyburide (Oral Hypoglycemics); acarbose, troglitazone (Oral Antihyperglycemics)

GENERAL DESCRIPTION
Glucophage is a brand-name form of metformin, an antidiabetic drug used to treat excess blood sugar in people with non-insulin-dependent (Type 2) diabetes when diet, weight loss, and exercise do not produce sufficient control but insulin is not required. It helps lower blood sugar, apparently by decreasing the production of sugar in the liver and by increasing the body's sensitivity to insulin. It promotes uptake of blood sugar by the body's cells.

Glucophage can be combined with a sulfonylurea drug for more effective blood sugar control.

PRECAUTIONS

WARNING
In patients with kidney, liver, or heart disease, Glucophage can cause a rare, serious metabolic disorder called lactic acidosis. These persons should not use Glucophage.

An overdose of Glucophage can cause hypoglycemia, or low blood sugar, with symptoms of unusual weakness, shakiness, stomach pain, nausea or excessive hunger, rapid heartbeat, cold sweats or chills, confusion, anxiety, convulsions, and unconsciousness. For mild symptoms of hypoglycemia, consume something that contains sugar as soon as possible. For more severe symptoms seek emergency care immediately.

Consume alcohol moderately when taking Glucophage. The risk of lactic acidosis is increased when alcohol is consumed with Glucophage.

Glucophage may cause dizziness or drowsiness. Avoid driving and other dangerous activities until you see how the drug affects you.

Glucophage should be discontinued 48 hours prior to a CT scan or any x-ray study involving the administration of intravascular radiocontrast, as the radiocontrast may cause kidney damage and raise the risk of lactic acidosis.

Other oral antidiabetic drugs (tolbutamide and phenformin) have been shown to increase the risk of cardiovascular death. Though Glucophage has not been shown to carry the same risk, the same caution could possibly apply. Discuss any concerns you have about this with your doctor.

SPECIAL INFORMATION
- Consult your doctor before beginning to take Glucophage if you have allergies, a kidney or liver dysfunction, hyper- or hypothyroidism, or a heart or circulatory disease. Tell your doctor also if you are planning surgery or if you have a history of intestinal disorders, megaloblastic anemia, alcoholism, or acid in the blood (metabolic acidosis or ketoacidosis).
- The somewhat common gastrointestinal side effects of Glucophage will often lessen over time. Taking the drug with food may minimize nausea or diarrhea.
- If you develop an illness or infection, contact your doctor. You may need a tempo-

CONTINUED

GLUCOPHAGE

rary change of medications.

- Glucophage should not be used during pregnancy or by nursing mothers.
- Before taking Glucophage, tell your doctor if you are a premenopausal, anovulatory woman, as this drug may cause a resumption of ovulation, increasing the possibility of pregnancy.
- Diabetes and its treatment are complex, requiring patient participation as well as periodic monitoring. Consult with your doctor regularly in order to determine the continuing effectiveness and safety of treatment.
- It is a good idea to wear medical identification containing the information that you take Glucophage for diabetes management.

POSSIBLE INTERACTIONS

Alcohol: increased effect of Glucophage; increased risk of acid in the blood or hypoglycemia.

ACE inhibitors, amiloride, calcium channel blockers, cimetidine, digoxin, furosemide, hypoglycemics, morphine, procainamide, quinidine, quinine, ranitidine, triamterene, trimethoprim, vancomycin: increased effect of Glucophage.

Beta blockers: may slow recovery from low blood sugar or mask the warning signs of low blood sugar.

Contraceptives (estrogen-containing), corticosteroids, thiazide diuretics, estrogens, isoniazid, nicotinic acid, phenytoin, sympathomimetics, thyroid hormones: may raise blood sugar levels, necessitating increased dose of Glucophage.

Clofibrate, monoamine oxidase (MAO) inhibitors, probenecid, propranolol, rifabutin, rifampin, salicylates, long-acting sulfonamides, sulfonylureas: may lower blood sugar, necessitating decreased dose of Glucophage.

Itraconazole, other azole antifungal medications: increase Glucophage's hypoglycemic effects.

TARGET AILMENTS

Type 2 diabetes mellitus

SIDE EFFECTS

NOT SERIOUS

- Stomach pain; gas; diarrhea; nausea; vomiting
- Changes in taste; decreased appetite; weight loss
- Headache; dizziness; nervousness; fatigue
- Rash

CALL YOUR DOCTOR IF THESE EFFECTS PERSIST.

SERIOUS

- Diarrhea, chills, muscle pain, weakness and sleepiness, slow heartbeat, and difficulty breathing (lactic acidosis)
- Unusual weakness, shakiness, stomach pain, nausea or excessive hunger, rapid heartbeat, cold sweats or chills, confusion, anxiety, convulsions, and unconsciousness (hypoglycemia)
- Vitamin B_{12} deficiency anemia (extremely rare)

CALL YOUR DOCTOR IMMEDIATELY.

Glucosamine Sulfate

Vital Statistics

GENERAL DESCRIPTION

Glucosamine is a natural compound that plays a role in forming bones, nails, tendons, skin, and ligaments. It also acts to maintain and repair the cartilage surrounding bone joints. It's considered the building block of this cartilage. Glucosamine sulfate is an artificially synthesized substance made up of glucose, nitrogen, hydrogen, and sulfur.

Studies in Europe and in Japan suggest that glucosamine sulfate can be effective in treating at least one type of arthritis, osteoarthritis. Osteoarthritis develops when the cartilage around the joints breaks down. The joints gradually deteriorate and become painful and stiff. In one study in Italy, osteoarthritis patients treated with injectable glucosamine sulfate, followed by an oral form of the supplement, reported relief from pain at rest and pain during movement. Another study showed that osteoarthritis patients' pain, joint tenderness, and swelling were relieved after six to eight weeks of treatment with glucosamine sulfate.

The supplement is believed to work by stimulating cells to synthesize proteoglycans and glycosaminoglycans, two substances that play a role in building cartilage. Proponents of glucosamine sulfate say the supplement also has anti-inflammatory qualities, but without the potentially dangerous side effects associated with aspirin and nonsteroidal anti-inflammatory drugs (NSAIDs).

Critics say none of the studies to date have shown any long-term benefits of glucosamine sulfate, either for relieving symptoms or for preventing further deterioration of the cartilage and the joints. They also argue there is little known about any potential long-term side effects.

PREPARATIONS

Glucosamine sulfate is sold in the United States in capsule form as a dietary supplement.

Precautions

SPECIAL INFORMATION

Some books and media reports have touted glucosamine sulfate as a cure for osteoarthritis, but experts warn consumers not to rely on the supplement as a treatment for the disease. They advise checking with a physician for advice on effective lifestyle changes and proven treatments.

TARGET AILMENTS
Joint pain
Joint stiffness
Osteoarthritis

SIDE EFFECTS

NOT SERIOUS

- Stomach upset; heartburn; diarrhea; nausea; indigestion

CALL YOUR DOCTOR IF THESE SYMPTOMS PERSIST.

GLUCOTROL

VITAL STATISTICS

DRUG CLASS
Antidiabetic Drugs [Oral Hypoglycemics]

GENERIC NAME
glipizide

OTHER DRUGS IN THIS CLASS
acarbose, glyburide, insulin, metformin, troglitazone

GENERAL DESCRIPTION
Glucotrol is a brand-name form of glipizide, which treats a form of non-insulin-dependent (Type 2) diabetes that cannot be controlled by diet and exercise alone. It stimulates the release of existing insulin in people whose bodies are capable of producing it. See Oral Hypoglycemics for information about side effects and possible drug interactions. For visual characteristics of Glucotrol XL, see the Color Guide to Prescription Drugs and Herbs.

PRECAUTIONS

SPECIAL INFORMATION

- An overdose can result in hypoglycemia. Signs of hypoglycemia include excessive hunger, cold sweats, shakiness, nervousness or anxiety, rapid pulse, headache, drowsiness, confusion, nausea, and cool, pale skin. Keep hard candy, fruit juice, or glucose tablets handy to raise your blood sugar level and counteract hypoglycemia. Call your doctor.
- Tell your doctor if you are allergic to other sulfa drugs; you may also be allergic to oral hypoglycemics.
- People who are elderly, debilitated, or malnourished, as well as those with adrenal, thyroid, pituitary, kidney, or liver problems, have an increased susceptibility to the hypoglycemic action of antidiabetic drugs and should use them with caution.
- It is important to self-monitor your glucose level when taking these drugs.
- Strict adherence to your prescribed regimen of diet and exercise is required for these medications to be effective.

TARGET AILMENTS

Non-insulin-dependent (Type 2) diabetes

SIDE EFFECTS

NOT SERIOUS

- Constipation or diarrhea; nausea, vomiting, or stomach pain; dizziness; mild drowsiness; headache; heartburn; appetite change; skin allergies; weakness; tingling of hands and feet

CALL YOUR DOCTOR IF THESE SYMPTOMS CONTINUE.

SERIOUS

- Sore throat and unusual bleeding or bruising; water retention (edema); weight gain; yellowing of skin or eyes (jaundice); abnormally light-colored stools; low-grade fever, fatigue, chills

CONTACT YOUR DOCTOR IMMEDIATELY. ALSO SEE OVERDOSE SYMPTOMS AT LEFT.

Rx GLYBURIDE

VITAL STATISTICS

DRUG CLASS
Antidiabetic Drugs [Oral Hypoglycemics]

BRAND NAMES
DiaBeta, Glynase, Micronase

OTHER DRUGS IN THIS CLASS
acarbose, glipizide, insulin, metformin, troglitazone

GENERAL DESCRIPTION
Glyburide, used to treat a form of non-insulin-dependent (Type 2) diabetes that cannot be controlled by diet and exercise alone, stimulates the release of existing insulin in people whose bodies are capable of producing it. See Oral Hypoglycemics for more information, including facts about side effects and possible drug interactions. For visual characteristics of glyburide and the brand-name drugs DiaBeta, Glynase, and Micronase, see the Color Guide to Prescription Drugs and Herbs.

PRECAUTIONS

SPECIAL INFORMATION
- An overdose can cause hypoglycemia. Signs include excessive hunger, cold sweats, shakiness, anxiety, rapid pulse, headache, drowsiness, confusion, nausea, and cool, pale skin. Keep hard candy, fruit juice, or glucose tablets handy to raise your blood sugar level. Call your doctor.
- Tell your doctor if you are allergic to other sulfa drugs; you may also be allergic to oral hypoglycemics.
- People who are elderly, debilitated, or malnourished, as well as those with adrenal, thyroid, pituitary, kidney, or liver problems, have an increased susceptibility to the hypoglycemic action of antidiabetic drugs and should use them with caution.
- It is important to self-monitor your glucose level when taking these drugs.
- Strict adherence to your prescribed regimen of diet and exercise is required for these medications to be effective.

TARGET AILMENTS

Non-insulin-dependent (Type 2) diabetes

SIDE EFFECTS

NOT SERIOUS
- Constipation or diarrhea; nausea, vomiting, or stomach pain; dizziness; mild drowsiness; headache; heartburn; appetite change; skin allergies; weakness; tingling of hands and feet

CALL YOUR DOCTOR IF THESE SYMPTOMS CONTINUE.

SERIOUS
- Sore throat and unusual bleeding or bruising; water retention (edema); weight gain; yellowing of the skin or eyes (jaundice); abnormally light-colored stools; low-grade fever, fatigue, chills

CONTACT YOUR DOCTOR IMMEDIATELY. ALSO SEE OVERDOSE SYMPTOMS AT LEFT.

GOLDENSEAL

LATIN NAME
Hydrastis canadensis

G

VITAL STATISTICS

GENERAL INFORMATION

Herbalists use goldenseal to treat several respiratory and skin infections. The herb acts as a stimulant and seems to affect the body's mucous membranes by drying up secretions, reducing inflammation, and fighting infection through the mild antimicrobial action of its active ingredient, berberine. Goldenseal also aids digestion by promoting the production of digestive enzymes. In addition it may control postpartum bleeding by its astringent action. For visual characteristics, see the Color Guide to Prescription Drugs and Herbs.

PREPARATIONS

Over the counter:
Available in dry bulk, capsules, and tincture.

At home:

TEA: Pour 1 cup boiling water onto 2 tsp goldenseal; steep covered for 10 to 15 minutes. Drink three times daily.

DOUCHE: Simmer covered 1 tbsp powdered herb in 1 pt water for 10 minutes. The liquid should be as warm as is tolerable. Douche daily, up to two weeks.

Consult a practitioner for the dosage appropriate for you and your specific condition.

SIDE EFFECTS

NOT SERIOUS

IN HIGH DOSES, GOLDENSEAL CAN IRRITATE THE SKIN, MOUTH, THROAT, AND VAGINA. IT MAY ALSO CAUSE NAUSEA AND DIARRHEA. IF ANY OF THESE DEVELOP, STOP TAKING IMMEDIATELY.

PRECAUTIONS

SPECIAL INFORMATION

- Do not use goldenseal if you are pregnant.
- Do not use without consulting a physician if you have had heart disease, diabetes, glaucoma, a stroke, or high blood pressure.
- Do not give to children under two; give small doses to older ones and adults over 65. Use by children for more than seven days should be monitored by a healthcare practitioner.

POSSIBLE INTERACTIONS

Combining goldenseal with other herbs may necessitate a lower dosage.

TARGET AILMENTS

Take internally for:

Infectious diarrhea; gastritis

Ulcers; gallstones; jaundice

Sinusitis; ear infections

Laryngitis; sore throat

Infected gums

Postpartum uterine bleeding

Vaginal yeast infections

Apply externally for:

Eczema; impetigo

Ringworm; athlete's foot

Contact dermatitis

Gotu Kola

LATIN NAME
Centella asiatica

Vital Statistics

GENERAL INFORMATION

The gotu kola plant grows in marshy areas in many parts of the world. Its fan-shaped leaves contain the soothing agent known as asiaticoside. As a result they have been used to treat burns, skin grafts, and episiotomies (a surgical technique designed to prevent tearing of the vagina during childbirth). Gotu kola may also help heal outbreaks of psoriasis.

There is some evidence that in addition gotu kola may help decrease edema (the retention of fluid by the body) and promote blood circulation in the legs by strengthening the veins and capillaries. It may therefore be useful in treating phlebitis (inflammation of the leg veins).

For visual characteristics, see the Color Guide to Prescription Drugs and Herbs.

PREPARATIONS

Over the counter:
Available in dry bulk, capsules, and tincture.

At home:

Tea: Use 1 to 2 tsp dried gotu kola per cup of boiling water; steep covered 10 to 15 minutes. Drink twice daily to improve circulation in the legs.

Compress: Soak a pad in gotu kola tea or in a tincture to help treat wounds or psoriasis. Start with a weak solution and increase the concentration of gotu kola if necessary.

Consult a qualified practitioner for the dosage appropriate for you and the specific condition being treated.

Precautions

SPECIAL INFORMATION

- Do not use gotu kola if you are pregnant or nursing or are using tranquilizers or sedatives.
- For adults over 65, start with low-strength doses and increase if necessary.
- This herb should not be used with children unless it is specifically prescribed by a healthcare practitioner who is knowledgeable about herbs.

POSSIBLE INTERACTIONS

Combining gotu kola with other herbs may necessitate a lower dosage.

TARGET AILMENTS

Take internally for:

Poor circulation in the legs

Edema

Use an external compress for:

Burns

Cuts and other skin injuries

Psoriasis

SIDE EFFECTS

NOT SERIOUS

- Skin rash; headache

LOWER YOUR DOSAGE OF GOTU KOLA OR STOP TAKING.

G

Grains-of-Paradise Fruit

LATIN NAME
Amomum villosum
(or A. xanthioides)

Vital Statistics

GENERAL DESCRIPTION

The fragrant, acrid-tasting grains-of-paradise fruit is known as cardamom, of which there are several types. This herb is prescribed for a variety of abdominal complaints. Grains-of-paradise fruit is considered a stimulant, and great value is placed on its aroma. Chinese herbalists often add it to fruits such as baked pears to reduce the production of mucus in the body. The shell of the fruit is believed to have medicinal properties similar to but weaker than the fruit itself. The choicest fruits are large, solid, and extremely aromatic. Classified in traditional Chinese medicine as an acrid, warm herb, grains-of-paradise fruit grows in the Chinese provinces of Guangdong and Guanxi and in several areas of Southeast Asia, where it is harvested in August and September.

Chinese medicine takes a holistic approach to healthcare, fashioning remedies to treat the entire being as well as the specific parts or areas. Single herbs may be used alone or in combination with other herbs to prevent and combat disease, which is thought to arise from disturbances in the flow of a bodily energy called chi (pronounced "chee") and blood, or from a lack of balance in the complementary states of yin and yang.

PREPARATIONS

Cardamom is available in bulk or powder from Chinese pharmacies, Asian markets, and some Western health food stores.

Combinations: Mixed with atractylodes (white) and codonopsis root, it is used to treat morning sickness. For other types of discomfort during pregnancy, herbalists prescribe a mixture with mulberry mistletoe stems. It is generally added to combinations near the end of the cooking period and should be crushed before it is used.

Precautions

SPECIAL INFORMATION

Chinese practitioners avoid the use of cardamom in patients with what they call a yin deficiency, a condition marked by symptoms of excessive heat such as fever, thirst, and sweating. Consult your practitioner for advice.

TARGET AILMENTS

Take internally for:

- Nausea and vomiting
- Abdominal pain, diarrhea, indigestion, gas, or loss of appetite
- Morning sickness
- Pain and discomfort during pregnancy
- Involuntary urination

SIDE EFFECTS

NONE EXPECTED IF USED PRECISELY IN THE PRESCRIBED DOSAGE.

GUAIFENESIN

VITAL STATISTICS

DRUG CLASS
Expectorants

BRAND NAMES
Rx: Entex LA
OTC: Primatene Dual Action Formula, Robitussin-CF, Robitussin-DM, Triaminic Expectorant, Vicks DayQuil LiquiCaps, Vicks DayQuil Liquid

GENERAL DESCRIPTION
Guaifenesin is an expectorant drug, used to provide symptomatic relief from coughs, particularly those associated with the common cold or flu. The medication works by thinning and loosening mucus or phlegm from the upper respiratory tract, making it easier to cough up and expel the secretions.

This drug is used in many over-the-counter and prescription cough preparations, often in combination with a decongestant, an antihistamine, or some other medication. Guaifenesin is available in tablet, capsule, or liquid form.

PRECAUTIONS

SPECIAL INFORMATION
- If you are using the extended-release tablet form of this medication, swallow it whole; do not crush or chew the tablet before swallowing it.
- This medication is most effective when taken on an empty stomach.
- To help guaifenesin loosen mucus from the lungs, drink eight to 10 glasses of fluid each day, including a glass of water after each dose.
- If you are pregnant or nursing, check with your doctor before using this medication.
- Do not give this medication to a child under the age of two without first consulting the child's pediatrician.
- Do not take this drug for persistent cough due to smoking, asthma, bronchitis, or emphysema.
- If your cough does not improve within seven days, see your doctor.

POSSIBLE INTERACTIONS
None expected.

TARGET AILMENTS

Coughs due to the common cold, flu, and other minor upper respiratory conditions

SIDE EFFECTS

NOT SERIOUS
- Stomach pain
- Diarrhea
- Nausea
- Drowsiness
- Mild weakness

CONTACT YOUR DOCTOR IF THESE SYMPTOMS PERSIST OR BECOME BOTHERSOME.

SERIOUS
- Skin rash
- Persistent headache
- Vomiting
- High fever

CONTACT YOUR DOCTOR AT ONCE.

GUANFACINE

VITAL STATISTICS

DRUG CLASS
Antihypertensive Drugs

BRAND NAME
Tenex

GENERAL DESCRIPTION
Introduced in 1980, guanfacine is used alone or in combination with a thiazide diuretic to help manage mild-to-moderate high blood pressure (hypertension). It decreases both systolic and diastolic blood pressure.

Guanfacine works by stimulating the alpha$_2$-adrenergic receptors in the brain, which causes a reduction in nerve impulses to the heart, kidneys, and arteries. With fewer of these impulses, the blood vessel walls relax and blood flows through them more easily, thus reducing heart rate and lowering blood pressure.

This drug does not cure high blood pressure, but it helps to control it. Because untreated hypertension can have serious consequences, you may need to take the medication for the rest of your life. Like other blood-pressure-lowering drugs, guanfacine is most effective when combined with regular exercise, stress reduction, weight loss, and a salt-restricted diet. For more information, see Antihypertensive Drugs, Alpha$_1$-Adrenergic Blockers, Angiotensin-Converting Enzyme (ACE) Inhibitors, Beta-Adrenergic Blockers, Calcium Channel Blockers, Diuretics, and the entry for the generic drug losartan.

PRECAUTIONS

SPECIAL INFORMATION
- Do not take guanfacine if you have had an allergic reaction to this drug in the past.
- Tell your doctor if you are pregnant or planning a pregnancy; are nursing; have heart, kidney, or liver disease; have coronary insufficiency or cerebrovascular disease; or are suffering from depression.
- Tell your doctor if you are taking sedatives, hypnotics, or antidepressants, or are planning surgery requiring general anesthesia.
- Be sure to check with your doctor before taking any other medications, especially over-the-counter antihistamines; appetite-control pills; medicines for colds, coughs, sinus, or hay fever; pain pills; or muscle relaxants. Some of these medications may increase your blood pressure; others will result in excessive drowsiness.
- Because guanfacine can act as a sedative, it may impair your mental alertness, judgment, and coordination. Until you know how the drug will affect you, be cautious about driving, using machines, or engaging in any potentially dangerous activity. To reduce daytime drowsiness, take the drug at bedtime.
- Be sure you always have an adequate supply of guanfacine to tide you over during holidays and vacations. You may want to carry a backup prescription for emergency use.

GUANFACINE

- Pay special attention to dental hygiene. Guanfacine can cause mouth dryness, which may increase the likelihood of dental disease. Check with your dentist or doctor if dry mouth continues for more than two weeks.
- It usually takes four to six weeks to know if guanfacine will control your high blood pressure. Do not abruptly stop taking the drug: You may experience severe withdrawal effects.

POSSIBLE INTERACTIONS

Alcohol and other central nervous system depressants, such as antihistamines and muscle relaxants: may increase drowsiness and guanfacine's blood-pressure-lowering effect.

Food: avoid excessive salt.

TARGET AILMENTS

High blood pressure (hypertension)

SIDE EFFECTS

NOT SERIOUS

- Drowsiness
- Dry mouth and nose
- Constipation
- Headache
- Dizziness
- Fatigue
- Insomnia
- Decreased sex drive
- Dry, itching, or burning eyes
- Nausea or vomiting

CALL YOUR DOCTOR IF THESE SYMPTOMS PERSIST OR ARE BOTHERSOME.

SERIOUS

- Confusion
- Mental depression

CONTACT YOUR DOCTOR AS SOON AS POSSIBLE.

HAWTHORN

LATIN NAME
Crataegus laevigata
(or Crataegus oxyacantha)

VITAL STATISTICS

GENERAL INFORMATION
Herbalists use the flowers, fruit, and leaves of the hawthorn, a European shrub with thorny branches. They prescribe the herb as a mild heart tonic. It is thought to dilate the blood vessels, thereby facilitating the flow of blood through the arteries and lowering blood pressure. Hawthorn is also believed to increase the pumping force of the heart muscle and to eliminate arrhythmias. Some practitioners think hawthorn may have a calming effect on the nervous system, and they sometimes recommend it as a remedy for insomnia. Identified by crimson berries and blue-green leaves, hawthorn is also called mayflower, because its delicate white flowers bloom primarily in May.

For visual characteristics, see the Color Guide to Prescription Drugs and Herbs.

PREPARATIONS
Hawthorn is available as fluidextract, dried berries and leaves, or capsules.

Consult a qualified practitioner for the dosage appropriate for you and the specific condition being treated.

PRECAUTIONS

WARNING
Use hawthorn as a heart tonic only if you have been diagnosed with angina, cardiac arrhythmias, or congestive heart failure, and only in consultation with a physician. Do not practice self-diagnosis.

Children and pregnant or nursing women should use hawthorn only under the direction of a medical herbalist or a licensed healthcare professional.

POSSIBLE INTERACTIONS
Combining hawthorn with other herbs may necessitate a lower dosage.

TARGET AILMENTS

Take internally in conjunction with conventional medical treatment for:

High blood pressure

Clogged arteries

Heart palpitations

Angina

Inflammation of the heart muscle

Take internally for:

Insomnia and nervous conditions

Use as a gargle for:

Sore throat

SIDE EFFECTS

SERIOUS

TAKING VERY LARGE AMOUNTS OF HAWTHORN MAY RESULT IN A DRAMATIC DROP IN BLOOD PRESSURE, WHICH IN TURN MAY CAUSE YOU TO FEEL FAINT.

H

Rx HEPARIN

VITAL STATISTICS

DRUG CLASS
Anticoagulant and Antiplatelet Drugs

OTHER DRUGS IN THIS CLASS
aspirin, dalteparin, dipyridamole, warfarin

GENERAL DESCRIPTION
Heparin, a very powerful drug, is the anticoagulant of choice when an instant effect is required. It works by inhibiting the formation of blood clots at various sites throughout the body. Heparin is administered by injection or intravenous infusion in a hospital, clinic setting, or at home by a trained healthcare professional. If you are receiving heparin at home, it is essential that the medicine be administered exactly as directed and that you have regular blood tests to determine how fast your blood is clotting. See Anticoagulant and Antiplatelet Drugs for additional information on side effects, special information, and drug interactions.

PRECAUTIONS

WARNING
Do not use heparin without telling your physician if you have had a heart attack, uncontrolled high blood pressure, ulcers, or a stroke.

SPECIAL INFORMATION
- Because heparin is derived from animal tissue, individuals with a history of asthma or allergies should try a test dose before starting treatment.
- Pregnant and nursing women should check with a physician before taking heparin.
- Avoid dangerous activities that might cause injuries. Be sure to report all falls and blows to your doctor. Internal bleeding may occur without symptoms.

TARGET AILMENTS
Prevention and treatment of blood clots

SIDE EFFECTS

SERIOUS
- Hemorrhaging
- Chest pain
- Severe headache
- Low blood pressure
- Rash
- Breathing problems
- Wheezing
- Runny nose
- Tightness in the chest

CALL YOUR DOCTOR IMMEDIATELY IF YOU EXPERIENCE ANY OF THESE SYMPTOMS.

H

HEPAR SULPHURIS

LATIN NAME
Hepar sulphuris calcareum

VITAL STATISTICS

GENERAL DESCRIPTION

The flaky inner layer of oyster shells provides the calcium used in this homeopathic remedy, also called *Hepar sulph* and commonly known as calcium sulfide. Once an antidote for mercury poisoning, calcium sulfide is now used by homeopathic physicians to treat patients with conditions that tend to involve infection and often produce pus. These disorders are accompanied by symptoms that include mental and physical hypersensitivity and an intolerance of pain and cold.

To make the homeopathic remedy, finely ground oyster shell and sulfur are mixed together and then heated in an airtight container. The resulting powder is dissolved in hot hydrochloric acid, then combined with lactose (milk sugar) in a pharmaceutical process of dilution called trituration. When a patient exhibits a set of symptoms that matches the cataloged symptoms brought on by calcium sulphide, the homeopathic practitioner then prescribes it in an extremely dilute form. For more information on homeopathic medicine, see page 14.

PREPARATIONS

Hepar sulph is available in various potencies, in both liquid and tablet form, at selected stores and pharmacies. Consult your practitioner for more precise information.

PRECAUTIONS

SPECIAL INFORMATION

- When a remedy is administered, no one but the patient should touch the pills. If tablets are spilled, throw them away.
- The mouth should be clear of flavors 15 minutes before and after taking a remedy, and strong flavors and aromas, such as coffee, camphor, and heavily scented perfumes, should be avoided for the duration of treatment.

TARGET AILMENTS

Abscesses that are swollen and painful but have not yet opened

Colds, sore throat, and earache

Inflamed cuts and wounds that may be taking longer than normal to heal

Aching joints

Fits of coughing with chest pain

Hoarseness

Asthma

Emphysema

Croup

Genital herpes

Constipation

SIDE EFFECTS

NONE EXPECTED

HIBISCUS

LATIN NAME
Hibiscus sabdariffa

VITAL STATISTICS

GENERAL INFORMATION

Hibiscus, a widespread category of annuals whose lush, showy flowers are nearly synonymous with tropical beauty, includes more than 200 species of plants. Most of them are believed to have some medicinal properties; different species are used in Ayurvedic (Hindu), Chinese, and Western herbal medicines. *Hibiscus sabdariffa,* also known as roselle or Jamaica sorrel, is valued for its mild laxative effect and for its ability to increase urination, attributed to two diuretic ingredients, ascorbic acid and glycolic acid. Because it contains citric acid, a refrigerant, it is used as a cooling herb, providing relief during hot weather by increasing the flow of blood to the skin's surface and dilating the pores to cool the skin.

Hibiscus seeds, leaves, fruits, and roots are used in various folk remedies, and tea is made from the flowers, in particular the calyx, the leaflike segment that makes up the outermost part of the flower. Its flowers are also used in jams and jellies to impart a tart, refreshing taste. The tart flavor of hibiscus tea may clash with that of other strong-tasting herbs, such as chamomile or dandelion; mix with mint or rose hip tea instead.

PREPARATIONS

Over the counter:

Fresh or dried hibiscus flowers and teas are available in health food stores.

At home:

TEA: Use 2 tsp crumbled dried blossom or 1 tbsp fresh chopped blossom per cup of boiling water; steep covered 10 minutes. Drink up to 3 cups per day. Iced hibiscus tea is also refreshing.

Consult a qualified practitioner for the dosage appropriate for you and the specific condition being treated.

PRECAUTIONS

SPECIAL INFORMATION

Because many types of hibiscus are sold, check with an herbal practitioner to determine if the species you are using is an appropriate treatment. Some species may not be recommended for pregnant women.

POSSIBLE INTERACTIONS

Combining hibiscus with other herbs may necessitate a lower dosage.

TARGET AILMENTS

Take internally for:

Constipation

Mild bladder infections

Mild nausea

Apply the herb or extract externally for:

Sunburn

SIDE EFFECTS

NOT SERIOUS

YOU MIGHT NOTICE A SLIGHTLY DRY SENSATION IN THE MOUTH, WHICH IS CAUSED BY THE HERB'S ASTRINGENT PROPERTY.

H

Rx

HISTAMINE H_2 BLOCKERS

VITAL STATISTICS

DRUG CLASS
Antiulcer Drugs

GENERIC NAMES
cimetidine, famotidine, nizatidine, ranitidine

GENERAL DESCRIPTION
A subclass of antiulcer drugs, histamine H_2 blockers help reduce the secretion of certain digestive juices in the stomach. For more information, including facts about side effects and possible interactions with other medications, see Cimetidine, Famotidine, Nizatidine, and Ranitidine.

TARGET AILMENTS
Duodenal ulcer
Gastric ulcer
Upper gastrointestinal bleeding associated with gastric ulcer or duodenal ulcer, or with gastritis
Zollinger-Ellison syndrome
Multiple endocrine neoplasia
Other conditions characterized by an overproduction of stomach acid
Gastroesophageal reflux
Acid indigestion and heartburn (OTC forms)

PRECAUTIONS

SPECIAL INFORMATION
- Inform your doctor if you have a history of arthritis, kidney or liver disease, organic brain syndrome, asthma, or low sperm count.
- Avoid if you are pregnant or nursing.
- These drugs may affect some medical tests.

SIDE EFFECTS

NOT SERIOUS
- Mild diarrhea
- Skin rash or hives
- Dizziness
- Headache
- Blurred vision
- Fatigue
- Muscle and joint pain

CONTACT YOUR DOCTOR IF THESE SYMPTOMS CONTINUE OR BECOME BOTHERSOME.

SERIOUS
- Confusion
- Nervousness
- Delirium and hallucinations
- Slowed or irregular heartbeat
- Abnormal bleeding or bruising
- Combined weakness, fever, and sore throat (signs of bone marrow depression)
- Hair loss
- Enlarged or painful breasts (in women or men)
- Male impotence
- Jaundice

CALL YOUR DOCTOR IMMEDIATELY.

Honeysuckle Flower

LATIN NAME
Lonicera japonica

Vital Statistics

GENERAL DESCRIPTION

This ornamental flower is prescribed for sores, swellings, fevers, colds, and flu. Chinese medicine practitioners use it as an antibiotic. In addition, the flower is believed to have some value in the treatment of chronic conjunctivitis and other eye conditions. Test-tube studies indicate a possible antibiotic effect. And injected into acupuncture points, preparations of the herb have been used to treat pneumonia and bacillary dysentery. In a laboratory test, honeysuckle flower seemed to lower cholesterol levels in rats. Practitioners have found the stem of the honeysuckle, when prepared in a soup, also useful in clearing up abscesses and sores.

The best variety of the plant has several large, pale yellow, unopened flowers. Considered a sweet, cold herb in traditional Chinese medicine, it grows throughout China and is harvested in May and June.

Chinese medicine takes a holistic approach to healthcare, fashioning remedies to treat the entire being as well as the specific parts or areas. Single herbs may be used alone or in combination with other herbs to prevent and combat disease, which is thought to arise from disturbances in the flow of a bodily energy called chi (pronounced "chee") and blood, or from a lack of balance in the complementary states of yin and yang.

PREPARATIONS

You can find honeysuckle flower in bulk at Asian markets and pharmacies, and Western health food stores. The herb is also available in tablet form.

Combinations: The flowers, together with platycodon and great burdock fruit, form a mixture used to treat pain and swelling in the throat. A preparation with skullcap and coptis is prescribed for high fever. When skullcap alone is added to honeysuckle flower, the blend is employed to discharge pus from boils.

For advice on other combinations and dosages, consult a Chinese medicine practitioner.

Precautions

SPECIAL INFORMATION

- Chinese medicine practitioners advise against using honeysuckle flower to treat sores exuding clear fluid; it should be used only in cases where there is a thick, yellow discharge.
- Chinese medicine practitioners do not prescribe this herb for the type of diarrhea associated with stomach rather than intestinal problems.

TARGET AILMENTS

Take honeysuckle flower internally for:

Sores and inflammations, particularly of the breast, throat, and eyes; heat rash; boils

Fevers; colds; flu

Salmonella and other microbial infections

Intestinal abscesses

Painful urination and dysentery

SIDE EFFECTS

None expected

HOPS

LATIN NAME
Humulus lupulus

VITAL STATISTICS

GENERAL INFORMATION

Hops has a long history as a remedy for insomnia and muscle cramps. Today it is prescribed primarily as a sedative. Because of its bitterness, which stimulates gastric juices and decreases gas, hops is also used as a digestive aid.

For visual characteristics, see the Color Guide to Prescription Drugs and Herbs.

PREPARATIONS

Over the counter:

Available as dried or fresh herbs and in the form of capsules, powder, or tincture.

At home:

TEA: Use 2 tsp dried herb per cup boiling water; steep covered 15 minutes. For insomnia, drink 1 cup at night; if a single dose doesn't bring sleep, or for general anxiety, take up to 3 cups a day. To aid digestion, drink cold an hour before meals or after a meal.

POULTICE: Pour boiling water over 1 to 2 cups dried herbs, steep covered 5 minutes, and wrap in a cloth. Apply warm to the affected area for facial pain or tension headache.

Consult a practitioner for the dosage appropriate for you and your specific condition.

PRECAUTIONS

SPECIAL INFORMATION

- For prolonged or daytime use, take under medical supervision. Do not take during the day if you operate heavy machinery or drive.
- Pregnant women and women with estrogen-dependent breast cancer should avoid hops; it may contain an estrogen-like chemical and has been known to induce menstruation.
- Use low-strength doses for adults over 65 or children from two to 12. Do not give to children under two at all or to older ones for more than seven to 10 days except in conjunction with a healthcare practitioner.

POSSIBLE INTERACTIONS

Use caution when taking hops with prescription sedatives or antianxiety medications.

Combining hops with other herbs may necessitate a lower dosage.

TARGET AILMENTS

Take internally for:

Insomnia

Anxiety; tension headache

Indigestion; low appetite

Apply externally for:

Neuralgia; tension headache

SIDE EFFECTS

NOT SERIOUS

- Sleepiness
- Upset stomach; diarrhea
- Constipation
- A skin rash or eye irritation

STOP TAKING AND CALL YOUR DOCTOR.

SERIOUS

HOPS CAN WORSEN DEPRESSION. SEEK PROFESSIONAL HELP.

HOREHOUND

LATIN NAME
Marrubium vulgare

VITAL STATISTICS

GENERAL DESCRIPTION

Horehound, a grayish white, hairy, flowering herb, has over the centuries been reputed to fend off a variety of ills, from asthma to witches' spells. Today it is most popular as a cough suppressant and throat soother. Until recently horehound was used in over-the-counter cough syrups, but in 1989 the Food and Drug Administration, claiming that horehound is ineffective, banned its use in these preparations. Studies indicate that the chemical marrubiin in horehound accounts for its effectiveness as an expectorant.

PREPARATIONS

Over the counter:
Available as a loose tea, a tincture, and in a sore-throat lozenge or candy.

At home:

TEA: For relief of cough, pour 1 cup boiling water over ½ to 2 tsp dried leaves; steep covered 10 to 15 minutes. Add honey or sugar if desired. Take up to three times a day.

TINCTURE: Take ⅛ to ¼ tsp up to three times a day.

COMBINATIONS: To make your own expectorant, combine 1 oz horehound, 2 oz licorice, 1 oz wild black cherry, 1 oz coltsfoot, and ⅛ oz lobelia. (WARNING: Lobelia can be poisonous; never use more than the prescribed amount, and never give to children or pregnant women.) Simmer 1 tbsp of the mixture in 1 cup water for 5 minutes; let steep covered 10 minutes, then strain into a clean container. Adults drink 1 cup every 2 hours.

Consult a qualified practitioner for the dosage appropriate for you and the specific condition being treated.

PRECAUTIONS

☠ *WARNING*

Persons over 65 should begin with mild doses and increase the strength gradually, if necessary.

Persons with heart disease should avoid using horehound.

SPECIAL INFORMATION

Horehound should be used for an acute cough only. If a cough does not improve within 10 days to two weeks, seek medical advice.

POSSIBLE INTERACTIONS

Combining horehound with other herbs may necessitate a lower dosage.

TARGET AILMENTS

Cough; cold; bronchitis; fever

Whooping cough

SIDE EFFECTS

NOT SERIOUS

- Upset stomach; diarrhea

DISCONTINUE USE AND CALL YOUR DOCTOR.

SERIOUS

- Persistent cough
- Brown, black, or bloody phlegm

CALL YOUR DOCTOR RIGHT AWAY.

H

HORSETAIL

LATIN NAME
Equisetum arvense

VITAL STATISTICS

GENERAL INFORMATION

Horsetail is rich in silica, which helps mend broken bones and form collagen. Herbalists prescribe horsetail for urinary problems, wounds, benign prostate disorders, and rheumatism and arthritis. For visual characteristics, see the Color Guide to Prescription Drugs and Herbs.

PREPARATIONS

Over the counter:
Available as dried or fresh herb, capsules, and tincture.

At home:
TEA: Steep covered 2 tsp dried herb or 1 tbsp fresh herb per cup of boiling water for 15 minutes. For bladder or kidney disorders, drink cold, up to 4 cups a day. To prevent kidney irritation during treatment, take 2 tbsp at a time. Apply tea externally to wounds, sores, or mouth irritations.
Consult a qualified practitioner for the dosage appropriate for you and your specific condition.

PRECAUTIONS

☠ *WARNING*

Use only under a doctor's care. Do not take internally for more than three consecutive days; do not exceed recommended dosage.

Pregnant women should not use this herb; people with cardiac disease or high blood pressure should use it with caution.

Use low-strength doses for adults over 65 and children from two to 12. Do not give to children under two at all or to older ones for more than seven to 10 days except in conjunction with a healthcare practitioner.

POSSIBLE INTERACTIONS

Combining horsetail with other herbs may necessitate a lower dosage.

TARGET AILMENTS

Take internally for:

Bladder infections; cystitis

Urethritis; prostatitis

Kidney stones, with caution

Pain of rheumatism or arthritis

Apply externally for:

Sores; wounds

Inflammations

SIDE EFFECTS

NOT SERIOUS

- Upset stomach; diarrhea
- Increased urination

DISCONTINUE AND CALL A DOCTOR.

SERIOUS

- Pain in the kidneys or lower back, or upon urination, with nausea or vomiting

MAY INDICATE KIDNEY DAMAGE; CALL YOUR DOCTOR AT ONCE.

- Cardiac problems

MAY OCCUR WITH EXTREME OVERUSE. CALL YOUR DOCTOR AT ONCE.

Hsiao Keh Chuan

Vital Statistics

ENGLISH NAME
Cough-Relieving Formula

GENERAL DESCRIPTION
Hsiao Keh Chuan, a Chinese medicine formula available in capsule and liquid form, is used to suppress coughs. It is particularly helpful when there is a lot of mucus. The herbal ingredient, rhododendron, acts as an expectorant and helps diminish the phlegm, thus relieving asthma, bronchitis, and coughs from colds.

Chinese medicine takes a holistic approach to healthcare, fashioning remedies to treat the entire being as well as the specific parts or areas. Precise combinations of herbs are used to prevent and combat disease, which is thought to arise from disturbances in the flow of a bodily energy called chi (pronounced "chee") and blood, or from a lack of balance in the complementary states of yin and yang. A patent formula, *Hsiao Keh Chuan* is made by using a standardized method of preparation.

INGREDIENTS
rhododendron root and branch

PREPARATIONS
This formula is sold in liquid and capsule form at many Chinese pharmacies and Oriental grocery stores.

Precautions

WARNING
Do not use for a dry cough.

TARGET AILMENTS
Cough with copious phlegm
Asthma
Bronchitis

SIDE EFFECTS
NONE EXPECTED

H

Huang Lien Shang Ching Pien

H

Vital Statistics

ENGLISH NAME
Coptis Upper-Body-Clearing Tablets

ALSO SOLD AS
Huang Lian Shang Qing Pian

GENERAL DESCRIPTION
The Chinese medicine formula *Huang Lien Shang Ching Pien* is used for a wide range of ailments that traditional Chinese medicine characterizes as "hot," "painful," or "red." The formula is said to clear inflammation in the upper body and thereby relieve fever, mouth ulcers, conjunctivitis, toothache, and bronchitis. *Huang Lien Shang Ching Pien* sends "heat" out through the lower part of the body by clearing it through the stool and thus also promotes bowel movements. A patent formula, *Huang Lien Shang Ching Pien* is made by using a standardized combination of herbs and method of preparation.

INGREDIENTS
coptis, ligusticum, schizonepeta, ledebouriella, scutellaria, platycodon, gypsum, chrysanthemum, angelica root, licorice *(Glycyrrhiza uralensis),* rhubarb root, vitex, forsythia, inula flower, phellodendron, mint, gardenia

PREPARATIONS
This formula is sold in tablet form in many Chinese pharmacies and Oriental grocery stores.

Precautions

WARNING
Avoid this formula during pregnancy.
Do not use if diarrhea is already present.

TARGET AILMENTS
Fever
Ear infections
Mouth ulcers
Sore gums or throat
Conjunctivitis, or pinkeye
Toothache
Tonsillitis or swollen glands in the neck
Sores or boils
Acute bronchitis
Early stages of pneumonia
Constipation

SIDE EFFECTS

NOT SERIOUS

- Loose stools

DISCONTINUE IF THIS PROVES TOO UNCOMFORTABLE.

HUMULIN

VITAL STATISTICS

DRUG CLASS
Antidiabetic Drugs [Insulin]

BRAND NAMES
Humalog, Humulin L, Humulin N, Humulin R, Humulin U, Humulin 50/50, Humulin 70/30

GENERAL DESCRIPTION
Humulin is a brand name for insulin, a hormone naturally produced by the pancreas that helps regulate the body's levels of glucose (blood sugar) and is involved in the metabolism of fats, carbohydrates, and proteins. The biosynthetically produced Humulin is structurally identical to the insulin produced by the human pancreas; it is manufactured from a special strain of the *Escherichia coli* bacteria to which the gene for human insulin production has been added. Humulin is called human insulin to distinguish it from other brands that are derived from beef or pork.

The drug is injected directly beneath the skin of insulin-dependent (Type 1) diabetics, whose bodies are unable to produce the hormone on their own. Humulin is also used to treat some non-insulin-dependent (Type 2) diabetics whose diabetes is not controlled by oral antidiabetic drugs. Humulin may be used temporarily to treat high blood sugar due to pregnancy, infection, stress, or certain medications.

Humulin comes in several varieties. Humalog, the brand name for rapid-acting insulin, starts working within 15 minutes after injection, reaches its peak effect after 30 to 90 minutes, and lasts three to four hours. Humulin R is a short-acting, "regular" insulin that takes effect within 30 to 40 minutes and lasts for six hours. The intermediate-acting insulins, Humulin N and Humulin L, take effect in two to four hours and last up to 24 hours. Humulin U, a long-acting insulin, takes effect in six to eight hours and lasts up to 28 hours. Humulin 70/30 combines Humulin N (70 percent) with Humulin R (30 percent). Humulin 50/50 is another combination of Humulin N and Humulin R.

PRECAUTIONS

SPECIAL INFORMATION
- Humulin, like all insulins, is not active when taken orally; it must be injected.
- An overdose of insulin can result in low blood sugar (hypoglycemia). Symptoms include excessive hunger, cold sweats, shakiness, nervousness or anxiety, rapid pulse, headache, drowsiness, confusion, nausea, and cool or pale skin. Keep hard candy, fruit juice, glucose tablets, or an emergency glucagon injection kit handy to counteract hypoglycemia, which, untreated, can lead to coma or seizures.
- An underdose of insulin can result in high blood sugar (hyperglycemia). Symptoms include drowsiness, dry mouth, fruity breath, increased frequency of urination, loss of appetite, stomach pain, nausea or vomiting, unusual thirst, trouble breathing, fatigue, and flushed or dry skin. Hyperglycemia can lead to ketoacidosis or a life-threatening diabetic coma. Take a dose of insulin as soon as you realize you have missed one, or as soon as you begin to experience symptoms. Make advance preparations for a friend, colleague, or family member to administer the dose if you are unable.
- Insulin is considered safe for pregnant and nursing women, since the drug does not pass into breast milk.

HUMULIN

- Illness and exercise can alter your insulin requirements.
- Monitor blood glucose regularly. Check for ketones in urine in special circumstances such as pregnancy, illness, or episodes of high blood glucose levels. Do not change the brand or type of insulin you use or stop taking the drug without consulting your doctor.
- Be prepared for a diabetic emergency and discuss a plan of action with your doctor, family members, friends, and co-workers. It is a good idea to carry a card or wear a medical identification bracelet or tag indicating that you have diabetes.
- Smoking affects insulin requirements. If you stop smoking cigarettes or begin wearing a nicotine patch while taking insulin, your blood sugar level may change. You may need to adjust your dosage.
- Humulin causes fewer allergic reactions than insulin derived from animals.

POSSIBLE INTERACTIONS

Humulin can interact with a number of other drugs. Check with your doctor or pharmacist before taking any other medications and be sure to read all labels for sugar content.

Alcohol, anabolic steroids, clofibrate, fenfluramine, guanethidine, MAO inhibitors, nonsteroidal anti-inflammatory drugs (NSAIDs), phenylbutazone, salicylates, sulfinpyrazone, tetracycline: these drugs decrease blood sugar levels and may affect insulin dosages.

Amphetamines, baclofen, corticosteroids, corticotropin (ACTH), danazol, dextrothyroxine, epinephrine, estrogens, ethacrynic acid, furosemide, glucagon, molindone, phenytoin, thiazide diuretics, thyroid hormones, and triamterene: may raise blood sugar levels, increasing the risk of hyperglycemia.

Beta-adrenergic blockers: may mask symptoms of hypoglycemia when used with insulin.

TARGET AILMENTS

Insulin-dependent (Type 1) diabetes

Non-insulin-dependent (Type 2) diabetes that is not properly controlled by diet, exercise, and weight reduction

Severe blood sugar imbalances occurring in nondiabetics as a result of pregnancy, surgery, acute stress, or shock

SIDE EFFECTS

NOT SERIOUS

- Allergic reactions; breakdown of fatty tissue at the site of the injection, which may cause a depression in the skin; accumulation of fat under the skin as a result of an overdependence on the same site for injection

LET YOUR DOCTOR KNOW ABOUT THESE SYMPTOMS.

SERIOUS

- Diabetic coma or hyperglycemia (high blood sugar) from underdosing
- Hypoglycemia (low blood sugar) from overdosing

CALL YOUR DOCTOR IMMEDIATELY IF YOU EXPERIENCE INTENSE ITCHING, HIVES, OR RASH OR FEEL FAINT AFTER A DOSE. SEE OVERDOSE AND UNDERDOSE SYMPTOMS IN SPECIAL INFORMATION.

HUO HSIANG CHENG CHI PIAN

VITAL STATISTICS

ENGLISH NAME
Agastaches Qi-Correcting Pills

ALSO SOLD AS
Lophanthus Antifebrile Pills or *Huo Xiang Zheng Qi Wan*

GENERAL DESCRIPTION
This Chinese medicine formula is used most often to treat intestinal flu (gastroenteritis) when the primary symptom is diarrhea. The formula is used to relieve other accompanying symptoms such as fever, vomiting, headache, and lack of appetite. It can also be used for motion sickness or morning sickness. Traditionally, *Huo Hsiang Cheng Chi Pian* was used to treat acute diarrhea that occurs in the summer and to treat cholera.

Chinese medicine takes a holistic approach to healthcare, fashioning remedies to treat the entire being as well as the specific parts or areas. Precise combinations of herbs are used to prevent and combat disease, which is thought to arise from disturbances in the flow of a bodily energy called qi or chi (pronounced "chee") and blood, or from a lack of balance in the complementary states of yin and yang. A patent formula, *Huo Hsiang Cheng Chi Pian* is made by using a standardized combination of herbs and method of preparation.

INGREDIENTS
agastache, angelica root, areca husk, perilla leaves, poria, atractylodes, magnolia bark, platycodon, aged mandarin orange peel, licorice *(Glycyrrhiza uralensis)*

PREPARATIONS
Over the Counter
This formula is sold in pill form and also in a slightly different form as liquid in many Chinese pharmacies and Oriental grocery stores.

PRECAUTIONS

WARNING
Do not use when there is dry mouth, thirst, and a yellow coating on the tongue. Consult with a Chinese practitioner for more information.

TARGET AILMENTS
Acute diarrhea
Acute gastroenteritis, or intestinal flu
Morning sickness
Motion sickness with nausea
Cholera

SIDE EFFECTS
NONE EXPECTED

H

Rx HYDROCHLOROTHIAZIDE

VITAL STATISTICS

DRUG CLASS
Diuretics

BRAND NAMES
Aldactazide, Dyazide, Maxzide-25

OTHER DRUGS IN THIS CLASS
amiloride, bumetanide, furosemide, indapamide, spironolactone, triamterene

GENERAL DESCRIPTION
Introduced in 1959, hydrochlorothiazide is a diuretic used to treat hypertension (high blood pressure), diabetes insipidus (extreme thirst and excessive production of urine), and excess fluid retention associated with congestive heart failure or cirrhosis.

This drug acts by promoting urine production. It also has the effect of increasing the loss of potassium and other minerals from the body. This effect is particularly pronounced with hydrochlorothiazide. To prevent potassium loss, the drug is frequently combined with the potassium-sparing diuretic triamterene. (Unlike other diuretics, hydrochlorothiazide appears to decrease the body's loss of calcium.)

For more information, see Diuretics. See Triamterene and Amiloride for information about potassium-sparing diuretics often combined with this drug. For visual characteristics of hydrochlorothiazide and the brand-name drug Dyazide, see the Color Guide to Prescription Drugs and Herbs.

PRECAUTIONS

SPECIAL INFORMATION
- Because excess sodium and potassium loss appears more likely with hydrochlorothiazide than with some other diuretics, a higher risk of cardiovascular side effects is associated with this drug.
- Tell your doctor if you have gout; hydrochlorothiazide increases uric acid levels and may cause gout attacks.
- Tell your doctor if you are allergic to sulfa drugs, such as sulfonamide antibiotics or sulfonylurea antidiabetics; hydrochlorothiazide is chemically related to these medications and may trigger similar allergic reactions.
- Tell your doctor if you have diabetes. Dose adjustment of insulin or oral diabetic medication may be necessary.
- Let your doctor know if you have liver or kidney disease.
- Hydrochlorothiazide may increase your sensitivity to sunlight.
- Take this drug with food or milk.

TARGET AILMENTS

Hypertension (high blood pressure)

Diabetes insipidus (extreme thirst and excessive production of urine)

Excess fluid retention

HYDROCHLOROTHIAZIDE

POSSIBLE INTERACTIONS

Alcohol: increased action of hydrochlorothiazide.

Amantadine: possible amantadine toxicity.

Amiodarone: low blood potassium levels and subsequent heart arrhythmias.

Cholestyramine, colestipol: decreased effectiveness of hydrochlorothiazide. Take hydrochlorothiazide one hour before or four hours after these drugs.

Digitalis glycosides: the potassium loss from hydrochlorothiazide can increase the risk of digitalis toxicity and heart-rhythm problems. Your doctor will closely monitor your progress.

Lithium: the combination may increase the risk of lithium toxicity.

Nonsteroidal anti-inflammatory drugs (NSAIDs): reduced effectiveness of hydrochlorothiazide.

Other blood pressure drugs, including angiotensin-converting enzyme (ACE) inhibitors: although hydrochlorothiazide is frequently taken with medications to lower blood pressure, caution should be exercised to ensure that blood pressure does not go too low.

SIDE EFFECTS

NOT SERIOUS

- Mild nausea or diarrhea
- Loss of appetite
- Dizziness or lightheadedness when getting up (orthostatic hypotension)
- Fatigue
- Increased risk of sunburn
- Increased frequency of urination

LET YOUR DOCTOR KNOW IF THESE SYMPTOMS CONTINUE OR BECOME TROUBLESOME.

SERIOUS

- Hypokalemia, or abnormally low blood potassium levels (nausea or vomiting, fatigue or weakness, irregular or weak pulse, increased thirst, dry mouth, mood changes)
- Abnormally low blood sodium levels (muscle pain or cramps, mental confusion, fatigue, irritability)
- Jaundice
- Bleeding disorder (blood in urine or stools, unusual bruising or bleeding)
- Allergic skin rash

TELL YOUR DOCTOR IMMEDIATELY IF YOU EXPERIENCE ANY OF THESE SYMPTOMS. YOU MAY BE ADVISED TO LOWER YOUR DOSAGE AND INCREASE YOUR INTAKE OF FLUIDS AND MINERALS.

HYDROCODONE

VITAL STATISTICS

DRUG CLASS
Analgesics [Opioid Analgesics]

BRAND NAMES
Hycodan, Hycomine, Lorcet 10/650, Lorcet Plus, Lortab 7.5/500

OTHER DRUGS IN THIS SUBCLASS
codeine, oxycodone, propoxyphene, tramadol

H

GENERAL DESCRIPTION
Hydrocodone is a type of pain reliever that acts on the central nervous system to alter the perception of pain. Like other opioids, it is often combined with acetaminophen. Hydrocodone may be prescribed for moderate to severe pain relief and cough suppression. For further information, see Opioid Analgesics.

PRECAUTIONS

WARNING
Seek emergency medical care if you overdose on hydrocodone. Symptoms include pinpoint pupils; slow, shallow, or troubled breathing, and slow heartbeat; extreme dizziness or weakness; confusion; convulsions.

Some hydrocodone-containing drugs also contain a nonnarcotic analgesic, such as acetaminophen. Before taking any other medication, read the label carefully to avoid accidental overdose.

SPECIAL INFORMATION
- Hydrocodone can lead to addiction, both physical and psychological.
- Hydrocodone may cause drowsiness; do not drive or operate machinery until you know how it affects you.
- Do not drink alcoholic beverages while you are taking this drug.
- Tell your doctor if you notice the following symptoms after you stop taking this drug: fever, runny nose, or sneezing; diarrhea; goose flesh; unusually large pupils; nervousness or irritability; fast heartbeat.

TARGET AILMENTS

Moderate to severe pain, especially from acute trauma or surgery

Nonproductive cough in bronchial disorders

SIDE EFFECTS

NOT SERIOUS

- Dry mouth; dizziness; lethargy; drowsiness
- Anxiety
- Difficulty in urination; frequent urge to urinate
- Mild nausea or constipation

CONSULT YOUR DOCTOR IF SYMPTOMS CONTINUE OR ARE BOTHERSOME.

SERIOUS

- Slow or shallow breathing
- Somnolence
- Fast heartbeat with increased sweating and shortness of breath
- Severe constipation; nausea; vomiting

DISCONTINUE USE AND CALL YOUR DOCTOR.

HYDROCORTISONE

VITAL STATISTICS

DRUG CLASS
Corticosteroids

BRAND NAMES
Cortaid, Cortizone

OTHER DRUGS IN THIS CLASS
Rx: beclomethasone, betamethasone, fluticasone, methylprednisolone, mometasone furoate, prednisone, triamcinolone

GENERAL DESCRIPTION
Hydrocortisone cream is used for temporary relief of minor skin problems, including inflammation and rashes caused by eczema, poison ivy, poison oak, poison sumac, insect bites, psoriasis, soaps, detergents, cosmetics, and jewelry. The drug treats only the symptoms, not the underlying causes.

Like other corticosteroids, hydrocortisone is a powerful drug. It can affect almost all parts of the body, so it should be used with caution. For more information, see Corticosteroids.

TARGET AILMENTS
Rash
Inflammation
Itching
Psoriasis
Eczema
Sunburn

PRECAUTIONS

SPECIAL INFORMATION

- Hydrocortisone should not be used for rosacea, acne, viral skin infections such as herpes, or fungal infections such as athlete's foot.
- Do not use this medication near your eyes; with prolonged use, doing so can cause a number of problems, including glaucoma or cataracts.
- If you have diabetes, check with your doctor before using hydrocortisone.
- These creams may sting slightly when they are first applied.
- Do not use excessive quantities of this medication or bind dressings tightly over the treated area.
- Corticosteroid topical creams may be absorbed into your system after prolonged use. Tell your doctor if you are taking any other medication and watch for any significant side effects or possible drug interactions.
- Hydrocortisone should be used with caution if you are allergic to other corticosteroids; if you have an infection or thin skin at the treatment site; or if you have or have had cataracts, glaucoma, diabetes, or tuberculosis.
- Ask your doctor about the risks and benefits of corticosteroid treatment if you have or have had any of the following conditions: HIV infection or AIDS, heart disease, hypertension, ulcerative colitis, diabetes, diverticulitis, gastritis or peptic ulcers, recent chickenpox or measles, candidiasis or other fungal infections, glaucoma, herpes simplex, liver or kidney disease, myasthenia gravis, osteoporosis, anastomoses, lupus, tuberculosis, recent intestinal problems, or any infection, such as a cold or flu.
- One of the actions of corticosteroids is to

H

CONTINUED

HYDROCORTISONE

suppress your immune system, thereby making you more susceptible to opportunistic infections. Corticosteroids can also mask symptoms of infection that occur while you are taking the drugs; because the symptoms will not appear, an infection may worsen without your being aware of it.

- Prolonged use of corticosteroids can cause birth defects. Pregnant and nursing women should avoid these drugs.
- Prolonged use of corticosteroids increases the risk of osteoporosis, cataracts, glaucoma, Cushing's syndrome (moon face), and diabetes. It can also reactivate tuberculosis.
- Check with your doctor before you stop using corticosteroids. It may be necessary to reduce the dosage gradually to avoid serious consequences.

SIDE EFFECTS

NOT SERIOUS

- Mild and transient skin rash
- Burning
- Irritation
- Dryness
- Redness
- Itchiness
- Scaling

CALL YOUR DOCTOR IF THESE SYMPTOMS PERSIST OR BECOME BOTHERSOME.

SERIOUS

- Eye pain
- Loss of or blurred vision
- Stomach pain or burning
- Black, tarry stools
- Severe and lasting skin rash, hives, or burning, itching, or painful skin
- Blisters, acne, or other skin problems
- Nausea or vomiting
- High blood pressure
- Foot or leg swelling
- Rapid weight gain
- Fluid retention (edema)
- Prolonged sore throat, fever, cold, or other signs of infection

CONTACT YOUR DOCTOR IMMEDIATELY.

Hydroxyurea

Vital Statistics

BRAND NAME
Hydrea

GENERAL DESCRIPTION
Hydroxyurea is a cytotoxic agent used to treat several types of cancers and to decrease the frequency of painful crises in sickle cell disease. Because hydroxyurea affects bone marrow, it can increase the risk of infections, mouth ulcers, and decreased blood counts, which can cause unusual bruising or bleeding.

Hydroxyurea is safe and effective for patients aged 18 to 60 years and older; dosages and administration schedules are determined for each patient individually. Cancer patients take hydroxyurea on a regular schedule for up to 16 weeks or perhaps even longer; sickle cell patients take the drug at the lowest effective dose on a continual, indefinite basis.

Precautions

WARNING
Call your doctor immediately if you develop a fever or chills, or if you have a seizure.

Hydroxyurea use requires constant monitoring by a physician. Hemoglobin levels, total leukocyte counts, and platelet counts should be checked weekly.

Do not take hydroxyurea if you are pregnant or breast-feeding.

SPECIAL INFORMATION
- This medication should be taken on an empty stomach. If vomiting occurs shortly after ingestion, call your doctor.
- Do not take hydroxyurea if you have ever had an allergic reaction to it in the past, or if you have depressed bone marrow, evidenced by low white blood cell, platelet, or hemoglobin counts.
- Before taking hydroxyurea, inform your physician if you are considering pregnancy (male or female); have previously had chemotherapy or radiation therapy; have shingles; have recently been exposed to chickenpox; are having unusual bleeding or bruising; or take other prescription or nonprescription medications.
- While taking hydroxyurea, avoid contact with anyone with a bacterial or viral infection. Report any signs of infection to your doctor immediately.
- Avoid contact with anyone who has taken a live poliovirus vaccine recently.
- Do not have any vaccinations without your doctor's approval while taking this drug.
- Since this drug may cause dizziness or hallucinations, restrict driving or hazardous activity as necessary.
- If radiation therapy is administered simultaneously, hydroxyurea dosages may need to be reduced to avoid excessive bone marrow depression.
- Let your doctor know if you have impaired kidney function. You may need a lower dosage of hydroxyurea.
- Exercise caution in exposure to the sun while taking this medication.
- Necessary dental work should be completed prior to using hydroxyurea, if possible.
- See your dentist for regular dental checkups while you are taking this medication.

H

CONTINUED

HYDROXYUREA

POSSIBLE INTERACTIONS

Alcohol: may cause increased risk of gastrointestinal bleeding. Do not drink alcohol while taking hydroxyurea.

Antigout drugs, including probenecid and sulfinpyrazone: dosages may need to be adjusted since hydroxyurea may raise uric acid concentrations in the blood, increasing the risk of kidney damage or gout attacks.

Live virus vaccines: may prevent the development of immunity to these vaccines; the virus may spread in the body and cause diesease. Wait three months to one year after discontinuation of hydroxyurea before getting a live virus vaccine, such as some poliovirus vaccines.

Other medications that cause bone marrow depression, such as fluorouracil: may cause increased inhibition of blood cell production. Reduction in dose may be required if these drugs are taken with hydroxyurea.

TARGET AILMENTS
Cancers of the head and neck
Chronic myelocytic leukemia
Melanoma
Ovarian cancer
Prostatic cancer, advanced
Sickle cell disease

SIDE EFFECTS

NOT SERIOUS

- Hair loss
- Loss of appetite
- Nausea, vomiting, or diarrhea
- Sun sensitivity
- Skin rash and itching

CALL YOUR DOCTOR IF THESE EFFECTS PERSIST OR BECOME TROUBLESOME.

SERIOUS

- Painful mouth sores
- Fever or chills, cough or hoarseness; lower back or side pain; painful or difficult urination (anemia)
- Unusual bruising or bleeding; black, tarry stools; blood in urine or stools; pinpoint red spots on skin (bone marrow depression)
- Skin ulcerations

DISCONTINUE USE AND CALL YOUR DOCTOR IMMEDIATELY.

HYDROXYZINE

VITAL STATISTICS

DRUG CLASS
Anti-Itch Drugs

BRAND NAMES
Atarax, Vistaril

GENERAL DESCRIPTION
Introduced in 1953, hydroxyzine is an antihistamine that appears to depress the central nervous system. It also has antipruritic, or anti-itch, properties. This medication is used to treat tension, restlessness, and some types of anxiety, and to relieve itching due to allergic reactions. Hydroxyzine has also been prescribed for the treatment of motion sickness, as a sedative, and as an antinausea medication.

Like other antihistamines, hydroxyzine blocks the action of histamine, a natural substance the body releases when fighting infection and in allergic reactions. Histamine causes the runny nose, watery eyes, congestion, and hives or itching associated with allergies.

TARGET AILMENTS
Tension
Restlessness
Some types of anxiety
Itching due to allergic reactions

PRECAUTIONS

SPECIAL INFORMATION
- Do not take hydroxyzine if you have had an unusual or allergic reaction to this drug or to another antihistamine in the past.
- If you are pregnant, consult your doctor before using this medication.
- Hydroxyzine may pass into breast milk; avoid using it while nursing.
- Do not drink alcohol while using this drug.
- If hydroxyzine gives you an upset stomach, nausea, diarrhea, or other gastrointestinal problems, take the medication with meals or with milk.
- To help relieve dry mouth (a common side effect), chew gum or suck on hard candy, and drink plenty of water.
- Because hydroxyzine can make you drowsy, avoid driving, operating hazardous machinery, or engaging in other potentially dangerous activities that require intense concentration.
- To avoid drowsiness, take less of the drug. Drowsiness is usually temporary and may disappear after a few days or after reduction of the dose.
- The body develops a tolerance to hydroxyzine after prolonged use, reducing the drug's effectiveness.
- Do not take hydroxyzine with any other prescription medication or over-the-counter drug without first consulting your doctor.

HYDROXYZINE

POSSIBLE INTERACTIONS

Attapulgite: a decrease in the effect of hydroxyzine.

Antianxiety drugs; barbiturates or other sedatives: do not take with hydroxyzine, as the combination may result in excessive sedation.

Central nervous system depressants (such as alcohol, antidepressants, antipsychotics, narcotics, pain relievers, sedatives and hypnotics, sleep inducers, and tranquilizers): increased effects of both combined drugs.

Clozapine: increased side effects of clozapine.

Nonprescription cold or allergy medications that contain antihistamines: increased drowsiness.

Monoamine oxidase (MAO) inhibitors: can cause hypotension and dryness of the respiratory passages when taken with hydroxyzine. Do not combine these drugs with hydroxyzine.

SIDE EFFECTS

NOT SERIOUS

- Dry mouth
- Drowsiness
- Difficulty in urinating
- Headache (rare)

NOTIFY YOUR DOCTOR IF THESE SYMPTOMS PERSIST OR BECOME BOTHERSOME.

SERIOUS

- Wheezing
- Chest tightness
- Difficulty breathing

YOU MAY BE HAVING AN ADVERSE REACTION TO THE DRUG. CALL YOUR DOCTOR IMMEDIATELY.

- Excessive drowsiness
- Unsteadiness
- Tremors
- Convulsions

CALL YOUR DOCTOR IMMEDIATELY.

HYPERICUM

LATIN NAME
Hypericum perforatum

VITAL STATISTICS

GENERAL DESCRIPTION

Also known as St.-John's-wort, *Hypericum* grows in woodlands across Europe, Asia, and the United States, blooming with a profusion of yellow flowers from June to September. The flowers, if bruised, bleed a reddish juice. The dark green leaves of the plant are dotted with oil-producing pores. According to ancient healing wisdom, because *Hypericum* seemed to resemble skin, with its pores and its simulation of bleeding on injury, it was considered ideal for all manner of flesh wounds *(see St.-John's-Wort, page 709).* In homeopathy, the remedy *Hypericum* is often prescribed for bodily injuries, among other conditions; but it is selected for the soothing effect it is said to have on injured nerves rather than for any traditional reason.

The entire plant is harvested for homeopathic use in summer, when its yellow flowers are in full bloom. It is pounded to a pulp and soaked in an alcohol solution before being brought to the desired potencies through a vigorous dilution process.

Like most homeopathic prescriptions, *Hypericum* was developed as a remedy by observation of the reactions of healthy individuals to doses of various strengths. The mental, emotional, and physical changes induced by *Hypericum* were then cataloged. When a patient exhibits a set of symptoms that matches the cataloged symptoms brought on by *Hypericum,* the homeopathic practitioner then prescribes it in an extremely dilute form. It is presumed that in this highly dilute dosage, *Hypericum* can counter symptoms that are similar to the ones it induces when it is at full strength. For more information on homeopathic medicine, see page 14.

PREPARATIONS

Hypericum is available in various strengths, in both liquid and tablet form, at selected stores and pharmacies. Consult your practitioner for more precise information.

PRECAUTIONS

SPECIAL INFORMATION

- When a remedy is administered, no one but the patient should touch the pills. If tablets are spilled, throw them away.
- The mouth should be clear of flavors 15 minutes before and after taking a remedy, and strong flavors and aromas, such as coffee, camphor, and heavily scented perfumes, should be avoided for the duration of treatment.

TARGET AILMENTS

Backaches centered along the lower spine that may include shooting pains

Bites and stings from animals and insects, especially when they have become inflamed or include nerve damage

Cuts and wounds to nerve-rich parts of the body, like the fingers and lips, caused by accidents or surgery

SIDE EFFECTS

NONE EXPECTED

HYSSOP

LATIN NAME
Hyssopus officinalis

VITAL STATISTICS

GENERAL INFORMATION

Hyssop is used as an expectorant, digestive aid, sedative, and muscle relaxant. Volatile oils in the leaves and flowers help loosen mucus and stimulate coughing, and decrease gas. Hyssop is also used as an antiseptic; its oils may heal wounds and herpes simplex sores.

PREPARATIONS

Over the counter:
Available dried or fresh and as tincture.

At home:

TEA: Steep covered 2 tsp dried herb per cup boiling water for 10 to 15 minutes. Drink three times daily for cough (honey or lemon improves the flavor); gargle three times a day for sore throat. Apply to burns and wounds.

COMPRESS: Steep covered 1 oz dried herb in 1 pt boiling water for 15 minutes; soak clean cloth in solution and apply warm to cold sores or genital herpes sores; place on the chest to relieve congestion.

COMBINATIONS: Used with white horehound and coltsfoot for coughs and bronchitis; with boneset, elder flower, and peppermint for cold symptoms.

Consult a qualified practitioner for the dosage appropriate for your specific condition.

SIDE EFFECTS

NOT SERIOUS

- Upset stomach or diarrhea

DISCONTINUE USE AND CALL YOUR DOCTOR.

H

PRECAUTIONS

SPECIAL INFORMATION

- Use hyssop only under medical supervision if you use it for more than three consecutive days.
- Pregnant women should avoid hyssop; it was once used to induce abortion.
- Use low-strength preparations for adults over 65 and children from two to 12. Do not give to children under two at all or to older ones for more than seven to 10 days except in conjunction with a healthcare practitioner.

POSSIBLE INTERACTIONS

Combining hyssop with other herbs may necessitate a lower dosage.

TARGET AILMENTS

Take internally for:

- Coughs; common colds
- Bronchitis
- Indigestion; gas
- Anxiety; hysteria
- Petit mal (a form of epilepsy)

Apply externally for:

- Cold sores
- Genital herpes sores
- Burns; wounds; skin irritations

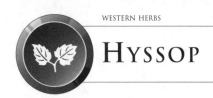

Rx HYTRIN

VITAL STATISTICS

DRUG CLASS
Alpha$_1$-Adrenergic Blockers

GENERIC NAME
terazosin

OTHER DRUGS IN THIS CLASS
doxazosin

GENERAL DESCRIPTION
Hytrin is the brand name of the generic drug terazosin. Introduced in 1987, this drug is one of several alpha$_1$-adrenergic blocking agents used in the treatment of high blood pressure. It can be used alone or in conjunction with other drugs, such as beta-adrenergic blockers or diuretics, depending on the degree of hypertension. For more information, including possible drug interactions, see Alpha$_1$-Adrenergic Blockers. For visual characteristics of Hytrin, see the Color Guide to Prescription Drugs and Herbs.

PRECAUTIONS

SPECIAL INFORMATION

- You should not take Hytrin if you have ever had an allergic or unusual reaction to it, or to doxazosin or prazosin.
- Avoid driving and hazardous tasks for 24 hours after the first dose, after a dosage increase, or after resumption of treatment.
- The effects of Hytrin on pregnant women, nursing mothers, and children under 12 years of age are not yet known. Use only if directed by your physician.
- Before taking Hytrin, tell your doctor if you have previously experienced an unusual or allergic reaction to doxazosin, prazosin, terazosin or Hytrin, or have encountered dizziness, faintness, or lightheadedness with other drugs. Inform your doctor if you have a history of mental depression, stroke, or impaired circulation to the brain; coronary artery disease; impaired liver function or active liver disease; impaired kidney function; or any plans to undergo surgery in the near future.
- To minimize dizziness, take the first Hytrin dose at bedtime. Dosages must be adjusted on an individual basis.
- Hytrin may affect some laboratory tests. Effects may include a mild decrease in white blood cell counts, certain cholesterol ratios, and blood sugar levels.
- The symptoms of prostate cancer are similar to those of benign prostate enlargement. Ask your doctor to test for prostate cancer before starting Hytrin treatment.

H

TARGET AILMENTS

High blood pressure

Benign prostatic hyperplasia (benign enlargement of the prostate)

SIDE EFFECTS

NOT SERIOUS

ALTHOUGH RARE, A SLIGHT (TWO- TO THREE-POUND) WEIGHT GAIN IS POSSIBLE WITH USE OF THIS DRUG.

FOR ADDITIONAL SIDE EFFECTS, SEE ALPHA$_1$-ADRENERGIC BLOCKERS.

Rx IBUPROFEN

VITAL STATISTICS

DRUG CLASS
Analgesics [Nonsteroidal Anti-Inflammatory Drugs (NSAIDs)]

BRAND NAMES
Rx: Children's Motrin Ibuprofen Suspension, various forms of Motrin for adults
OTC: Advil, Advil Cold and Sinus, Children's Motrin Ibuprofen Suspension, Midol-200, Motrin IB, Nuprin, Pamprin

GENERAL DESCRIPTION
Introduced in 1969, ibuprofen became available for the over-the-counter (OTC) market in 1984. The drug is used to relieve headaches, menstrual cramps, muscle aches, rheumatoid arthritis, osteoarthritis, and minor aches and pains of the common cold. It also reduces inflammation and fever. This drug is used by people who cannot take aspirin, or when acetaminophen or aspirin is not effective. For further information, see Nonsteroidal Anti-Inflammatory Drugs (NSAIDs). For visual characteristics of the brand-name drug Motrin, see the Color Guide to Prescription Drugs and Herbs.

TARGET AILMENTS

Inflammation, especially related to arthritis

Pain, especially from inflammation, dental and other surgeries, menstruation, and migraines

Fever

PRECAUTIONS

WARNING
Do not take ibuprofen during the last three months of pregnancy.

SPECIAL INFORMATION
- Do not use ibuprofen if allergic to NSAIDs or to aspirin. It may cause bronchoconstriction or anaphylaxis in aspirin-sensitive asthmatics.
- Avoid this drug or consult your doctor before using it if you have asthma, peptic ulcer, enteritis, heart disease, high blood pressure, bleeding problems, or liver or kidney impairment.

SIDE EFFECTS

- Dizziness, drowsiness, or headache
- Mild abdominal pain; constipation or diarrhea; heartburn or nausea

CONSULT YOUR DOCTOR IF THESE SYMPTOMS PERSIST.

SERIOUS
- Anaphylactic reaction (hives, rash, intense itching, and trouble breathing)
- Gastrointestinal bleeding; ulceration; stomach perforation (black or tarry stools)
- Angina; irregular heartbeat
- Diminished hearing or ringing in the ears
- Fluid retention
- Jaundice; blood in urine

CALL YOUR DOCTOR IMMEDIATELY.

IGNATIA

LATIN NAME
Ignatia amara

VITAL STATISTICS

GENERAL DESCRIPTION

The beans of this plant, sometimes called St. Ignatius bean, are in fact seeds from the fruit of a small tree native to China and the Philippines. Seventeenth-century Spanish missionaries in the Philippines were introduced to the seeds by the locals, who wore them as amulets to ward off disease. Small doses of the seed can produce mild but unpleasant symptoms of poisoning, including increased salivation, pounding headache, cramps, giddiness, twitching, and trembling; large doses can be fatal. Homeopaths may prescribe *Ignatia,* a dilute solution of the seed, for ailments that include symptoms like those associated with mild poisoning.

For the homeopathic preparation, the seeds are collected and ground to a powder, then mixed with alcohol. When the powder is thoroughly saturated, the mixture is strained and diluted until it becomes a nontoxic substance. When a patient exhibits a set of symptoms that matches the cataloged symptoms brought on by *Ignatia,* the homeopathic practitioner then prescribes it in an extremely dilute form. For more information on homeopathic medicine, see page 14.

PREPARATIONS

Ignatia is available in various potencies, in both liquid and tablet form, at selected stores and pharmacies. Consult a homeopathic practitioner for more precise information.

PRECAUTIONS

SPECIAL INFORMATION

- Only the patient should touch the pills. If tablets are spilled, throw them away.
- The mouth should be clear of flavors 15 minutes before and after taking a remedy, and strong flavors and aromas, such as coffee, camphor, and heavily scented perfumes, should be avoided for the duration of treatment.

TARGET AILMENTS
Anxiety
Dry, tickling coughs
A sore throat that feels as if there is a lump in it
Tension headaches
Indigestion
Insomnia
Irritable bowel syndrome
Painful hemorrhoids
Effects of grief, shock, or disappointment; or depression where the patient tends to sigh frequently

SIDE EFFECTS

NONE EXPECTED

INDAPAMIDE

VITAL STATISTICS

DRUG CLASS
Diuretics

BRAND NAME
Lozol

OTHER DRUGS IN THIS CLASS
amiloride, bumetanide, furosemide, hydrochlorothiazide, spironolactone, triamterene

GENERAL DESCRIPTION
Indapamide is a relatively new diuretic prescribed to treat hypertension (high blood pressure) and excess fluid retention. Among the group of drugs known as nonpotassium-sparing diuretics, indapamide increases the loss of potassium and other minerals from the body as it promotes urine production. For more information, see Diuretics. For visual characteristics of the brand-name drug Lozol, see the Color Guide to Prescription Drugs and Herbs.

PRECAUTIONS

SPECIAL INFORMATION
- Tell your doctor if you are allergic to sulfa drugs, such as sulfonamide antibiotics or sulfonylurea antidiabetics; indapamide is chemically related to these medications and may trigger similar reactions.
- Taking diuretics in hot weather or while engaged in heavy exertion can cause a dangerous loss of fluids or minerals. Watch for signs of dehydration (fatigue, dizziness, headache, nausea).
- Your doctor will closely monitor your potassium levels to prevent heart-rhythm problems. If you are taking indapamide, you may be given a potassium supplement (such as potassium chloride).
- Because diuretics have both known and suspected effects on glucose (blood sugar) levels, people with diabetes or who have been diagnosed with borderline diabetes should have their blood sugar levels monitored closely.
- Tell your doctor if you have kidney or liver disease before taking this drug.

Indapamide

POSSIBLE INTERACTIONS

Alcohol: increased action of diuretics.

Anticoagulants: decreased or increased anti-coagulant effect.

Cholestyramine and colestipol: decreased absorption of indapamide.

Digitalis and other heart drugs: increased risk of potassium loss and additional heart-rhythm problems. Your doctor will closely monitor your progress.

Lithium: increased risk of lithium toxicity.

Oral antidiabetic drugs, insulin: in rare cases, diuretics may raise blood glucose levels and interfere with these medicines.

Other blood pressure drugs, including angiotensin-converting enzyme (ACE) inhibitors: although diuretics are frequently taken with medications to lower blood pressure, caution should be exercised to ensure that blood pressure does not go too low.

TARGET AILMENTS

Hypertension (high blood pressure)

Excess fluid retention associated with congestive heart failure

SIDE EFFECTS

NOT SERIOUS

- Headache
- Blurred vision
- Diarrhea
- Dizziness or lightheadedness when getting up (orthostatic hypotension)
- Loss of appetite
- Increased risk of sunburn

LET YOUR DOCTOR KNOW IF THESE SYMPTOMS CONTINUE OR BECOME TROUBLESOME.

SERIOUS

- Nausea or vomiting
- Fatigue or weakness
- Irregular or weak pulse
- Increased thirst and dry mouth
- Muscle pain or cramps
- Mood changes
- Mental confusion
- Blood in urine or stools
- Unusual bruising
- Skin rash; itching

TELL YOUR DOCTOR IMMEDIATELY IF YOU EXPERIENCE ANY OF THESE SYMPTOMS. YOU MAY BE ADVISED TO LOWER YOUR DOSAGE AND INCREASE YOUR INTAKE OF FLUIDS AND MINERALS.

INDOLE-3-CARBINOL

VITAL STATISTICS

GENERAL DESCRIPTION

Cruciferous vegetables, or crucifers, have long been praised for their vitamin content, and now they are receiving even greater acclaim as cancer-fighting foods. Indole-3-carbinol is one of several phytonutrients, or plant nutrients, found in the crucifers, a group that includes broccoli, cauliflower, Brussels sprouts, cabbage, and kale. Some studies reveal that indoles can disable carcinogens and thus protect against cancer. Indole-3-carbinol appears to suppress or help regulate the distribution of estrogen in the body and is especially noted for helping to prevent breast cancer, a disease associated with estrogen. Other indoles may prove effective in fending off cancers of the stomach, intestines, and lungs. The speculated positive effects of indoles also include an increased energy level, improved skin, hair, and nails, and healthier cells. Like other vegetables, the crucifers are most valuable when fresh and only lightly cooked. Steam, blanch, or eat them raw to receive their vitamins and cancer-fighting benefits. In 1995 the American Institute for Cancer Research demonstrated interest in indole-3-carbinol by granting funding for further research into its potential health benefits.

NATURAL SOURCES

broccoli and other cruciferous vegetables

PREPARATIONS

Available as an extract.

TARGET AILMENTS

Breast cancer (prevention)

SIDE EFFECTS

NONE EXPECTED

Rx INSULIN

VITAL STATISTICS

DRUG CLASS
Antidiabetic Drugs

GENERIC NAMES
insulin lispro, lente insulin, NPH insulin, regular insulin, semilente insulin, ultralente™ insulin

BRAND NAMES
Humalog, Humulin, Iletin, Novolin, Velosulin

GENERAL DESCRIPTION
Insulin, a hormone naturally produced by the pancreas, helps regulate the body's levels of glucose (blood sugar) and is involved in the metabolism of fats, carbohydrates, and protein. The insulin used today in the treatment of diabetes is manufactured synthetically or is extracted from beef or pork pancreases.

The drug is injected directly beneath the skin of insulin-dependent (Type 1) diabetics, whose bodies are unable to produce the hormone. In Type 1 diabetics, this imbalance can lead to ketoacidosis—in which a buildup of ketones (by-products of metabolism) causes the blood to become increasingly acidic—and possibly to a life-threatening diabetic coma. Insulin is also used to treat some non-insulin-dependent (Type 2) diabetics when the condition is not controlled by oral antidiabetic drugs. Insulin therapy may be required temporarily to treat high blood sugar due to pregnancy, infection, stress, or certain medications.

Insulin comes in four varieties: rapid-acting (lispro), short-acting (regular), intermediate-acting (NPH and lente), and long-acting (ultralente™ or semilente). Rapid-acting insulin starts working within 15 minutes after injection, reaches its peak effect after 30 to 90 minutes, and lasts three to four hours. Short-acting takes effect within 30 to 40 minutes and lasts six hours. Intermediate-acting takes effect in two to four hours and lasts up to 24 hours. Long-acting takes effect in six to eight hours and last up to 28 hours.

PRECAUTIONS

SPECIAL INFORMATION

- Insulin is not active when taken orally. The drug must be injected to be effective.
- An overdose of insulin can result in low blood sugar (hypoglycemia). Symptoms include excessive hunger, cold sweats, shakiness, nervousness or anxiety, rapid pulse, headache, drowsiness, confusion, nausea, and cool or pale skin. Keep hard candy, fruit juice, glucose tablets, or an emergency glucagon injection kit handy to counteract hypoglycemia, which, untreated, can lead to coma or seizures.
- An underdose of insulin can result in high blood sugar (hyperglycemia). Symptoms include drowsiness, dry mouth, fruity breath, increased frequency of urination, loss of appetite, stomach pain, nausea or vomiting, unusual thirst, trouble breathing, fatigue, and flushed or dry skin. Hyperglycemia can lead to ketoacidosis or a life-threatening diabetic coma. Take a dose of insulin as soon as you realize you have missed one, or as soon as you begin to experience symptoms. Make advance preparations for a friend, colleague, or family member to administer the dose if you are unable to do so.
- Insulin is considered safe for pregnant and nursing women.
- Strict adherence to a prescribed regimen of diet and exercise is essential to controlling the disease.
- Illness and exercise can alter your insulin requirements.

CONTINUED

INSULIN

- Monitor blood glucose regularly. Check for ketones in urine in special circumstances such as pregnancy, illness, or high blood glucose levels. Do not change the brand or type of insulin you use or stop taking the drug without consulting your doctor.
- Be prepared for a diabetic emergency and discuss a plan of action with your doctor, family members, friends, and co-workers. It is a good idea to carry a card or wear a medical identification bracelet or tag indicating that you have diabetes.
- Smoking affects insulin requirements. If you stop smoking cigarettes or begin wearing a nicotine patch while taking insulin, you may need to adjust your dosage.
- Most insulin in use today is processed synthetically. It causes fewer allergic reactions than insulin derived from animals.

POSSIBLE INTERACTIONS

Insulin can interact with a number of other drugs. Check with your doctor or pharmacist before taking any other medications and be sure to read all labels for sugar content.

Alcohol, anabolic steroids, clofibrate, fenfluramine, guanethidine, monoamine oxidase (MAO) inhibitors, nonsteroidal anti-inflammatory drugs (NSAIDs), phenylbutazone, salicylates, sulfinpyrazone, tetracycline: these drugs decrease blood sugar levels and may affect insulin dosages.

Amphetamines, baclofen, corticosteroids, corticotropin (ACTH), danazol, dextrothyroxine, epinephrine, estrogens, ethacrynic acid, furosemide, glucagon, molindone, phenytoin, thiazide diuretics, thyroid hormones, triamterene: may raise blood sugar levels, increasing the risk of hyperglycemia.

Beta-adrenergic blockers: may mask the symptoms of hypoglycemia when used concurrently with insulin.

TARGET AILMENTS

Insulin-dependent (Type 1) diabetes

Non-insulin-dependent (Type 2) diabetes that is not properly controlled by diet, exercise, and weight reduction

Severe blood sugar imbalances occurring in nondiabetics as a result of pregnancy, surgery, acute stress, or shock

SIDE EFFECTS

- Allergic reactions
- Breakdown of fatty tissue at the site of the injection, which may cause a depression in the skin
- Accumulation of fat under the skin as a result of an overdependence on the same site for injection

LET YOUR DOCTOR KNOW ABOUT THESE SYMPTOMS.

SERIOUS

- Diabetic coma or hyperglycemia (high blood sugar) from underdosing
- Hypoglycemia (low blood sugar) from overdosing

CALL YOUR DOCTOR AT ONCE IF YOU EXPERIENCE INTENSE ITCHING, HIVES, OR RASH OR IF YOU FEEL FAINT AFTER A DOSE. SEE OVERDOSE AND UNDERDOSE SYMPTOMS IN SPECIAL INFORMATION.

IODINE

VITAL STATISTICS

GENERAL DESCRIPTION

Iodine was one of the first minerals recognized as essential to human health. For centuries, it has been known to prevent and treat goiter—enlargement of the thyroid gland. As part of several thyroid hormones, iodine strongly influences nutrient metabolism; nerve and muscle function; skin, hair, tooth, and nail condition; and physical and mental development. Iodine may also help convert beta carotene into vitamin A, and it is an effective antiseptic and water sterilizer.

Iodine deficiency is now uncommon; besides goiter, the effects of deficiency include weight gain, hair loss, listlessness, insomnia, and some forms of mental retardation.

RDA

Adults: 150 mcg
Pregnant women: 175 mcg

NATURAL SOURCES

Kelp, seafood, and vegetables grown in iodine-rich soils are excellent sources of this mineral. More than half of all the salt consumed in the United States is iodized, supplying sufficient iodine in a regular diet.

PRECAUTIONS

SPECIAL INFORMATION

- Supplements are usually unnecessary, but pregnant women should ensure sufficient intake for themselves and their babies to prevent potential mental retardation or cretinism, a form of dwarfism in infants.
- Most excess iodine is excreted by the kidneys, but an extremely high intake may cause nervousness, hyperactivity, headache, rashes, a metallic taste in the mouth, and goiter—in this case due to hyperactivity of the thyroid gland.
- In rare cases, iodine may inhibit thyroid hormone secretion.

TARGET AILMENTS
Goiter
Skin problems

SIDE EFFECTS

NONE EXPECTED

IPECAC

LATIN NAME
Cephaelis ipecacuanha

VITAL STATISTICS

GENERAL DESCRIPTION

The *ipecacuanha* shrub, native to Central and South America, was named by Portuguese colonists, who called it "roadside sick-making plant" in recognition of its ability to induce vomiting. Varying doses of its root can produce a variety of symptoms that includes mild appetite stimulation, sweating, expectoration, vomiting, gastritis, inflammation of the lungs, and cardiac failure. Other health disorders can display symptoms similar to those of mild ipecac poisoning, and it is these symptoms that homeopathic practitioners hope to counteract when they prescribe *Ipecac.*

The homeopathic remedy is made from the root, the most potent part of the plant. The root is dried and then ground into a coarse powder, which is diluted either in milk sugar as a dry substance or in a water-alcohol base. Both preparations are brought to a nontoxic level.

Like most homeopathic prescriptions, *Ipecac* was developed as a remedy by observation of the reactions of healthy individuals to doses of various strengths. The mental, emotional, and physical changes induced by *Ipecac* were then cataloged. When a patient exhibits a set of symptoms that matches the cataloged symptoms brought on by *Ipecac,* the homeopathic practitioner then prescribes it in an extremely dilute form. For more information on homeopathic medicine, see page 14.

PREPARATIONS

Ipecac is available in various potencies, in both liquid and tablet form, at selected stores and pharmacies. Consult your practitioner for more precise information.

PRECAUTIONS

SPECIAL INFORMATION

- Only the patient should touch the pills. If tablets are spilled, throw them away.
- The mouth should be clear of flavors 15 minutes before and after taking a remedy, and strong flavors and aromas, such as coffee and heavy perfume, should be avoided for the duration of treatment.

TARGET AILMENTS
Persistent nausea
Vomiting
Motion sickness
Menstrual problems
Asthma
Dry, irritating cough accompanied by wheezing
Diarrhea
Flu with nausea
Colic
Gastroenteritis

SIDE EFFECTS

NONE EXPECTED

Ipratropium

Vital Statistics

DRUG CLASS
Bronchodilators

BRAND NAMES
Atrovent, Combivent

OTHER DRUGS IN THIS CLASS
Rx: albuterol, epinephrine, salmeterol, terbutaline, theophylline
OTC: ephedrine, epinephrine, theophylline

GENERAL DESCRIPTION
Ipratropium is prescribed as an oral inhalant to prevent and relieve the symptoms of chronic bronchitis and emphysema by opening up the bronchial tubes. Unlike many other bronchodilators, ipratropium is not used to treat acute bronchial asthma attacks because it is not a fast-acting medication. Ipratropium is also available as a nasal spray for runny nose associated with hay fever and the common cold. For more information, see Bronchodilators.

Precautions

WARNING
Your body can build up tolerance to bronchodilators used as inhalants, causing them to become less effective. If this happens, tell your doctor. Do not increase the dose. Increasing the dose can lead to serious, perhaps fatal bronchial constriction.

SPECIAL INFORMATION
If you are pregnant or breast-feeding, consult a doctor before using this drug. Tell your doctor if you have narrow-angle glaucoma, prostatic hypertrophy, urinary retention, or bladder-neck obstruction before using ipratropium.

POSSIBLE INTERACTIONS
See Bronchodilators.

TARGET AILMENTS

Chronic bronchitis (aerosol)

Emphysema (aerosol)

Runny nose (nasal spray)

SIDE EFFECTS

NOT SERIOUS

- Mild nausea; mild insomnia; nervousness; restlessness; dry mouth and throat (oral inhalant)
- Nasal dryness; bleeding from the nose (nasal spray)

CALL YOUR DOCTOR IF THESE EFFECTS BECOME BOTHERSOME.

SERIOUS

- Change in blood pressure; change in heartbeat (irregular or pounding, for example)
- Breathing problems
- Anxiety; dizziness; rash; headache
- Nausea

LET YOUR DOCTOR KNOW RIGHT AWAY IF YOU EXPERIENCE THESE SIDE EFFECTS.

IRON

VITAL STATISTICS

GENERAL DESCRIPTION

Iron is found in hemoglobin, the protein in red blood cells that transports oxygen from the lungs to body tissues. It is also a component of myoglobin, a protein that provides extra fuel to muscles during exertion.

Lack of iron deprives body tissues of oxygen and may cause iron deficiency anemia; warning signs include fatigue, paleness, dizziness, sensitivity to cold, listlessness, irritability, poor concentration, and heart palpitations. Because iron strengthens immune function, iron deficiency also may increase susceptibility to infection. Women need more iron before menopause than after, because menstruation causes iron loss each month.

On a doctor's recommendation, adults can augment their iron intake by means of a multinutrient supplement. Straight iron supplements should be taken only under a doctor's supervision.

RDA

Adults: 10 mg
Premenopausal women: 15 mg
Pregnant women: 30 mg

NATURAL SOURCES

Dietary iron exists in two forms: heme iron, found in red meat, chicken, seafood, and other animal products; and nonheme iron, found in dark green vegetables, whole grains, nuts, dried fruit, blackstrap molasses, and other plant foods. Many flour-based food products are fortified with iron. Heme iron is easier to absorb, but eating foods containing nonheme iron along with foods that have heme iron or vitamin C will maximize iron absorption.

PRECAUTIONS

☠ *WARNING*

Though uncommon, severe iron poisoning can result in coma, heart failure, and death.

Children should never be given adult iron supplements. If your pediatrician recommends an iron supplement, make sure it is a specific, child-formulated variety.

SPECIAL INFORMATION

- Coffee, tea, soy-based foods, antacids, and tetracycline inhibit iron absorption, as do excessive amounts of calcium, zinc, and manganese.
- People who have special iron-intake needs include menstruating or pregnant women, children under age two, vegetarians, and anyone with bleeding conditions such as hemorrhoids or bleeding stomach ulcers.
- Excess iron inhibits absorption of phosphorus, interferes with immune function, and may increase your risk of developing cancer, cirrhosis, or heart attack.
- Symptoms of iron toxicity include diarrhea, vomiting, headache, dizziness, fatigue, stomach cramps, and weak pulse.
- Excess iron may cause constipation.

TARGET AILMENTS
Anemia
Fatigue

SIDE EFFECTS

NONE EXPECTED

ISOCARBOXAZID

VITAL STATISTICS

DRUG CLASS
Antidepressants [Monoamine Oxidase (MAO) Inhibitors]

BRAND NAME
Marplan

OTHER DRUGS IN THIS SUBCLASS
phenelzine, tranylcypromine

GENERAL DESCRIPTION
Isocarboxazid belongs to the subclass of antidepressants known as monoamine oxidase (MAO) inhibitors. Like other MAO inhibitors, this drug is used to treat depression when other antidepressant drugs have failed. See Monoamine Oxidase (MAO) Inhibitors for more information, including side effects and possible drug interactions.

TARGET AILMENTS

Major depression, especially if the condition has not responded to other drugs

Panic disorder

Prevention of vascular headache (including migraine) or tension headache

SIDE EFFECTS

SEE MONOAMINE OXIDASE (MAO) INHIBITORS.

PRECAUTIONS

WARNING
Isocarboxazid reacts with many drugs and foods. Following are substances you should avoid when taking this drug: high-protein foods that are aged, fermented, or pickled, including (but not limited to) aged or processed cheeses; sour cream; alcohol, especially wine and beer (including alcohol-free wine and beer); pickled fish; dry sausages (salami); soy sauce; bean curd; yogurt; liver; figs; raisins; bananas; avocados; chocolate; papaya; meat tenderizers; and fava beans. Also avoid caffeine. But beware: This is only a partial list. Talk to your doctor and pharmacist about other drugs and foods you should avoid.

SPECIAL INFORMATION
- Let your doctor know if you have diabetes, epilepsy, hyperthyroidism, or manic or suicidal tendencies, or if you have had a stroke.
- Isocarboxazid may suppress heart pain, thereby masking heart problems. Let your doctor know if you have any history of angina or other heart disease.
- The full effects of isocarboxazid may not be felt until after several weeks of therapy.
- Use this drug during pregnancy or breast-feeding only if your doctor says that the benefits outweigh the risks.

Rx ISOSORBIDE DINITRATE

VITAL STATISTICS

DRUG CLASS
Nitrates

BRAND NAME
Isordil

OTHER DRUGS IN THIS CLASS
isosorbide mononitrate, nitroglycerin

GENERAL DESCRIPTION
Like other drugs in its class, isosorbide dinitrate is used to control angina. In some cases it is also used as a complementary treatment for congestive heart failure. Introduced in 1959, isosorbide dinitrate is available in a variety of forms. Sublingual (those that are dissolved under the tongue) and chewable tablets are prescribed for immediate relief from angina, while standard and extended-use tablets are offered for long-term management of the condition. For more information, including possible food and drug interactions, see Nitrates.

PRECAUTIONS

SPECIAL INFORMATION
- If you are pregnant or nursing, consult your doctor before using this drug.
- Tolerance to isosorbide dinitrate may occur, requiring an adjustment (increase) of dosage over time. Consult your doctor.
- Tell your doctor if you have severe anemia, recent head trauma, glaucoma, an overactive thyroid, or a digestive absorption problem. Your doctor may decide not to use this drug or to give you a smaller dose.
- Isosorbide dinitrate may cause the Zlatkis-Zak cholesterol test to show a lower-than-actual cholesterol level.

TARGET AILMENTS

Angina pectoris (chronic or acute)

Congestive heart failure

SIDE EFFECTS

NOT SERIOUS

- Lightheadedness when changing position (orthostatic hypotension)
- Flushing of face and neck
- Nausea or vomiting
- Rapid heartbeat

CALL YOUR DOCTOR IF THESE PROBLEMS PERSIST.

SERIOUS

- Blurred vision (rare)
- Severe or prolonged headache
- Fever
- Convulsions
- Dizziness or fainting
- Weakness or change in heartbeat
- Bluish tinge to lips, fingernails, or palms of hands
- Skin rash not from an ointment or patch

CONTACT YOUR DOCTOR IMMEDIATELY.

Isosorbide Mononitrate

Vital Statistics

DRUG CLASS
Nitrates

BRAND NAMES
Imdur (extended release), Ismo, Monoket

OTHER DRUGS IN THIS CLASS
isosorbide dinitrate, nitroglycerin

GENERAL DESCRIPTION
Isosorbide mononitrate is used to prevent attacks of angina pectoris, the crushing chest pain caused when the heart's blood supply is restricted. This drug works by relaxing blood vessel walls, lightening the heart's work load. Isosorbide mononitrate is not effective for acute angina but is taken to help prevent attacks. For information about possible drug interactions, see Nitrates. For visual characteristics of the brand-name drug Imdur, see the Color Guide to Prescription Drugs and Herbs.

Precautions

WARNING
An overdose of isosorbide mononitrate can be fatal. Contact a poison control center or seek emergency care if you've taken more than the amount prescribed.

Because isosorbide mononitrate can cause dizziness and other symptoms of low blood pressure, restrict your activities as necessary; do not drive or operate machinery until you know how the drug will affect you.

SPECIAL INFORMATION
- Isosorbide mononitrate should not be used if you have certain kinds of heart disease, severe anemia, or an overactive thyroid. Be sure to consult your doctor about any medical conditions or allergies you have before you take this drug.
- Isosorbide mononitrate must be taken on a precise, sometimes asymmetric schedule to avoid developing tolerance to the drug.
- If you suffer from headaches while taking this medication, they may be treated with aspirin or acetaminophen. Contact your doctor if the headaches become worse, but do not stop taking the drug.
- Isosorbide mononitrate might affect some medical tests. Be sure any doctor you consult knows you are taking the drug.
- Consult your doctor before using this drug if you are pregnant or breast-feeding.

I

TARGET AILMENTS
Angina

SIDE EFFECTS

NOT SERIOUS
- Headache (often disappears after a few days)
- Dizziness; fainting
- Nausea; vomiting; diarrhea
- Rash
- Cough
- Mild to moderate chest pain

SERIOUS
- Abnormally low blood pressure (dizziness, fainting)
- Rapid heartbeat
- Severe headache; migraine
- Severe skin rash

ISRADIPINE

VITAL STATISTICS

DRUG CLASS
Calcium Channel Blockers

BRAND NAME
DynaCirc

OTHER DRUGS IN THIS CLASS
amlodipine, diltiazem, nifedipine, verapamil

GENERAL DESCRIPTION
Like other calcium channel blockers, isradipine inhibits the passage of calcium into muscle cells, thus relaxing the muscles that control the walls of arteries. It also reduces the work load on the heart. The combined effect of these two actions lowers blood pressure.

This drug is used primarily in the treatment of mild to moderate high blood pressure (hypertension); in some cases it is prescribed to help manage angina. For more information, including possible drug interactions, see Calcium Channel Blockers.

PRECAUTIONS

SPECIAL INFORMATION
- Some healthcare professionals are concerned about the safety of calcium channel blockers. Before using this drug, discuss this matter thoroughly with your doctor. If you are already taking it, do not stop the medication without first consulting your doctor.
- Pregnant or nursing women should use isradipine only if it is clearly needed.
- Tell your doctor if you have low blood pressure (hypotension); heart, liver, or kidney disease; or congestive heart failure, especially if you are using a beta-blocking drug.

TARGET AILMENTS

Angina

High blood pressure

Migraine headache (prevention)

SIDE EFFECTS

NOT SERIOUS

- Weight gain
- Increased appetite
- Drowsiness
- Dizziness
- Lightheadedness
- Headache
- Flushing
- Nausea; diarrhea; constipation (rare)

CALL YOUR DOCTOR IF THESE EFFECTS BECOME TROUBLESOME.

SERIOUS

- Heart problems, such as congestive heart failure, heart-rhythm irregularities, or increased angina (heart pain)
- Low blood pressure
- Swelling of the lower extremities
- Allergic reaction, such as skin rash

CONTACT YOUR DOCTOR IMMEDIATELY.

Jasmine Absolute

LATIN NAME
Jasminum officinale
(or J. grandiflorum)

Vital Statistics

GENERAL DESCRIPTION

Jasmine is a hardy evergreen vine and shrub native to India, China, and, in earlier times, ancient Persia. The white flower, from which jasmine absolute is made, produces a scent that is both spicy and sweet. A mild analgesic, jasmine is also valued as an anti-inflammatory, antiseptic, antispasmodic, and expectorant.

Since the late 1980s, jasmine has been rendered for use not as an oil but as a highly concentrated substance known as an absolute. Production of an absolute requires huge quantities of flowers and the use of a solvent such as alcohol or petroleum. Jasmine absolute is dark orange in color, with a rich, floral, tealike scent.

PREPARATIONS

Jasmine absolute can simply be worn as perfume, sprinkled on a handkerchief and inhaled, or used with a diffuser to scent a room.

TO APPLY TO THE SKIN, blend 4 drops in 1 tbsp vegetable or nut oil, or aloe gel.

FOR BATHING, mix 5 drops jasmine absolute in the bathwater.

Precautions

WARNING

Do not buy any jasmine product labeled "essential oil." Essential oils are produced by distillation, which ruins the delicate perfume.

SPECIAL INFORMATION

- To ensure the highest quality and least amount of solvent residue, buy jasmine absolute only from a reputable source.
- Some experts do not recommend using jasmine absolute on the skin because the solvent residue or other ingredients can cause irritation.

TARGET AILMENTS
Migraine headache
Depression
Anxiety and stress
Coughing
Laryngitis
Menstrual symptoms
Irritated or dry skin (skin application, baths)
Muscle spasms and sprains (skin application, baths)
Low sex drive

SIDE EFFECTS

NOT SERIOUS

- Allergic reactions, such as dermatitis or skin irritation
- Insomnia

DISCONTINUE USE.

JUNIPER

LATIN NAME
Juniperus communis

VITAL STATISTICS

GENERAL DESCRIPTION

The berrylike juniper cone, a purple fruit, is produced by female varieties of an evergreen shrub that can grow six to 25 feet tall. Juniper is known for giving gin its tart bite. Because it also acts as a diuretic, juniper is used to treat high blood pressure and bladder infections. Juniper oil is thought to have anti-inflammatory properties considered useful for treating arthritis and gout. Juniper teas can be taken for digestive problems.

PREPARATIONS

Over the counter:
Available in whole berries, bulk, capsules, and tinctures.

At home:
TEA: Steep covered 1 tsp crushed juniper berries in 1 cup boiling water for 20 minutes. Drink at least two times daily. Do not use for more than 6 weeks at a time.

PRECAUTIONS

WARNING

Juniper can irritate the kidneys and urinary tract and is suitable for short-term use only.

Do not use juniper if you have a kidney infection or a history of kidney problems.

Do not use juniper if you are pregnant; it may stimulate contraction of the uterus.

Juniper should not be used by children unless it is prescribed by a healthcare practitioner who is knowledgeable about herbs.

POSSIBLE INTERACTIONS

Combining juniper with other herbs may necessitate a lower dosage.

TARGET AILMENTS

Take internally for:

Bladder infections

Cystitis

Digestive problems

High blood pressure

Apply externally for:

Arthritis

Gout

SIDE EFFECTS

NOT SERIOUS

- Allergy symptoms, such as nasal congestion

STOP TAKING JUNIPER AND CALL YOUR DOCTOR.

SERIOUS

- Signs of kidney or urinary tract damage (diarrhea, intestinal pain, kidney pain, blood in the urine, purplish urine, a faster heartbeat)

STOP TAKING JUNIPER IMMEDIATELY AND SEE YOUR DOCTOR AS SOON AS POSSIBLE.

Kai Kit Pills

Vital Statistics

ENGLISH NAME
Dispel Swelling Pills

GENERAL DESCRIPTION
Kai Kit Pills are used to ease pain and promote urination in cases where the prostate gland is enlarged and the swelling is pronounced and chronic.

Chinese medicine takes a holistic approach to healthcare, fashioning remedies to treat the entire being as well as the specific parts or areas. Precise combinations of herbs are used to prevent and combat disease, which is thought to arise from disturbances in the flow of a bodily energy called chi (pronounced "chee") and blood, or from a lack of balance in the complementary states of yin and yang. A patent formula, Kai Kit Pills are made by using a standardized combination of herbs and method of preparation.

INGREDIENTS
rehmannia, astragalus, codonopsis, ligustrum fruit, plantago seeds, achyranthes, salvia root, cuscuta seeds, mantis egg case

PREPARATIONS
This formula is sold in pill form in many Chinese pharmacies and Oriental grocery stores.

Precautions

WARNING
Do not take Kai Kit Pills if you have an acute inflammation of the prostate.

TARGET AILMENTS

Painful and difficult urination due to chronic enlarged prostate gland

SIDE EFFECTS

None expected

KALI BICHROMICUM

LATIN NAME
Kali bichromicum

VITAL STATISTICS

GENERAL DESCRIPTION

Kali bichromicum is potassium bichromate, a chemical compound that may be acquired from chromium iron ore or by processing potassium chromate with one of a number of strong acids. A highly corrosive substance, it is used primarily in textile dyeing, in the staining of wood, and as a component in electric batteries. It is also a powerful poison.

Homeopathic practitioners believe the remedy *Kali bichromicum,* or *Kali bi,* works best for conditions that are accompanied by the symptom of pain in a distinct spot, where the ache is easily located with a fingertip. For homeopathic use, this caustic chemical is diluted to nontoxic levels with large amounts of milk sugar, a pharmaceutical process called trituration.

Like most homeopathic prescriptions, *Kali bi* was developed as a remedy by observation of the reactions of healthy individuals to doses of various strengths. The mental, emotional, and physical changes induced by *Kali bi* were then cataloged. When a patient exhibits a set of symptoms that matches the cataloged symptoms brought on by *Kali bi,* the homeopathic practitioner then prescribes it in an extremely dilute form. It is presumed that in this highly dilute dosage, *Kali bi* can counter symptoms that are similar to the ones it induces when at full strength. For more information on homeopathic medicine, see page 14.

PREPARATIONS

Kali bichromicum is available in various potencies, in both liquid and tablet form, at selected stores and pharmacies. Consult your practitioner for more precise information.

PRECAUTIONS

SPECIAL INFORMATION

- When a remedy is administered, no one but the patient should touch the pills. If tablets are spilled, throw them away.
- The mouth should be clear of flavors 15 minutes before and after taking a remedy, and strong flavors and aromas, such as coffee, camphor, and heavily scented perfumes, should be avoided for the duration of treatment.

TARGET AILMENTS

- Acute bronchitis
- Colds in which there is a thick mucus discharge and a heavy cough that produces pain in the chest
- Croup
- Sinusitis and resulting headaches
- Indigestion
- Pains in the joints

SIDE EFFECTS

NONE EXPECTED

K

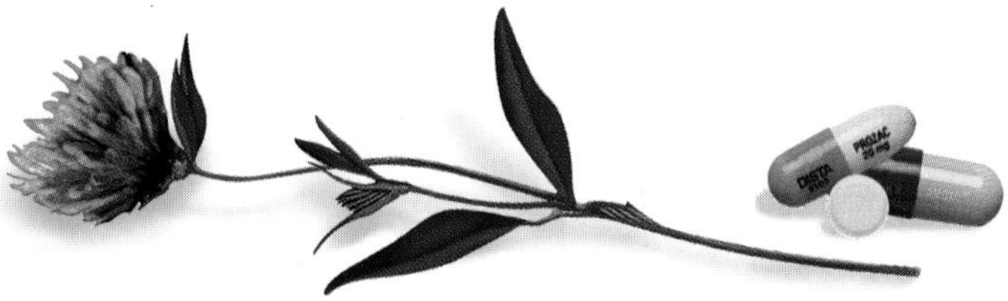

COLOR GUIDE TO PRESCRIPTION DRUGS & HERBS

Be advised that although every effort has been made to ensure accurate reproduction of the prescription drugs in this guide, variations in color can result from the printing process, and pills are not shown actual size. Take care not to confuse brand-name drugs with their generic counterparts. Do not depend only on the images in this book to identify a given drug or herb; consult a physician, pharmacist, or qualified healthcare practitioner for proper identification.

Prescription Drugs

The following are the most common brand-name and generic prescription drugs.

ACCUPRIL	ACETAMINOPHEN/ CODEINE	ADALAT CC	ALLEGRA
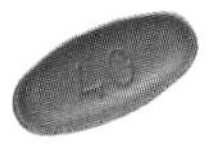	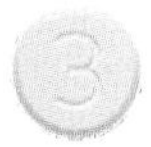	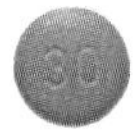	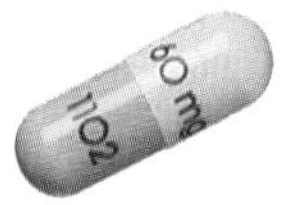
40 MG	300 MG ACETAMINOPHEN/ 30 MG CODEINE	30 MG	60 MG
PAGE 20	PAGE 22	PAGE 544	PAGE 35
ALLOPURINOL	ALPRAZOLAM	ALTACE	AMBIEN
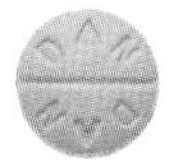	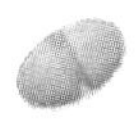	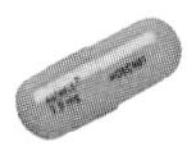	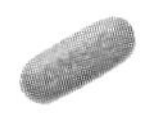
300 MG	1 MG	5 MG	5 MG
PAGE 37	PAGE 42	PAGE 652	PAGE 45

AMITRIPTYLINE

100 MG
PAGE 49

AMOXICILLIN
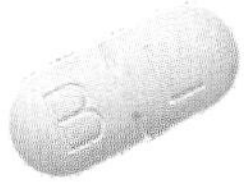
250 MG
PAGE 51

AMOXIL
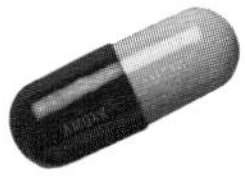
250 MG
PAGE 53

ANAPROX
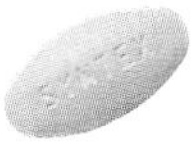
275 MG
PAGE 533

ATENOLOL

50 MG
PAGE 108

ATIVAN

1 MG
PAGE 482

AUGMENTIN
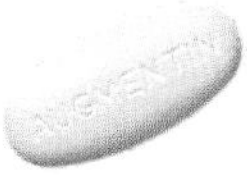
500 MG AMOXICILLIN/
125 MG CLAVULANATE
PAGE 112

AXID
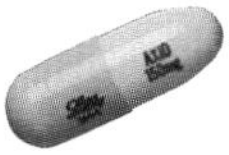
150 MG
PAGE 550

BACTRIM DS
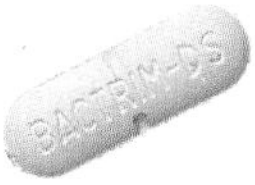

800 MG SULFAMETHOXAZOLE/
160 MG TRIMETHOPRIM
PAGE 115

BENTYL
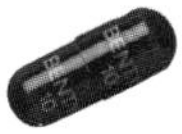
10 MG
PAGE 281

BIAXIN
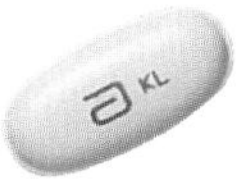
500 MG
PAGE 136

BRETHINE
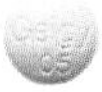
5 MG
PAGE 735

BUMETANIDE
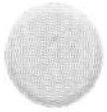
1 MG
PAGE 158

BUSPAR

10 MG
PAGE 162

CALAN SR
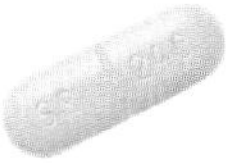
240 MG
PAGE 794

CAPOTEN

25 MG
PAGE 181

CARAFATE
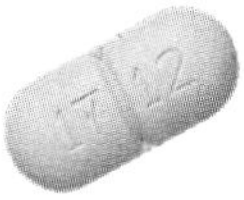
1 GRAM
PAGE 710

CARBAMAZEPINE

200 MG
PAGE 183

CARDIZEM CD
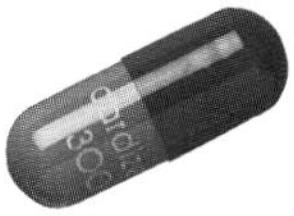
300 MG
PAGE 186

CARDURA
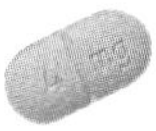
4 MG
PAGE 297

CARISOPRODOL
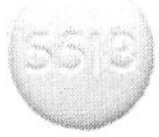
350 MG
PAGE 187

CATAPRES

0.2 MG
PAGE 237

CECLOR
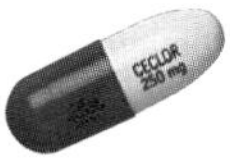

250 MG
PAGE 192

CEDAX
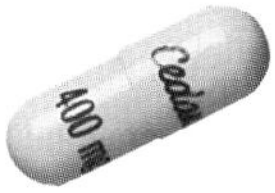
400 MG
PAGE 192

CEFACLOR	CEFTIN	CEFZIL	CEPHALEXIN
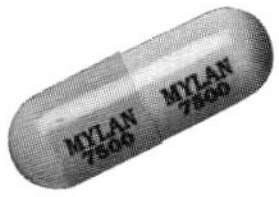	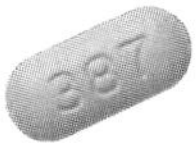	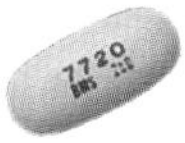	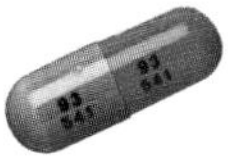
500 mg	250 mg	250 mg	250 mg
Page 192	Page 192	Page 192	Page 192
CIMETIDINE	CIPRO	CLARITIN	CLARITIN-D 12 HOUR
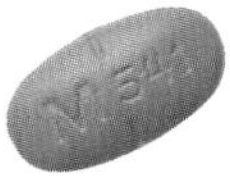	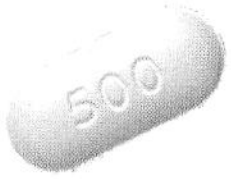		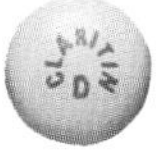
800 mg	500 mg	10 mg	5 mg loratadine/ 120 mg pseudoephedrine
Page 220	Page 225	Page 228	Page 229
CLONIDINE	COLCHICINE	COUMADIN	COZAAR
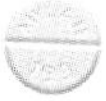		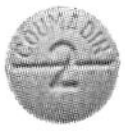	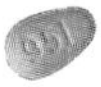
0.3 mg	0.6 mg	2 mg	25 mg
Page 237	Page 247	Page 260	Page 484
CYCLOBENZAPRINE	CYCRIN	DARVOCET-N 100	DAYPRO
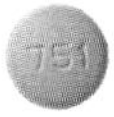	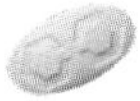	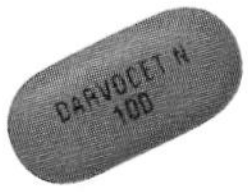	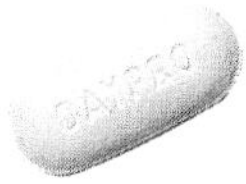
10 mg	100 mg	100 mg propoxyphene napsylate /650 mg acetaminophen	600 mg
Page 264	Page 644	Page 640	Page 573
DELTASONE	DEMULEN 1/35	DEPAKENE	DESOGEN
		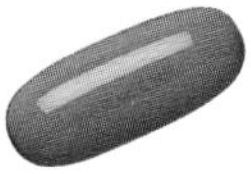	
10 mg	1 mg ethynodiol diacetate/ 35 mcg ethinyl estradiol	250 mg	0.15 mg desogestrel/ 0.03 mg ethinyl estradiol
Page 630	Page 318	Page 784	Page 318
DIABETA	DIAZEPAM	DICLOFENAC SODIUM	DICYCLOMINE
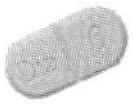		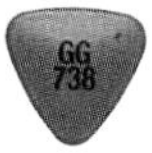	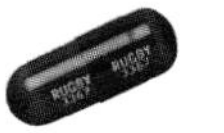
5 mg	5 mg	50 mg	10 mg
Page 381	Page 278	Page 280	Page 281

DIFLUCAN

200 MG
PAGE 343

DILACOR XR

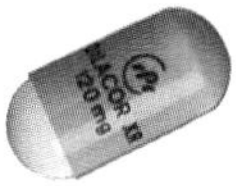

120 MG
PAGE 287

DILANTIN

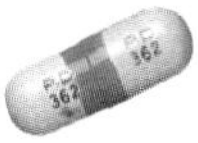

100 MG
PAGE 285

DORYX

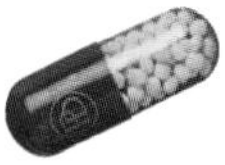

100 MG
PAGE 299

DOXYCYCLINE

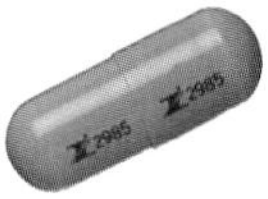

100 MG
PAGE 299

DYAZIDE

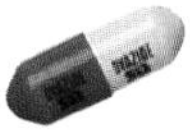

25 MG HYDROCHLOROTHIAZIDE/
37.5 MG TRIAMTERENE
PAGE 759

EFFEXOR

100 MG
PAGE 792

ELAVIL

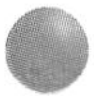

10 MG
PAGE 49

ENTEX LA

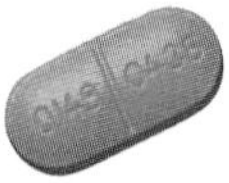

75 MG PHENYLPROPANOLAMINE/
400 MG GUAIFENESIN
PAGE 605

EPIVIR

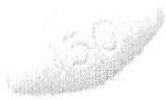

150 MG
PAGE 27

ERY-TAB

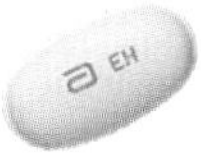

333 MG
PAGE 314

ERYTHROCIN STEARATE

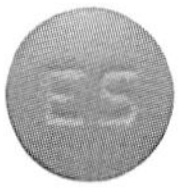

250 MG
PAGE 314

ESTRACE TABS

2 MG
PAGE 316

FIORINAL WITH CODEINE

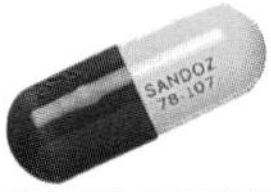

MULTIPLE INGREDIENTS
PAGE 341

FLEXERIL

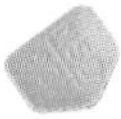

10 MG
PAGE 264

FLOXIN

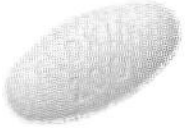

250 MG
PAGE 560

FOSAMAX

10 MG
PAGE 32

FUROSEMIDE

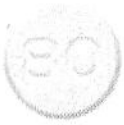

80 MG
PAGE 356

GEMFIBROZIL

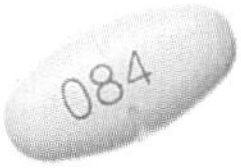

600 MG
PAGE 365

GENORA 1/35

1 MG NORETHINDRONE/
35 MCG ETHINYL ESTRADIOL
PAGE 318

GLIPIZIDE

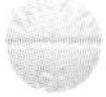

5 MG
PAGE 376

GLUCOPHAGE

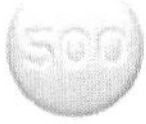

500 MG
PAGE 377

GLUCOTROL XL

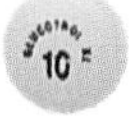

10 MG
PAGE 380

GLYBURIDE

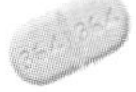

5 MG
PAGE 381

GLYNASE PRESTAB

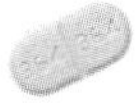

3 MG

PAGE 381

HISMANAL

10 MG

PAGE 103

HYDROCHLOROTHIAZIDE

25 MG

PAGE 402

HYDROCODONE/APAP

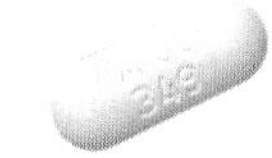

5 MG HYDROCODONE/
500 MG ACETAMINOPHEN

PAGE 404

HYTRIN

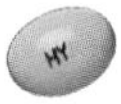

2 MG

PAGE 413

HYZAAR

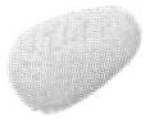

50 MG LOSARTAN/
12.5 MG HYDROCHLOROTHIAZIDE

PAGE 484

IBUPROFEN

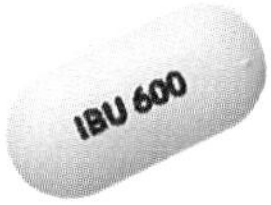

600 MG

PAGE 414

IMDUR

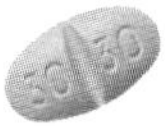

30 MG

PAGE 427

IMITREX

25 MG

PAGE 719

IMODIUM

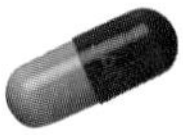

2 MG

PAGE 478

K-DUR

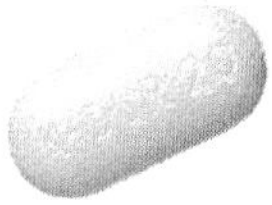

20 MEQ

PAGE 434

KEFTAB

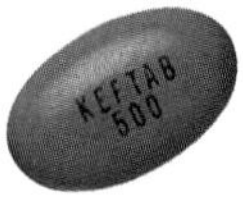

500 MG

PAGE 192

KLONOPIN

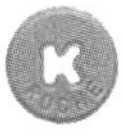

1 MG

PAGE 444

KLOR-CON

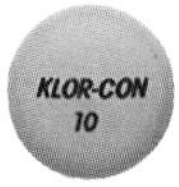

10 MEQ

PAGE 626

LANOXIN

0.125 MG

PAGE 448

LASIX

20 MG

PAGE 452

LESCOL

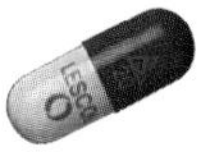

20 MG

PAGE 351

LEVORA

0.15 MG LEVONORGESTREL/
30 MCG ETHINYL ESTRADIOL

PAGE 318

LEVOXYL

0.05 MG

PAGE 466

LODINE

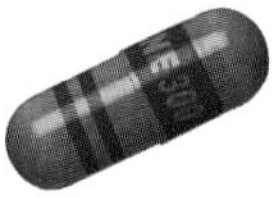

300 MG

PAGE 321

LOESTRIN 1/5/30

1.5 MG NORETHINDRONE/
30 MCG ETHINYL ESTRADIOL

PAGE 318

LO/OVRAL

0.3 MG NORGESTREL/
30 MCG ETHINYL ESTRADIOL

PAGE 318

LOPID

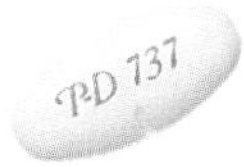

600 MG

PAGE 365

LOPRESSOR

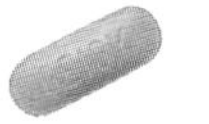

50 MG

PAGE 511

COLOR GUIDE TO PRESCRIPTION DRUGS & HERBS

LORABID 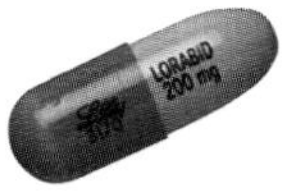 200 MG PAGE 479	LORAZEPAM  0.5 MG PAGE 482	LORCET PLUS  7.5 MG HYDROCODONE/ 650 MG ACETAMINOPHEN PAGE 404	LORCET 10/650 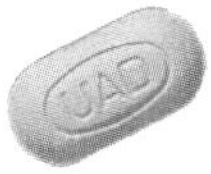 10 MG HYDROCODONE/ 650 MG ACETAMINOPHEN PAGE 404
LOTENSIN 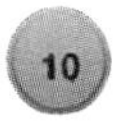 10 MG PAGE 486	LOZOL  2.5 MG PAGE 416	MACROBID 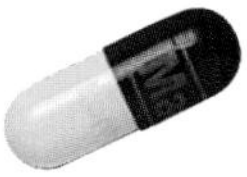 75 MG NITROFURANTOIN MONO- HYDRATE/25 MG MACROCRYSTALS PAGE 547	MEDROXYPROGES- TERONE TABS 20 MG PAGE 644
METHYLPHENIDATE  10 MG PAGE 506	METHYLPREDNISO- LONE TABS 4 MG PAGE 508	METOPROLOL TARTRATE 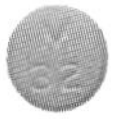 50 MG PAGE 511	MEVACOR 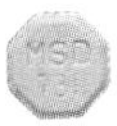 20 MG PAGE 512
MICRO-K 10 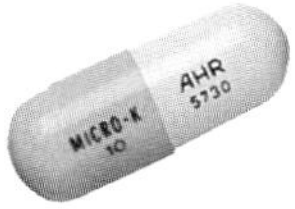 10 MEQ PAGE 626	MICRONASE  5 MG PAGE 381	MONOPRIL 10 MG PAGE 353	MOTRIN  600 MG PAGE 414
NAPROSYN 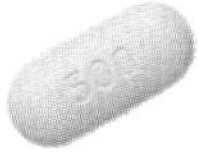 500 MG PAGE 533	NAPROXEN  500 MG PAGE 533	NITROSTAT  0.4 MG PAGE 549	NIZORAL 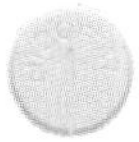 200 MG PAGE 438
NORTRIPTYLINE 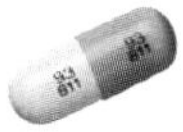 25 MG PAGE 554	NORVASC  5 MG PAGE 555	ORTHO-CEPT  0.15 MG DESOGESTREL/ 30 MCG ETHINYL ESTRADIOL PAGE 318	ORTHO-CYCLEN  0.25 MG NORGESTIMATE/ 35 MCG ETHINYL ESTRADIOL PAGE 318

ORTHO-NOVUM 1/35

1 MG NORETHINDRONE/ 35 MCG ETHINYL ESTRADIOL

PAGE 569

ORTHO-NOVUM 7/7/7

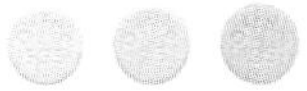

NORETHINDRONE AND ETHINYL ESTRADIOL IN DIFFERENT DOSAGES

PAGE 569

ORTHO TRI-CYCLEN

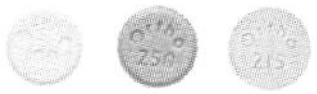

NORGESTIMATE AND ETHINYL ESTRADIOL IN DIFFERENT DOSAGES

PAGE 318

ORUVAIL

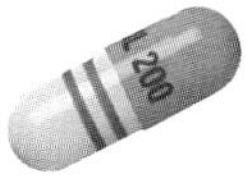

200 MG

PAGE 440

PAXIL

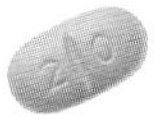

20 MG

PAGE 583

PEPCID

20 MG

PAGE 331

PHENERGAN

25 MG

PAGE 639

PHENTERMINE

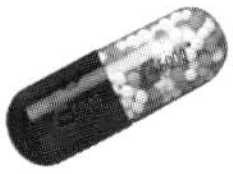

30 MG

PAGE 602

PHENYLPROPANOL-AMINE/GUAIFENESIN

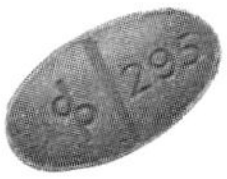

75 MG PHENYLPROPANOLAMINE/ 400 MG GUAIFENESIN

PAGE 605

PONDIMIN

20 MG

PAGE 333

POTASSIUM CHLORIDE

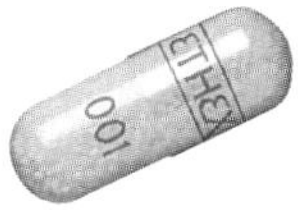

10 MEQ

PAGE 626

PRAVACHOL

20 MG

PAGE 628

PREDNISONE ORAL

5 MG

PAGE 630

PREMARIN TABS

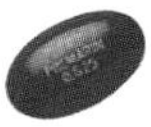

0.625 MG

PAGE 632

PREMPRO

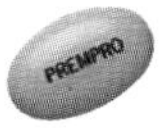

0.625 MG CONJUGATED ESTROGENS/ 2.5 MG MEDROXYPROGESTERONE

PAGE 633

PREVACID

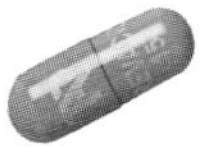

15 MG

PAGE 450

PRILOSEC

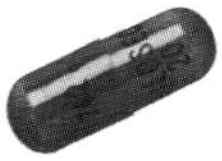

20 MG

PAGE 634

PRINCIPEN

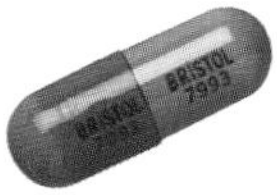

500 MG

PAGE 54

PRINIVIL

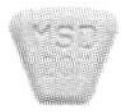

20 MG

PAGE 635

PROCARDIA XL

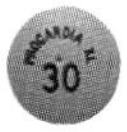

30 MG

PAGE 637

PROPOXYPHENE HCL/ APAP

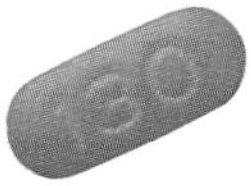

65 MG PROPOXYPHENE HCL/ 650 MG ACETAMINOPHEN

PAGE 640

PROPOXYPHENE NAPSYLATE /ACETAMINOPHEN

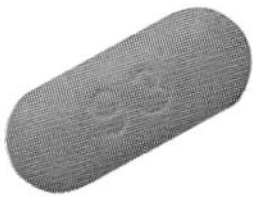

100 MG PROPOXYPHENE NAPSYLATE /650 MG ACETAMINOPHEN

PAGE 640

PROPULSID

10 MG

PAGE 226

PROVERA

5 MG

PAGE 644

COLOR GUIDE TO PRESCRIPTION DRUGS & HERBS

PROZAC
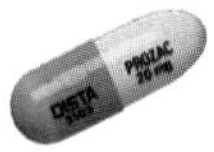
20 MG
PAGE 645

RELAFEN
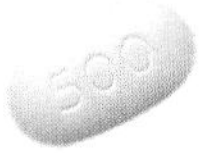
50 MG
PAGE 657

RESTORIL
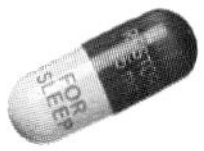
15 MG
PAGE 732

RETROVIR
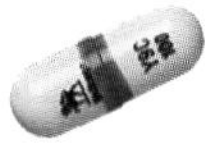
100 MG
PAGE 27

RISPERDAL

1 MG
PAGE 659

RITALIN

5 MG
PAGE 661

ROXICET
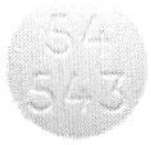
5 MG OXYCODONE/
325 MG ACETAMINOPHEN
PAGE 574

SELDANE

60 MG
PAGE 737

SELDANE-D

60 MG TERFENADINE/
10 MG PSEUDOEPHEDRINE
PAGE 737

SLOW-K
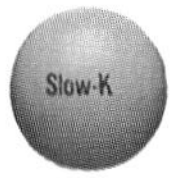

8 MEQ
PAGE 626

SOMA

350 MG
PAGE 187

SULFAMETHOXAZOLE/ TRIMETHOPRIM
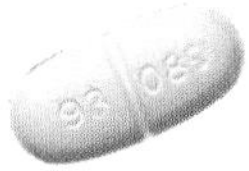
800 MG SULFAMETHOXAZOLE/
160 MG TRIMETHOPRIM
PAGE 712

SUMYCIN
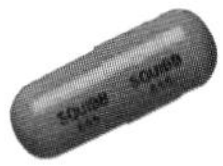
250 MG TETRACYCLINE
PAGE 738

SUPRAX
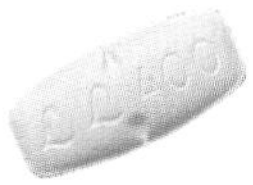
400 MG
PAGE 192

SYNTHROID

100 MCG
PAGE 723

TAGAMET
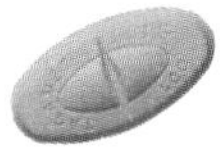
400 MG
PAGE 220

TEGRETOL
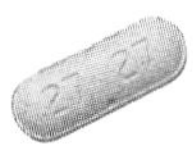
200 MG
PAGE 183

TEMAZEPAM
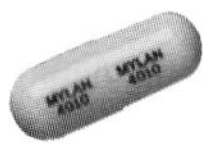
15 MG
PAGE 732

TENORMIN

50 MG
PAGE 108

THEO-DUR
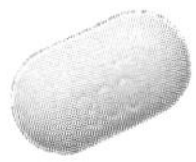
300 MG
PAGE 740

TOPROL-XL
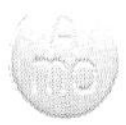
50 MG
PAGE 511

TORADOL ORAL
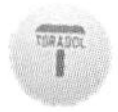
10 MG
PAGE 442

TRENTAL
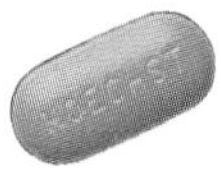
400 MG
PAGE 589

TRI-LEVLEN
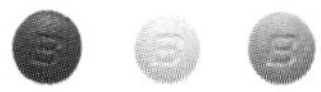
LEVONORGESTREL AND ETHINYL ESTRADIOL IN DIFFERENT DOSAGES
PAGE 318

COLOR GUIDE TO PRESCRIPTION DRUGS & HERBS

TRIAMTERENE/HCTZ

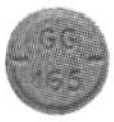

37.5 MG TRIAMTERENE/
25 MG HYDROCHLOROTHIAZIDE

PAGE 759

TRIMOX

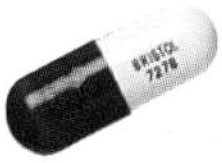

250 MG

PAGE 765

TRIPHASIL

LEVONORGESTREL AND ETHINYL
ESTRADIOL IN DIFFERENT DOSAGES

PAGE 766

ULTRAM

50 MG

PAGE 773

VALIUM

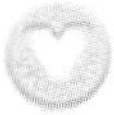

2 MG

PAGE 782

VALTREX

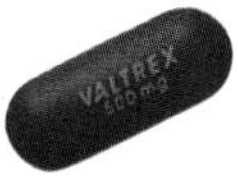

500 MG

PAGE 780

VASOTEC

5 MG

PAGE 789

VEETIDS

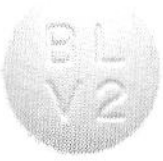

500 MG

PAGE 790

VENTOLIN TABLETS

2 MG

PAGE 793

VERAPAMIL SR

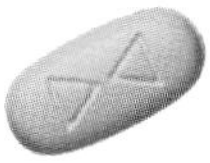

240 MG

PAGE 794

VERELAN

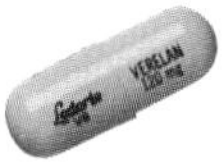

120 MG

PAGE 794

VICODIN

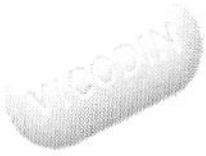

5 MG HYDROCODONE/
500 MG ACETAMINOPHEN

PAGE 795

VOLTAREN

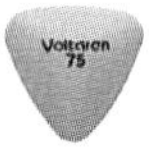

75 MG

PAGE 280

XANAX

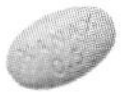

0.5 MG

PAGE 42

ZANTAC 150

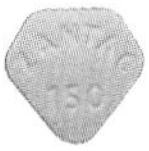

150 MG

PAGE 822

ZESTRIL

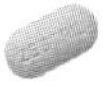

5 MG

PAGE 823

ZIAC

2.5 MG

PAGE 142

ZITHROMAX

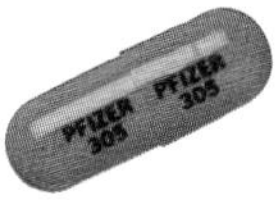

250 MG

PAGE 829

ZOCOR

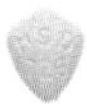

5 MG

PAGE 830

ZOLOFT

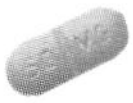

50 MG

PAGE 831

ZOVIA 1/35

1 MG ETHYNODIOL DIACETATE/
35 MCG ETHINYL ESTRADIOL

PAGE 318

ZOVIRAX

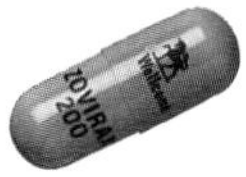

200 MG

PAGE 25

ZYRTEC

10 MG

PAGE 194

Herbs

The following are 50 commonly used herbs shown in their plant form.

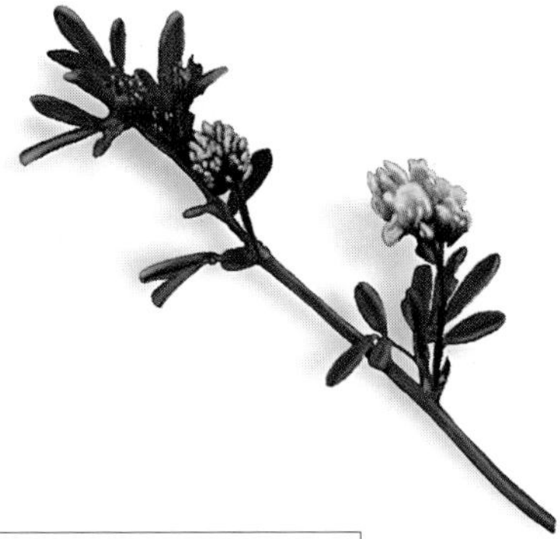

ALFALFA
Medicago sativa
PAGE 34

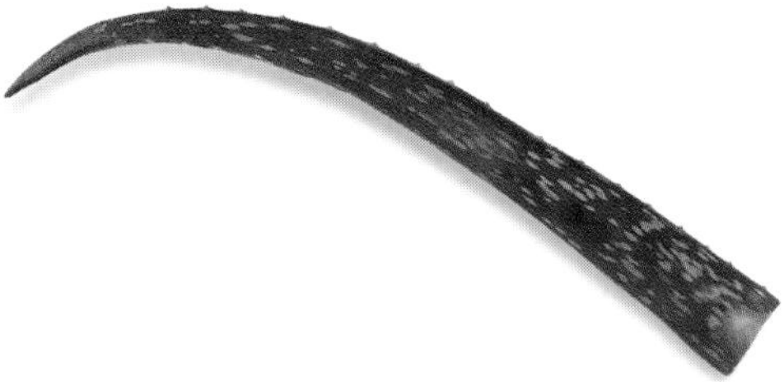

ALOE
Aloe barbadensis
PAGE 39

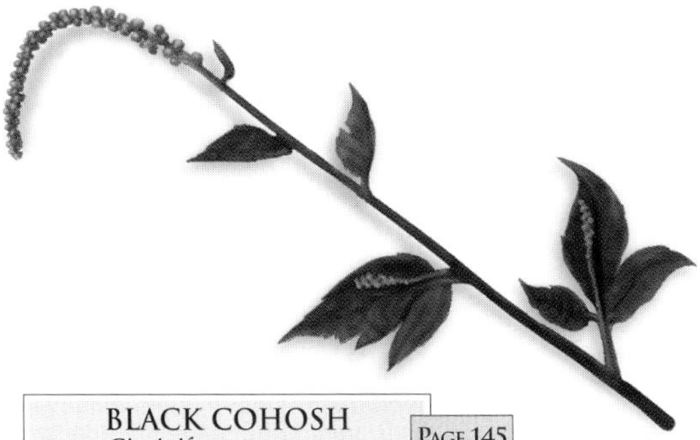

BLACK COHOSH
Cimicifuga racemosa
PAGE 145

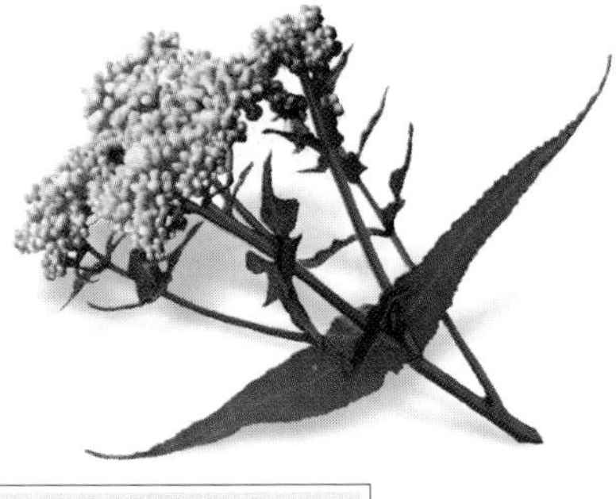

BONESET
Eupatorium perfoliatum
PAGE 150

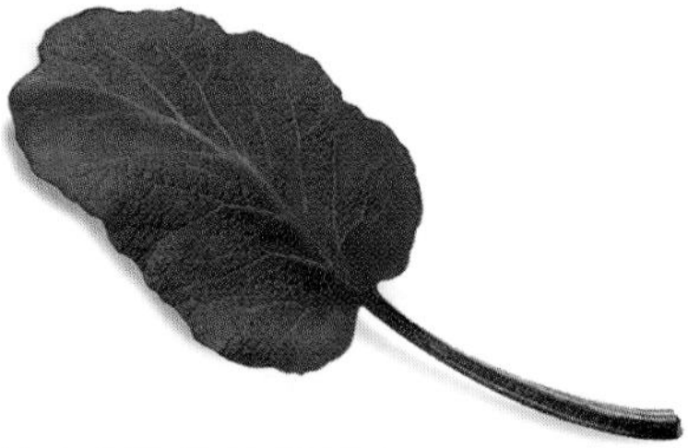

BURDOCK
Arctium lappa
PAGE 161

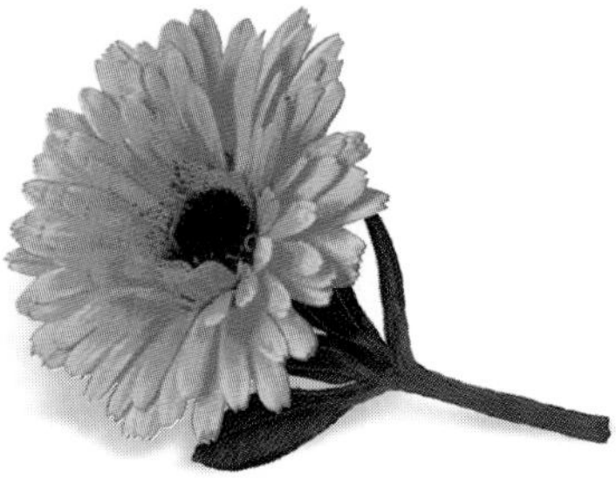

CALENDULA
Calendula officinalis
PAGE 176

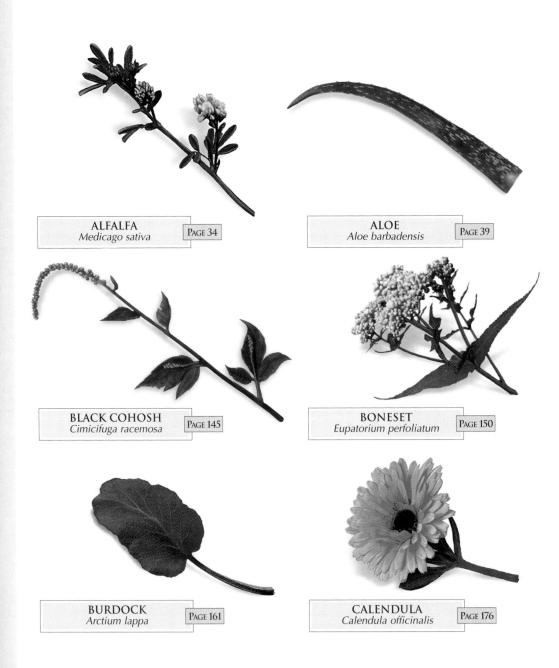

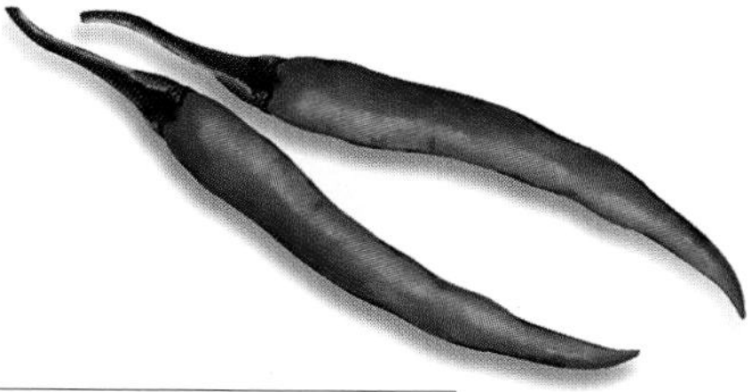

CAYENNE
Capsicum annuum var. annuum
PAGE 191

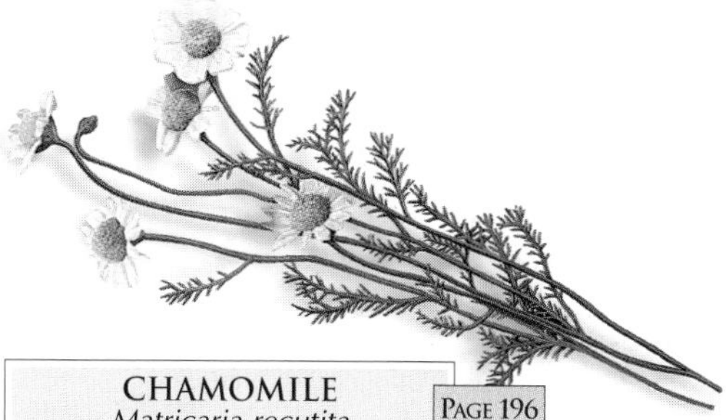

CHAMOMILE
Matricaria recutita
PAGE 196

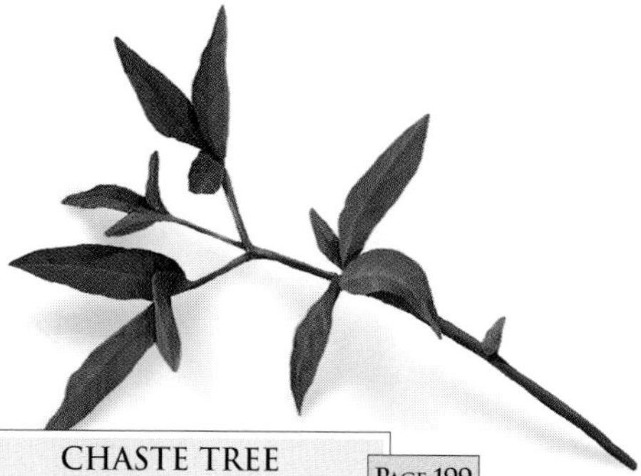

CHASTE TREE
Vitex agnus-castus
PAGE 199

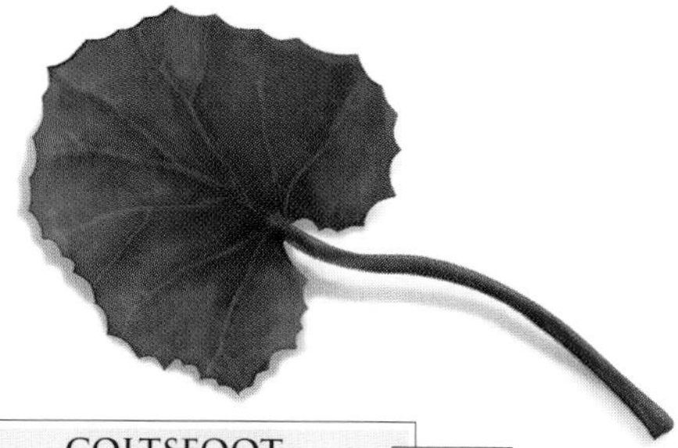

COLTSFOOT
Tussilago farfara
PAGE 251

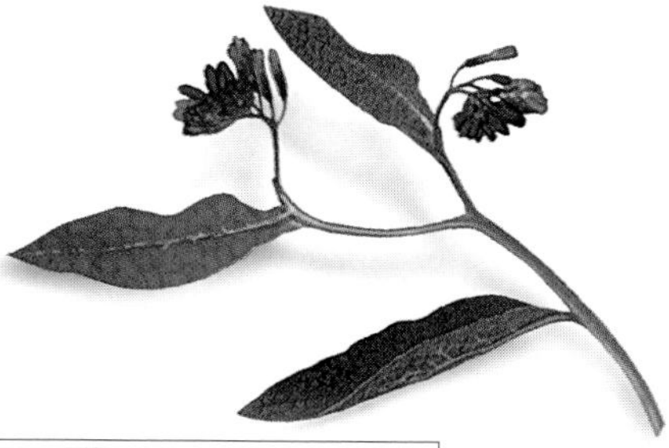

COMFREY
Symphytum officinale
PAGE 252

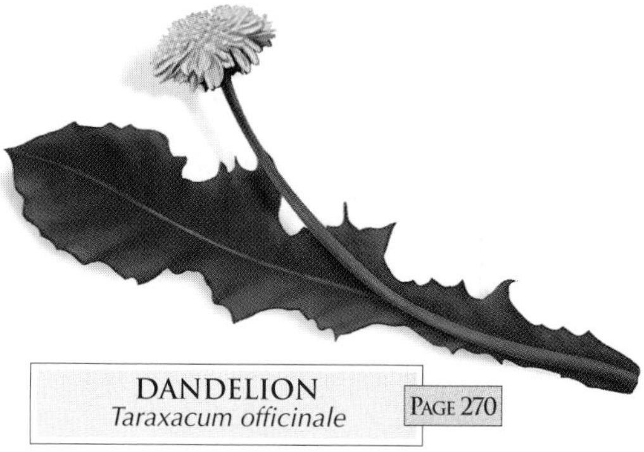

DANDELION
Taraxacum officinale
PAGE 270

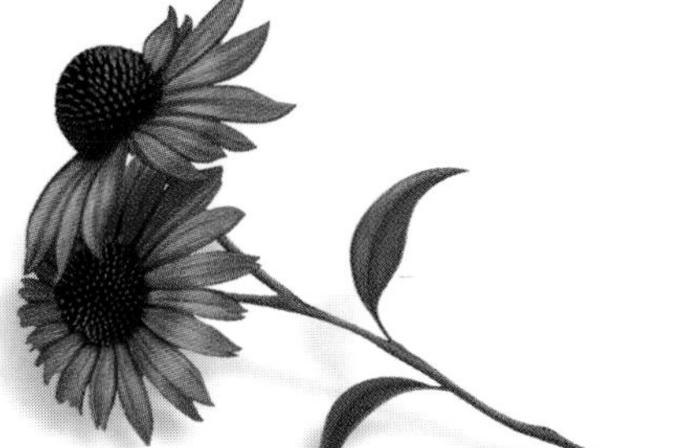

ECHINACEA
Echinacea spp.
PAGE 304

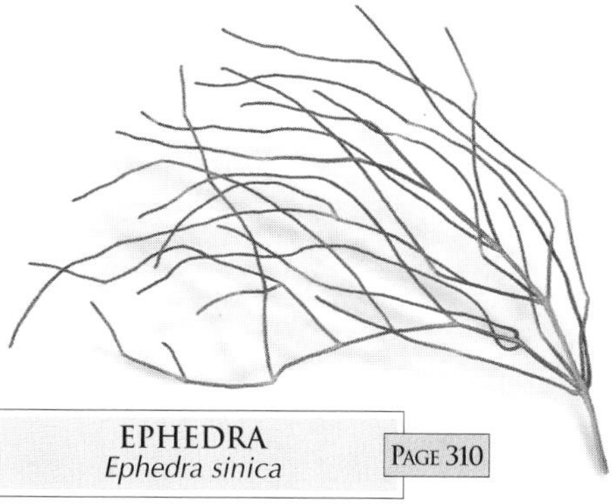

EPHEDRA
Ephedra sinica
PAGE 310

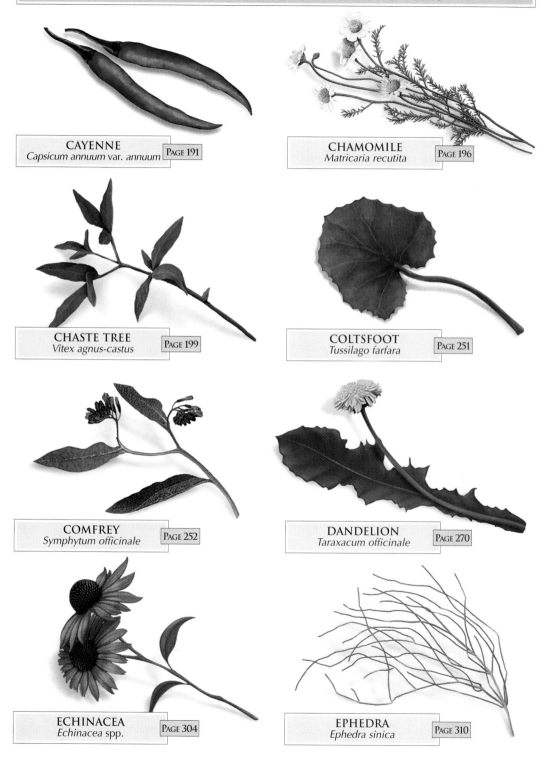

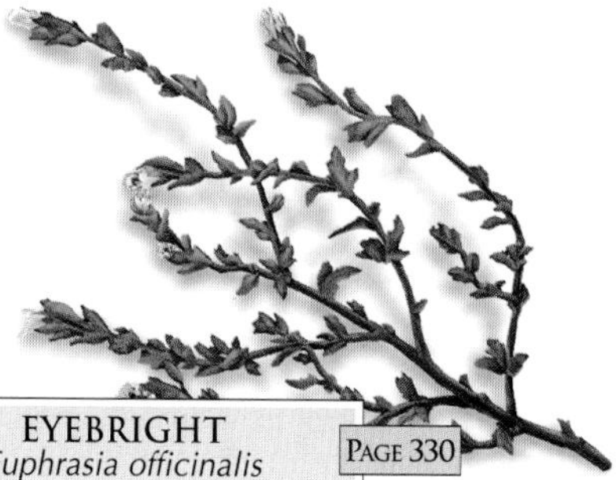

EYEBRIGHT
Euphrasia officinalis
PAGE 330

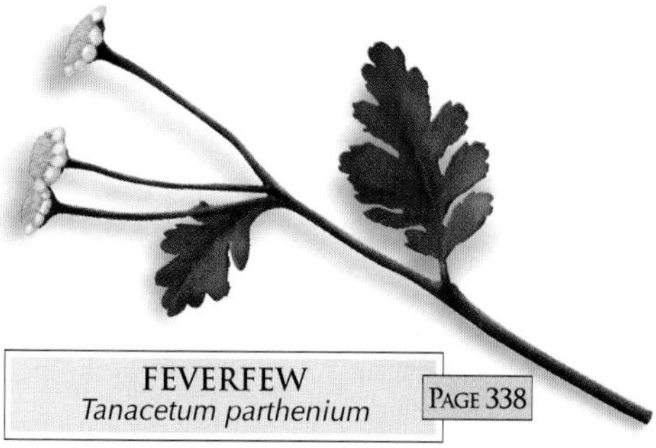

FEVERFEW
Tanacetum parthenium
PAGE 338

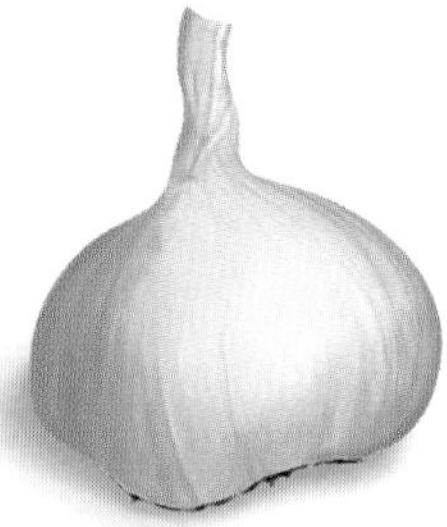

GARLIC
Allium sativum
PAGE 362

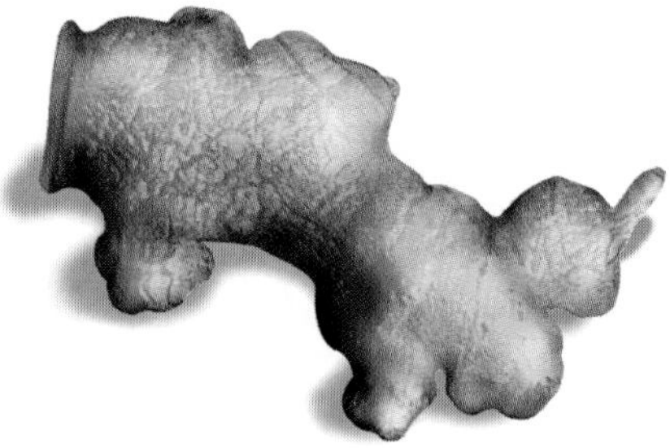

GINGER
Zingiber officinale
PAGE 370

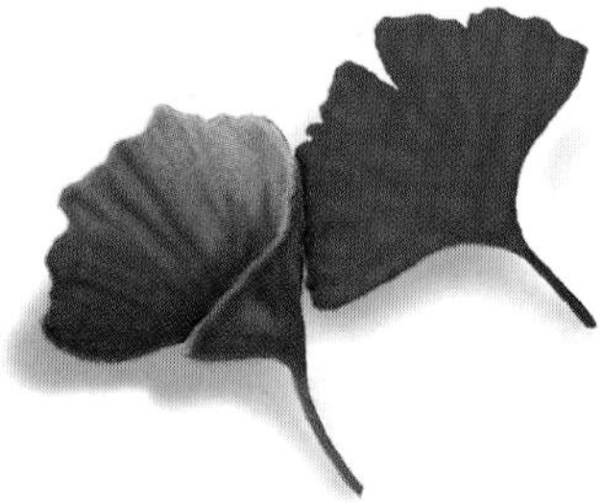

GINKGO
Ginkgo biloba
PAGE 371

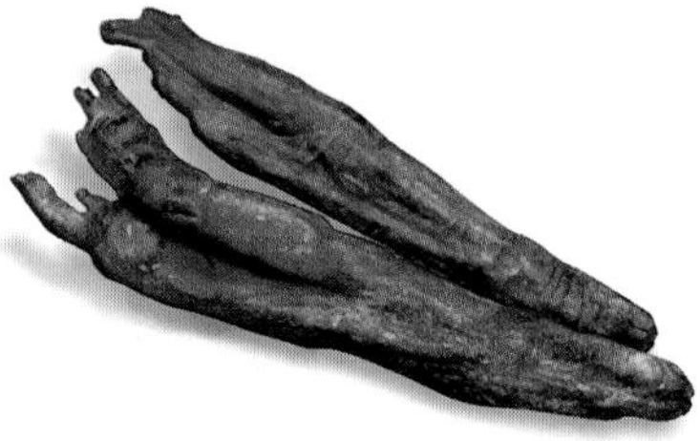

GINSENG
Panax ginseng
PAGE 373

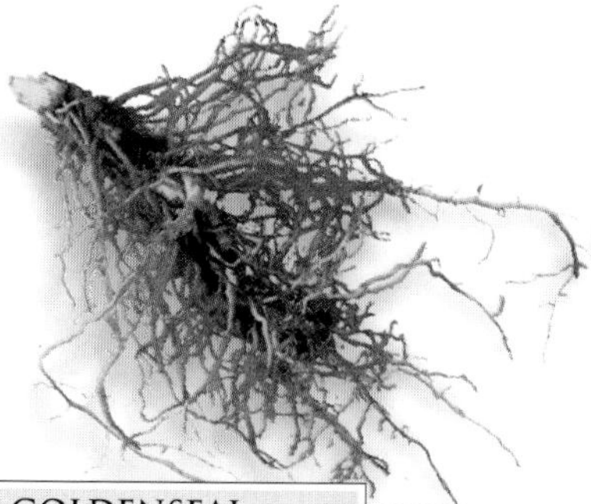

GOLDENSEAL
Hydrastis canadensis
PAGE 382

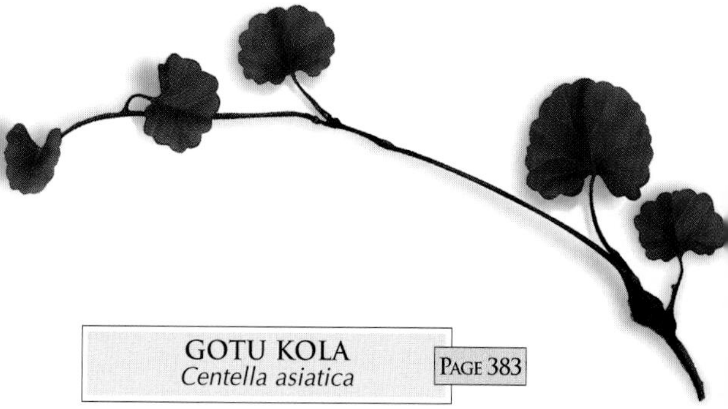

GOTU KOLA
Centella asiatica
PAGE 383

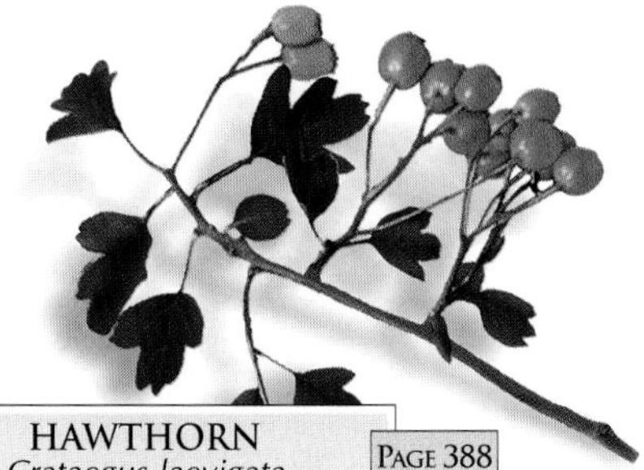

HAWTHORN
Crataegus laevigata
PAGE 388

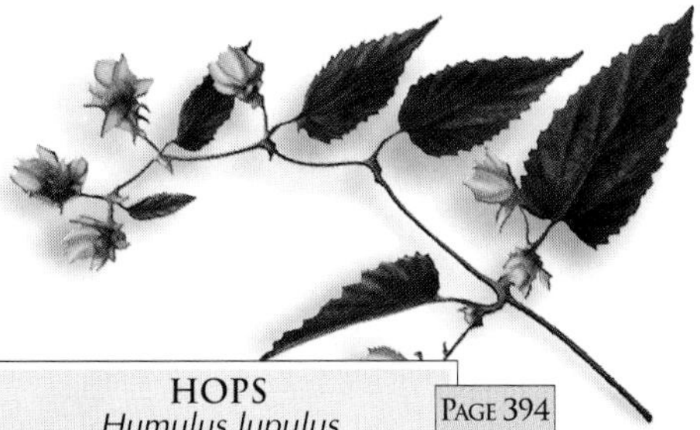

HOPS
Humulus lupulus
PAGE 394

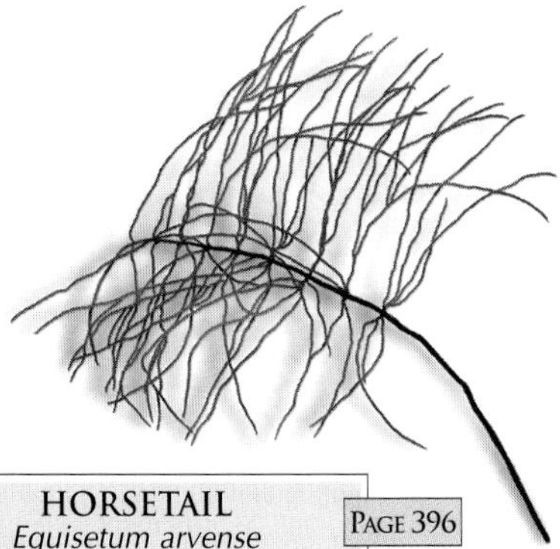

HORSETAIL
Equisetum arvense
PAGE 396

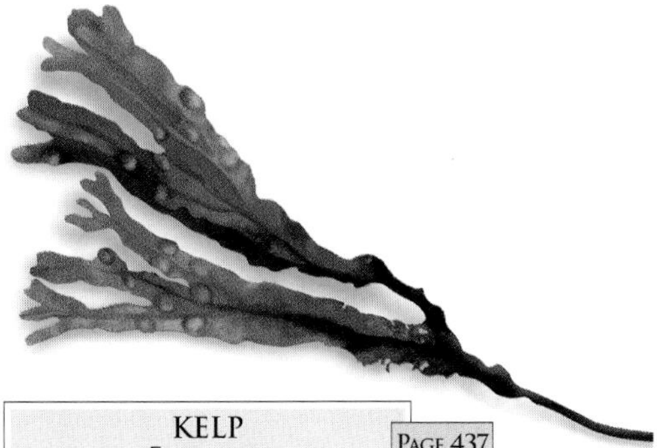

KELP
Fucus spp.
PAGE 437

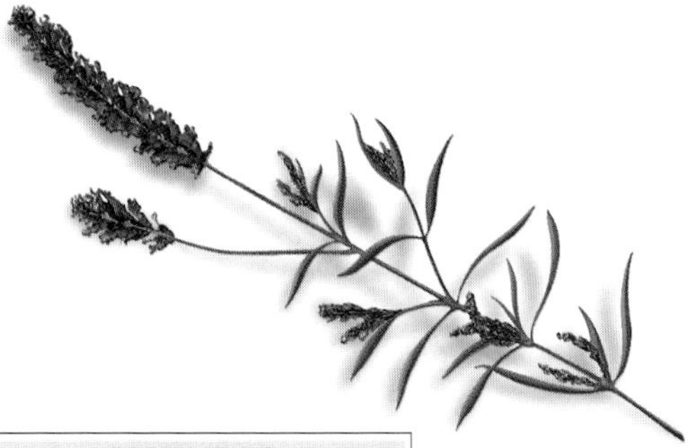

LAVENDER
Lavandula officinalis
PAGE 454

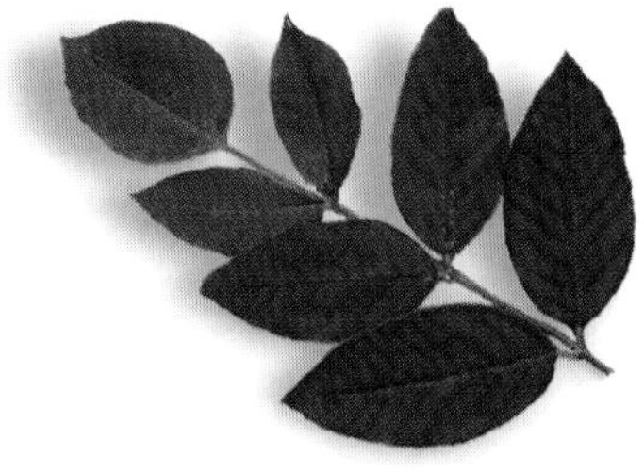

LICORICE
Glycyrrhiza glabra
PAGE 469

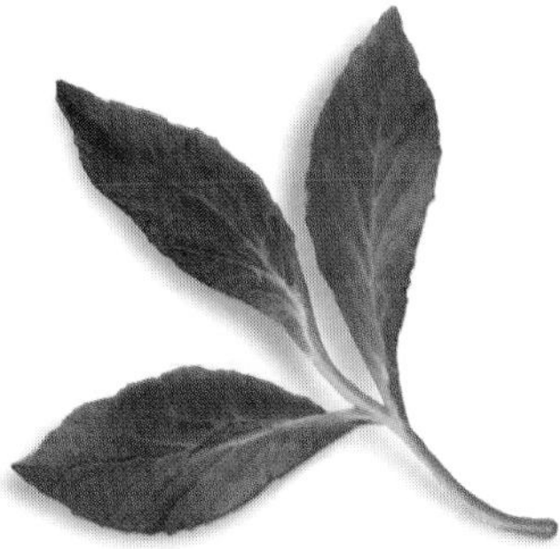

LOBELIA
Lobelia inflata
PAGE 476

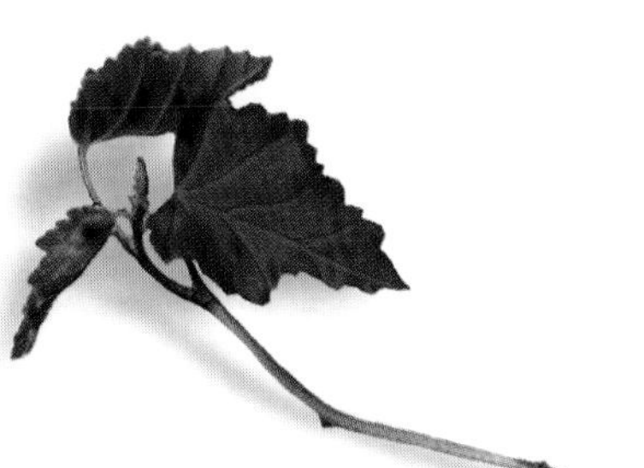

MARSH MALLOW
Althaea officinalis
PAGE 497

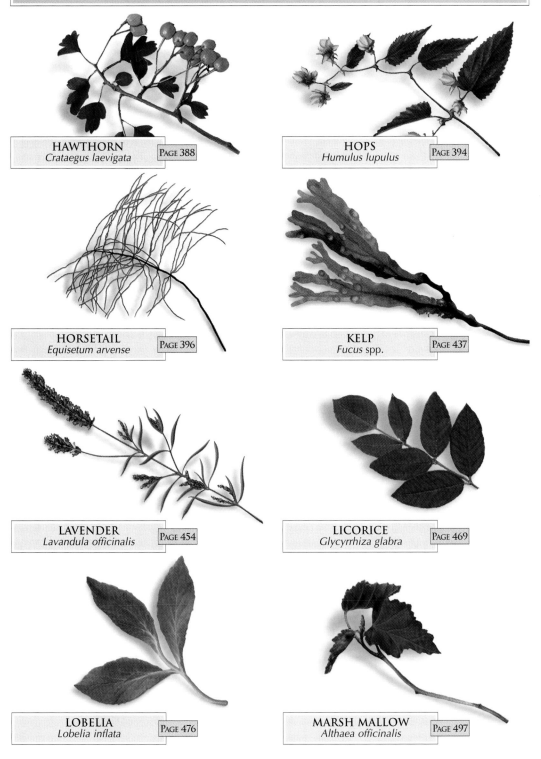

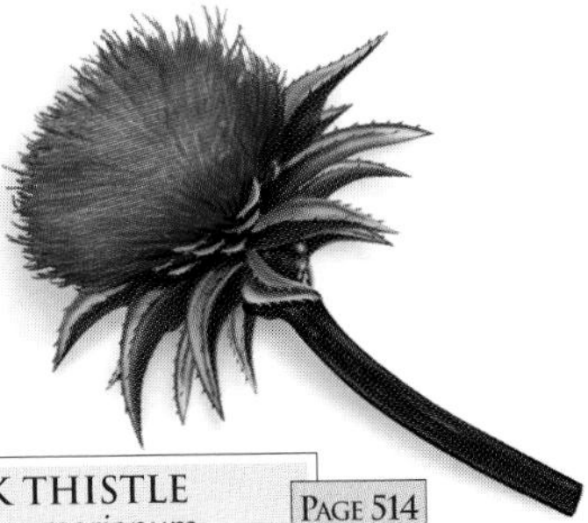

MILK THISTLE
Silybum marianum
PAGE 514

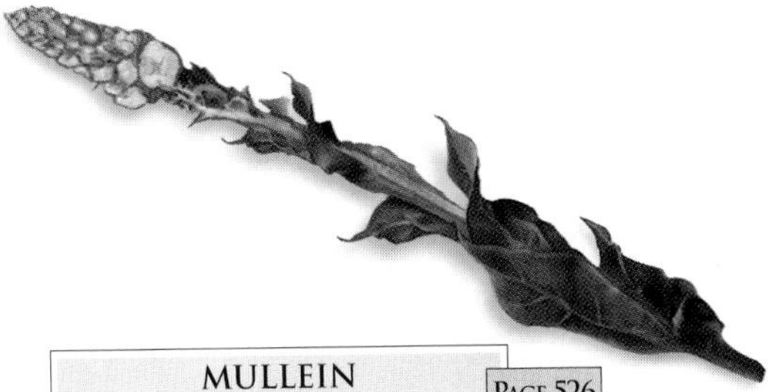

MULLEIN
Verbascum thapsus
PAGE 526

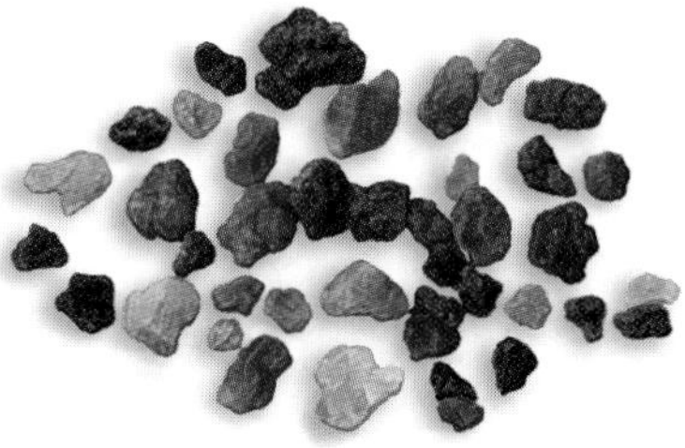

MYRRH
Commiphora molmol
PAGE 530

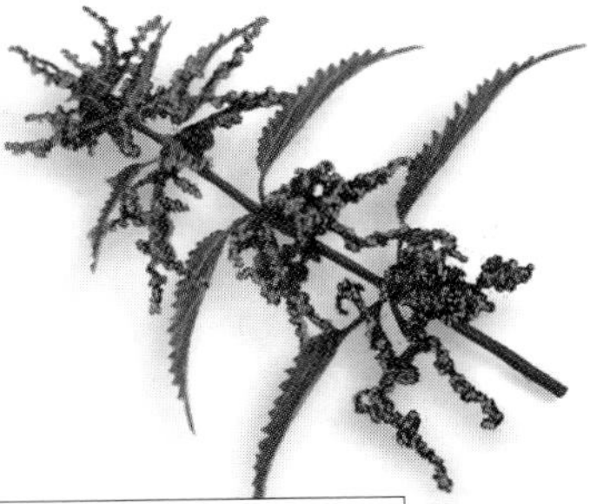

NETTLE
Urtica dioica
PAGE 538

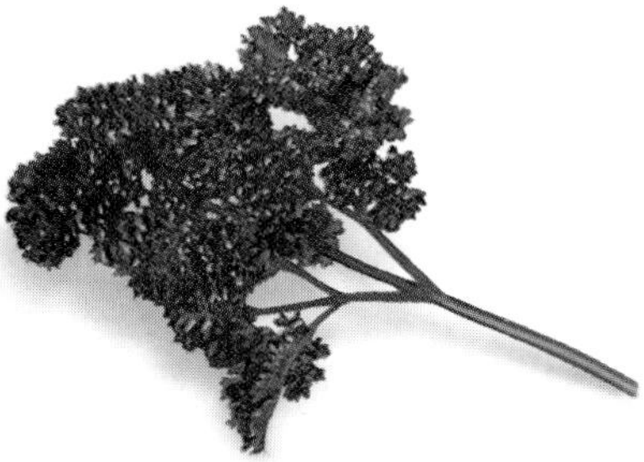

PARSLEY
Petroselinum crispum
PAGE 579

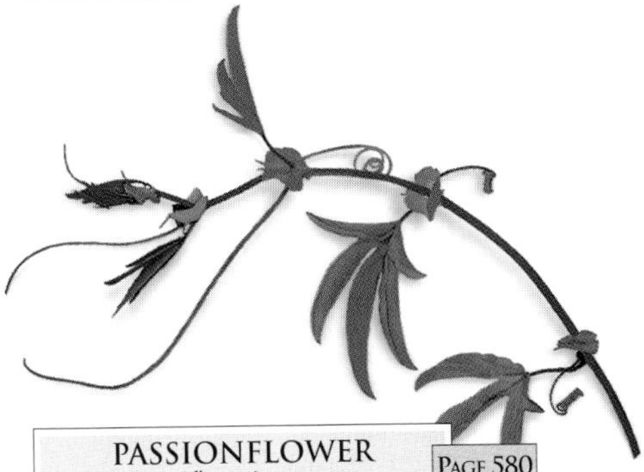

PASSIONFLOWER
Passiflora incarnata
PAGE 580

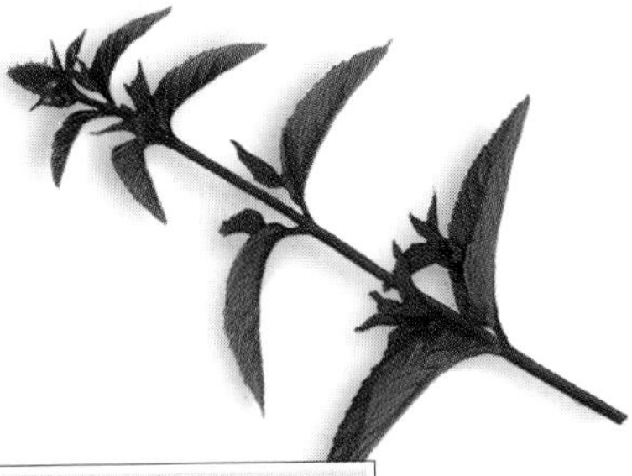

PEPPERMINT
Mentha x piperita
PAGE 594

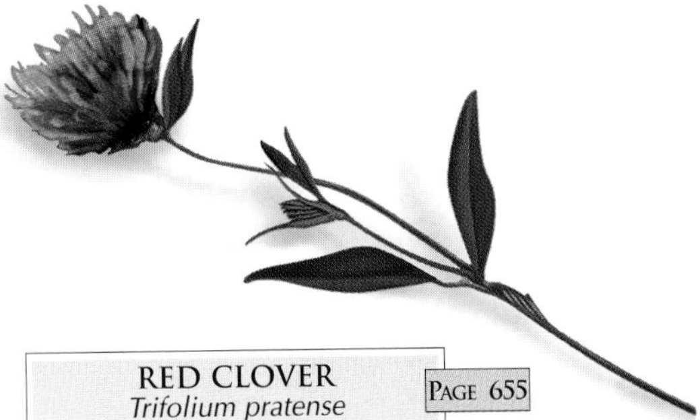

RED CLOVER
Trifolium pratense
PAGE 655

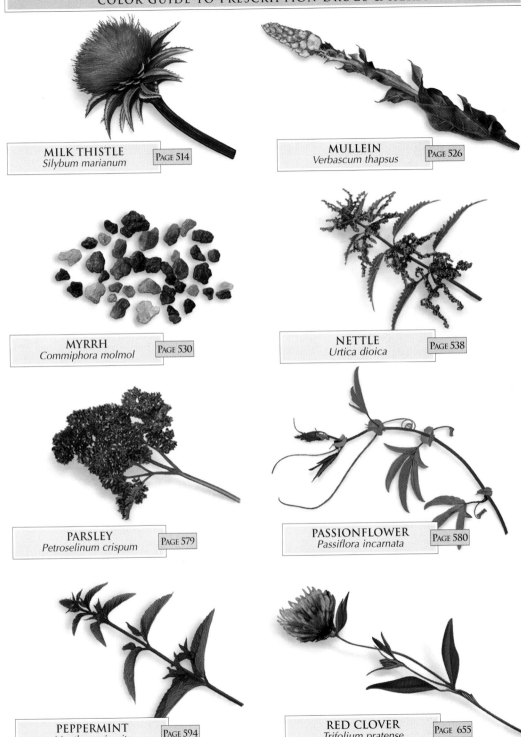

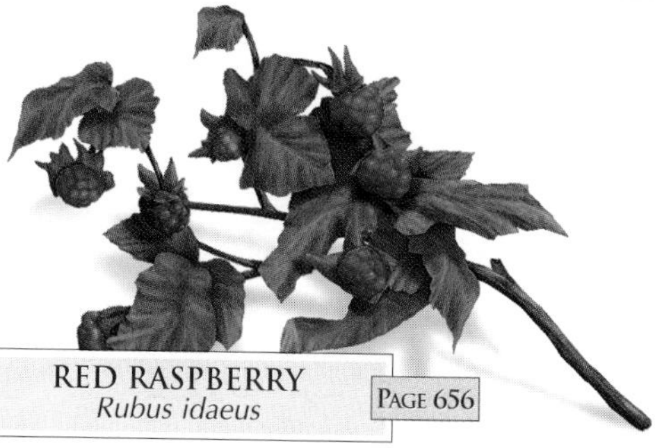

RED RASPBERRY
Rubus idaeus
PAGE 656

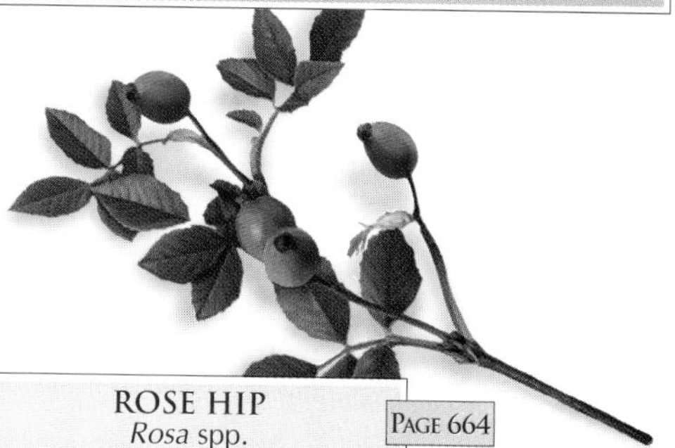

ROSE HIP
Rosa spp.
PAGE 664

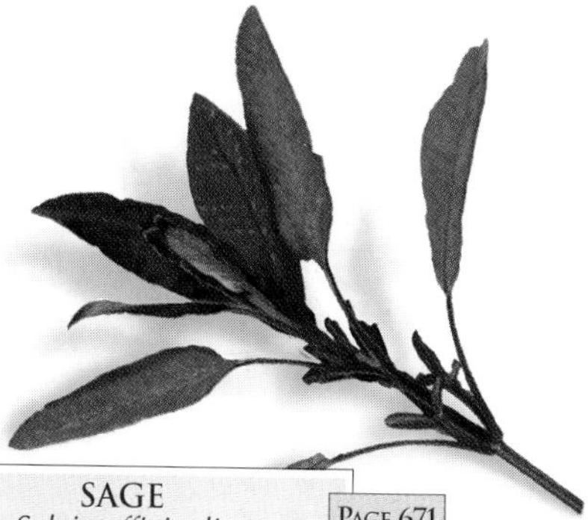

SAGE
Salvia officinalis
PAGE 671

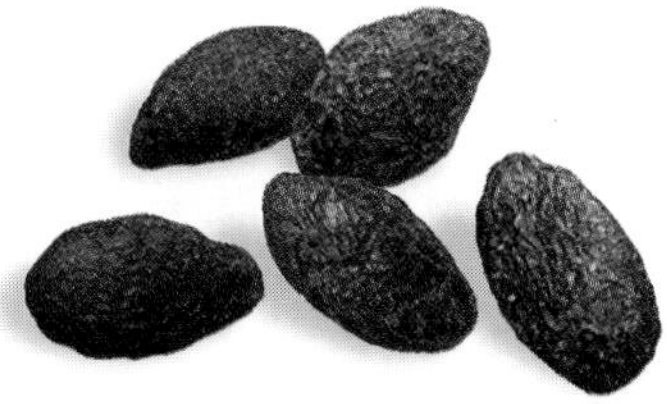

SAW PALMETTO
Serenoa repens
PAGE 677

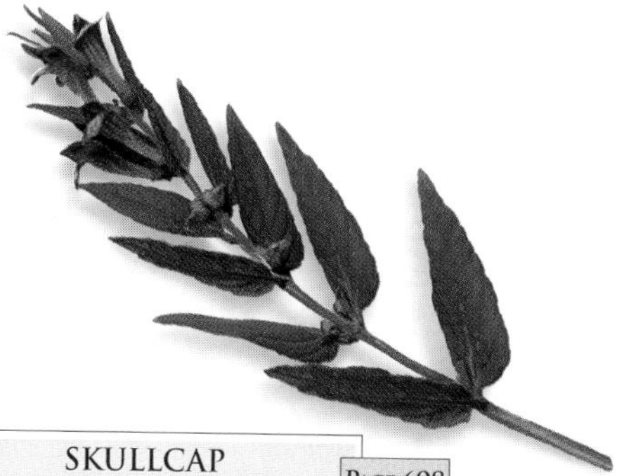

SKULLCAP
Scutellaria lateriflora
PAGE 698

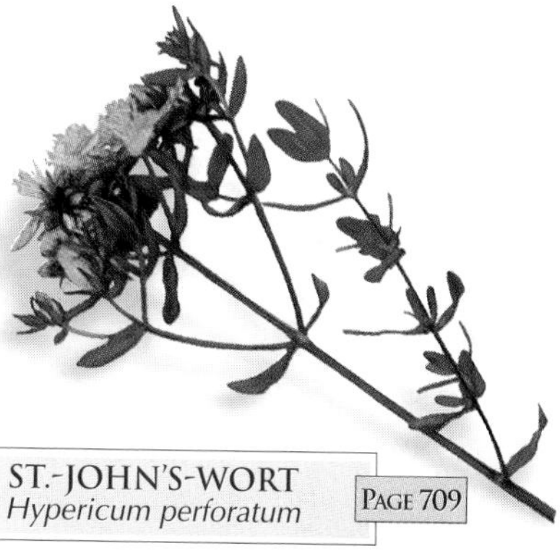

ST.-JOHN'S-WORT
Hypericum perforatum
PAGE 709

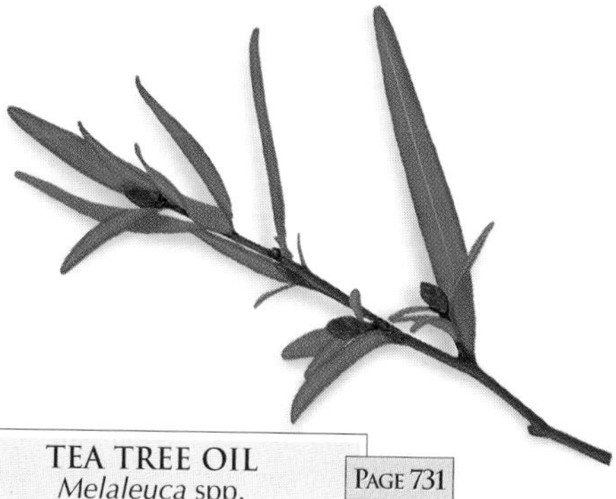

TEA TREE OIL
Melaleuca spp.
PAGE 731

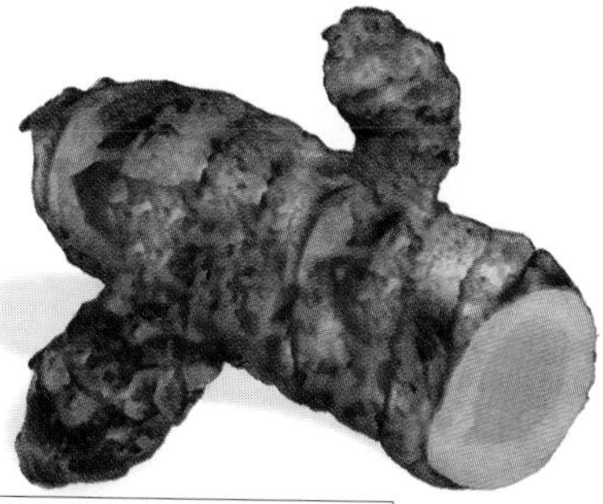

TURMERIC
Curcuma longa
PAGE 770

UVA URSI
Arctostaphylos uva-ursi
PAGE 778

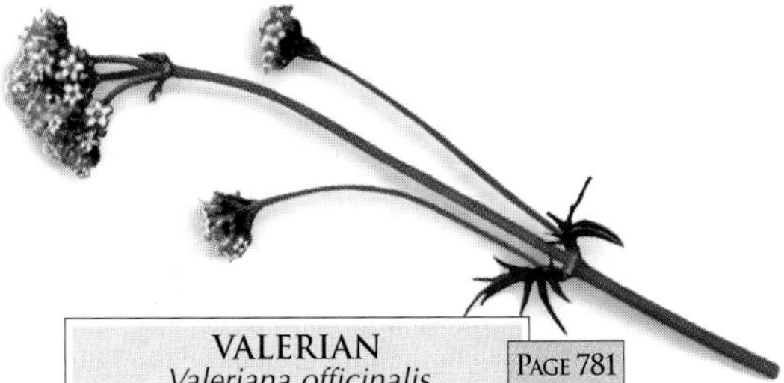

VALERIAN
Valeriana officinalis
PAGE 781

WILD YAM
Dioscorea villosa
PAGE 813

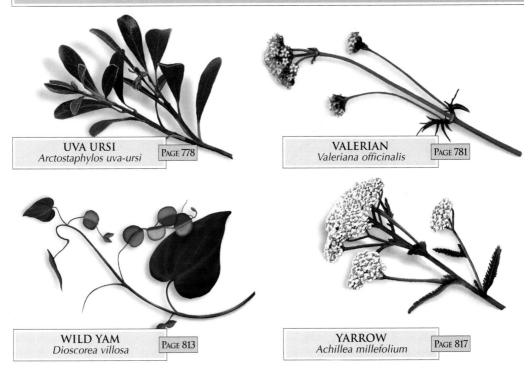

YARROW
Achillea millefolium
PAGE 817

KAVA

LATIN NAME
Piper methysticum

VITAL STATISTICS

GENERAL DESCRIPTION

Drinking kava, a beverage brewed from the dried roots and rhizomes of an indigenous pepper plant, has been a feature of some South Pacific religious rituals for many centuries. Today kava is frequently prescribed, for that same euphoric effect, as an antidepressant; practitioners find it useful for treating anxiety and tension. Because of its diuretic action, it is also used to treat gout and rheumatism. In addition, kava is believed to act as an antiseptic and anti-inflammatory agent in the urinary tract, making it suitable for treating urinary tract infections such as cystitis; it is also used for prostatitis (inflammation of the prostate gland) that may arise from bacteria traveling from the urethra.

Western herbalists recommend kava for its sedative properties, which do not seem to impair mental alertness. The active ingredients, called kavalactones, act on the stem and other parts of the brain to yield kava's mild tranquilizing effect. While kava compounds do not seem to be addictive, the herb still must be used with caution.

PREPARATIONS

Available in dry bulk, capsules, and tinctures. Consult a qualified practitioner for the dosage appropriate for you and the specific condition being treated.

PRECAUTIONS

☠ *WARNING*

Long-term, constant use of kava in large doses has been associated with damage to the liver, skin, eyes, and even the spinal cord.

SPECIAL INFORMATION

Use of this herb by children for more than seven to 10 days should be done in conjunction with a healthcare practitioner.

POSSIBLE INTERACTIONS

Combining kava with other herbs may necessitate a lower dosage.

TARGET AILMENTS

Take internally for:

- Urinary disorders
- Prostate inflammations
- Gout
- Rheumatism
- Insomnia; fatigue
- Depression
- Muscle spasms

SIDE EFFECTS

NOT SERIOUS

Chronic use can cause a type of dermatitis that will clear up when you stop taking kava.

SERIOUS

Too much kava can cause intoxication or drowsiness. If this happens, lower your dosage or stop taking kava.

K

K-DUR

VITAL STATISTICS

DRUG CLASS
Diuretics [Adjunct Therapy]

GENERIC NAME
potassium chloride

GENERAL DESCRIPTION
K-Dur is a brand name for potassium chloride, a mineral supplement prescribed for the prevention and treatment of potassium depletion. Such depletion usually results from the use of drugs known as nonpotassium-sparing diuretics, which promote the excretion of minerals through increased urine flow. For more information, see Diuretics. For visual characteristics, see the Color Guide to Prescription Drugs and Herbs.

PRECAUTIONS

SPECIAL INFORMATION
- Tell your doctor if you have stomach ulcers; K-Dur can cause stomach irritation.
- Do not use K-Dur if you are taking potassium-sparing diuretics or salt substitutes.

POSSIBLE INTERACTIONS
Angiotensin-converting enzyme (ACE) inhibitors: elevated potassium chloride levels.
Digoxin: increased digoxin levels.
Potassium-sparing diuretics (such as amiloride or triamterene): increased potassium chloride levels.

TARGET AILMENTS

Potassium depletion

SIDE EFFECTS

NOT SERIOUS

- Gastrointestinal upset (to help alleviate this discomfort, take the medication with meals)
- Muscle cramps

CALL YOUR DOCTOR IF THESE SYMPTOMS PERSIST OR BECOME BOTHERSOME.

SERIOUS

- Black stools (a symptom of gastrointestinal bleeding)
- Severe vomiting
- Heart-rhythm problems
- Mental confusion

IF YOU EXPERIENCE AN IRREGULAR HEARTBEAT OR FEEL CONFUSED, CALL YOUR DOCTOR IMMEDIATELY. ELEVATED POTASSIUM LEVELS IN THE BLOOD CAN ALSO CAUSE MUSCLE CRAMPS, A LESS SERIOUS SIDE EFFECT BUT ONE THAT ALSO WARRANTS CONSULTATION WITH YOUR DOCTOR.

KEFLEX

VITAL STATISTICS

DRUG CLASS
Antibiotics [Cephalosporins]

GENERIC NAME
cephalexin

OTHER DRUGS IN THIS SUBCLASS
cefaclor, cefadroxil, cefixime, cefprozil, ceftibuten, cefuroxime, cephalexin hydrochloride

GENERAL DESCRIPTION
Keflex is a brand name of the generic drug cephalexin, a cephalosporin antibiotic used to treat respiratory tract infections and ear infection (otitis media) as well as bacterial infections of the skin, bones and joints, and genitourinary tract.

Cephalosporins act by destroying growing bacteria. They do not kill fungi or viruses, such as those responsible for colds and the flu. Your doctor may prescribe these drugs if you have an infection caused by bacteria resistant to penicillins. For visual characteristics of Keflex, see the Color Guide to Prescription Drugs and Herbs.

PRECAUTIONS

SPECIAL INFORMATION
- Let your doctor know if you have ever had an allergic reaction to a cephalosporin drug or to penicillins, penicillamine, or a penicillin derivative. Your doctor may decide to prescribe a different drug. About 10 percent of people with allergies to penicillin are also allergic to cephalosporins. Reactions range from mild rashes and fever to life-threatening anaphylaxis.
- Tell your doctor if you have kidney or liver impairment, phenylketonuria, or a history of bleeding disorders or gastrointestinal disease; Keflex can make these conditions worse.
- Take the full course of your prescription, even if you feel better before finishing the medication; otherwise, the infection may return.
- This drug may cause false-positive results for the Clinitest urine glucose test. (It does not affect results of Clinistix or Tes-Tape.)
- Although Keflex may be taken on a full or an empty stomach, it is absorbed more quickly on an empty stomach.
- If possible, avoid taking this drug if you are pregnant or breast-feeding.
- Cephalosporins also kill "good" intestinal bacteria that keep harmful fungi and intestinal bacteria in check. Eating yogurt containing *Lactobacillus acidophilus* culture or taking acidophilus tablets may help restore the body's normal bacteria.
- Prolonged use of any antibiotic drug can lead to fungal infections, including candidiasis, or to bacterial infections such as pseudomembranous colitis.

CONTINUED

KEFLEX

POSSIBLE INTERACTIONS

Aminoglycosides (amikacin, gentamicin, kanamycin, neomycin, netilmicin, streptomycin, tobramycin): risk of kidney failure.

Bacteriostatic drugs (tetracycline, erythromycin, chloramphenicol, sulfonamides): may impair the bacteria-killing action of Keflex.

Loop diuretics: risk of kidney failure.

Nephrotoxic drugs (vancomycin, colistin, polymyxin B): risk of kidney failure.

Probenecid: decreases the kidneys' ability to excrete cephalosporins; possible cephalosporin toxicity. However, this combination is sometimes prescribed to treat serious infections that require high, prolonged serum levels of cephalosporins.

TARGET AILMENTS

Otitis media

Infections of the respiratory tract, genitourinary tract, skin, or soft tissue

Serious infections of the blood, bones, joints, abdomen, lungs, or heart

SIDE EFFECTS

NOT SERIOUS

- Mild nausea or diarrhea
- Yeast infections of the mouth (sore mouth or tongue)
- Vaginal yeast infections (vaginal itching or discharge)

TELL YOUR DOCTOR WHEN CONVENIENT.

SERIOUS

- Dizziness
- Serum sickness (fever accompanied by joint pains and rash)
- Severe diarrhea
- Severe allergic reaction
- Unusual bruising or bleeding
- Severe stomach cramps

CALL YOUR DOCTOR IMMEDIATELY.

KELP

LATIN NAME
Fucus spp.

VITAL STATISTICS

GENERAL DESCRIPTION
Extracts of iodine-rich kelp, one of the many forms of seaweed, provided an effective goiter remedy for many years. Today some herbalists rely on another component of kelp's stemlike and leaflike parts, an agent known as sodium alginate. Because of its action, kelp is prescribed to aid in the treatment of the effects on the body of heavy-metal environmental pollutants, such as barium and cadmium, and to prevent the body from absorbing strontium 90, a radioactive substance created in nuclear power plants.

Some practitioners of alternative medicine also recommend taking kelp supplements for thyroid disorders such as mild hypothyroidism (underactive thyroid).

For visual characteristics of kelp, see the Color Guide to Prescription Drugs and Herbs.

PREPARATIONS
Over the counter:
Available in dry bulk, capsules, and tinctures.

At home:
INFUSION: Steep covered 2 to 3 tsp dried kelp in 1 cup boiling water for 10 minutes; drink three times a day.
Consult a qualified practitioner for the dosage appropriate for you and the specific condition being treated.

PRECAUTIONS

WARNING
If you are already taking medication for hyperthyroidism (overactive thyroid), kelp supplements could worsen the condition.

Do not gather your own wild kelp for use; coastal colonies may be contaminated by offshore pollutants.

Check with your practitioner before using kelp if you have a history of thyroid problems or high blood pressure.

SPECIAL INFORMATION
This herb should not be used with children unless it is specifically prescribed by a health-care practitioner who is knowledgeable about herbs.

POSSIBLE INTERACTIONS
Combining kelp with other herbs may necessitate a lower dosage.

TARGET AILMENTS
- Goiter
- Hypothyroidism
- Radiation exposure
- Effects of heavy-metal environmental pollutants

SIDE EFFECTS
NONE EXPECTED

Rx KETOCONAZOLE

VITAL STATISTICS

DRUG CLASS
Antifungal Drugs

BRAND NAME
Nizoral

OTHER DRUGS IN THIS CLASS
Rx: clotrimazole, fluconazole, miconazole, terconazole
OTC: clotrimazole, miconazole, tolnaftate, undecylenate

GENERAL DESCRIPTION
Ketoconazole, introduced in 1981, is a powerful antifungal medication that is used to treat a wide variety of skin, lung, and systemic fungal infections, including yeast infections (candidiasis) and ringworm (tinea). The drug works by preventing the growth and reproduction of fungal cells; in high concentrations, ketoconazole actually destroys fungal cells. This medication is available in cream, shampoo, oral suspension, or tablet form.

Ketoconazole is also an antiadrenal drug. Because it suppresses the excess production of adrenal corticosteroid hormones and testosterone, ketoconazole is occasionally used in the treatment of prostate cancer and Cushing's syndrome, in which the body produces excessive amounts of corticosteroid hormones. For more information, see Antifungal Drugs.

PRECAUTIONS

SPECIAL INFORMATION
- Do not take this drug if you have an active liver disease.
- Weigh the risks and benefits of this drug with your doctor if you have hypochlorhydria, a history of alcoholism, impaired liver function, or liver disease.
- Tell your doctor if you are allergic to other antifungal drugs or are taking any other medications.
- In some cases, this drug can be severely toxic to the liver; your doctor may want to perform periodic liver function tests.
- While you are taking this medicine, your skin may burn more readily when exposed to sunlight. To protect your skin, wear sunblock and avoid prolonged exposure to the sun and sunlamps.
- Avoid taking this drug if you are pregnant or nursing.
- High doses of this drug can suppress corticosteroid secretion in your body, reduce testosterone levels, decrease male libido, and cause breast enlargement or impotence in men and menstrual irregularities in women.
- Take ketoconazole with food to increase absorption of the drug into the body and lessen stomach irritation.
- Some infections require that ketoconazole be taken for many months. If you are undergoing long-term treatment with this drug, be sure to contact your doctor for periodic evaluations and monitoring. Do not stop taking ketoconazole without consulting your doctor.

KETOCONAZOLE

POSSIBLE INTERACTIONS

Alcohol and hepatotoxic (liver) medications: increased risk of stomach ulceration and liver damage.

Antacids, histamine H_2 blockers, and other medications that reduce stomach acid: these medicines may counteract the effects of antifungal drugs by preventing their full absorption into the body.

Anticholinergics and omeprazole: may decrease the effectiveness of antifungal drugs.

Astemizole, terfenadine, and oral corticosteroids: ketoconazole may increase the blood levels of these drugs, which may lead to potentially fatal heart arrhythmias.

Cyclosporine: ketoconazole may increase the absorption of cyclosporine to potentially toxic levels.

Didanosine: both ketoconazole and didanosine, when taken together, may be absorbed into the body less efficiently. Take these medications two hours apart.

Phenytoin: blood levels of phenytoin may rise and those of the antifungal drug may decrease when these two medications are taken together.

Rifampin, isoniazid: may decrease blood levels, and thus the effectiveness, of ketoconazole.

Sucralfate: decreased absorption of ketoconazole. Take sucralfate two hours after taking ketoconazole.

Theophylline: blood levels of theophylline (which is used to treat asthma) may decrease when taken with antifungal drugs, possibly precipitating an asthma attack.

Warfarin: the anticoagulant effects of warfarin may increase when taken with an antifungal drug.

TARGET AILMENTS

Fungal diseases of the lungs

Yeast infections (candidiasis) of the mouth, skin, and internal organs

Chromomycosis (a chronic, usually tropical skin infection)

Ringworm (tinea) of the body, skin, groin (jock itch), and feet (athlete's foot); seborrheic dermatitis; dandruff

Cushing's syndrome and prostate cancer (occasionally)

SIDE EFFECTS

NOT SERIOUS

- Dizziness; drowsiness; headache; abdominal pain; diarrhea, mild nausea or vomiting; skin irritation

CALL YOUR DOCTOR IF THESE SYMPTOMS BECOME BOTHERSOME.

SERIOUS

- Signs of liver disease, including nausea, loss of appetite, dark urine, light-colored stools, jaundice (yellow eyes and skin)
- Depression

CALL YOUR DOCTOR IF YOU EXPERIENCE ANY OF THESE SYMPTOMS.

Rx KETOPROFEN

VITAL STATISTICS

DRUG CLASS
Analgesics [Nonsteroidal Anti-Inflammatory Drugs (NSAIDs)]

BRAND NAMES
Actron, Orudis KT, Orudis, Orudis SR, Oruvail

OTHER DRUGS IN THIS SUBCLASS
Rx: diclofenac, etodolac, flurbiprofen, ibuprofen, ketorolac, nabumetone, naproxen, oxaprozin
OTC: ibuprofen, naproxen

GENERAL DESCRIPTION
Like other nonsteroidal anti-inflammatory drugs (NSAIDs), ketoprofen is a nonnarcotic analgesic used to reduce pain, inflammation, and fever. NSAIDs are used by people who cannot take aspirin or are used when aspirin or acetaminophen is not effective. Ketoprofen is thought to act by reducing the body's production of prostaglandins and other substances that cause inflammation and pain.

Ketoprofen is available in tablet and capsule form at various dosage levels. The extended-release form is intended for the treatment of chronic pain, such as that associated with arthritis, and not for the treatment of acute pain. For visual characteristics of the brand-name drug Oruvail, see the Color Guide to Prescription Drugs and Herbs.

PRECAUTIONS

WARNING
Ketoprofen may cause drowsiness. Do not drive or operate machinery until you know how the drug will affect you.

Do not take more than the recommended dose, and seek emergency help in case of overdose. Symptoms include drowsiness, dizziness, ringing in the ears, increased sweating, rapid heartbeat, abdominal pain, vomiting, nausea, gastrointestinal bleeding, and disorientation.

SPECIAL INFORMATION
- Tell your doctor before using ketoprofen if you have any bleeding disorder, severe impairment of kidney function, an allergy to aspirin or to aspirin substitutes, impaired liver function, asthma, ulcers, enteritis (intestinal inflammation), epilepsy, Parkinson's disease, high blood pressure, or a history of heart failure, or if you are taking any aspirin substitutes or anticoagulants.
- The safety and effectiveness of this drug have not been established for children under the age of 12.
- Ketoprofen may affect some medical tests. Notify any doctor or dentist you consult that you are taking this drug.
- Ketoprofen may cause oversensitivity to sunlight, and it can mask the early signals of infection, such as fever.
- Anemia can occur commonly in patients with rheumatoid arthritis. It can be aggravated by ketoprofen and other NSAIDs. Patients on long-term treatment should have their hematocrit monitored.

POSSIBLE INTERACTIONS
Because NSAIDs interact with many substances, check with your doctor or pharmacist before taking in combination with other drugs. NSAIDs can affect liver and kidney function, thereby increasing the toxicity of other drugs.

Acetaminophen: can increase the effects of acetaminophen and increase the risk of kidney or liver damage.

KETOPROFEN

Alcohol: increased risk of stomach irritation, ulceration, or bleeding.

Anticoagulants: increased effects of anticoagulants; increased risk of bleeding.

Anticonvulsant drugs (phenytoin): increased blood levels of anticonvulsant drugs.

Antidiabetic drugs and insulin: can increase the hypoglycemic effect of these drugs.

Aspirin, dipyridamole, enoxaparin, indomethacin, sulfinpyrazone, valproic acid, and other drugs that inhibit platelet aggregation: ketoprofen when taken in combination with any of these drugs can increase the risk of bleeding.

Beta-adrenergic blockers: decreased effects of some beta blockers.

Cimetidine: this drug may increase or decrease the effect of ketoprofen.

Colchicine: possibility of bleeding and ulcers when this drug is combined with certain NSAIDs.

Corticosteroids: possible bleeding and ulcers. Don't combine ketoprofen and these drugs unless directed by your doctor.

Cyclosporine: increased risk of kidney damage.

Diuretics: decreased effect of diuretics; may increase the risk of renal failure.

Methotrexate: can increase the effects of methotrexate and cause major toxicity.

Potassium supplements: increased risk of gastrointestinal bleeding.

Probenecid: increased NSAID effect; possible NSAID toxicity.

Sulfonamides: possible sulfonamide toxicity.

Verapamil: decreased effectiveness of verapamil, possibly leading to inadequate control of blood pressure.

TARGET AILMENTS

Mild to moderate pain

Rheumatoid arthritis; osteoarthritis

Painful menstruation

SIDE EFFECTS

NOT SERIOUS

- Fluid retention
- Skin rash; itching
- Headache; dizziness, blurred vision; drowsiness
- Mouth sores; indigestion; nausea; vomiting; constipation; diarrhea

CONTACT YOUR DOCTOR IF THESE SYMPTOMS PERSIST.

SERIOUS

- Anaphylactic reaction (hives, intense itching, fainting, trouble breathing, swelling of the eyes)

SEEK EMERGENCY HELP.

- Diminished hearing or ringing in the ears; trouble breathing; stomach cramps
- Fluid retention; black or tarry stools; painful or reduced urination, or blood in urine
- Hypersensitivity to sunlight
- Jaundice

DISCONTINUE USE AND SEEK MEDICAL ASSISTANCE.

Rx KETOROLAC

VITAL STATISTICS

DRUG CLASS

Analgesics [Nonsteroidal Anti-Inflammatory Drugs (NSAIDs)]

BRAND NAMES

Toradol, Acular (ophthalmic)

OTHER DRUGS IN THIS SUBCLASS

diclofenac, etodolac, flurbiprofen, ibuprofen, ketoprofen, nabumetone, naproxen, oxaprozin

GENERAL DESCRIPTION

A new, nonnarcotic NSAID, ketorolac may be used by people who cannot take aspirin (unless they are allergic to aspirin), or in cases when aspirin or acetaminophen is not effective. Unlike many other NSAIDs, ketorolac is used for short-term pain management only; it is not used for treatment of chronic conditions such as arthritis. This drug is also available in ophthalmic form for relief of itching due to allergic conjunctivitis. For more information, including possible drug interactions, see Nonsteroidal Anti-Inflammatory Drugs (NSAIDs). For visual characteristics of the brand-name drug Toradol Oral, see the Color Guide to Prescription Drugs and Herbs.

PRECAUTIONS

SPECIAL INFORMATION

- Do not use ketorolac if you are allergic to NSAIDs or to aspirin.
- Avoid ketorolac or consult your doctor before using it if you have asthma, peptic ulcer, enteritis (intestinal inflammation), high blood pressure, bleeding problems, or impaired liver or kidney function.
- Do not take more than the recommended dose. Seek emergency help in case of overdose. Possible symptoms include drowsiness, increased sweating, rapid heartbeat, abdominal pain, vomiting, nausea, gastrointestinal bleeding, and disorientation.

TARGET AILMENTS

Pain, especially from inflammation, dental and other surgeries

Allergic conjunctivitis; ocular itching (ophthalmic form)

SIDE EFFECTS

NOT SERIOUS

- Dizziness; drowsiness; headache; abdominal pain or cramps; constipation; diarrhea; indigestion; nausea

CONSULT YOUR DOCTOR.

SERIOUS

- Anaphylactic reaction (hives, rash, intense itching, trouble breathing)

SEEK EMERGENCY HELP.

- Heart palpitations; high blood pressure
- Diminished hearing or ringing in the ears; trouble breathing; fluid retention
- Black or tarry stools; blood in urine; jaundice

DISCONTINUE USE AND CALL YOUR DOCTOR IMMEDIATELY.

K

King To's Natural Herb Loquat Flavored Syrup

Vital Statistics

CHINESE NAME
Mi Lian Chuan Bei Pi Pa Gao

GENERAL DESCRIPTION
King To's Natural Herb Loquat Flavored Syrup is a basic, pleasant-tasting cough syrup that helps loosen phlegm, halt coughing, and even relieve sinus congestion.

Chinese medicine takes a holistic approach to healthcare, fashioning remedies to treat the entire being as well as the specific parts or areas. Precise combinations of herbs are used to prevent and combat disease, which is thought to arise from disturbances in the flow of a bodily energy called chi (pronounced "chee") and blood, or from a lack of balance in the complementary states of yin and yang. A patent formula, King To's syrup is made by using a standardized combination of herbs and method of preparation.

INGREDIENTS
fritillary bulb, loquat leaf, aged citrus peel, mint, trichosanthes seed, licorice, balloon-flower, pinellia, almond, ginger-root, honey, sugar

PREPARATIONS
This formula is sold as a syrup and can be found in many Chinese pharmacies and Oriental grocery stores.

TARGET AILMENTS

- Cough
- Sinus congestion
- Acute bronchitis
- Emphysema

SIDE EFFECTS
None expected

KLONOPIN

VITAL STATISTICS

DRUG CLASS
Antianxiety Drugs [Benzodiazepines]

GENERIC NAME
clonazepam

OTHER DRUGS IN THIS SUBCLASS
alprazolam, diazepam, lorazepam, temazepam, triazolam

GENERAL DESCRIPTION
Klonopin is a brand name for the generic drug clonazepam. Introduced in 1977, clonazepam is a benzodiazepine that is prescribed alone or in combination with other drugs to control epileptic absence (petit mal) seizures as well as myoclonic and akinetic seizures. The effects of this drug start after the first dose. See Benzodiazepines for other information, including side effects and possible drug interactions. For visual characteristics of Klonopin, see the Color Guide to Prescription Drugs and Herbs.

TARGET AILMENTS

Convulsions or seizures

SIDE EFFECTS

SEE BENZODIAZEPINES.

PRECAUTIONS

WARNING
Never combine alcohol with Klonopin; the combination can cause dangerous central nervous system and respiratory depression.

Do not abruptly stop taking Klonopin. Sudden cessation can provoke withdrawal symptoms, including seizures; irritability; insomnia; confusion; mental depression; hypersensitivity to pain, noise, or light; and feelings of suspicion and distrust. Slowly reduce the dosage under your doctor's guidance.

SPECIAL INFORMATION
- Do not confuse the brand name Klonopin with the generic name clonidine. Clonidine is used to treat high blood pressure.
- Klonopin can impair your alertness, judgment, and coordination. Avoid driving and performing hazardous activities until you know how the drug affects you.
- Let your doctor know if you have narrow-angle glaucoma, a liver or kidney impairment, chronic respiratory disease, myasthenia gravis, depression, sleep apnea, or a history of drug abuse or addiction. Klonopin may exacerbate these conditions.
- This drug can cause sleep apnea in people with chronic respiratory disease, such as emphysema.
- Klonopin can cause physical and psychological dependence, sometimes after only one or two weeks but usually after prolonged use.
- Tolerance may increase with prolonged use; as your body adjusts to Klonopin, the drug becomes less effective. Never increase the dose without consulting your doctor, because the risk of Klonopin dependence increases with higher doses.
- Do not take Klonopin if you are pregnant or breast-feeding.

KOLA

LATIN NAME
Cola vera
(or C. nitada)

VITAL STATISTICS

GENERAL DESCRIPTION

The seed of the 40-foot kola tree, source of the world's most popular soft drink flavoring, is a stimulant that herbalists prescribe for overall mental fatigue or depression. In addition, it is used to treat diarrhea caused by nervousness; headaches; motion sickness; and loss of appetite. Medical evidence suggests that the herb may also open the bronchial passages, helping asthmatics to breathe more easily. The effective ingredient in kola is caffeine; kola nuts contain more in proportion than do coffee beans, although cola beverages generally contain considerably less caffeine than does coffee.

Kola has a long history of medicinal use in West Africa. Brought to the Americas by slaves, it earned a reputation among 19th-century practitioners as a treatment for depression, diarrhea, pneumonia, migraine headaches, morning sickness, and typhoid fever.

PREPARATIONS

Over the counter:
Available in dry bulk, capsules, and tinctures.

At home:
Soft drinks containing kola (or cola) syrups are probably the easiest way to use the herb medicinally, especially for children.

DECOCTION: Bring to a boil and simmer covered ½ tsp powdered seeds in 1 cup water for 10 minutes; drink three times a day.

COMBINATIONS: For depression, use kola mixed with any or all of the following: oats, damiana, or skullcap.

Consult a qualified practitioner for the dosage appropriate for you and the specific condition being treated.

PRECAUTIONS

SPECIAL INFORMATION

Kola should not be used with children unless it is specifically prescribed by a healthcare practitioner who is knowledgeable about herbs.

POSSIBLE INTERACTIONS

Combining kola with other herbs may necessitate a lower dosage.

TARGET AILMENTS
Depression
Migraine headache
Poor appetite
Diarrhea caused by nervousness
Motion sickness
Fluid retention
Respiratory problems, such as asthma

SIDE EFFECTS

NOT SERIOUS

KOLA MAY BE TOO STRONG A STIMULANT FOR INDIVIDUALS WHO ARE SENSITIVE TO CAFFEINE. IF YOU FEEL NERVOUS OR HAVE TROUBLE SLEEPING, DECREASE YOUR DOSE OR STOP TAKING KOLA.

LACHESIS

LATIN NAME
Lachesis

VITAL STATISTICS

GENERAL DESCRIPTION

The South American bushmaster snake grows to a length of seven feet and kills its prey, both animal and human, by constriction or by injection of its highly poisonous venom, known as lachesis, from which this homeopathic remedy is derived. Small doses of the venom can destroy red blood cells and impair the clotting of blood. Larger amounts of lachesis poison the heart. Homeopathic practitioners believe that the conditions best treated with *Lachesis* are those with symptoms similar to the ones induced by the venom. To prepare the homeopathic remedy, venom is extracted from the snake and diluted in large quantities of lactose (milk sugar).

Like most homeopathic prescriptions, *Lachesis* was developed as a remedy by observation of the reactions of healthy individuals to doses of various strengths. The mental, emotional, and physical changes induced by *Lachesis* were then cataloged. When a patient exhibits a set of symptoms that matches the cataloged symptoms brought on by *Lachesis,* the homeopathic practitioner then prescribes it in an extremely dilute form. For more information on homeopathic medicine, see page 14.

PREPARATIONS

Lachesis is available in various potencies, in both liquid and tablet form, at selected stores and pharmacies. Consult your practitioner for more precise information.

SIDE EFFECTS

NONE EXPECTED

PRECAUTIONS

SPECIAL INFORMATION

- When a remedy is administered, no one but the patient should touch the pills. If tablets are spilled, throw them away.
- The mouth should be clear of flavors 15 minutes before and after taking a remedy. Avoid strong flavors and aromas, such as coffee, camphor, and heavily scented perfumes, for the duration of treatment.

TARGET AILMENTS
Choking coughs
Croup
A constricted feeling in the throat
Earaches that are worse during swallowing
Left-sided sore throats
Indigestion
Throbbing headaches, especially those that appear during menopause
Insomnia
Hot flashes
Heart arrhythmias
Hemorrhoids
Sciatica

LACTOBACILLUS ACIDOPHILUS

VITAL STATISTICS

OTHER NAME
acidophilus

DAILY DOSAGE
One or two capsules twice a day before meals (or as directed)

GENERAL DESCRIPTION
Bacteria are usually something to avoid. But *Lactobacillus acidophilus* is one type of bacteria you may want to seek out. Acidophilus resembles certain bacteria that occur naturally in our bodies. These natural bacteria inhabit the colon and vagina, where they play an important role in digestion and in controlling the overgrowth of fungi and other organisms. For many people, taking antibiotics can upset this delicate balance. This is because antibiotics cannot distinguish between "good" bacteria and harmful bacteria. When populations of "helpful" bacteria diminish, the result can be intestinal problems and, for women, vaginal yeast infections. Ingesting acidophilus during and after a course of antibiotics can help restore populations of good bacteria.

Acidophilus can help in other ways as well. For example, these bacteria have been found to help reduce the incidence of yeast infections in susceptible women. By helping to break down lactose (milk sugar), acidophilus can make it easier for people who are lactose intolerant to digest milk, and it may help relieve symptoms of spastic colon.

Several studies suggest that acidophilus may one day be useful in treating or reducing the risk of colon cancer. Some proponents believe that these bacteria may also help lower cholesterol levels, boost immunity, and help in the treatment of allergies, although these benefits have not been proved.

PREPARATIONS
Acidophilus is sold in capsules, tablets, powders, and liquids. It is also added to some yogurt, kefir, and milk products. Check the label carefully to make sure acidophilus is listed as an ingredient.

PRECAUTIONS

WARNING
People who have serious, medically treated intestinal problems should consult their doctor before taking acidophilus.

SPECIAL INFORMATION
High temperatures can kill acidophilus. Any products containing these bacteria should be kept in the refrigerator.

TARGET AILMENTS
Canker sores
Constipation; diarrhea; indigestion; gas
Lactose intolerance; postantibiotic therapy; spastic colon
Yeast infections; urinary tract infections

SIDE EFFECTS
NONE EXPECTED

L

LANOXIN

VITAL STATISTICS

DRUG CLASS
Digitalis Preparations

GENERIC NAME
digoxin

GENERAL DESCRIPTION
Lanoxin is a brand name for the generic drug digoxin, a digitalis preparation that has been used since 1934 to strengthen the heart and to treat heart arrhythmias. Digitalis preparations are effective, but toxicity is a major concern with their use, since the effective dose is often only slightly smaller than a toxic dose. Additionally, digoxin interacts with many over-the-counter and prescription drugs.

For visual characteristics of Lanoxin, see the Color Guide to Prescription Drugs and Herbs.

PRECAUTIONS

SPECIAL INFORMATION

- Do not discontinue this medication without your doctor's knowledge; to do so might cause heart problems.
- Check your pulse if directed by your doctor; be sure to report any low pulse rate (less than 60 beats per minute) to your doctor immediately.
- Lanoxin can cross the placenta and affect the fetus, and it can pass to infants through breast milk. Pregnant and nursing women should therefore use caution when taking this medication. The dosage often must be reduced for women who have given birth recently (within six weeks).
- Avoid all over-the-counter antacids as well as cough, cold, allergy, and diet medications, except when advised otherwise by your doctor.
- Foods high in fiber may interfere with the absorption of Lanoxin.
- Heart failure may cause potassium levels in your body to drop. Talk with your doctor about adding potassium-rich foods (such as bananas and oranges) to your diet, since digoxin toxicity is increased if serum potassium is low.
- Patients with kidney failure require lower doses of Lanoxin.

LANOXIN

POSSIBLE INTERACTIONS

Following is a partial list of the drugs and other substances that can interact with Lanoxin. To compensate for these interactions, your doctor may have to adjust the dosages of Lanoxin and any other drugs you may be taking.

Amiodarone (an antiarrhythmia drug): increased amounts of Lanoxin circulating in the blood, which can lead to heart-rhythm problems.

Other antiarrhythmia drugs, calcium supplements, rauwolfia (an antihypertensive drug): increased heart arrhythmias.

Antacids, antidiarrheal drugs (such as kaolin and pectin), antiulcer drugs (including sulfasalazine), dietary fiber, laxatives: inhibited absorption of Lanoxin, reducing its effectiveness.

Calcium channel blockers: increased amounts of Lanoxin circulating in the blood, possibly leading to heart-rhythm problems.

Diuretics: may increase or decrease the effects of Lanoxin.

Erythromycin: increased absorption of Lanoxin into the body, thereby increasing its actions and side effects.

Fluoxetine: increased Lanoxin effects.

Indomethacin, a nonsteroidal anti-inflammatory drug (NSAID): increased amounts of Lanoxin circulating in the blood.

Potassium supplements (salts): increased risk of excess potassium, possibly leading to heart-rhythm problems; do not take potassium supplements with Lanoxin.

Quinidine or quinine: increased blood concentration of Lanoxin.

Stimulant drugs, such as amphetamines or over-the-counter decongestants: increased risk of heart-rhythm problems.

TARGET AILMENTS

Congestive heart failure (all degrees)

Prevention and treatment of heart arrhythmias (atrial fibrillation and flutter, atrioventricular tachycardia, and paroxysmal nodal tachycardia)

SIDE EFFECTS

NOT SERIOUS

NONE EXPECTED. ALL SIDE EFFECTS ARE POTENTIALLY SERIOUS.

SERIOUS

- Slow or irregular heartbeat; in children, fast heartbeat
- Visual disturbances, such as blurred vision or halos around objects
- Drowsiness, confusion, or depression
- Headache
- Fainting
- Digestive problems, such as pain in the lower stomach, diarrhea, nausea, vomiting, or loss of appetite
- Unusual tiredness or weakness
- Allergic reactions, such as skin rash or hives (rare)

CALL YOUR DOCTOR IMMEDIATELY IF YOU EXPERIENCE ANY OF THESE EFFECTS.

Rx LANSOPRAZOLE

VITAL STATISTICS

DRUG CLASS
Antiulcer Drugs

BRAND NAME
Prevacid

OTHER DRUGS IN THIS CLASS
omeprazole, sucralfate
Histamine H_2 Blockers: cimetidine, famotidine, ranitidine, nizatidine

GENERAL DESCRIPTION
Lansoprazole is used for short-term treatment of duodenal and stomach ulcers and inflammation of the esophagus, and for the long-term treatment of other conditions, such as Zollinger-Ellison syndrome, that involve excessive production of stomach acid. Called a proton-pump inhibitor, the drug reduces production of stomach acid by blocking an enzyme system in certain cells of the stomach lining, an action that both removes the corrosive acid and creates an environment conducive to healing.

The drug may be taken for up to four weeks for duodenal ulcer and up to eight weeks for stomach ulcer; these patients may experience decreased symptoms in about a week. Patients with esophagitis may take two eight-week courses of the drug, if necessary, and can expect improvement in one to four weeks.

Recently, development of duodenal and stomach ulcers has been strongly associated with the presence of a bacterium, *Helicobacter pylori,* in the gastrointestinal tract. Lansoprazole works in conjunction with appropriate antibiotics that rid the body of the organism.

Lansoprazole is best taken in the morning, on an empty stomach. To be effective, the capsules should be taken whole, without chewing or crushing. Because alcohol stimulates the secretion of stomach acid, it is preferable to restrict or stop alcohol consumption while taking this drug. It is also a good idea to stop smoking—for overall better health, and also because smoking stimulates production of stomach acid, reducing the effectiveness of this medicine.

PRECAUTIONS

WARNING
Tell your doctor before taking this drug if you have a history of liver disease. Your doctor may recommend a reduced dosage or a different drug. Also, let your doctor know if you are a smoker with no plans to quit.

SPECIAL INFORMATION
- Because this drug may cause drowsiness in some people, limit potentially hazardous activities, such as driving, until you know how this drug will affect you.
- Follow your doctor's orders concerning the length of time you take this medication, and take it exactly as prescribed. See your physician for follow-up as advised.
- If you are over 60 years of age, this drug may make you dizzy. Be cautious until you know if it has this effect on you.
- It is not yet known whether lansoprazole is safe to take during pregnancy.
- Because it is not known whether lansoprazole passes into human breast milk, it's best to avoid this drug if you are nursing a baby.
- The safety and efficacy have not been established in children younger than 18.
- Your physician may want to monitor your health with blood tests and liver function tests while you are taking this drug. Lansoprazole has been associated with ulcerative

colitis, protein in the urine, liver toxicity, and a decreased blood platelet level.
- Discuss with your doctor any plan to discontinue taking this medicine. If you stop too soon, your ulcer may not heal.
- If you miss a dose of this drug, do not double the next dose; take the next dose as soon as possible.
- An overdose of lansoprazole may cause nausea, vomiting, dizziness, lethargy, and abdominal pain. Contact a poison control center.
- It is not known whether this medication is safe for use in long-term maintenance of duodenal or stomach ulcer. It has been approved for long-term (one year) therapy to maintain healing in erosive esophagitis.
- While you are taking lansoprazole, your blood will contain increased amounts of gastrin (a hormone secreted by the stomach). Doctors do not know the significance of this increase. The levels will return to normal within four weeks of stopping therapy.
- Long-term therapy with lansoprazole may increase the risk of a tumor of the stomach, although this has not been established.

POSSIBLE INTERACTIONS

Ampicillin esters, digoxin, iron salts, ketoconazole: lansoprazole may interfere with the absorption of these medications.

Cyanocobalamin: decreased absorption of cyanocobalamin.

Diazepam, phenytoin: increased effect of these drugs.

Sucralfate: may lessen the body's absorption of lansoprazole. Take sucralfate at least 30 minutes after lansoprazole.

Theophylline: diminished levels of theophylline in the blood. Patients may require changes in their theophylline dosage when lansoprazole is started or stopped.

TARGET AILMENTS

Duodenal ulcer

Stomach ulcer

Esophagitis

Zollinger-Ellison syndrome and other conditions involving increased stomach acid

Mastocytosis

Endocrine adenoma

SIDE EFFECTS

NOT SERIOUS

- Skin rash; itching
- Headache; fatigue; dizziness
- Diarrhea; nausea
- Cold-like or flulike symptoms; muscle pain

CALL YOUR DOCTOR IF THESE PROBLEMS PERSIST.

SERIOUS

- Abdominal or stomach pain
- Anxiety; depression
- Unusual bleeding or bruising

CONTACT YOUR DOCTOR IMMEDIATELY.

LASIX

VITAL STATISTICS

DRUG CLASS
Diuretics

GENERIC NAME
furosemide

OTHER DRUGS IN THIS CLASS
amiloride, bumetanide, hydrochlorothiazide, indapamide, potassium chloride (adjunct therapy), spironolactone, triamterene

GENERAL DESCRIPTION
Lasix is a brand name for the generic drug furosemide, a fast-acting and powerful diuretic used to treat high blood pressure (hypertension) and excess fluid retention. The drug acts by increasing urine production, thereby removing water from the body and reducing swelling and blood volume. In the process, however, salts containing sodium, potassium, calcium, and other vital minerals are also eliminated, sometimes leading to muscle cramps and serious cardiovascular side effects. For more information, including possible drug interactions, see Furosemide; also see Diuretics. For visual characteristics, see the Color Guide to Prescription Drugs and Herbs.

TARGET AILMENTS

General edema (swelling caused by water retention)

Edema associated with various medical conditions, including congestive heart failure and cirrhosis of the liver

High blood pressure

PRECAUTIONS

SPECIAL INFORMATION
- While you are taking this medicine, your skin will burn more readily when exposed to sunlight. To protect your skin, use a sunblocking lotion when outside and avoid prolonged exposure to the sun or sunlamps.
- Taking this drug in hot weather or while engaged in heavy exertion can cause a dangerous loss of fluids or minerals. Watch for signs of dehydration (fatigue, dizziness, headache, nausea).

SIDE EFFECTS

NOT SERIOUS
- Headache; blurred vision; diarrhea; dizziness or lightheadedness when getting up (orthostatic hypotension)

LET YOUR DOCTOR KNOW IF THESE SYMPTOMS PERSIST.

SERIOUS
- Nausea or vomiting
- Fatigue or weakness
- Irregular or weak pulse
- Increased thirst; dry mouth
- Ringing in ears; hearing loss
- Muscle pain or cramps
- Mood changes; confusion
- Blood in urine or stools
- Unusual bruising; skin rash

CALL YOUR DOCTOR IMMEDIATELY. YOU MAY BE ADVISED TO LOWER YOUR DOSAGE AND INCREASE YOUR INTAKE OF FLUIDS AND MINERALS.

LAVENDER

LATIN NAME
Lavandula angustifolia

VITAL STATISTICS

GENERAL DESCRIPTION

This evergreen shrub, native to the Mediterranean but now grown worldwide, is the most versatile of the aromatic oils. Lavender is valued for its calming, soothing, and balancing effects. Well known for its ability to ease skin disorders, the plant is also said to have analgesic and antiseptic properties.

The flowering tops of the lavender shrub are used to produce the essential oil, which is clear or yellow green. The oil glands are easily accessible on the outside of the leaves; to release the familiar aroma, rub a flower or leaf between your fingers.

PREPARATIONS

To treat minor burns, apply the pure oil to the affected area and cover with gauze.

To relieve a tension headache, moisten your index finger with 2 drops lavender oil and rub gently over the temples, behind the ears, and across the back of the neck. The oil can also be used on small wounds and insect bites.

For larger areas, dilute the oil by mixing 15 drops with 2 tbsp vegetable or nut oil or aloe gel. This mixture can be useful in treating a variety of ailments, including skin problems, muscle or joint pain, headache, and insomnia. Nearly all complaints, except skin problems, can be relieved by simply inhaling lavender oil. Use a room diffuser to scent the air or place drops on a tissue or pillow. For a therapeutic bath, mix 10 drops lavender oil in the bathwater.

PRECAUTIONS

SPECIAL INFORMATION

- Do not apply lavender oil near the eyes.
- Buy from a reputable source. Lavender is often adulterated with other oils.
- Other species of lavender are used to produce another type of oil that is sometimes sold as lavender. This other oil has different properties, however, and will not produce the same good results.

TARGET AILMENTS
Headache; depression; stress; insomnia
Muscular and joint pain; menstrual pain
Digestive problems and nausea; colds and flu
Athlete's foot
Cuts and wounds; burns and sunburn; insect bites
Acne; eczema; dermatitis

SIDE EFFECTS

NONE EXPECTED. LAVENDER IS NONTOXIC AND NONIRRITATING.

LAVENDER

LATIN NAME
Lavandula officinalis

VITAL STATISTICS

GENERAL DESCRIPTION
Herbalists prescribe lavender tea and the essential oil of lavender, both made from the plant's flowers, to treat common minor ailments such as insomnia, headaches, nausea, and flatulence. Years of anecdotal evidence suggest that lavender has a calming effect that relieves anxiety and promotes gastrointestinal relaxation. Its aroma is thought to stimulate mental processes and help alleviate depression, especially when it is used with other herbs. Lavender oil also has antiseptic qualities that may kill several types of disease-causing bacteria, and herbalists use it to treat skin ailments such as fungus, burns, wounds, eczema, and acne. For visual characteristics, see the Color Guide to Prescription Drugs and Herbs.

PREPARATIONS
Over the counter:
Available in dried bulk, capsules, oils, tinctures.

At home:
Tea: Steep covered 1 tsp dried flowers in 1 cup boiling water for 10 minutes; drink three times a day.
Oil: To relax, use 1 to 4 drops of the essential oil in a bath; rub the oil on your skin to mitigate rheumatism, or use 1 to 2 drops in a steam inhalation for coughs, colds, and flu.
Combinations: For depression, lavender can be used with rosemary, skullcap, or kola.
Consult a qualified practitioner for the dosage appropriate for your specific condition.

SIDE EFFECTS
None expected

PRECAUTIONS

☠ ***WARNING***
Do not use oil of lavender internally.

POSSIBLE INTERACTIONS
Combining lavender with other herbs may necessitate a lower dosage.

TARGET AILMENTS
Take internally for:
Insomnia; depression
Headache, especially when caused by stress
Poor digestion
Nausea
Flatulence
Colic
Apply externally for:
Burns
Wounds
Eczema
Acne
Fungal infections such as candidiasis or ringworm
Rheumatism

LAXATIVES

VITAL STATISTICS

GENERIC NAMES

Bulk: calcium polycarbophil, methylcellulose, psyllium hydrophilic mucilloid
Stimulant: phenolphthalein, sennosides
Stool softener: docusate

GENERAL DESCRIPTION

Laxatives are used for the temporary relief of occasional constipation and other bowel problems, and to prevent straining during bowel movements. The drugs can be taken orally in powder, liquid, granular, wafer, or pill form, or rectally as suppositories or enemas.

The bulk-forming types, considered the safest, work by absorbing water and expanding, thus increasing the moisture content of the stool to make passage easier. Increased bulk also encourages the bowels' motility. Stimulant laxatives are believed to promote evacuation by increasing peristalsis (waves of contractions) in the intestinal muscles. Stool softeners add to the bowels' liquid content, softening the stool. For more information, see entries for the individual generic drugs listed above.

PRECAUTIONS

SPECIAL INFORMATION

- If you experience a sudden change in bowel habits that lasts longer than two weeks, you should consult your doctor before using a laxative.
- If you are pregnant or nursing, consult your doctor before using any kind of laxative.
- Unless prescribed by your physician, laxatives should not be given to children under the age of six.
- Bulk-forming laxatives are best for geriatric patients with poorly functioning colons.
- Do not use laxatives if you have symptoms of appendicitis, including abdominal pain, nausea, or vomiting, or if you think you may have an intestinal obstruction.
- If you have congestive heart failure or rectal bleeding of unknown cause, do not use laxatives without your doctor's consent.
- If you are diabetic, avoid sennosides and psyllium-type laxatives that contain large amounts of sugar; instead, use sugar-free types that contain the artificial sweetener aspartame.
- If you have hypertension or are on a low-sodium diet, avoid laxatives containing sodium.
- If you have difficulty swallowing—as with dysphagia—do not take bulk-forming laxatives, which can cause an esophageal obstruction.

CONTINUED

LAXATIVES

- Chronic use of laxatives may cause excessive loss of potassium in the body.
- Laxatives can be habit forming. Use them infrequently, at the lowest effective dosage, and for no longer than one week at a time. Long-term use, particularly of stimulant laxatives, can cause physical dependence, resulting in loss of normal bowel function and chronic constipation.
- Call your doctor if the laxative fails to have the desired effect after one week of use.

POSSIBLE INTERACTIONS

Antacids, histamine H_2 blockers (cimetidine, famotidine, nizatidine, ranitidine), milk: if taken within an hour of a dosage of some types of stimulant laxatives, these medications may cause gastric upset by dissolving the outer coating of the laxative too quickly.

Laxatives that may contain danthron, mineral oil, or phenolphthalein: increased absorption of these substances, increasing the possibility of toxic effects.

Oral anticoagulants, digitalis, salicylate, tetracycline: these drugs may be less effective when taken concurrently with bulk-forming laxatives. After taking any of these medications, wait two hours before taking a laxative.

TARGET AILMENTS

Constipation

Diarrhea (bulk-forming types)

Irritable bowel syndrome, or spastic colon (bulk-forming types)

Straining during bowel movements following rectal surgery, heart attacks, childbirth, or when hemorrhoids are present

SIDE EFFECTS

NOT SERIOUS

- Harmless urine discoloration from dyes in some laxatives
- Rectal irritation (from suppositories)
- Intestinal cramping, nausea, belching, or diarrhea (from stimulant laxatives)
- Stomach cramps or throat irritation (from liquid stool softeners)

SERIOUS

- Rectal bleeding or infection (from suppositories)
- Skin rash

IF YOU DEVELOP A RASH, DISCONTINUE USE AND SEE YOUR DOCTOR.

L-Carnitine

Vital Statistics

GENERAL DESCRIPTION

An amino acid synthesized in the kidneys and liver, L-carnitine works continually to rebuild body tissue, helps in the metabolism of fatty acids, contributes to muscle growth, and enhances the antioxidant properties of vitamins E and C. Although it has not officially achieved vitamin status or been assigned a recommended daily allowance, L-carnitine is gaining recognition as a necessary ingredient for good health, particularly for cardiovascular health. Studies reveal that L-carnitine is often depleted in heart patients and that these patients respond well to supplements, experiencing increased physical endurance. Chronic alcoholics also exhibit low levels of L-carnitine, and in these patients supplements may help prevent liver damage. L-carnitine can promote weight loss, because it helps build muscles that in turn use energy and burn fat. Others who may benefit from L-carnitine supplements include vegan vegetarians (those who eat no animal products).

A "nonessential" amino acid, L-carnitine is produced by the body and does not have to be acquired from dietary sources. At this time no evidence suggests that persons within their normal weight who are not vegan and who have healthy heart function necessarily benefit from supplements. In such cases the body's own production is considered sufficient.

NATURAL SOURCES

avocados; tempeh (small amounts)
dairy products; red meat (highest amounts)

PREPARATIONS

Available as tablets, in natural or synthetic over-the-counter preparations. Sometimes administered intravenously for heart patients.

Precautions

WARNING

DL-carnitine supplements have caused harmful side effects. Use L-carnitine only.

SPECIAL INFORMATION

1,500 mg to 4,000 mg is an average daily dose. Consult your healthcare practitioner for dosages.

TARGET AILMENTS
High cholesterol; atherosclerosis
Heart, liver, or kidney disease
Obesity or anorexia nervosa
Diabetes; muscular dystrophy

SIDE EFFECTS

NOT SERIOUS

- Gastrointestinal complaints
- Body odor

CONSULT YOUR DOCTOR FOR DECREASED DOSAGE.

SERIOUS

- Muscle weakness (DL-carnitine only)

DISCONTINUE USE AND CONSULT YOUR DOCTOR.

L

LECITHIN

VITAL STATISTICS

GENERAL DESCRIPTION

Lecithin is an essential natural compound found throughout the body. It's one of the main components of cell membranes, and it helps prevent these membranes from hardening. Lecithin is made up of various elements, including fatty acids, phosphorus, and choline, a B vitamin. Choline is involved in the production of the neurotransmitter acetylcholine, which is essential for the proper function of the nervous system. It is also an important component of the myelin sheaths that cover nerve fibers. Choline plays a role in processing fat and cholesterol and protects against atherosclerosis and heart disease. By emulsifying and transporting fat, choline helps to maintain the health of the liver and kidneys.

Lecithin is found in soybeans, cabbage, cauliflower, chickpeas, green beans, lentils, corn, calves' liver, and eggs. Its fat- and cholesterol-processing qualities are found only in the polyunsaturated forms of lecithin, such as those found in soybeans and vegetables. Eggs contain its saturated form. Lecithin is used as a thickener in foods such as mayonnaise, margarine, and ice cream. Most people who eat a healthy, well-balanced diet do not need to take lecithin supplements. People who take niacin or nicotinic acid for treatment of high cholesterol often are advised to take lecithin supplements because niacin can deplete the body's choline supply.

Lecithin supplements can help people with the neurological disorder tardive dyskinesia, which is characterized by involuntary, abnormal facial movements. This is a common side effect in people taking antipsychotic medications. The choline in the lecithin may help stabilize the acetylcholine neurotransmitter system in these people. Because of its role in maintaining the nervous system, lecithin supplements are being studied in combination with various drugs for treatment of Alzheimer's disease, Parkinson's disease, and Huntington's chorea, as well as Tourette's syndrome. Lecithin supplements may also be useful in preventing and treating gallstones.

PREPARATIONS

Lecithin is sold in the United States as a dietary supplement in tablet or liquid form.

L

TARGET AILMENTS
Dizziness; fatigue; headache
Liver disorders; high cholesterol
Bipolar depression
Insomnia
Memory loss; Alzheimer's disease

SIDE EFFECTS

SERIOUS

- Nausea; vomiting; diarrhea; bloating; abdominal pain
- Dizziness

DISCONTINUE USE AND CALL YOUR DOCTOR.

LEDUM

LATIN NAME
Ledum palustre

VITAL STATISTICS

GENERAL DESCRIPTION

Ledum, sometimes called marsh tea, can be found in bogs across northern Europe, Canada, and the United States. The herb has an antiseptic smell, and its upper branches are covered with a coat of tiny brown hairs. These may have given ledum its name; in Greek, *ledos* means "woolly robe." Once used in Scandinavia for insect control, ledum has also served as a tea substitute and replaced hops in beer, although overconsumption has resulted in dizziness and a splitting headache—even before the hangover. Homeopathic practitioners consider dilute doses of *Ledum* helpful for conditions that may be accompanied by signs of infection or inflammation.

The homeopathic remedy is prepared from the whole plant, which is gathered, dried, and crushed to a powder. This is diluted to nontoxic levels in a water-alcohol mix.

Like most homeopathic prescriptions, *Ledum* was developed as a remedy by observation of the reactions of healthy individuals to doses of various strengths. The mental, emotional, and physical changes induced by *Ledum* were then cataloged. When a patient exhibits a set of symptoms that matches the cataloged symptoms brought on by *Ledum,* the homeopathic practitioner then prescribes it in an extremely dilute form. It is presumed that in this highly dilute dosage, *Ledum* can counter the symptoms that are similar to those it induces when it is at full strength. For more information on homeopathic medicine, see page 14.

PREPARATIONS

Ledum is available over the counter in various potencies, in both liquid and tablet form, at selected stores and pharmacies. Consult your practitioner for further information.

PRECAUTIONS

SPECIAL INFORMATION

- When a remedy is administered, no one but the patient should touch the pills. If tablets are spilled, throw them away.
- The mouth should be clear of flavors 15 minutes before and after taking a remedy, and strong flavors and aromas, such as coffee, camphor, and heavily scented perfumes, should be avoided for the duration of treatment.

TARGET AILMENTS
Animal bites or insect stings
Bruises that have already discolored the skin
Deep cuts or puncture wounds where there is danger of infection
Gout or aching joints, where the pain is relieved by cold applications and aggravated by heat

SIDE EFFECTS

NONE EXPECTED

LEMON

LATIN NAME
Citrus limon

VITAL STATISTICS

GENERAL DESCRIPTION

The essential oil of lemon is pressed from the rind of the fruit. The juice is rich in vitamins A, B, and C. Lemon's healing properties make it a good all-purpose cure-all.

Probably native to Southeast Asia, the lemon tree is now cultivated worldwide. It is used extensively in the food and beverage, perfume, and pharmaceutical industries. Lemon essence is second only to orange essence in its world production and use.

PREPARATIONS

Fresh lemon oil is pale yellow, sometimes green; as it ages, it turns cloudy and brown. The oil can be applied externally and is used for a range of skin disorders and circulatory and respiratory problems.

To ease a cold or other upper respiratory discomfort, put a few drops of lemon oil on a tissue and bring the tissue to your nose to inhale. Alternatively, put a few drops on the front of the shirt the patient is wearing; this is an especially effective way to treat children's colds. Inhalation is the preparation of choice for all lemon's target ailments except skin problems.

For circulatory problems, massage the oil all over the body. Mix 6 drops lemon oil into 4 tsp almond oil to make a pleasing massage oil. For a soothing bath, add 3 to 5 drops to bathwater. Both lemon oil and lemon juice can be used internally to soothe a sore throat. The oil, however, should not be ingested. To make a gargle, add 3 drops oil to ½ cup warm water, or add pure lemon juice to hot water.

PRECAUTIONS

☠ *WARNING*

Lemon is highly phototoxic. Always dilute before using and do not apply to the skin before long periods of exposure to the sun or before entering a tanning booth.

SPECIAL INFORMATION

Lemon oil does not keep well. Check the expiration date when buying, and don't buy oil that looks cloudy.

TARGET AILMENTS
Anxiety; depression
Headache; insomnia
Throat infections, bronchitis, laryngitis, colds, and flu
High blood pressure
Varicose veins; broken capillaries
Palpitations
Dandruff; eczema; psoriasis
Premenstrual syndrome; irregular periods

SIDE EFFECTS

LEMON OIL CAN BE IRRITATING TO THE SKIN; USE IN DILUTION ONLY.

L

LEMON BALM

LATIN NAME
Melissa officinalis

VITAL STATISTICS

GENERAL DESCRIPTION

As an antiviral agent, lemon balm is useful in treating mumps, cold sores, and other viral ailments. Both its antiviral and its antihistaminic properties make it useful in treating colds and flu. The herb's antidepressant properties, along with the sedative effect of its volatile oils, make it effective in treating anxiety, nervousness, depression, insomnia, headaches, and anxiety-induced heart palpitations. Its carminative and antispasmodic properties make it useful in treating indigestion and other digestive upsets. Lemon balm has also been shown to have antibacterial and antioxidant properties.

PREPARATIONS

Over the counter:
Available as tincture, tea, lip balm, dried bulk.

At home:

INFUSION: Pour 1 cup boiling water over 2 to 3 tsp dried herb or 4 to 6 fresh leaves. Steep covered 10 minutes. Drink 1 cup in the morning and another in the evening, or as needed. For infusions, fresh or freeze-dried leaves are best; drying greatly reduces the volatile oils available in the leaves.

TINCTURE: Take 1/8 to 1/2 tsp three times a day or 1 tsp at bedtime for insomnia.

COMBINATIONS: Combine with hops, chamomile, or meadowsweet to treat digestive ailments; with lavender and linden to reduce stress.

Consult a qualified practitioner for the dosage appropriate for your specific condition.

SIDE EFFECTS

NONE EXPECTED

PRECAUTIONS

WARNING

People who have thyroid-related conditions should take lemon balm only with a doctor's permission.

SPECIAL INFORMATION

When applied externally for skin ailments, tincture may burn. Use tea or salve instead.

POSSIBLE INTERACTIONS

May increase efficacy of other diaphoretic medicines. Combining lemon balm with other herbs may necessitate a lower dosage.

TARGET AILMENTS

Take internally for:

- Depression
- Digestive disorders, especially when induced by anxiety, stress, or depression
- Tension; migraines and tension-induced headaches
- Neuralgia
- Anxiety-induced palpitations, insomnia, or high blood pressure
- Fever, colds, and flu

Apply tea or balm externally for:

- Skin lesions of herpes simplex
- Eczema

LEMONGRASS

LATIN NAME
Cymbopogon citratus

VITAL STATISTICS

GENERAL DESCRIPTION

Lemongrass, a tropical plant that can grow as high as five feet in dry soils, has uses that extend beyond its tangy role in Thai cuisine. Tea made from blades of lemongrass is a traditional Caribbean remedy for fevers, and Brazilians have a long history of using the herb for gastrointestinal and nervous disorders. Natives of the Amazon also hold that lemongrass is an effective contraceptive. And the oils from several closely related species of lemongrass are used to make citronella candles to repel insects.

The results of a clinical study to pinpoint the herb's therapeutic properties suggest that myrcene, one of the active ingredients isolated in the essential oil of lemongrass, may serve as a site-specific painkiller, or one that affects particular parts of the body; herbalists differentiate this type from systemic painkillers, such as aspirin. This analgesic action of myrcene may also explain the apparent sedative effect of lemongrass tea, a tart beverage long enjoyed in the Amazon region.

Some practitioners use the oil of lemongrass as a rub to treat circulatory problems and to enhance muscle tone by increasing the blood flow to the affected area.

PREPARATIONS

Over the counter:
Available in dried bulk.

At home:
TEA: Use 1 to 2 tsp fresh or dried blades in 1 cup boiling water and steep covered for 10 to 15 minutes; drink as often as needed until symptoms improve.
Consult a qualified practitioner for the dosage appropriate for you and the specific condition being treated.

PRECAUTIONS

POSSIBLE INTERACTIONS

Combining lemongrass with other herbs may necessitate a lower dosage.

TARGET AILMENTS
Take internally for:
Diarrhea and stomachache
Headache
Fever
Influenza
Apply externally for:
Athlete's foot
Acne
Circulatory problems

SIDE EFFECTS
NONE EXPECTED

LEMON-SCENTED EUCALYPTUS

LATIN NAME
Eucalyptus citriodora

VITAL STATISTICS

GENERAL DESCRIPTION
This tall evergreen, sometimes called a gum tree, is native to Australia. Its colorless or pale yellow oil has long been used for sachets in linen closets. Because of its lemon scent, it is also an especially effective insect repellent. The leaves and twigs are used to produce the essential oil. To release the oil, the leaves must first be bruised because the glands are not accessible to the distillation process.

Lemon-scented eucalyptus has sedative, anti-inflammatory, antiseptic, and deodorant action. It also can kill bacteria, viruses, and fungi.

PREPARATIONS
For most ailments, the oil can be diluted and rubbed directly on the problem area. Dilute by mixing 10 to 15 drops essential oil with 2 tbsp aloe gel or a carrier oil, such as vegetable or almond oil. Apply to the chest area to relieve respiratory ailments.

To prepare a healing bath, add 10 drops essential oil to bathwater.

Inhaling the oil can be especially useful for treating stress, colds, and flu. Place a few drops on a cloth, or use a diffuser to scent the entire room.

For sore throat, prepare a gargle by mixing 3 drops essential oil in a half-cup water.

PRECAUTIONS

WARNING
Do not take internally.

TARGET AILMENTS
Mosquito bites and skin irritations
Athlete's foot
Herpes sores
Muscle tension
Stress
Asthma
Laryngitis
Colds and flu
Sore throat

SIDE EFFECTS

NOT SERIOUS
- May cause irritation to extremely sensitive skin

DISCONTINUE USE.

LEVODOPA

VITAL STATISTICS

DRUG CLASS
Anti-Parkinsonism Drugs

BRAND NAME
Sinemet

GENERAL DESCRIPTION
Levodopa is used to treat the trembling, stiffness, indistinct speech, and other symptoms that characterize Parkinson's disease. In the brain, levodopa is converted into dopamine, a chemical necessary for proper transmission of the nerve impulses that control muscle movement. People with Parkinson's disease have a shortage of dopamine due to degeneration of the cells that produce the chemical. The disease can be brought on by viral infections or by exposure to environmental poisons such as carbon monoxide and manganese, but in most cases the cause is unknown.

Sinemet is a combination of levodopa and carbidopa, a chemical that prevents levodopa from breaking down in the system before reaching the brain. Carbidopa and levodopa may also be prescribed separately.

PRECAUTIONS

SPECIAL INFORMATION

- Levodopa may interfere with normal fetal development; if you are pregnant, discuss the risk-to-benefit ratio with your doctor before using the drug. Do not take levodopa if you are nursing.
- Inform your doctor if you have a history of any of the following ailments: diabetes, epilepsy, urine retention, peptic ulcer, heart or lung disease, melanoma, glaucoma, asthma, psychosis, heart attack, kidney disease, or liver disease. You should also tell your physician if you are planning surgery.
- If levodopa upsets your stomach, try taking it with food, although this will slow the drug's absorption.
- Levodopa may cause drowsiness; use caution when driving or operating machinery.
- It may take several weeks or months for the medication to reach maximum effectiveness.
- Laboratory tests that may be affected by levodopa include complete blood cell counts, blood thyroxine levels, urine sugar or ketone tests.
- Dosages must be determined on an individual basis. Adjustments in quantity and dosing frequency are unavoidable.

LEVODOPA

POSSIBLE INTERACTIONS

Antacids, metoclopramide: increased levodopa effect.

Anticholinergics, methionine, papaverine, phenothiazines, phenytoin, pyridoxine, tricyclic antidepressants: decreased levodopa effect.

Some monoamine oxidase (MAO) inhibitors: may cause a severe rise in body temperature and blood pressure; these medications should be discontinued two to four weeks prior to your taking levodopa.

TARGET AILMENTS

Parkinson's disease

SIDE EFFECTS

NOT SERIOUS

- Headache
- Urine discoloration
- Loss of appetite
- Dry mouth and drooling
- Decreased attention span or intellectual functioning
- Mental confusion
- Insomnia
- Skin rash
- Drowsiness
- Fatigue

CONSULT YOUR DOCTOR IF THESE SYMPTOMS PERSIST OR BECOME BOTHERSOME.

SERIOUS

- A sudden drop in blood pressure upon standing
- Uncontrollable movements of the hands, arms, legs, neck, face, eyelids, mouth, or tongue
- Double or blurred vision
- Marked changes in mood or mental state
- Irregular or rapid heartbeat
- Difficulty urinating
- Severe or persistent nausea or vomiting
- Weight change
- Bitter taste or burning sensation on tongue
- Stomach bleeding or ulcer

CONTACT YOUR DOCTOR PROMPTLY.

Levothyroxine

Vital Statistics

DRUG CLASS
Thyroid Hormones

BRAND NAMES
Levoxine, Levoxyl, Synthroid

OTHER DRUGS IN THIS CLASS
thyroid USP

GENERAL DESCRIPTION
Introduced in 1953, synthetically produced levothyroxine is the drug of choice for thyroid replacement therapy because of its standard hormone content and predictable effect. Hormones produced by the thyroid gland regulate functions such as metabolism and protein synthesis, general body growth, and development of the bones and central nervous system. They also affect the heart rate. Thyroid hormone therapy usually must be maintained throughout the patient's life unless it is prescribed for a transient condition affecting thyroid function. Because these hormones are so critical to normal growth and development, children should be tested to ensure that their thyroid glands are functioning normally; those whose bodies are not producing sufficient quantities must be given supplemental thyroid hormones as soon as possible. Thyroid medications are sometimes used diagnostically to check for thyroid disease.

For visual characteristics of levothyroxine and the brand-name drugs Levoxyl and Synthroid, see the Color Guide to Prescription Drugs and Herbs.

Precautions

SPECIAL INFORMATION
- Your doctor may tell you to continue using levothyroxine while you're pregnant or nursing. Although small amounts of this drug may cross the placenta or be present in breast milk, no studies have shown harm to the fetus or breast-feeding baby.
- Tell your doctor if you have cardiovascular disease, or if you have diabetes or other hormone problems, such as low pituitary gland secretions. Your doctor may decide not to use levothyroxine or to lower the dosage.
- Absorption of levothyroxine through the digestive tract may be affected by food. Take on an empty stomach (one hour before or two hours after a meal).
- The dosage for older people and for people with severe hypothyroidism or cardiovascular problems must be monitored closely. Dosages for older patients are usually lower than those prescribed for younger ones.
- In rare cases after long-term use at high dosages, levothyroxine may cause bone loss.

TARGET AILMENTS
Hypothyroidism (underactive or nonfunctioning thyroid) or as treatment following removal of thyroid gland
Goiter (enlargement of thyroid)
Some types of thyroid cancer, for prevention and treatment, especially after radiation therapy to the neck

LEVOTHYROXINE

POSSIBLE INTERACTIONS

Anticoagulant and antiplatelet drugs (such as warfarin): increased anticlotting action. Your doctor may have to adjust the dosage of anticlotting drugs.

Antidepressants, including tricyclic antidepressants such as amitriptyline: increased action and side effects of both combined drugs, leading to heart-rhythm problems and other signs of excess stimulation.

Antidiabetic drugs (such as insulin): increased need for insulin or other diabetic drugs, perhaps leading to higher blood sugar levels. Your doctor may need to adjust your insulin dose.

Cholesterol-reducing drugs (such as cholestyramine): blocked or delayed absorption of levothyroxine, decreasing its effectiveness. Take levothyroxine one hour before or four to five hours after taking cholesterol-reducing drugs.

Heart-stimulating drugs (such as epinephrine or pseudoephedrine): increased effects of both combined drugs, potentially causing heart problems or increased chance of levothyroxine overdose.

Other hormones (such as estrogen): may interfere with levothyroxine action, necessitating higher doses.

SIDE EFFECTS

NOT SERIOUS

- Changes in menstrual periods (short-term)
- Clumsiness
- Coldness
- Constipation
- Dry, puffy skin
- Headache
- Sleepiness, tiredness, or weakness
- Heart palpitations
- Muscle aches
- Weight gain
- Temporary hair loss in children

THESE PROBLEMS ARE RARE BUT MAY OCCUR AT THE BEGINNING OF TREATMENT. CALL YOUR DOCTOR IF THE PROBLEMS PERSIST.

SERIOUS

- Allergic reactions such as skin rash or hives
- Severe persistent and continuing headache
- Menstrual irregularity
- Changes in appetite
- Chest pain
- Irregular heartbeat; tremors
- Fever or sweating
- Nervousness; irritability
- Leg cramps
- Sensitivity to heat
- Weight loss

THESE PROBLEMS ARE RARE. IF YOU EXPERIENCE ANY OF THEM TELL YOUR DOCTOR RIGHT AWAY. YOUR DOCTOR MAY NEED TO ADJUST YOUR DOSAGE.

LICORICE

LATIN NAME
Glycyrrhiza uralensis

VITAL STATISTICS

GENERAL DESCRIPTION

The licorice root is often used to flavor herbal formulas, but it has important medicinal properties of its own. Chinese herbalists prescribe it for several digestive and stomach problems and for coughs and colds. Licorice is also considered an anti-inflammatory medication, useful in treating skin diseases, and it is prescribed as well for ulcers. Practitioners speculate that an extract made from licorice may prevent tooth decay and gum disease. The best form of the herb is powdery, with a thin, unwrinkled, reddish brown outer skin and a white cross section. The raw form is characterized as neutral in traditional Chinese medicine; when fried in honey it is believed to be a warm herb. See also the species of licorice known as *Glycyrrhiza glabra,* regarded as a Western herb.

Chinese medicine takes a holistic approach to healthcare, fashioning remedies to treat the entire being as well as the specific parts or areas. Single herbs may be used alone or in combination with other herbs to prevent and combat disease, which is thought to arise from disturbances in the flow of a bodily energy called chi (pronounced "chee") and blood, or from a lack of balance in the complementary states of yin and yang.

PREPARATIONS

Available in bulk or combined with other herbs in tablet form at Chinese pharmacies and Asian markets.

COMBINATIONS: Mixed with ephedra stem and apricot seed, licorice is prescribed for coughing and wheezing. Combined with honeysuckle flower, it treats rashes or acne. For details on dosages and preparations, check with a Chinese medicine practitioner.

PRECAUTIONS

☠ *WARNING*

Licorice taken in large amounts long term can affect the body's electrolyte balance, leading to high blood pressure and edema.

SPECIAL INFORMATION

- Pregnant women and individuals with edema, kidney disease, glaucoma, or high blood pressure should avoid the herb.
- Licorice affects the body's balance between salt and potassium, retaining salt while depleting potassium. You may need potassium supplements when using this herb. Consult a Chinese medicine practitioner for advice.

POSSIBLE INTERACTIONS

Some practitioners consider licorice incompatible with euphorbia, genkwa flower, kansui root, sargassum seaweed, and polygala.

TARGET AILMENTS
Take internally for:
Cough, colds, and sore throat
Asthma and wheezing
Poor digestion; ulcers; abdominal pains and spasms
Carbuncles and sores

SIDE EFFECTS

NONE EXPECTED WHEN USED IN THE SMALL AMOUNTS FOUND IN CHINESE MEDICINE PREPARATIONS.

LICORICE

LATIN NAME
Glycyrrhiza glabra

VITAL STATISTICS

GENERAL DESCRIPTION

Licorice is one of the most widely used medicinal herbs. Its taste, alleged to be 50 times sweeter than sugar, masks the bitterness in any herbal mixture. Western herbalists use licorice root as a cough suppressant and also to treat digestive disorders, believing that it acts as a mild laxative and prevents ulcers by forming a protective coating on the stomach wall. Applying licorice as an external antibiotic, practitioners think it relieves ulcerated skin conditions, such as herpes sores. For visual characteristics of licorice, see the Color Guide to Prescription Drugs and Herbs.

PREPARATIONS

Over the counter:

Available as dried root, liquid extract, capsules.

At home:

TEA: Simmer covered 1 tbsp licorice root in 1 cup water for 10 minutes. Drink up to 2 cups per day.

ANTI-INFLAMMATORY: Sprinkle licorice powder directly on the infection or sore.

Consult a qualified practitioner for the dosage appropriate for you and your specific condition.

SIDE EFFECTS

NOT SERIOUS

- Upset stomach; diarrhea
- Headache
- Edema (fluid retention)
- Grogginess; weakness

DISCONTINUE USE AND CALL YOUR DOCTOR.

PRECAUTIONS

WARNING

Though safe in moderate, short-term doses, licorice taken in large amounts long term can affect the body's electrolyte balance, leading to high blood pressure and edema. Consult your practitioner for advice, and do not use licorice root if you have edema, high blood pressure, kidney disease, or glaucoma.

Avoid licorice if you are pregnant. It causes increased production of aldosterone, a hormone that regulates the salt and water balance of the body, resulting in a rise in blood pressure.

SPECIAL INFORMATION

Use of this herb by children for more than seven to 10 days should be done in conjunction with a healthcare practitioner.

POSSIBLE INTERACTIONS

Combining licorice with other herbs may necessitate a lower dosage.

TARGET AILMENTS
Take internally for:
Cough; sore throat
Constipation; heartburn; colic
Stomach ulcers
Arthritis
Hepatitis; cirrhosis
Apply externally for:
Skin ulcerations; herpes sores

LIGUSTICUM

LATIN NAME
Ligusticum chuanxiong

VITAL STATISTICS

GENERAL DESCRIPTION

Ligusticum, or cnidium root as it is also known, is used for what Chinese medicine calls "stagnant blood." This condition is diagnosed in such gynecological problems as painful menstruation, lack of menstruation, or difficult labor. Stagnant blood may also manifest itself as sharp stabbing pains in the chest.

Traditional Chinese medicine classifies ligusticum as a very "light" herb, which means it is useful for conditions at the top or surface of the body, such as headache, dizziness, and certain skin conditions. In separate laboratory experiments, ligusticum has lowered blood pressure and has inhibited disease-causing bacteria.

Chinese medicine takes a holistic approach to healthcare, fashioning remedies to treat the entire being as well as the specific parts or areas. Single herbs may be used alone or in combination with other herbs to prevent and combat disease, which is thought to arise from disturbances in the flow of a bodily energy called chi (pronounced "chee") and blood, or from a lack of balance in the complementary states of yin and yang.

PREPARATIONS

Over the counter:

Ligusticum is available in Chinese pharmacies in dried bulk or in combination with other herbs in pill form.

At home:

Simmer with other herbs for 10 to 20 minutes.

COMBINATIONS: Ligusticum is used in combination with ledebouriella and schizonepeta for headaches with colds or flu. Dong quai and ligusticum is a very common combination for menstrual irregularities and pain.

PRECAUTIONS

SPECIAL INFORMATION

- Do not give to a person who has a red tongue, night sweats, or afternoon fevers.
- Do not use for violent headaches or migraines when the person has a red tongue.
- This herb should not be used if there is excessive menstrual bleeding.

POSSIBLE INTERACTIONS

Some herbalists say that ligusticum is an antagonist to cornus and astragalus, counteracts talc and coptis, and is incompatible with veratrum root and rhizome.

TARGET AILMENTS

Painful, irregular, or absent menstrual periods; difficult labor

Pain and soreness in the chest area

Headache and dizziness

SIDE EFFECTS

NOT SERIOUS

- Vomiting and dizziness (with overdose)

L

LINDEN

LATIN NAME
Tilia x europaea

VITAL STATISTICS

GENERAL DESCRIPTION

Linden, also known as lime blossoms, lime flowers, linden flowers, or tilia, comes from the tall-growing lime tree and has been used in herbal therapy since the late Middle Ages. Its diaphoretic (sweat-inducing) properties make it useful for reducing fever in colds and flu. It can also be helpful for clearing excess mucus from the bronchial passages. The herb has a relaxing effect on the nervous system and is therefore taken as a tea for insomnia, nervous tension, migraine headaches, and cramps. Some herbalists recommend it for preventing high blood pressure and atherosclerosis and for treating high blood pressure, kidney stones, and gout. Traditionally, linden was used to treat epileptic patients and was thought to help calm overactive children. The herb is also considered helpful for promoting digestion and makes a pleasant after-dinner drink.

PREPARATIONS

Over the counter:
Available as a tea.

At home:

Tea: Pour 1 cup boiling water over 1 tsp blossoms; steep covered 10 minutes. Drink three times a day. To help break a fever, use 2 to 3 tsp blossoms.

Tincture: Take 1/8 to 1/4 tsp three times a day.

Combinations: To calm nerves, mix with hops. To relieve a cold, combine with elder flower. For migraines brought on by stress, combine with equal parts hawthorn, wood betony, skullcap, and cramp bark; take three times a day as a tea or tincture. To treat mild high blood pressure, combine with hawthorn and valerian.

Consult a qualified practitioner for the dosage appropriate for you and the specific condition being treated.

PRECAUTIONS

WARNING

People with heart problems should use linden only in consultation with or upon the advice of a doctor.

SPECIAL INFORMATION

Use of this herb by children for more than seven to 10 days should be done in conjunction with a healthcare practitioner.

POSSIBLE INTERACTIONS

Combining linden with other herbs may necessitate a lower dosage.

TARGET AILMENTS
Fever
Colds
Influenza
Nervous tension
Insomnia
Headache

SIDE EFFECTS
None expected

Rx LISINOPRIL

VITAL STATISTICS

DRUG CLASS
Angiotensin-Converting Enzyme (ACE) Inhibitors

BRAND NAMES
Prinivil, Zestril

OTHER DRUGS IN THIS CLASS
benazepril, captopril, enalapril, fosinopril, quinapril, ramipril

GENERAL DESCRIPTION
Introduced in 1988, the ACE inhibitor lisinopril relaxes arterial walls, thereby lowering blood pressure. It is used in the management of hypertension (high blood pressure) and congestive heart failure. For increased blood-pressure-lowering action, lisinopril may be combined with hydrochlorothiazide, a diuretic that reduces water retention. For further information, see Angiotensin-Converting Enzyme (ACE) Inhibitors. For visual characteristics of the brand-name drugs Prinivil and Zestril, see the Color Guide to Prescription Drugs and Herbs.

PRECAUTIONS

WARNING
Get medical attention immediately if you notice swelling of your face, tongue, or vocal cords or have difficulty swallowing or breathing; this reaction can be life threatening.

This drug should not be taken during pregnancy; it has been associated with death of the fetus and newborn.

SPECIAL INFORMATION
- Lisinopril increases blood potassium levels. Do not use potassium-rich products without first consulting your doctor. The potassium in your blood could rise to dangerous levels, leading to heart-rhythm problems.
- Do not abruptly stop taking this drug. Your doctor must reduce the dosage gradually.

TARGET AILMENTS

High blood pressure

Congestive heart failure (in conjunction with digitalis preparations and diuretics)

Heart attacks (used within 24 hours to improve survival)

SIDE EFFECTS

NOT SERIOUS
- Dry, persistent cough
- Headache; fatigue
- Nausea, mild diarrhea
- Loss of sense of taste
- Temporary skin rash

CALL YOUR DOCTOR IF THESE EFFECTS BECOME BOTHERSOME.

SERIOUS
- Fainting or dizziness
- Persistent skin rash
- Fever or chills; joint pain
- Numbness and tingling
- Abdominal pain; vomiting
- Chest pain or palpitations

CALL YOUR DOCTOR IMMEDIATELY.

LITHIUM

VITAL STATISTICS

DRUG CLASS
Antimanic Drugs

BRAND NAMES
Eskalith, Lithobid, Lithonate, Lithotabs

GENERAL DESCRIPTION
Introduced in 1949, lithium is the drug of choice for the management of bipolar disorder, an illness characterized by severe mood swings from depression to mania. Symptoms of mania include elation, unusual talkativeness, inflated self-esteem, hyperactivity, decreased need for sleep, and aggressiveness. Lithium treats and controls the manic episodes of manic-depressive illness and reduces the frequency and intensity of mood swings.

PRECAUTIONS

SPECIAL INFORMATION
- Tell your doctor if you have impaired kidney function or kidney disease. Since lithium is eliminated through the kidneys, people with impaired kidney function who take the drug have a higher risk of lithium toxicity.
- Tell your doctor if you have cardiovascular disease, diabetes, hypothyroidism, Parkinson's disease, psoriasis, schizophrenia, or a history of leukemia or epilepsy or other seizure disorder; lithium may exacerbate these conditions.
- Drink plenty of water or decaffeinated beverages and avoid activities that cause you to sweat heavily. Loss of water can lead to lithium toxicity.
- Lithium should not be used by pregnant or breast-feeding women.
- Call your doctor immediately if you experience overdose symptoms: diarrhea, vomiting, muscle weakness or clumsiness, trembling, slurred speech, blurred vision, confusion, dizziness, convulsions.

POSSIBLE INTERACTIONS
Alcohol: increased intoxicating effect; possible lithium toxicity.
Lithium interacts with many other drugs. Tell your doctor about any prescription or over-the-counter medications you are using.

TARGET AILMENTS

Bipolar disorder (manic-depression)

SIDE EFFECTS

NOT SERIOUS
- Mild nausea or diarrhea
- Urinary incontinence
- Slight hand tremors

CALL YOUR DOCTOR IF THESE SYMPTOMS CONTINUE.

SERIOUS
- Irregular heartbeat; difficulty breathing; unusual tiredness; weight gain
- Hypothyroidism (dry skin, hair loss, depression, goiter, edema, constipation)

IF YOU EXPERIENCE THESE EFFECTS OR THE OVERDOSE SYMPTOMS LISTED IN SPECIAL INFORMATION, CALL YOUR DOCTOR RIGHT AWAY.

Liu Wei Di Huang Wan

Vital Statistics

ENGLISH NAME
Six-ingredient Pills with Rehmannia

GENERAL DESCRIPTION
Liu Wei Di Huang Wan is an herbal formula used to enhance what in Chinese medicine is called the yin aspect. Yin and yang are a pair of dual expressions of the universe. The yin aspect is the cooler, darker, quieter, more receptive and the yang is the warmer, brighter, more active aspect of the world. According to Chinese medicine, the yin aspects of our bodies are most available when we are very young, and a natural part of aging is the diminishing of yin as seen in the drying out of bones and joints, hot flashes in women, and diminished hearing. Illness, overwork, and other factors can accelerate the diminishing of yin. Practitioners of traditional Chinese medicine believe that this formula restores what we lose over time, and thereby helps make aging a more graceful process.

Chinese medicine takes a holistic approach to healthcare, fashioning remedies to treat the entire being as well as the specific parts or areas. Precise combinations of herbs are used to prevent and combat disease, which is thought to arise from disturbances in the flow of a bodily energy called chi (pronounced "chee") and blood, or from a lack of balance in the complementary states of yin and yang. A patent formula, *Liu Wei Di Huang Wan* is made by using a standardized combination of herbs and method of preparation.

INGREDIENTS
cooked rehmannia, cornus fruit, wild mountain yam, poria, tree peony, alisma

PREPARATIONS
This formula is sold as pills in many Chinese pharmacies and Oriental grocery stores.

Precautions

SPECIAL INFORMATION
Do not use unless the tongue is red, nor if there is a heavy coating on the tongue. Consult a Chinese practitioner for more information.

TARGET AILMENTS

- Night sweats or afternoon fevers; fatigue from chronic overwork; weakness of the lower back and legs
- Diabetes (yin-deficient type)
- Hyperthyroidism
- Symptoms of tuberculosis and AIDS
- Some kinds of weakened eyesight; some kinds of tinnitus or hearing loss
- Some chronic kidney problems

SIDE EFFECTS

NOT SERIOUS
- Loose stools if used inappropriately

DISCONTINUE AND CALL YOUR CHINESE MEDICAL PRACTITIONER.

L-LYSINE

VITAL STATISTICS

DAILY DOSAGE
General, 50 mg
To help control herpes, 500 mg per day. (During outbreaks, increase to 6,000 mg per day.)
For shingles, take 500 mg one to three times a day for one week or until resolved.

GENERAL DESCRIPTION
The body continually draws on proteins to produce and rejuvenate cells, particularly for muscles and bones. Of the 21 amino acids needed to build protein, lysine is one of the 10 that are known as essential amino acids, meaning that they cannot be produced in the body and must be obtained through the diet. Signs that the body may be low in lysine include fatigue, moodiness, bloodshot eyes, anemia, poor concentration, slow development, and reproductive problems.

Supplements of lysine may be helpful for athletes recovering from pulled muscles or for patients recovering from surgery. Growing children should be sure to eat foods containing lysine, although synthetic supplements should not be given to children except upon the advice of a physician.

Recently, L-lysine (as supplements of the amino acid are called) has received considerable attention as a treatment for the herpesvirus. Low doses are sometimes used on a long-term basis to keep herpes symptoms at bay. Larger doses can be used for shorter periods to help control and heal outbreaks. L-lysine may also be used to treat shingles and canker sores. Arginine, another amino acid, triggers herpes outbreaks, so while herpes patients are encouraged to maintain their intake of lysine, they are also advised to avoid foods high in arginine, such as chocolate, peanut butter, nuts, and seeds.

NATURAL SOURCES
kidney beans, lima beans, soybeans, split peas, corn, red meat, fish, milk, cheese, potatoes

PREPARATIONS
Available as a supplement in capsule form.

PRECAUTIONS

WARNING
Do not take L-lysine if you are pregnant or breast-feeding, except on the advice of your doctor.

Avoid taking L-lysine or other amino-acid supplements for a long period of time. Consult your doctor for guidance.

TARGET AILMENTS
- Herpes
- Shingles
- Cold sores
- Sports injuries

SIDE EFFECTS

SERIOUS
- Increased blood levels of cholesterol and triglycerides

SEEK GUIDANCE FROM YOUR PHYSICIAN.

LOBELIA

LATIN NAME
Lobelia inflata

VITAL STATISTICS

GENERAL DESCRIPTION

Lobelia, sometimes called Indian tobacco, is used for both respiratory ailments and external conditions, but it can be extremely toxic. Two of lobelia's active ingredients, lobeline and isolobelanine, may give the plant the ability to act as a relaxant for the entire body even while it stimulates the respiratory system. Lobeline mildly mimics the effect of nicotine; this has prompted people who are trying to quit smoking to use it as a temporary substitute.

Lobelia is most widely used to treat respiratory illnesses such as asthma and bronchitis. Lobelia compresses have also been used to treat skin problems and muscle strains. For visual characteristics of lobelia, see the Color Guide to Prescription Drugs and Herbs.

PREPARATIONS

Over the counter:

Available in dried bulk, capsules, tinctures.

At home:

Tea: Steep covered 1/4 to 1/2 tsp dried leaves in 1 cup boiling water for 10 to 15 minutes; drink three times daily.

Compress: Soak a piece of fabric in an infusion for several minutes; wring out and apply.

Consult a qualified practitioner for the dosage appropriate for your specific condition.

PRECAUTIONS

WARNING

Use lobelia only in doses prescribed by your practitioner.

This herb should not be used with children, unless it is specifically prescribed by a healthcare practitioner who is knowledgeable about herbs. Monitor the child frequently for the development of any side effects.

POSSIBLE INTERACTIONS

Combining lobelia with other herbs may necessitate a lower dosage.

TARGET AILMENTS

Take internally for:

Pneumonia; asthma

Bronchitis; smoking

Apply externally for:

Insect bites; poison ivy

Fungus infections

Muscle strains

SIDE EFFECTS

SERIOUS

SYMPTOMS OF TOXIC DOSES OF LOBELIA INCLUDE:

- Nausea; vomiting
- Excessive salivation
- Diarrhea
- Hearing and vision problems
- Weakness; mental confusion

IF NOT TREATED PROMPTLY, ACUTE CASES OF POISONING CAN BRING ON RESPIRATORY FAILURE AND EVEN DEATH. IF YOU DEVELOP ANY SIDE EFFECTS, CALL YOUR DOCTOR IMMEDIATELY.

L

Long Dan Xie Gan Wan

Vital Statistics

ENGLISH NAME

Gentiana Drain the Liver Pills

GENERAL DESCRIPTION

Long Dan Xie Gan Wan is used to treat a condition known in Chinese medicine as Damp Heat of the Liver. In Chinese medicine, the function of the liver involves not only the action of the organ itself but also the eyes and the emotion anger. This formula, therefore, is used to treat red, sore eyes, and irritability or a short temper. It is also used to treat herpes, hepatitis, and infections (a type of damp heat) of the eyes, ears, urinary tract, genitals, and vagina.

Chinese medicine takes a holistic approach to healthcare, fashioning remedies to treat the entire being as well as specific parts or areas. Precise combinations of herbs are used to prevent and combat disease, which is thought to arise from disturbances in the flow of a bodily energy called chi (pronounced "chee") and blood, or from a lack of balance in the complementary states of yin and yang. A patent formula, *Long Dan Xie Gan Wan* is made by using a standardized combination of herbs and method of preparation.

INGREDIENTS

gentiana, scutellaria, gardenia, akebia, plantain seeds, alisma, bupleurum, raw rehmannia, dang gui, licorice

PREPARATIONS

This formula is sold in pill form at many Chinese pharmacies and Oriental grocery stores.

Precautions

SPECIAL INFORMATION

This formula should be used only for acute conditions and stopped when the symptoms have improved. It should not be used for long periods of time.

TARGET AILMENTS
Conjunctivitis or red, painful eyes
Otitis media
Herpes; shingles
Some migraine headaches
Hepatitis with jaundice
Acute gallstone attack
Cystitis; urethritis; vaginal discharge; itchy, swollen genitals
Some kinds of bad temper
Hyperthyroidism or Graves' disease

SIDE EFFECTS

None expected

L

Rx LOPERAMIDE

VITAL STATISTICS

DRUG CLASS
Antidiarrheal Drugs

BRAND NAMES
Rx: Imodium
OTC: Imodium A-D

OTHER DRUGS IN THIS CLASS
attapulgite, bismuth subsalicylate

GENERAL DESCRIPTION
Introduced in 1977, loperamide is used primarily for symptomatic control of diarrhea and cramping. It is available in both over-the-counter and prescription strength. Loperamide should be taken on an empty stomach. See Antidiarrheal Drugs for more information. For visual characteristics of the brand-name prescription-strength drug Imodium, see the Color Guide to Prescription Drugs and Herbs.

L

PRECAUTIONS

WARNING
Do not use loperamide if:
- diarrhea is accompanied by high fever (101°F or higher).
- blood or mucus is present in stool.
- you have a rash or other allergic reaction to the drug.
- you are taking antibiotics or have a history of liver disease or colitis.
- you are pregnant or nursing a baby. Consult a doctor before using this drug.

POSSIBLE INTERACTIONS
Alcohol, sleeping pills, and tranquilizers: may increase depressant and sedative effects.
Antibiotics and narcotic pain medicine: may cause severe constipation if taken with antidiarrheals.

TARGET AILMENTS
Symptomatic relief of diarrhea

SIDE EFFECTS

NOT SERIOUS
- Mild constipation

CHECK WITH YOUR DOCTOR IF THE CONSTIPATION CONTINUES OR IF YOU DEVELOP A FEVER.

WHEN USED AT THE RECOMMENDED DOSAGE FOR NO MORE THAN TWO DAYS, LOPERAMIDE AND OTHER ANTIDIARRHEAL MEDICATIONS RARELY CAUSE SIDE EFFECTS. BUT IF THE DIARRHEA DOES NOT DECREASE WITHIN ONE OR TWO DAYS, CHECK WITH YOUR DOCTOR.

LORACARBEF

VITAL STATISTICS

DRUG CLASS
Antibiotics [Carbacephems]

BRAND NAME
Lorabid

GENERAL DESCRIPTION
Loracarbef, introduced in 1992, is the first of the carbacephem antibiotics, a subclass of drugs that work in much the same way as penicillins and cephalosporins to kill growing bacteria.

For visual characteristics of the brand-name drug Lorabid, see the Color Guide to Prescription Drugs and Herbs.

PRECAUTIONS

SPECIAL INFORMATION

- Tell your doctor if you are allergic to penicillins or cephalosporins; if so, you are likely to be allergic to loracarbef as well. Allergic reactions to these drugs can be life threatening.
- Tell your doctor if your kidneys are impaired; you may require a smaller dose of loracarbef, or you may need a different drug altogether.
- Take this drug one hour before or two hours after a meal.
- If this drug causes severe diarrhea, consult your doctor before taking any antidiarrheal medicine. For mild diarrhea, use only antidiarrheal preparations containing kaolin or attapulgite.
- To prevent reinfection, take the full course of your prescription, even if you feel better before you've taken all the medicine.

TARGET AILMENTS
Bronchitis
Otitis media
Strep throat
Some forms of pneumonia
Sinusitis
Infections of the skin and soft tissue
Urinary tract infections
Other bacterial infections

CONTINUED

LORACARBEF

- Carbacephems kill not only harmful bacteria but also "good" intestinal bacteria that keep harmful fungi and intestinal bacteria in check. Eating yogurt containing *Lactobacillus acidophilus* culture or taking acidophilus tablets may help restore the body's normal bacteria.
- Prolonged use of any antibiotic can lead to fungal infections, including candidiasis, or to bacterial infections such as pseudomembranous colitis.
- Unless it is clearly needed, avoid taking loracarbef if you are pregnant or breastfeeding.

POSSIBLE INTERACTIONS

Probenecid: decreases the kidneys' ability to excrete loracarbef; possible loracarbef toxicity.

See entries for two similar antibiotic subclasses, Penicillins and Cephalosporins, for other possible drug interactions.

SIDE EFFECTS

NOT SERIOUS

- Nausea
- Abdominal pain
- Mild diarrhea
- Loss of appetite

CONSULT YOUR DOCTOR IF THESE SYMPTOMS CONTINUE FOR MORE THAN TWO DAYS OR ARE BOTHERSOME.

SERIOUS

- Severe itching, rash, or difficulty breathing (possibly indicating an anaphylactic reaction)
- Severe diarrhea
- Severe abdominal pain
- Stomach cramps

CALL YOUR DOCTOR IMMEDIATELY; YOU MAY NEED TO ALTER YOUR CURRENT PRESCRIPTION OR SWITCH TO A DIFFERENT MEDICINE.

- Dizziness
- Headache
- Drowsiness
- Insomnia
- Nervousness
- Vaginal itching and discharge

CONSULT YOUR DOCTOR IF THESE SYMPTOMS CONTINUE OR BECOME SEVERE.

Rx LORATADINE

VITAL STATISTICS

DRUG CLASS
Antihistamines

BRAND NAMES
Claritin, Claritin-D 12 Hour, Claritin-D 24 Hour

OTHER DRUGS IN THIS CLASS
Rx: astemizole, cetirizine, diphenhydramine, fexofenadine, promethazine, terfenadine
OTC: brompheniramine, chlorpheniramine, clemastine, dexbrompheniramine, diphenhydramine, doxylamine, triprolidine

GENERAL DESCRIPTION
A newer, relatively nonsedating antihistamine, loratadine is commonly prescribed for seasonal allergies. It generally doesn't cause the drowsiness, jitters, or dry mouth associated with other drugs of its kind. Loratadine is combined with pseudoephedrine in the brand-name drugs Claritin-D 12 Hour and Claritin-D 24 Hour. See Antihistamines for additional side effects and interaction information. For visual characteristics of the brand-name drugs Claritin and Claritin-D 12 Hour, see the Color Guide to Prescription Drugs and Herbs.

PRECAUTIONS

SPECIAL INFORMATION
- If your liver is impaired, loratadine can build up in your body and provoke serious heart problems. Depending on the severity of your liver condition, your doctor may prescribe a different antihistamine.
- Check with your doctor before using loratadine if you have asthma, liver disease, or kidney disease; loratadine may exacerbate these conditions.
- Let your doctor know if you are pregnant or breast-feeding. Your doctor may advise you to stop using loratadine or to stop breast-feeding while you're using the drug.

POSSIBLE INTERACTIONS
Azithromycin, cimetidine, clarithromycin, erythromycin, itraconazole, ketoconazole, ranitidine, theophylline, and troleandomycin: may interfere with the body's metabolism of loratadine, possibly causing life-threatening cardiac effects.

TARGET AILMENTS

Nasal and respiratory allergies, including hay fever; chronic hives; asthma induced by exercise (adjunct treatment)

SIDE EFFECTS

NOT SERIOUS
- Sedation; insomnia; dry nose, mouth, or throat

CALL YOUR DOCTOR IF THESE SYMPTOMS CONTINUE.

SERIOUS
- Fainting; heart palpitations or change in heartbeat; cardiac arrest

CALL YOUR DOCTOR RIGHT AWAY. THESE EFFECTS ARE RARE BUT MAY OCCUR IF PROPER DOSAGE IS EXCEEDED OR IF YOU HAVE LIVER DAMAGE.

Rx LORAZEPAM

VITAL STATISTICS

DRUG CLASS
Antianxiety Drugs [Benzodiazepines]

BRAND NAME
Ativan

OTHER DRUGS IN THIS SUBCLASS
alprazolam, clonazepam, diazepam, temazepam, triazolam

GENERAL DESCRIPTION
Introduced as an injectable drug in 1963 and as a tablet in 1984, lorazepam is a benzodiazepine prescribed for the treatment of anxiety, severe nervous tension, and insomnia. In injection form, it is also used to relieve presurgery anxiety. For more information, see Benzodiazepines. For visual characteristics of lorazepam and the brand-name drug Ativan, see the Color Guide to Prescription Drugs and Herbs.

PRECAUTIONS

WARNING
Never combine alcohol with lorazepam; the combination can cause dangerous central nervous system and respiratory depression.

Do not abruptly stop taking lorazepam. Sudden cessation can provoke withdrawal symptoms, including seizures; irritability; insomnia; confusion; mental depression; hypersensitivity to pain, noise, or light; and feelings of suspicion and distrust. Slowly reduce the dosage under your doctor's guidance.

SPECIAL INFORMATION
- Lorazepam can impair your alertness, judgment, and coordination. Avoid driving and performing hazardous activities until you know how the drug affects you.
- Let your doctor know if you have narrow-angle glaucoma, a liver or kidney impairment, chronic respiratory disease, myasthenia gravis, depression, sleep apnea, or a history of drug abuse or addiction. Lorazepam may exacerbate these conditions.
- This drug can cause sleep apnea in people with chronic respiratory disease, such as emphysema.
- Lorazepam can cause physical and psychological dependence, sometimes after only one or two weeks, but usually after prolonged use.
- People with a history of drug or alcohol abuse are at a greater risk of psychological dependence on lorazepam.
- Tolerance may increase with prolonged use; as your body adjusts to lorazepam, the drug becomes less effective. Never increase the dose without consulting your doctor, because the risk of lorazepam dependence increases with higher doses.
- Do not take lorazepam if you are pregnant or breast-feeding.

TARGET AILMENTS
Anxiety and panic disorders
Insomnia
Presurgery anxiety (an adjunct to anesthesia)

POSSIBLE INTERACTIONS

Alcohol, anticonvulsants, antihistamines that cause drowsiness (clemastine, diphenhydramine), barbiturates, monoamine oxidase (MAO) inhibitors, opioids, tricyclic antidepressants: increased sedative effects, such as excessive mental (central nervous system) depression, sleepiness, and slow or shallow breathing. Do not take lorazepam in combination with any of these drugs.

Antacids: may slow the absorption of lorazepam. Take antacids one hour before or after taking lorazepam.

Beta blockers, cimetidine, disulfiram, erythromycin, ketoconazole, omeprazole, oral contraceptives, probenecid: may prolong the amount of time lorazepam remains in your body, leading to increased lorazepam effects and possible toxicity.

Clozapine: risk of profound hypotension (low blood pressure), slow or shallow breathing, cessation of breathing, and cardiac arrest leading to death.

Isoniazid: possible increased effect and toxicity of lorazepam.

Levodopa: decreased levodopa effect.

Rifampin: possible decreased effect of lorazepam.

Tobacco (smoking): decreased lorazepam effects.

Valproic acid: increased lorazepam effects, including mental depression.

Zidovudine: risk of zidovudine toxicity.

SIDE EFFECTS

NOT SERIOUS

- Clumsiness or unsteadiness; drowsiness; dizziness
- Blurred vision
- Lethargy
- Dry mouth; nausea
- Change in bowel habits
- Temporary amnesia (especially "traveler's amnesia" when taken to treat insomnia associated with jet lag)

TELL YOUR DOCTOR IF THESE SYMPTOMS PERSIST, PARTICULARLY IF YOU ARE HAVING DIFFICULTY WITH YOUR MEMORY.

SERIOUS

- Persistent or severe headache
- Confusion; depression
- Changes in behavior (outbursts of anger, difficulty concentrating)
- Hallucinations
- Uncontrolled movement of body or eyes
- Muscle weakness
- Chills or fever
- Sore throat
- Allergic reaction, such as rash or itching (rare)
- Jaundice (rare)
- Low blood pressure (rare)
- Anemia (rare)
- Unusual bruising or bleeding (rare)

TELL YOUR DOCTOR ABOUT THESE SYMPTOMS RIGHT AWAY.

LOSARTAN

VITAL STATISTICS

DRUG CLASS
Antihypertensive Drugs

BRAND NAMES
Cozaar, Hyzaar

OTHER DRUGS IN THIS CLASS
guanfacine

GENERAL DESCRIPTION
Introduced in 1995, losartan treats high blood pressure by relaxing blood vessels to improve blood flow. It works by preventing the effects of a protein that causes blood vessels to constrict. The brand-name drug Hyzaar is losartan in combination with hydrochlorothiazide, a thiazide diuretic, which lowers blood pressure by promoting excretion of salt and water. Like other blood-pressure-lowering drugs, losartan is most effective when combined with regular exercise, stress reduction, weight loss, and a salt-restricted diet.

For more information, see Antihypertensive Drugs. For visual characteristics of the brand-name drug Hyzaar, see the Color Guide to Prescription Drugs and Herbs.

PRECAUTIONS

☠ ***WARNING***
An overdose of losartan can cause faintness, dizziness, and slow or irregular heartbeat. Contact a poison control center or seek emergency treatment if you've taken too much.

Losartan can cause dizziness or confusion. Until you know how it will affect you, be cautious about driving, using machines, or engaging in any potentially dangerous activity.

SPECIAL INFORMATION

- Do not take this drug if you are pregnant, planning to become pregnant, or breastfeeding. If you become pregnant while taking losartan, discontinue the drug immediately and tell your doctor.
- Consult your doctor before taking losartan if you are allergic to any food, medicine (especially aspirin or penicillin), or other substance, or if you have any kidney or liver disease, anuria, asthma, or a history of coronary artery disease or circulation problems in the brain.
- Several weeks' treatment may be necessary to determine the effectiveness of this drug.
- Regular contact with your doctor is recommended in order to monitor the effectiveness of blood pressure control.
- Do not stop taking this medicine without the advice of your doctor, even if you feel well. High blood pressure can cause problems without any symptoms and usually requires treatment for the rest of your life.
- This drug may affect some lab tests; notify any healthcare practitioner you consult that you are taking losartan.
- Extreme heat can cause dehydration and lower blood pressure; use caution in hot weather and while exercising to avoid feeling dizzy or faint.
- Discuss with your doctor any over-the-counter or prescription medications you consider taking while taking losartan, especially antihistamines; appetite-control pills; medicines for colds, coughs, sinus, or hay fever; painkillers; or muscle relaxants. Some of these medications can increase your blood pressure; others may cause excess drowsiness.

LOSARTAN

POSSIBLE INTERACTIONS

Alcohol, barbiturates, narcotic analgesics: higher risk of lowered blood pressure upon standing up when taken with Hyzaar. Use alcohol with caution when taking this drug.

Antidiabetic agents: Hyzaar may increase blood glucose concentrations.

Anti-inflammatory drugs, nonsteroidal: decreased effect of losartan.

Cholestyramine, colestipol: may inhibit absorption of the hydrochlorothiazide component of Hyzaar.

Corticosteroids: may increase electrolyte depletion when taken with Hyzaar.

Cyclosporine; low-salt milk; potassium-sparing diuretics; potassium-containing medications, salt substitutes, or supplements: elevated potassium levels.

Diuretics: increased effect of losartan.

Food: avoid excessive salt.

Lithium: increased risk of toxicity.

Other blood-pressure-lowering drugs: excessively low blood pressure.

Sympathomimetics: decreased effect of both combined drugs.

TARGET AILMENTS

High blood pressure

SIDE EFFECTS

NOT SERIOUS

- Headache
- Fatigue
- Diarrhea
- Back pain
- Muscle cramps; leg pain
- Skin rash
- Stuffy nose; dry cough (rare)
- Insomnia (rare)
- Nausea; stomach pain (rare)
- Increased sensitivity to sunlight (rare)

CALL YOUR DOCTOR IF THESE EFFECTS PERSIST OR BECOME BOTHERSOME.

SERIOUS

- Dizziness
- Electrolyte imbalance (dry mouth, increased thirst, irregular heartbeat, weak pulse, nausea or vomiting, muscle cramps or pain, unusual fatigue)
- Cough; fever; sore throat
- Swelling of face and lips
- Severe headaches (rare)

CONTACT YOUR DOCTOR IMMEDIATELY IF YOU NOTICE ANY OF THESE SYMPTOMS.

Rx LOTENSIN

VITAL STATISTICS

DRUG CLASS
Angiotensin-Converting Enzyme (ACE) Inhibitors

GENERIC NAME
benazepril

OTHER DRUGS IN THIS CLASS
captopril, enalapril, fosinopril, lisinopril, quinapril, ramipril

GENERAL DESCRIPTION
Lotensin is the brand name for the generic drug benazepril, an ACE inhibitor introduced in 1991. Benazepril is prescribed for control of high blood pressure. It works by blocking a body enzyme that is essential for the production of a substance that causes blood vessels to constrict. This action relaxes arterial walls, lowering blood pressure. For further information, see the entries Benazepril and Angiotensin-Converting Enzyme (ACE) Inhibitors.

PRECAUTIONS

WARNING
Get medical attention immediately if you notice swelling of your face, tongue, or vocal cords or have difficulty swallowing or breathing; this reaction can be life threatening.

This drug should not be taken during pregnancy because it has been associated with malformations and death of the fetus and newborn baby.

SPECIAL INFORMATION
- Lotensin causes an increase in blood levels of potassium. Do not use potassium-rich products, including salt substitutes and low-salt milk, without first consulting your doctor. The potassium in your blood could rise to dangerous levels, leading to heart-rhythm problems.
- Do not abruptly stop taking this drug. Your doctor may tell you to reduce the dosage gradually.
- Because your first dose of an ACE inhibitor may cause a sudden drop in blood pressure, your doctor may recommend that you take the first dose at bedtime; you may also need to increase your dose gradually.
- Lotensin can cause an increased sensitivity to the sun that may result in serious, unexpected sunburn.
- Use caution during hot weather or while exercising; excessive perspiration can lead to dehydration and reduced blood pressure in people taking ACE inhibitors.
- Let your doctor know if you have arthritis or kidney disease, or if you are on a strict low-sodium diet or are taking diuretics.

LOTENSIN

POSSIBLE INTERACTIONS

Alcohol: increased ACE inhibitor effects, leading to much lower blood pressure.

Central nervous system stimulants (including pseudoephedrine, an over-the-counter decongestant): reduced ACE inhibitor effect.

Diuretics: combining ACE inhibitors with diuretics may initially cause a significant drop in blood pressure.

Estrogens: fluid retention, possibly raising blood pressure.

Lithium: lithium toxicity, which can lead to stupor, coma, and seizures.

Nonsteroidal anti-inflammatory drugs [NSAIDs] (especially indomethacin), salicylates (such as aspirin): may decrease the effects of ACE inhibitors and prevent the drugs from lowering blood pressure.

Other medications that lower blood pressure, such as beta-adrenergic blockers, calcium channel blockers, diuretics, levodopa, nitrates, and opioid analgesics: increased hypotensive (blood-pressure-lowering) effect of both combined medications.

Potassium products and diuretics that do not eliminate potassium from the body (such as amiloride, spironolactone, and triamterene): increased blood potassium levels, leading to heart-rhythm problems.

TARGET AILMENTS

High blood pressure

SIDE EFFECTS

NOT SERIOUS

- Dry, persistent cough
- Headache
- Fatigue
- Nausea or diarrhea
- Loss of sense of taste
- Temporary skin rash
- Low blood pressure or dizziness on suddenly rising or changing position

CALL YOUR DOCTOR IF THESE SIDE EFFECTS BECOME BOTHERSOME.

SERIOUS

- Fainting
- Persistent skin rash
- Joint pain
- Drowsiness
- Numbness and tingling
- Abdominal pain
- Vomiting
- Diarrhea
- Fever
- Chills
- Chest pain; heart palpitations
- Jaundice (yellowing of skin or eyes)

CALL YOUR DOCTOR RIGHT AWAY.

Rx LOVASTATIN

VITAL STATISTICS

DRUG CLASS
Cholesterol-Reducing Drugs

BRAND NAME
Mevacor

OTHER DRUGS IN THIS CLASS
cholestyramine, colestipol, fluvastatin, gemfibrozil, niacin, pravastatin, simvastatin

GENERAL DESCRIPTION
Introduced in 1987, lovastatin is one of several so-called HMG-CoA reductase inhibitors, which lower levels of cholesterol and other blood fats. These drugs work by blocking a liver enzyme needed in the production of cholesterol. For more information, see Cholesterol-Reducing Drugs.

PRECAUTIONS

SPECIAL INFORMATION
- If you become pregnant while taking this drug, stop using it immediately and inform your doctor.
- Lovastatin works better when taken with food.

POSSIBLE INTERACTIONS
Erythromycin, immunosuppressants, and niacin: severe muscle pain, kidney failure.

TARGET AILMENTS

The major types of cholesterol disorders, particularly those in which high levels of blood fats (cholesterol and triglycerides) have been linked to an increased risk of heart disease

Coronary atherosclerosis in patients with coronary heart disease

SIDE EFFECTS

NOT SERIOUS
- Constipation
- Gas
- Decreased sex drive
- Insomnia

CALL YOUR DOCTOR IF THESE EFFECTS PERSIST OR BECOME TROUBLESOME.

SERIOUS
- Fever
- Muscle aches
- Cramps
- Blurred vision

CALL YOUR DOCTOR RIGHT AWAY.

L

LYCIUM FRUIT

LATIN NAME
Lycium barbarum
(or Lycium chinense)

VITAL STATISTICS

GENERAL DESCRIPTION

Two varieties of lycium are used in Chinese herbal medicine: The more common *Lycium barbarum* grows in a number of Chinese provinces, while *Lycium chinense* occurs largely in the Hebei province. Both produce large, soft, red berries, sometimes called wolfberries, that are similar in appearance and in action. They ripen in the summer and have thick flesh and small seeds. The herbs are classified as sweet and neutral. Lycium given to rabbits in lab tests appeared to reduce blood pressure and calm labored breathing.

Chinese medicine takes a holistic approach to healthcare, fashioning remedies to treat the entire being as well as the specific parts or areas. Single herbs may be used alone or in combination with other herbs to prevent and combat disease, which is thought to arise from disturbances in the flow of a bodily energy called chi (pronounced "chee") and blood, or from a lack of balance in the complementary states of yin and yang.

PREPARATIONS

Lycium fruit can be purchased from Chinese pharmacies, Asian markets, and some Western health food stores. It is usually added to other ingredients of an herbal formula during the last five minutes of cooking.

COMBINATIONS: When mixed with cuscuta, eucommia bark, and Chinese foxglove root cooked in wine, lycium fruit is prescribed for impotence, dizziness, and tinnitus (ringing in the ears). Practitioners also combine lycium fruit with ophiopogon tuber, anemarrhena, and fritillaria to treat consumptive coughs.

For further information on appropriate preparations and dosages, check with a practitioner.

PRECAUTIONS

SPECIAL INFORMATION

You should not take this herb if you have an inflammatory ailment, weak digestion, or a tendency to become bloated.

TARGET AILMENTS

Take internally for:

- Night blindness
- Tinnitus (ringing in the ears)
- Dizziness; blurred vision
- Consumptive coughs
- Diabetes
- Sore back, knees, and legs
- Impotence and nocturnal emission

SIDE EFFECTS

NONE EXPECTED

LYCOPODIUM

LATIN NAME
Lycopodium clavatum

VITAL STATISTICS

GENERAL DESCRIPTION

Lycopodium, also known as club moss, grows in pastures and woodlands throughout Great Britain, northern Europe, and North America. Its spores contain a highly flammable pollen that was once used in fireworks. Powder made from its ground-up spores has been used for internal complaints like diarrhea and dysentery since the 17th century. Homeopathic physicians use dilute doses of *Lycopodium* for complaints that are accompanied by symptoms of digestive upset, ailments that seem to develop on the right side of the body, a strong desire for sweets, anxiety, and symptoms that worsen in the early evening.

To create the homeopathic remedy, pollen is extracted from the spores and diluted with milk sugar. For more information on homeopathic medicine, see page 14.

PREPARATIONS

Lycopodium is available in various potencies, in both liquid and tablet form, at selected stores and pharmacies. Consult your homeopathic physician for more precise information.

PRECAUTIONS

SPECIAL INFORMATION

- When a remedy is administered, no one but the patient should touch the pills. If tablets are spilled, throw them away.
- The mouth should be clear of flavors 15 minutes before and after taking a remedy, and strong flavors and aromas, such as coffee, camphor, and heavily scented perfumes, should be avoided for the duration of treatment.

TARGET AILMENTS

Backache with stiffness and soreness in the lower back

Bedwetting

Colds with stuffy nose

Constipation

Coughs with mucus present

Cystitis

Headache with throbbing pain that is at its worst between 4 and 8 p.m.

Gout

Indigestion accompanied by abdominal cramps

Gas

Heartburn

Joint pain

Sciatica

Right-sided sore throat

Eczema

SIDE EFFECTS

NONE EXPECTED

L

MAGNESIA PHOSPHORICA

LATIN NAME
Magnesia phosphorica

VITAL STATISTICS

GENERAL DESCRIPTION

This remedy is made from magnesium phosphate. Magnesium and phosphate are important in muscle and nervous function and, paradoxically, can both cause and cure nerve pain and muscle cramps. In fact, a toxic overdose of magnesium phosphate can cause numbness or paralysis. Sometimes called homeopathic aspirin, the remedy *Magnesia phosphorica,* or *Mag phos,* relieves minor aches and pains, especially those that are improved by heat. To prepare the remedy, magnesium sulfate and sodium phosphate are combined and mixed with water, left to crystallize, and then ground with milk sugar. For more information on homeopathic medicine, see page 14.

PREPARATIONS

Mag phos is available over the counter in various potencies, in both liquid and tablet form, at selected stores and pharmacies. *Mag phos* is best administered dissolved in warm water. Boil and partially cool a glass of water, dissolve four pills in it, and stir vigorously. Sip the water frequently until symptom relief is obtained. Wash glass and spoon in scalding water so that others who use them after you won't be affected by the remedy. Consult your homeopathic physician for more information.

PRECAUTIONS

SPECIAL INFORMATION

- Only the patient should touch the pills. If tablets are spilled, throw them away.
- The mouth should be clear of flavors 15 minutes before and after taking a remedy, and strong flavors and aromas should be avoided for the duration of treatment.

TARGET AILMENTS

Headaches worsened by mental exertion or chill

Dizziness following movement

Involuntary spastic movements; weak or twitching muscles

Neuralgia in right eye or right ear, worsened by cold water

Toothache made better by heat

Teething pains

Cramping nerve pain or sciatica made better by warmth and worsened by cold and exercise

Spasmodic earache

Writer's cramp

Abdominal pain and gas or menstrual cramps, improved with warmth and pressure

Infant colic with hiccups, relieved by warmth

Difficulty thinking clearly

SIDE EFFECTS

NONE EXPECTED

MAGNESIUM

VITAL STATISTICS

GENERAL DESCRIPTION

Magnesium contributes to health in many ways. Along with calcium and phosphorus, it is a main ingredient of bone. A proper balance of calcium and magnesium is essential for healthy bones and teeth, reduces the risk of osteoporosis, and may alleviate existing osteoporosis. Calcium and magnesium also help regulate muscle activity; calcium stimulates contraction, magnesium induces relaxation. Magnesium is essential for metabolism and for building proteins. Adequate blood levels of magnesium protect the body from cardiovascular disease, heart arrhythmias, and possibly, stroke due to blood clotting in the brain.

The body's need for magnesium increases with stress or illness. Given as a supplement, magnesium may treat insomnia, muscle cramps, premenstrual syndrome, and cardiovascular problems including hypertension, angina due to coronary artery spasm, and pain and cramping due to insufficient blood flow to the legs. Studies indicate that giving magnesium immediately to a heart attack patient greatly increases the chance of survival.

The body processes magnesium efficiently; the kidneys conserve it as needed and excrete any excess amounts, so the incidences of both severe deficiency and toxicity are rare. These conditions are dangerous when they do occur, however.

Many over-the-counter antacids, laxatives, and analgesics contain magnesium, but these medications should not be used as magnesium supplements. A multinutrient supplement is a relatively safe way to augment your magnesium intake. Of the supplemental forms, magnesium citrate-malate is the easiest to absorb, while magnesium glycinate is the least likely to cause diarrhea at high doses.

RDA

Men: 350 mg
Women: 280 mg
Pregnant women: 320 mg

NATURAL SOURCES

On average, people get enough (or nearly enough) magnesium in their diet. Fish, green leafy vegetables, milk, nuts, seeds, and whole grains are good sources.

PRECAUTIONS

WARNING

Take specific magnesium supplements only under a doctor's supervision. Magnesium toxicity can cause diarrhea, fatigue, muscle weakness, and in extreme cases, severely depressed heart rate and blood pressure, shallow breathing, loss of reflexes, coma, and even death. People who abuse laxatives or experience kidney failure are the most vulnerable to magnesium poisoning.

SPECIAL INFORMATION

Magnesium deficiency may cause nausea, vomiting, listlessness, muscle weakness, tremor, disorientation, and heart palpitations.

TARGET AILMENTS
Heart disease
Menstrual problems
Muscle cramps

SIDE EFFECTS

NONE EXPECTED

MAGNESIUM CARBONATE

VITAL STATISTICS

DRUG CLASS
Antacids

BRAND NAMES
Bayer Buffered Aspirin Tablets, Bufferin, Gaviscon (formula with aluminum hydroxide)

OTHER DRUGS IN THIS CLASS
aluminum hydroxide, calcium carbonate, magnesium hydroxide, sodium bicarbonate and citric acid

GENERAL DESCRIPTION
An active ingredient in some antacid medications, magnesium carbonate helps relieve symptoms of heartburn, sour stomach, acid indigestion, and upset stomach caused by diseases such as peptic ulcer, gastritis, esophagitis, and hiatal hernia. Magnesium carbonate is also used in combination with aspirin to increase the speed at which that drug dissolves, thereby reducing irritation in the gastrointestinal tract.

See Antacids for more information, including possible drug interactions and special information about this class of medications.

PRECAUTIONS

WARNING
Except under medical supervision, do not take magnesium carbonate (or any antacid containing a magnesium compound) if you have impaired kidney function. Doing so could result in reduced blood pressure, nausea and vomiting, respiratory distress, and even coma.

TARGET AILMENTS

Upset stomach; heartburn; acid indigestion; sour stomach

Ulcers; gastritis; esophagitis

Pain (when used as a buffering ingredient with aspirin)

SIDE EFFECTS

NOT SERIOUS

- Mild diarrhea or mild constipation
- Increased thirst
- Unpleasant taste in mouth
- Stomach cramps; belching; flatulence
- Change in stool color (white or speckled)

CALL YOUR DOCTOR IF THESE PROBLEMS PERSIST.

SERIOUS

- Muscle pain or weakness
- Frequent or urgent urination
- Nausea; vomiting; dizziness; loss of appetite
- Nervousness or change in mood
- Fatigue
- Swollen ankles and feet
- Headache
- Bone pain

CONTACT YOUR DOCTOR IMMEDIATELY.

M

MAGNESIUM HYDROXIDE

VITAL STATISTICS

DRUG CLASS
Antacids

BRAND NAMES
Phillips' Milk of Magnesia, Rolaids, some types of Maalox and Mylanta

OTHER DRUGS IN THIS CLASS
aluminum hydroxide, calcium carbonate, magnesium carbonate, sodium bicarbonate and citric acid

GENERAL DESCRIPTION
Magnesium hydroxide is a magnesium-containing antacid drug used to relieve symptoms of upset and sour stomach, acid indigestion, heartburn, and ulcers. It is most effective when taken on an empty stomach. The most common side effect of magnesium hydroxide is a laxative action or diarrhea. See Antacids for information about possible drug interactions and additional special information.

PRECAUTIONS

SPECIAL INFORMATION
- Magnesium-containing antacids increase the risk of magnesium toxicity; do not take these drugs if you have kidney disease.
- Notify your doctor if you develop symptoms such as black, tarry stools or vomit the consistency of coffee grounds. These are indications of bleeding in the stomach or intestines.

TARGET AILMENTS

Upset stomach; heartburn; acid indigestion; sour stomach

Ulcers

SIDE EFFECTS

NOT SERIOUS

- Mild constipation
- Laxative effect or diarrhea
- Chalky taste in the mouth
- Stomach cramps; nausea or vomiting
- Belching
- Flatulence
- White specks in the stool

CALL YOUR DOCTOR IF THESE PROBLEMS PERSIST.

SERIOUS

- Swelling of the wrist, foot, or lower leg
- Bone pain
- Severe constipation
- Dizziness
- Mood changes
- Muscle pain, weakness, or twitching
- Nervousness or restlessness
- Slow breathing
- Irregular heartbeat
- Fatigue
- Pain upon urinating or frequent need to urinate
- Change in appetite

CONTACT YOUR DOCTOR IMMEDIATELY.

M

Magnolia Flower

LATIN NAME
Magnolia liliiflora
(or M. denudata)

Vital Statistics

GENERAL DESCRIPTION

More accurately described as magnolia buds, this herb is the unopened magnolia flower. Chinese medicine practitioners prescribe it for blocked nasal and sinus passages. In test-tube studies, magnolia flowers seemed to inhibit the growth of several fungi on the skin. The best-quality buds are green and dry; they should include none of the stems or branches. The herb is characterized in traditional Chinese medicine as acrid and warm. Growing in several Chinese provinces, magnolia is harvested in early spring, before the flowers unfold.

Chinese medicine takes a holistic approach to healthcare, fashioning remedies to treat the entire being as well as the specific parts or areas. Single herbs may be used alone or in combination with other herbs to prevent and combat disease, which is thought to arise from disturbances in the flow of a bodily energy called chi (pronounced "chee") and blood, or from a lack of balance in the complementary states of yin and yang.

PREPARATIONS

Magnolia buds are available in bulk at Chinese pharmacies, Asian markets, and some Western health food stores. When you buy magnolia buds in bulk at a Chinese pharmacy, the buds will be broken and the hairy outer layer removed; this must be done before cooking in order for the herb to be effective.

Combinations: Magnolia flowers are mixed with xanthium, angelica *(Angelica dahurica),* and field mint to treat nasal congestion and sinus headaches, and with chrysanthemum flowers *(Chrysanthemum morifolium)* and siegesbeckia for frontal sinusitis.

Consult an herbal practitioner for details of other mixtures and doses.

Precautions

SPECIAL INFORMATION

Overdoses can cause dizziness and red eyes.

TARGET AILMENTS

Take internally for:

Nasal congestion, discharge

Sinus headaches, other sinus disorders

SIDE EFFECTS

None expected if taken as directed.

M

MANGANESE

VITAL STATISTICS

GENERAL DESCRIPTION

Manganese is essential for the proper formation and maintenance of bone, cartilage, and connective tissue; it contributes to the synthesis of proteins and genetic material; it helps produce energy from foods; it acts as an antioxidant; and it assists in normal blood clotting.

Manganese citrate, a dietary supplement, may help repair damaged tendons and ligaments. Excess dietary manganese is not considered toxic, and manganese deficiency is extremely rare.

EMDR

2.5 mg to 5 mg

NATURAL SOURCES

Most people get enough manganese through diet alone; for example, a breakfast of orange juice, a 1-oz serving of bran cereal, and a banana provides just over 2.5 mg of manganese. Other food sources include brown rice, nuts, seeds, wheat germ, beans, whole grains, peas, and strawberries.

TARGET AILMENTS

Sprains and strains

Inflammation

Diabetes

Epilepsy

SIDE EFFECTS

NONE EXPECTED

Marsh Mallow

LATIN NAME
Althaea officinalis

Vital Statistics

GENERAL DESCRIPTION

For centuries, people in Europe and the Middle East have eaten wild-growing marsh mallow when their crops failed. Today it is still recognized as a wilderness forage food. Herbalists use the roots, and sometimes the leaves, of this five-foot-high downy, erect perennial that grows in damp soils; they prescribe it for cuts and wounds, mouth sores, stomach distress, and other ailments. And teething, irritable babies and toddlers have traditionally found comfort in sucking on a root of marsh mallow.

The healing substance in marsh mallow is mucilage, a spongy root material that forms a gel when mixed with water and is especially soothing to inflamed mucous membranes. One study suggests that mucilage supports the immune system's white blood cells in their fight against invading microbes. Another trial, using animals, indicated that marsh mallow may help to lower blood sugar. For visual characteristics of marsh mallow, see the Color Guide to Prescription Drugs and Herbs.

PREPARATIONS

Over the counter:
Available in dried bulk, capsules, and tincture.

At home:

Decoction: Simmer covered 1 to 2 tsp finely chopped or crushed root in 1 cup water for 10 to 15 minutes; drink three times daily. Use the decoction as a gargle for mouth problems.

Gel: Add just enough water to the finely chopped root to give it a gel-like consistency. Use for skin problems.

Consult a qualified practitioner for the dosage appropriate for your specific condition.

Precautions

SPECIAL INFORMATION

- The candy named marshmallow contains none of the herb, although the marsh mallow plant was considered a delicacy by the Romans, who used it to make candy.
- Give marsh mallow only in low doses to infants and children.

POSSIBLE INTERACTIONS

Combining marsh mallow with other herbs may necessitate a lower dosage.

TARGET AILMENTS

Take marsh mallow internally for:

Sore throat; coughs; colds; flu; bronchitis; sinusitis

Upset stomach; peptic ulcers; gastritis; colitis

Cystitis; bladder infections; urethritis; kidney stones

Apply marsh mallow externally for:

Abscesses; boils; skin ulcers; cuts; burns; scrapes; other wounds

Varicose veins

Dental abscesses and gingivitis

SIDE EFFECTS

None expected

M

MEADOWSWEET

LATIN NAME
Filipendula ulmaria

VITAL STATISTICS

GENERAL DESCRIPTION

Meadowsweet was prized during the Middle Ages for its flowers, which were used to sweeten the air in the less-than-sanitary households. Today herbalists prescribe the herb for colds and flu, digestive upsets, muscle aches and pains, headaches, menstrual cramps, arthritis, and congestive heart failure.

PREPARATIONS

Over the counter:
Available as tincture and dried bulk.

At home:

INFUSION: Pour 1 cup boiling water over 2 tsp dried herb and steep covered for 10 minutes. Up to 3 cups a day may be consumed.

TINCTURE: Take 1/8 to 1/2 tsp up to three times a day. Take for no more than one week unless your doctor prescribes otherwise.

Consult a qualified practitioner for the dosage appropriate for your specific condition.

PRECAUTIONS

WARNING

Pregnant women and nursing mothers should not use any preparations containing salicylates without a doctor's knowledge.

Use of this herb by children for more than seven to 10 days should be done in conjunction with a healthcare practitioner. Do not give to children under two at all, or to children under 16 who show symptoms of colds, flu, or chickenpox; aspirin and aspirin-like substances increase their risk of developing Reye's syndrome.

Those with ulcers or gastritis should take meadowsweet only with a doctor's permission.

SPECIAL INFORMATION

- For children over two and adults over 65, start with a low-strength dose and gradually increase the dose if needed.
- People sensitive to salicylate should not use.

POSSIBLE INTERACTIONS

Do not take meadowsweet preparations if medications containing aspirin or salicylates are also being taken.

Combining meadowsweet with other herbs may necessitate a lower dosage.

TARGET AILMENTS
Headache
Pain; inflammation; muscle aches; arthritis; cramps
Colds; influenza
Digestive upsets including nausea, heartburn, and hyperacidity

SIDE EFFECTS

NOT SERIOUS

- Upset stomach
- Nausea or diarrhea

SERIOUS

- Bleeding of the stomach
- Respiratory paralysis

THESE EFFECTS MAY OCCUR IF DOSAGE IS EXCEEDED OR IF PATIENT IS VERY SENSITIVE TO SALICYLATES. DISCONTINUE USE AND CALL YOUR DOCTOR IMMEDIATELY.

M

MELATONIN

VITAL STATISTICS

GENERAL DESCRIPTION

Melatonin is a hormone that occurs naturally in the body. It helps to regulate the body's daily biological rhythms. The hormone is released in cyclical patterns during each 24-hour period. The level of melatonin is determined by the amount of light present. During the day, very little melatonin is present in the body. But at night, the pineal gland synthesizes and releases the hormone into the bloodstream. Melatonin plays a role in determining the quality and length of sleep. Nighttime levels of the hormone decrease significantly in the elderly, who often have trouble getting to sleep and tend to sleep for fewer hours.

Melatonin may help protect the immune system by minimizing the potentially damaging effects of high amounts of steroid hormones called corticosteroids. Chronic high levels of corticosteroids have been linked with glucose intolerance, impaired immune function, and clogged arteries—all factors associated with aging. Melatonin's effect on corticosteroids is one reason melatonin has been said to be able to combat aging. Animal research suggests the hormone also plays a role in suppressing the growth of certain cancer tumors.

Melatonin supplements were introduced in the U.S. market in the early 1990s. It is best known as a sleeping aid. Small amounts of the supplement taken after airplane flights that cross several time zones help alleviate jet lag. The supplements can also be effective in inducing sleep in people with insomnia, particularly the elderly, and in shift workers.

Proponents of melatonin claim the supplements boost the immune system, slow the aging process, and fight cancer, although these effects have not been proved in studies on human beings.

PREPARATIONS

In the United States, melatonin is sold as a dietary supplement in tablet and capsule form.

PRECAUTIONS

WARNING

Do not take melatonin if you are pregnant.

SPECIAL INFORMATION

Little is known about the effects of taking melatonin on a long-term basis. Because it is a potent hormone, some experts argue it should be regulated as a drug, as it is in Canada and Germany, and not as a dietary supplement, as it is in the United States. Animal research suggests melatonin can be harmful for people with autoimmune diseases, such as multiple sclerosis, or those with collagen-induced arthritis.

M

TARGET AILMENTS
Jet lag; insomnia; stress
Seasonal affective disorder (SAD)
Cancer (adjunct therapy)

SIDE EFFECTS

- Headache; rash; upset stomach
- Disruption of normal circadian rhythm

DISCONTINUE USE AND CALL YOUR DOCTOR.

MENTHOL

VITAL STATISTICS

BRAND NAMES

Ben-Gay, Halls Mentho-Lyptus Cough Drops, N'Ice Cough Drops, Ricola, Vicks VapoRub

GENERAL DESCRIPTION

Menthol, an aromatic oil from the peppermint plant, is a natural alcohol that is now usually produced synthetically. For centuries the drug has been used, either alone or in combination with other substances, in a wide variety of medicinal products, from rubs and liniments for itchy skin and aching muscles to gargles and lozenges for mouth and throat irritations. Menthol has been shown to be effective in relieving the itching and pain of hemorrhoids and minor skin irritations. It is also a useful medication for soothing a sore throat and suppressing coughs.

Menthol works by penetrating the skin or mucous membranes to calm nerve endings. It may also help kill some types of bacteria. The drug is available in many forms, including cough drops and lozenges, various topical preparations and rubs, and inhalants. Menthol is also used as an ingredient in mouthwashes, toothpastes, throat sprays, and foods such as candy and chewing gum.

PRECAUTIONS

SPECIAL INFORMATION

- Because instances of choking have been reported in very young children, menthol cough drops are not considered safe for children under five years old.
- Consult your doctor before using menthol liniments on children under the age of two.
- Because very little menthol is absorbed into the blood, low concentrations are generally considered safe for pregnant and nursing women. However, you should check with your doctor before using any medication that contains menthol.
- Menthol, when used alone, is considered safe in the doses available. However, when combined with methyl salicylate (as in some ointments for relieving sore muscles), the medication may cause redness of skin. Discontinue use if redness develops. Also, be aware that when applied to the skin or mucous membranes, high concentrations of menthol or pure peppermint oil (which contains a high concentration of menthol) can cause serious irritation that may require medical attention.

Menthol

TARGET AILMENTS
Itchy and painful skin
Hemorrhoids (to relieve itching and pain)
Cough
Minor sore throat and irritations of the throat
Arthritis; muscle strain (often in combination with methyl salicylate and camphor)
Congestion associated with colds or allergies (often in combination with camphor and desoxyephedrine)
Cold sores (to soothe and relieve pain)

SIDE EFFECTS

NOT SERIOUS

- Local irritation or a cooling sensation

YOU NEED NOT CALL YOUR DOCTOR UNLESS THESE SYMPTOMS BECOME BOTHERSOME. TO EASE THE SYMPTOMS, TRY USING LESS OF THE DRUG.

M

Mercurius vivus

LATIN NAME
Mercurius vivus

Vital Statistics

GENERAL DESCRIPTION

One of the metallic chemical elements, mercury, also called quicksilver, was known in ancient Chinese and Hindu civilizations and has had a long history of medicinal use. Ingesting certain mercury compounds can cause increased perspiration and salivation; and so in ancient medicine mercury was used, along with bloodletting and purging, as a means of ridding the body of impurities. Undilute mercury is toxic, however, and severe symptoms of mercury poisoning may include nausea, inflammation of the digestive tract, and kidney failure.

Homeopathic practitioners prescribe *Merc viv,* as the homeopathic preparation of mercury is called, for conditions accompanied by symptoms of shaking, hot and cold sweats, and restlessness. *Merc viv* is made from the chemical element mercury by dilution with large quantities of milk sugar. For more information on homeopathic medicine, see page 14.

PREPARATIONS

Merc viv is available in various potencies, in both liquid and tablet form, at selected stores and pharmacies. Consult a homeopathic physician for further information.

Precautions

SPECIAL INFORMATION

- When a remedy is administered, no one but the patient should touch the pills. If tablets are spilled, throw them away.
- The mouth should be clear of flavors 15 minutes before and after taking a remedy, and strong flavors and aromas, such as coffee, camphor, and heavily scented perfumes, should be avoided for the duration of treatment.

TARGET AILMENTS

Abscesses, especially dental or glandular

Backache with burning, shooting pains in the lower back

Chickenpox

Colds with an exceptionally runny nose and pain in the nostrils

Cystitis with slow urination

Painful diarrhea

Influenza

Earache with discharge of pus

Eye inflammation

Indigestion

Mouth ulcers

Burning sore throat

Toothache with increased salivation

SIDE EFFECTS

None expected

M

METFORMIN

VITAL STATISTICS

DRUG CLASS
Antidiabetic Drugs [Oral Antihyperglycemics]

BRAND NAME
Glucophage

OTHER DRUGS IN THIS CLASS
insulin; glipizide, glyburide (Oral Hypoglycemics); acarbose, troglitazone (Oral Antihyperglycemics)

GENERAL DESCRIPTION
Metformin is used to treat excess blood sugar in people with non-insulin-dependent (Type 2) diabetes when diet, weight loss, and exercise do not produce sufficient control but insulin is not required. It helps to lower blood sugar but does not cure diabetes. Metformin apparently works by decreasing the production of sugar in the liver and by increasing the body's sensitivity to insulin. It promotes uptake of blood sugar by the body's cells.

Metformin can be combined with a sulfonylurea drug for more effective blood sugar control. For visual characteristics of the brand-name drug Glucophage, see the Color Guide to Prescription Drugs and Herbs.

PRECAUTIONS

WARNING
In patients with kidney, liver, or heart disease, metformin can cause a rare, serious metabolic disorder called lactic acidosis. These persons should not use metformin.

An overdose of metformin can cause hypoglycemia, or low blood sugar, with symptoms of unusual weakness, shakiness, stomach pain, nausea or excessive hunger, rapid heartbeat, cold sweats or chills, confusion, anxiety, convulsions, or unconsciousness. For mild symptoms of hypoglycemia, consume something that contains sugar as soon as possible. For more severe symptoms seek emergency care immediately.

Consume alcohol moderately when taking metformin. The risk of lactic acidosis is increased when alcohol is consumed with this drug.

Metformin may cause dizziness or drowsiness. Avoid driving and other dangerous activities until you see how the drug affects you.

Metformin should be discontinued 48 hours prior to a CT scan or any x-ray study involving the administration of intravascular radiocontrast, as the radiocontrast may cause kidney damage and raise the risk of lactic acidosis.

Other oral antidiabetic drugs (tolbutamide and phenformin) have been shown to increase the risk of cardiovascular death. Although metformin has not been shown to carry the same risk, the same caution could possibly apply. Discuss any concerns you have about this with your doctor.

SPECIAL INFORMATION
- Consult your doctor before beginning to take metformin if you have allergies, a kidney or liver dysfunction, hyper- or hypothyroidism, or a heart or circulatory disease. Tell your doctor also if you are planning surgery or if you have a history of intestinal disorders, megaloblastic anemia, alcoholism, or acid in the blood (metabolic acidosis or ketoacidosis).
- The somewhat common gastrointestinal side effects of metformin will often lessen over time. Taking the drug with food may minimize nausea or diarrhea.
- If you develop an illness or infection, con-

CONTINUED

METFORMIN

tact your doctor. You may need a temporary change of medications.

- Metformin should not be used during pregnancy nor by nursing mothers.
- Before taking metformin, tell your doctor if you are a premenopausal, anovulatory woman, as this drug may cause a resumption of ovulation, increasing the possibility of pregnancy.
- Diabetes and its treatment are complex, requiring patient participation as well as periodic monitoring. Consult with your doctor regularly in order to determine the continuing effectiveness and safety of treatment.
- It is a good idea to wear medical identification containing the information that you take metformin for diabetes management.

POSSIBLE INTERACTIONS

Alcohol: increased effect of metformin; increased risk of acid in the blood or hypoglycemia.

ACE inhibitors, amiloride, calcium channel blockers, cimetidine, digoxin, furosemide, hypoglycemics, morphine, procainamide, quinidine, quinine, ranitidine, triamterene, trimethoprim, vancomycin: increased effect of metformin.

Beta blockers: may slow recovery from low blood sugar or mask the warning signs of low blood sugar.

Contraceptives (estrogen-containing), corticosteroids, thiazide diuretics, estrogens, isoniazid, nicotinic acid, phenytoin, sympathomimetics, thyroid hormones: may raise blood sugar levels, necessitating increased dose of metformin.

Clofibrate, monoamine oxidase (MAO) inhibitors, probenecid, propranolol, rifabutin, rifampin, salicylates, long-acting sulfonamides, sulfonylureas: may lower blood sugar, necessitating decreased dose of metformin.

Itraconazole, other azole antifungal medications: increase metformin's hypoglycemic effects.

TARGET AILMENTS

Type 2 diabetes mellitus

SIDE EFFECTS

NOT SERIOUS

- Stomach pain; gas; diarrhea; nausea; vomiting
- Changes in taste; decreased appetite; weight loss
- Headache; dizziness; nervousness; fatigue
- Rash

CALL YOUR DOCTOR IF THESE EFFECTS PERSIST OR BECOME BOTHERSOME.

SERIOUS

- Diarrhea, chills, muscle pain, weakness and sleepiness, slow heartbeat, and difficulty breathing (lactic acidosis)
- Unusual weakness, shakiness, stomach pain, nausea or excessive hunger, rapid heartbeat, cold sweats or chills, confusion, anxiety, convulsions, and unconsciousness (hypoglycemia)
- Vitamin B_{12} deficiency anemia (extremely rare)

CALL YOUR DOCTOR IMMEDIATELY.

METHYLCELLULOSE

VITAL STATISTICS

DRUG CLASS
Laxatives

BRAND NAME
Citrucel

OTHER DRUGS IN THIS CLASS
Bulk: calcium polycarbophil, psyllium hydrophilic mucilloid
Stimulant: phenolphthalein, sennosides
Stool softener: docusate

GENERAL DESCRIPTION
Methylcellulose is a bulk-forming laxative used for the temporary relief of both constipation and diarrhea, and to prevent straining during bowel movements. Bulk-forming laxatives work by absorbing water and expanding, thus softening the stool and stimulating normal contractions of the large intestine to make passage easier. They may be especially beneficial to people on low-fiber diets and patients with postpartum constipation, irritable bowel syndrome, diverticulitis, or hemorrhoids. You should experience results from this drug in 12 to 72 hours. See Laxatives for additional information.

TARGET AILMENTS

Constipation or diarrhea

Irritable bowel syndrome

Straining during bowel movements following rectal surgery, heart attacks, or childbirth, or when hemorrhoids are present

PRECAUTIONS

SPECIAL INFORMATION
- Be sure to drink plenty of water or other fluid to avoid throat or esophageal obstruction.
- Unless prescribed by a physician, laxatives should not be given to children under six.
- Do not use laxatives if you have symptoms of appendicitis, any undiagnosed abdominal pain, nausea, or vomiting, or if you think you have an intestinal obstruction.
- If you have congestive heart failure or rectal bleeding, do not use laxatives without your doctor's consent.
- If you have difficulty swallowing, do not take bulk-forming laxatives, which can cause an esophageal obstruction.
- Prolonged use is not recommended without a doctor's guidance.

POSSIBLE INTERACTIONS
Oral anticoagulants, digitalis, salicylate, and tetracycline may be less effective when taken concurrently with bulk-forming laxatives. Allow a two-hour interval between taking these drugs and a laxative.

SIDE EFFECTS

NOT SERIOUS
- Abdominal cramps; diarrhea; nausea; vomiting; intestinal obstruction (if taken dry)

SERIOUS
- Difficulty breathing (rare)
- Skin rash or itching (rare)
- Esophageal obstruction

CALL YOUR DOCTOR IMMEDIATELY.

M

METHYLPHENIDATE

VITAL STATISTICS

DRUG CLASS
Central Nervous System Stimulants

BRAND NAME
Ritalin

GENERAL DESCRIPTION
Methylphenidate is a mild central nervous system (CNS) stimulant that seems to work by activating the brainstem arousal system and cerebral cortex.

For some children with an attention deficit disorder, CNS stimulation decreases motor restlessness, increases attention span, and improves concentration. In adults, it can lead to increased motor activity and mental alertness, decreased fatigue, a cheerier outlook, and mild euphoria.

Because methylphenidate is an amphetamine-like drug, it can be habit forming, leading to marked tolerance and serious physical and psychological dependence. Dosages must be prescribed on an individual basis, and physician supervision is essential.

For visual characteristics of methylphenidate and of the brand-name drug Ritalin, see the Color Guide to Prescription Drugs and Herbs.

PRECAUTIONS

SPECIAL INFORMATION
- Seek immediate medical help for overdose. Signs of overdose include rapid, pounding, or irregular heartbeat; fever and sweating; confusion, convulsions, hallucinations, agitation, delirium, vomiting, dry mouth, trembling, muscle twitching, increased blood pressure, and loss of consciousness.
- Do not take if you have had an allergic reaction to this drug; have glaucoma or motor tics; or are suffering from severe tension, agitation, anxiety, or emotional depression.
- Before taking, tell your doctor if you have high blood pressure, epilepsy, angina, liver problems, or a history of alcoholism or drug dependence.
- Sleeping problems may be avoided if you take the last dose before 6 p.m.
- Although methylphenidate may be the primary agent in treating attention deficit disorders, its long-term effects are unknown. Your doctor may recommend occasional drug-free periods during treatment and discontinuance of the drug after puberty.

Methylphenidate

POSSIBLE INTERACTIONS

Anticholinergics, anticoagulants, anticonvulsants, and antidepressants (tricyclic): methylphenidate may increase the effects of these drugs.

Antihypertensives, guanethidine, minoxidil, and terazosin: methylphenidate may decrease the effects of these drugs.

Monoamine oxidase (MAO) inhibitors: methylphenidate should not be taken within two weeks of using MAO inhibitors. Concurrent use of the two drugs could cause dangerously high blood pressure and severe convulsions.

TARGET AILMENTS

Attention deficit disorders in children

Narcolepsy (uncontrollable spells of drowsiness or sleep)

Mild to moderate depression

In the elderly, apathy and withdrawal

Chronic pain (used with other drugs)

SIDE EFFECTS

NOT SERIOUS

- Nervousness
- Trouble sleeping
- Loss of appetite
- Headache
- Dizziness
- Nausea
- Stomach pains
- Mild skin rash
- Unusual fatigue

SEE YOUR DOCTOR IF THESE SYMPTOMS PERSIST.

SERIOUS

- Severe skin rash or hives
- Irregular or fast heartbeat
- Chest pain
- Unusual bruising
- Blurred vision
- Joint pain
- Sore throat and fever
- Weight loss
- Mood or mental changes
- Abnormal behavior patterns
- Psychotic reactions

CALL YOUR DOCTOR IMMEDIATELY.

Methylprednisolone

Vital Statistics

DRUG CLASS
Corticosteroids

BRAND NAMES
Medrol, Depo-Medrol (injectable)

OTHER DRUGS IN THIS CLASS
beclomethasone, betamethasone, fluticasone, hydrocortisone, mometasone furoate, prednisone, triamcinolone

GENERAL DESCRIPTION
One of a group of corticosteroid drugs, which are synthetic versions of the hormones produced by the adrenal glands, methylprednisolone is used principally as an anti-inflammatory agent and an immunosuppressant. It is effective against severe inflammations caused by a number of diseases, including arthritis, asthma, and some skin disorders. Methylprednisolone is also used to treat allergies, cancer, inflammation of the eyes, and other ailments. It reduces inflammation by blocking the normal defensive (or inflammatory) reactions of particular kinds of white blood cells.

In some diseases, methylprednisolone is used for its immunosuppressant effect, which means that it reduces the body's reaction to foreign proteins. In autoimmune diseases such as lupus and multiple sclerosis, the drug stops the body from producing an immune response against its own proteins. Methylprednisolone is also used to treat adrenal cortex insufficiency, in which the adrenal glands do not produce enough hormone. In this case, methylprednisolone replaces the missing hormone. See Corticosteroids for more information about this class of drugs. For visual characteristics of methylprednisolone tablets, see the Color Guide to Prescription Drugs and Herbs.

Precautions

WARNING
Do not take this drug if you have a fungal infection or are allergic to any corticosteroids. Before using this drug, let your doctor know if you have tuberculosis, bone disease, colitis, myasthenia gravis, heart disease, glaucoma, thyroid disease, diabetes, peptic ulcer, diverticulitis, liver or kidney disease, or herpes infection of the eyes, lips, or genitals.

Methylprednisolone suppresses the immune system and increases the susceptibility to infection. The drug can also mask signs of new infection.

Use of methylprednisolone for a long time may cause glaucoma, cataract, or eye infection. Dosage should be reduced gradually.

Sudden stopping of this medication can cause worsening of the underlying disease and may even be fatal.

TARGET AILMENTS
Inflammation caused by many diseases; eye inflammation; skin disorders
Adrenal cortex insufficiency
Allergy; asthma; arthritis; lupus
Anemia
Ulcerative colitis
Tuberculosis
Multiple sclerosis
Some cancers (adjunct)

METHYLPREDNISOLONE

SPECIAL INFORMATION

- Tell your doctor about any diseases you have or have had in the past. Let your doctor know if you have congestive heart failure, high blood pressure, or blood clots, or if you have had tuberculosis in the past.
- This drug can cause tuberculosis to recur in people who were cured.
- Normally, you should not use this drug if you have an uncontrolled bacterial or viral infection.
- Do not obtain immunizations while taking this drug; the combination may interfere with the development of immunity and cause problems with your nervous system.
- People over 60 may have more severe side effects, such as cataracts and osteoporosis.
- Long-term use of this drug in children can result in retarded growth.
- Tell your doctor if you have been exposed to measles or chickenpox or if you have plans to have surgery.
- Avoid methylprednisolone if you are pregnant or nursing.
- It is a good idea to carry medical identification stating that you use this drug if you use it for more than a week.

POSSIBLE INTERACTIONS

Alcohol: may cause stomach ulcers.
Amphotericin B: may cause loss of potassium.
Anticholinergic drugs: may cause glaucoma.
Anticoagulants: decreased anticoagulant effects.
Aspirin: increases the effect of methylprednisolone and decreases the effect of aspirin.
Carbamazepine (and other anticonvulsants), phenobarbital, rifampin: decreased effect of methylprednisolone.
Cyclosporine: risk of toxicity from both drugs.
Insulin or oral drugs for diabetes: decreased antidiabetic action.
Isoniazid: decreased isoniazid effect.
Loop diuretics (e.g., furosemide, bumetanide): may increase risk of potassium loss.
Nonsteroidal anti-inflammatory drugs: increased risk of peptic ulcer.
This list is not complete. Tell your doctor about any drugs you are taking.

SIDE EFFECTS

NOT SERIOUS

- Acne; headache; dizziness
- Increased thirst; change in appetite; weight gain; retention of salt and water
- Nausea; vomiting; constipation; gas; upset stomach
- Cough; hoarse throat
- Unpleasant taste; insomnia; nervousness; restlessness

CALL YOUR DOCTOR IF THESE PROBLEMS PERSIST.

SERIOUS

- Rash; hives; severe itching; serious allergic reaction
- Blurred vision; cataract; glaucoma
- Bone fractures; slow wound healing; peptic ulcers
- Convulsions; seizures
- Congestive heart failure; abnormal heartbeat; high blood pressure
- Growth retardation in children
- Severe emotional disturbance

CALL YOUR DOCTOR RIGHT AWAY.

Methyl Salicylate

Vital Statistics

DRUG CLASS
Analgesics [Topical Analgesics]

BRAND NAME
Ben-Gay

OTHER DRUGS IN THIS CLASS
acetaminophen, aspirin, nonsteroidal anti-inflammatory drugs (NSAIDs), opioid analgesics

GENERAL DESCRIPTION
Obtained from the leaves and bark of plants in the *Gaultheria,* birch, and poplar families, or produced synthetically, methyl salicylate is used as a topical medicine for relieving pain in muscles and joints. Sometimes called wintergreen oil, the substance works as a counterirritant; it stimulates skin receptors, providing temporary relief from aches and pains.

Methyl salicylate is available in a variety of gels, liniments, lotions, and ointments, usually in combination with menthol or camphor. The concentration of methyl salicylate in these products varies from 10 to 60 percent. Poisonous if ingested, methyl salicylate is relatively safe for external use.

Precautions

SPECIAL INFORMATION
- Heat and humidity increase the absorption of methyl salicylate through the skin, thus increasing the risk of salicylate toxicity. Do not exercise vigorously in hot, humid weather after application or use a heating pad immediately after application.
- To reduce risk of irritation, avoid contact with eyes; mucous membranes; or broken, irritated skin.

Target Ailments

Minor muscle and joint aches and pains from arthritis, sprains, strains, and bruises (use only if skin is intact)

Side Effects

Not Serious

- Local skin redness or irritation

DISCONTINUE USE AND CONTACT YOUR DOCTOR IF THESE EFFECTS BECOME TROUBLESOME.

Serious

- Salicylate toxicity (dizziness, ringing in ears, nausea, vomiting), a rare condition caused by absorption through the skin into the blood

DISCONTINUE USE AND CONTACT YOUR DOCTOR.

M

Rx METOPROLOL

VITAL STATISTICS

DRUG CLASS
Beta-Adrenergic Blockers

BRAND NAMES
Lopressor, Toprol-XL

OTHER DRUGS IN THIS CLASS
atenolol, bisoprolol, nadolol, propranolol, timolol

GENERAL DESCRIPTION
Metoprolol is prescribed to help manage hypertension, angina, and myocardial infarction. By blocking the action of certain parts of the nervous system, metoprolol slows the heart rate and relaxes blood vessels, thereby lowering blood pressure and easing the work load on the heart. See Beta-Adrenergic Blockers for more information, including possible interactions. Metoprolol may be combined with the diuretic hydrochlorothiazide. For visual characteristics of metoprolol and the brand-name drug Lopressor, see the Color Guide to Prescription Drugs and Herbs.

PRECAUTIONS

SPECIAL INFORMATION
- Metoprolol can make you drowsy, dizzy, and lightheaded. Avoid activities that require alertness, such as driving, until you know how you react to this drug.
- Tell your doctor if you are planning surgery or have any of the following conditions, which metoprolol may complicate: allergies; emphysema; congestive heart failure; diabetes mellitus; hyperthyroidism; impaired liver or kidneys; depression; myasthenia gravis; circulatory disease.
- Do not use metoprolol if you have a bronchospastic disease, bronchial asthma, or a severe chronic obstructive pulmonary disease.
- Suddenly stopping this drug may cause or increase heart problems. Dosage must be reduced gradually by your doctor.

TARGET AILMENTS

Heart disease, including angina (chest pain), heart attack, and abnormal heart rhythms

Hypertension

SIDE EFFECTS

NOT SERIOUS
- Decreased sexual ability
- Drowsiness or weakness
- Insomnia; nervousness
- Upset stomach; change in bowel habits

TELL YOUR DOCTOR IF THESE EFFECTS BECOME BOTHERSOME.

SERIOUS
- Trouble breathing
- Dizziness; depression
- Chest pain; fast or irregular heartbeat
- Prolonged reduced circulation; congestive heart failure
- Sudden shortness of breath
- Sweating, trembling, and weakness

CALL YOUR DOCTOR IMMEDIATELY.

Rx MEVACOR

VITAL STATISTICS

DRUG CLASS
Cholesterol-Reducing Drugs

GENERIC NAME
lovastatin

OTHER DRUGS IN THIS CLASS
cholestyramine, colestipol, fluvastatin, gemfibrozil, niacin, pravastatin, simvastatin

GENERAL DESCRIPTION
Mevacor is a brand name for the generic drug lovastatin. Introduced in 1987, this drug is one of several so-called HMG-CoA reductase inhibitors, which lower levels of cholesterol and other blood fats. These drugs work by blocking a liver enzyme needed in the production of cholesterol. For more information, see Cholesterol-Reducing Drugs.

TARGET AILMENTS

The major types of cholesterol disorders, particularly those in which high levels of blood fats (cholesterol and triglycerides) have been linked to an increased risk of heart disease

Coronary atherosclerosis in patients with coronary heart disease

PRECAUTIONS

SPECIAL INFORMATION
- Do not take this drug if you are pregnant or breast-feeding. If you become pregnant while taking this drug, stop using it immediately and inform your doctor.
- Do not take this drug if you have active liver disease or if you have had an allergic reaction to any other HMG-CoA reductase inhibitor.
- Liver function must be monitored while taking this drug.
- Mevacor works better when it is taken with food.

POSSIBLE INTERACTIONS
Erythromycin, immunosuppressants, gemfibrozil, and niacin: increased risk of severe muscle pain, kidney failure.

SIDE EFFECTS

NOT SERIOUS
- Constipation
- Gas
- Decreased sex drive
- Insomnia

CALL YOUR DOCTOR IF THESE EFFECTS PERSIST OR BECOME TROUBLESOME.

SERIOUS
- Fever
- Muscle aches
- Cramps
- Blurred vision

CALL YOUR DOCTOR RIGHT AWAY.

Rx MICONAZOLE

VITAL STATISTICS

DRUG CLASS
Antifungal Drugs

BRAND NAMES
Rx: Monistat-Derm, Monistat Dual-Pak, Monistat 3 Vaginal Suppositories
OTC: Monistat 7

OTHER DRUGS IN THIS CLASS
Rx: clotrimazole, fluconazole, ketoconazole, terconazole
OTC: clotrimazole, tolnaftate, undecylenate

GENERAL DESCRIPTION
Miconazole, available in topical and vaginal preparations, is used to treat a variety of fungal infections. See Antifungal Drugs for more information. For information about other medications commonly used to treat vaginal yeast infections, see Vaginal Antifungal Drugs.

PRECAUTIONS

SPECIAL INFORMATION
- Topical creams, lotions, and powders are applied directly to the skin to combat the fungi that cause body ringworm, jock itch, and athlete's foot. They can be used twice a day for up to one month.
- Vaginal creams and suppositories are inserted directly into the vagina, usually at bedtime, for a period of three to seven days.

POSSIBLE INTERACTIONS
No interactions are expected with most topical and vaginal forms of antifungal drugs. See Ketoconazole for a list of drugs and other substances you should avoid while taking systemic antifungal medications.

TARGET AILMENTS

Yeast infections (candidiasis) of the vulva and vagina, mouth, skin, hands, and internal organs

Ringworm (tinea) of the body, scalp, nails, hands, feet (athlete's foot), and groin (jock itch)

Tinea versicolor, a ringworm infection that produces white-brown patches on the skin

Fungal skin infections (topical)

SIDE EFFECTS

NOT SERIOUS
- Mild skin irritation in the infected area
- Headache; drowsiness
- Dizziness; nausea; vomiting
- Stomach pain
- Constipation or diarrhea

CALL YOUR DOCTOR IF THESE EFFECTS PERSIST.

SERIOUS
- Allergic skin reactions, such as a rash or hives (topical preparations)
- Redness, stinging, burning, or itching of the genitals; abdominal cramps or menstrual irregularities; or itching and burning of a sexual partner's penis (vaginal preparations)

CALL YOUR DOCTOR AT ONCE.

M

MILK THISTLE

LATIN NAME
Silybum marianum

VITAL STATISTICS

GENERAL DESCRIPTION

Milk thistle, a plant that reaches five feet in height and thrives both in the wild and in the garden, is used by herbalists to treat such liver disorders as cirrhosis and hepatitis. The active ingredient, silymarin, is found in the seeds. It is believed that silymarin prompts the manufacture of new, healthy liver cells without encouraging the growth of any malignant liver tissue that may be present. Silymarin, it is thought, also serves as an antioxidant, protecting liver cells from damage by free radicals, which are harmful by-products of many bodily processes, including cellular metabolism. The use of silymarin by healthy people can increase by as much as one-third the liver's content of glutathione, a key substance in detoxifying many potentially damaging hormones, chemicals, and drugs.

Extracts of silymarin appear to neutralize toxins from the death cup mushroom, which can inflict lethal injury on the liver. Milk thistle is also believed to ease outbreaks of psoriasis, since these may worsen when the liver fails to neutralize certain toxins that circulate in the bloodstream. For visual characteristics of milk thistle, see the Color Guide to Prescription Drugs and Herbs.

TARGET AILMENTS

- Liver problems, including cirrhosis and hepatitis
- Inflammation of the gallbladder duct
- Poisoning from ingestion of the death cup mushroom
- Psoriasis

SIDE EFFECTS

NOT SERIOUS

BECAUSE TAKING MILK THISTLE INCREASES BILE SECRETION, YOU MAY DEVELOP LOOSE STOOLS.

PREPARATIONS

Over the counter:
Available in dried bulk, capsules, and extract.

At home:
TEA: Steep covered 1 tsp freshly ground seeds in 1 cup boiling water for 10 to 15 minutes; drink three times daily. As an alternative to tea, eat 1 tsp freshly ground seeds. Milk thistle extract may be more effective than teas, since silymarin is only slightly soluble in water. See a herbalist for further information.
Consult a qualified practitioner for the dosage appropriate for your specific condition.

PRECAUTIONS

WARNING
If you think that you have a liver disorder, seek medical advice.

SPECIAL INFORMATION

Use of this herb by children for more than seven to 10 days should be done in conjunction with a healthcare practitioner.

POSSIBLE INTERACTIONS

Combining milk thistle with other herbs may necessitate a lower dosage.

M

Minor Blue Dragon Pills

Vital Statistics

CHINESE NAME
Xiao Qing Long Wan

GENERAL DESCRIPTION
Minor Blue Dragon Pills are used to treat colds, flu, and bronchitis accompanied by coughing and mucus. This formula is used if the patient feels a heaviness in the chest, has difficulty breathing, especially when lying down, and has a thick white coating on the tongue. Minor Blue Dragon Pills help dry the excess mucus in the lungs and relieve coughing and wheezing.

Chinese medicine takes a holistic approach to healthcare, fashioning remedies to treat the entire being as well as the specific parts or areas. Precise combinations of herbs are used to prevent and combat disease, which is thought to arise from disturbances in the flow of a bodily energy called chi (pronounced "chee") and blood, or from a lack of balance in the complementary states of yin and yang. Crucial to a practitioner's diagnosis is a careful examination of the tongue, considered an excellent barometer of the disharmonies in the body. A patent formula, Minor Blue Dragon Pills are made by using a standardized combination of herbs and method of preparation.

INGREDIENTS
ephedra, cinnamon twig, dry ginger, Chinese wild ginger, schisandra, white peony root, pinellia, licorice

PREPARATIONS
This formula is available from qualified herbal practitioners and some health food stores.

Precautions

WARNING
Do not use if the tongue coating is dark yellow. Consult with a Chinese practitioner for more information.

TARGET AILMENTS

Acute bronchitis

Coughing, with phlegm

Asthma or wheezing

Influenza

SIDE EFFECTS
None expected

MINOXIDIL

VITAL STATISTICS

DRUG CLASS
Hair Growth Stimulants

BRAND NAME
Rogaine

GENERAL DESCRIPTION
As a topical solution, minoxidil is used to treat baldness in both men and women. Under proper conditions, preparations containing 2 percent minoxidil may stimulate the growth of new hair on the scalp. These stimulating effects are more noticeable in younger people and in those with early male-pattern baldness. Although the exact mechanism of action is not established, researchers believe that minoxidil increases blood flow near the skin's surface, resulting in the stimulation of hair follicle cells. However, once treatment is stopped, new hair will fall out, which is why many people choose to use minoxidil indefinitely. Minoxidil preparations can also be used as supportive therapy in hair transplants.

Minoxidil was originally designed as an oral antihypertensive drug; as such, misuse or absorption of the drug into your system can have serious side effects. Those who use minoxidil as a topical hair growth stimulant should not have any heart problems, and they must have healthy scalps. When this drug is used as an oral antihypertensive, 4 out of 5 patients experience a side effect of thicker, longer, and darker body hair after three to six weeks.

PRECAUTIONS

WARNING
Do not take this medication if you have an adrenaline-producing tumor (pheochromocytoma).

SPECIAL INFORMATION
- Minoxidil topical preparations may be absorbed into your system after prolonged use. Possible side effects of systemic absorption include fast heartbeat, edema, and low blood pressure.
- Use this drug with caution if you have cardiovascular disease or hypertension. Talk with your doctor about the risks involved.
- The actual dosage and use of topical preparations should be individualized. In most cases, a thin application twice daily to the entire scalp will suffice. Follow package and doctor's instructions carefully.
- Skin abrasions or irritations such as psoriasis, sunburn, and flaking skin may worsen with use of topical minoxidil.
- Oral minoxidil crosses the placenta. Women should discontinue use of minoxidil at least one month before birth-control measures are discontinued. Pregnant women or nursing mothers should discuss the risks of using minoxidil with their doctor.

MINOXIDIL

POSSIBLE INTERACTIONS

Although no possible interactions are reported for the topical preparation, drug interactions are possible with other antihypertensive agents if systemic absorption occurs. Anyone taking antihypertensive drugs should be aware of the risks.

Oral minoxidil (concurrent use): toxicity may occur.

Topical adrenocorticoids, retinoids, and petrolatum products: may cause undesirable absorption of minoxidil.

TARGET AILMENTS
Baldness (alopecia)
Female androgenic baldness
Early male-pattern baldness (androgenic alopecia)

SIDE EFFECTS

NOT SERIOUS

- Allergic reaction, such as burning, itchy scalp, flaking, or reddening skin
- Increased baldness
- Dermatitis
- Headache; dizziness
- Sexual dysfunction
- Vision problems
- Increased hair growth in other areas
- Eczema; loss of hair; dry skin

CALL YOUR DOCTOR IF THESE EFFECTS PERSIST OR BECOME BOTHERSOME.

SERIOUS

- Chest pain; dizziness or faintness; fast, irregular heartbeat; hypotension; swelling in hands or feet from water retention; or vasodilation (signs of systemic absorption)
- Burning scalp; skin rash; unusual swelling or tingling in face, hands, feet; headache, flushing; rapid weight gain (rare)

DISCONTINUE USE AND SEEK EMERGENCY TREATMENT.

MISTLETOE

LATIN NAME
Viscum album

VITAL STATISTICS

GENERAL DESCRIPTION

Mistletoe was sacred to the Celtic Druids of Europe, who depended on this parasitic evergreen plant, found on the branches of deciduous trees, to guard them from evil. Today mistletoe is widely known as part of a Christmas kissing ritual. There is a great deal of controversy concerning mistletoe's medicinal value. Although the leaves are reputed to be an effective remedy for high blood pressure, the U.S. Food and Drug Administration has labeled this herb "unsafe" and does not approve of its use in treating any illness. The active constituents responsible for mistletoe's toxicity are proteins called viscotoxins, which slow and weaken the heartbeat and constrict the blood vessels.

Mistletoe is believed to be a poisonous plant, to be used, if at all, only under the supervision of a healthcare professional.

PREPARATIONS

Home remedies using mistletoe are not recommended. Check with a herbalist for other herbs that serve the same functions.

PRECAUTIONS

☠ *WARNING*

Mistletoe is a poisonous herb, potentially fatal. You should not take it unless instructed to do so by a healthcare professional.

According to a recent series of studies conducted over a period of 25 years in Germany, mistletoe impairs the growth of tumor cells in test tubes. No conclusions have been reached, although research is still being conducted to determine the herb's potential use in cancer chemotherapy.

POSSIBLE INTERACTIONS

Combining mistletoe with other herbs may necessitate a lower dosage.

TARGET AILMENTS
High blood pressure
Cancer (in conjunction with conventional medical treatment)

SIDE EFFECTS

SERIOUS

SYMPTOMS OF TOXICITY INCLUDE:

- Nausea; vomiting
- Diarrhea
- Headache
- Decreased heart rate
- Hallucinations
- Muscle spasms
- Convulsions

DISCONTINUE USE AND CALL YOUR DOCTOR IMMEDIATELY.

Molybdenum

Vital Statistics

GENERAL DESCRIPTION

The obscure mineral molybdenum is an enzyme component. It helps generate energy, process waste for excretion, mobilize stored iron for the body's use, and detoxify sulfites—chemicals used as food preservatives. As such, molybdenum is essential to normal development, particularly of the nervous system. It is also an ingredient of tooth enamel and may help prevent tooth decay.

People generally get enough molybdenum through diet; deficiency is virtually nonexistent. Toxicity is also rare in humans. Molybdenum is available in supplement form as molybdenum picolinate.

EMDR

Adults: 15 mcg to 250 mcg

NATURAL SOURCES

Molybdenum is present in peas, beans, cereals, pastas, green leafy vegetables, yeast, milk, and organ meats.

Precautions

SPECIAL INFORMATION

Prolonged intake of more than 10 mg of molybdenum picolinate daily can cause gout-like symptoms such as joint pain and swelling.

TARGET AILMENTS
Tooth decay
Sulfite sensitivities (sulfites are found in wine, restaurant salad bars)
Cancer prevention

SIDE EFFECTS

None expected

Rx MOMETASONE FUROATE

VITAL STATISTICS

DRUG CLASS
Corticosteroids

BRAND NAME
Elocon

OTHER DRUGS IN THIS CLASS
Rx: beclomethasone, betamethasone, fluticasone, methylprednisolone, prednisone, triamcinolone
OTC: hydrocortisone

GENERAL DESCRIPTION
Mometasone furoate is a topical corticosteroid, commonly used for the temporary relief of inflammation and itchiness associated with various common skin diseases. The drug is available in cream, lotion, or ointment form and, when used sparingly for a brief period, has minimal side effects. For more information, see Corticosteroids.

PRECAUTIONS

SPECIAL INFORMATION
- Do not use mometasone furoate if you are sensitive to this drug or to other corticosteroids.
- Prolonged use of mometasone furoate can cause birth defects. Pregnant and nursing women should avoid this drug.
- Mometasone furoate should not be used for treating acne, rosacea, or perioral dermatitis (lesions around the mouth and on the chin).
- Do not use this medication near your eyes; doing so can cause a number of problems, including glaucoma or cataracts with prolonged use.
- Unless your doctor advises otherwise, do not cover treated skin with a plastic bandage or other occlusive dressing.
- Corticosteroid topical creams may be absorbed into your system after prolonged use. Tell your doctor if you are taking any other medication, and watch for any significant side effects or possible interactions.

Mometasone Furoate

- Ask your doctor about the risks and benefits of corticosteroid treatment if you have or have had any of the following conditions: HIV infection or AIDS, heart disease, hypertension, ulcerative colitis, diabetes, diverticulitis, gastritis or peptic ulcers, recent chickenpox or measles, candidiasis or other fungal infections, glaucoma, herpes simplex, liver or kidney disease, myasthenia gravis, osteoporosis, anastomoses, lupus, tuberculosis, recent intestinal problems, or any infection, such as a cold or flu.

TARGET AILMENTS
Rash
Inflammation
Itching
Psoriasis
Eczema
Sunburn

SIDE EFFECTS

NOT SERIOUS

- Mild and transient skin rash
- Burning
- Irritation
- Dryness
- Redness
- Itchiness
- Scaling

CALL YOUR DOCTOR IF THESE EFFECTS PERSIST OR BECOME BOTHERSOME.

SERIOUS

- Severe and lasting skin rash or hives
- Severe burning, itching, or painful skin
- Stomach pain or burning
- Blisters, acne, or other skin problems
- High blood pressure
- Insomnia
- Unusual bruising
- Prolonged sore throat, fever, cold, or other sign of infection

CONTACT YOUR DOCTOR IMMEDIATELY.

Monoamine Oxidase (MAO) Inhibitors

Vital Statistics

GENERIC NAMES
isocarboxazid, phenelzine, tranylcypromine

GENERAL DESCRIPTION
MAO inhibitors, a subclass of antidepressant drugs, are generally used when other medications have failed. They are believed to work by stopping the breakdown of neurotransmitters in the brain, allowing these chemicals to maintain normal brain function. MAO inhibitors require more supervision by your doctor than do most drugs because they are known to have many side effects and adverse interactions with other drugs and even foods; they are not considered to be drugs of first choice in treating depression. For information about specific MAO inhibitors, see the entries for the generic drugs listed above; for information about other antidepressant medications, see Antidepressants.

TARGET AILMENTS
Major depression, especially if the condition has not responded to other drugs
Panic disorder (especially phenelzine)
Prevention of vascular headache (including migraine) or tension headache

Precautions

WARNING
Monoamine oxidase (MAO) inhibitors react with many drugs and foods. Following are some of the substances you should avoid when taking these drugs: high-protein foods that are aged, fermented, or pickled, including (but not limited to) aged or processed cheeses; sour cream; alcohol, especially wine and beer (including alcohol-free wine and beer); pickled fish; dry sausages (salami); soy sauce; bean curd; yogurt; liver; figs; raisins; bananas; avocados; chocolate; papaya; meat tenderizers; and fava beans. Also avoid caffeine. But beware: This is only a partial list. Talk to your doctor and pharmacist about other drugs and foods you should avoid.

SPECIAL INFORMATION
- Before taking these drugs, let your doctor know if you have diabetes, epilepsy, hyperthyroidism, or manic or suicidal tendencies, or if you have had a stroke.
- MAO inhibitors may suppress heart pain, thereby masking heart problems. Let your doctor know if you have any history of angina or other heart disease.
- The full effects of MAO inhibitors may not be seen until after several weeks of therapy.
- Use these drugs during pregnancy or breast-feeding only if your doctor says that the benefits outweigh the risks.

Monoamine Oxidase (MAO) Inhibitors

POSSIBLE INTERACTIONS

Amphetamines and other stimulant drugs (including prescription and OTC cold or hay fever products): can cause a serious rise in blood pressure.

Anticoagulants (such as warfarin): increased anticoagulant effect.

Antihistamines: increased action of MAO inhibitors. Taking these drugs with MAO inhibitors may increase the side effects of antihistamines, especially drowsiness. Report any gastrointestinal problems to your doctor immediately; they could be signs of paralytic ileus (lack of intestinal activity), which requires emergency treatment.

Caffeine: severe heart-rhythm problems or high blood pressure.

Drugs: MAO inhibitors are known to interact with many drugs and may interact with others. Contact your doctor and pharmacist before taking any drug (prescription or OTC) while you are taking MAO inhibitors. Also tell your doctor about any medication you take one or two weeks before you start MAO therapy and one or two weeks after you stop.

Food: see Warning, opposite.

Other antidepressants: taking these with or within a week of taking MAO inhibitors may cause an additive effect for either drug or both, possibly leading to serious side effects, including severe convulsions, changes in psychological states, severe hypertension, coma, and death.

Sedatives, including alcohol and barbiturates: high levels of sedation, very low blood pressure, possibly death.

SIDE EFFECTS

NOT SERIOUS

- Mild restlessness; insomnia
- Headache; blurred vision
- Shakiness or trembling; dizziness; weakness
- Drowsiness
- Decreased sexual ability
- Increased appetite; carbohydrate craving; weight gain or loss

LET YOUR DOCTOR KNOW IF THESE SYMPTOMS ARE BOTHERSOME. (SOME OF THESE EFFECTS MAY BE ALLEVIATED BY A LOWER DOSAGE.)

SERIOUS

- Severe blood pressure changes; severe dizziness or lightheadedness when changing position
- Skin rash or bruising; diarrhea; swelling of lower body; excessive stimulation (pounding heartbeat, unusual excitement, nervousness) (infrequent)
- Yellow skin; fever; sore throat; Parkinson's-like symptoms (slurred speech, difficulty walking) (rare)

CALL YOUR DOCTOR IMMEDIATELY.

- Severe headache; palpitations; neck stiffness or soreness (signs of overdose)

SEEK MEDICAL HELP IMMEDIATELY.

Motherwort

LATIN NAME
Leonurus cardiaca

Vital Statistics

GENERAL DESCRIPTION
Motherwort is used to treat disorders related to menstruation, childbirth, and menopause. Though a uterine stimulant and thus risky during pregnancy, the herb in fact both encourages and eases uterine contractions, making it useful during and after labor. The name *cardiaca* indicates another beneficial quality: Motherwort may help prevent blood clots that can lead to heart disease, and it can calm an overrapid heartbeat, especially one due to stress or hot flashes.

PREPARATIONS
Over the counter:
Available in bulk and as tincture and extract.

At home:
Tea: To stimulate the uterus during labor or help lower blood pressure, steep covered for 10 minutes 1 to 2 tsp dried herb in 1 cup boiling water. Drink up to 2 cups a day, 1 tbsp at a time. Add sugar, honey, or lemon for taste.
Tincture: Use ⅛ to ½ tsp up to three times daily.
Extract: Add 10 to 15 drops extract to warm liquid; take up to three times a day.
Consult a qualified practitioner for the dosage appropriate for your specific condition.

Precautions

☠ ***WARNING***
Always consult your doctor before using motherwort. Those over 65 should begin with low doses and increase gradually if needed.

Consult your doctor before using motherwort if you are pregnant; it may induce labor.

Do not use this herb if you have a blood or cardiac disorder unless it is prescribed and monitored by a healthcare practitioner.

This herb should not be used with children unless it is specifically prescribed by a healthcare practitioner knowledgeable about herbs. Do not give to children under two.

SPECIAL INFORMATION
If your symptoms do not improve in two weeks, consult your doctor.

POSSIBLE INTERACTIONS
For all conditions for which it is used, motherwort may interact with other medications. Consult your healthcare practitioner.

Combining motherwort with other herbs may necessitate a lower dosage.

TARGET AILMENTS

Delayed menstruation; PMS; menopausal problems

Insomnia related to menopause or PMS; anxiety

Use if prescribed and monitored by a healthcare practitioner for:

Rapid heartbeat

SIDE EFFECTS

NOT SERIOUS
- Rash
- Upset stomach; diarrhea

DISCONTINUE USE AND CALL YOUR DOCTOR.

M

MUGWORT LEAF

LATIN NAME
Artemisia argyi
(or A. vulgaris)

VITAL STATISTICS

GENERAL DESCRIPTION

The aromatic mugwort leaf is prescribed for a range of gynecological problems. In China, mugwort is harvested at the end of spring or in early summer, when the leaves are growing vigorously but flowers have not yet bloomed. Laboratory studies seem to indicate that the herb has an antibiotic effect. Crushed fresh mugwort leaves were placed over warts in a clinical trial; some of the warts fell off within 10 days. Traditional Chinese medicine characterizes the herb as bitter, acrid, and warm. The best leaves are grayish white in color, with a thick, hairy texture.

Chinese medicine takes a holistic approach to healthcare, fashioning remedies to treat the entire being as well as the specific parts or areas. Single herbs may be used alone or in combination with other herbs to prevent and combat disease, which is thought to arise from disturbances in the flow of a bodily energy called chi (pronounced "chee") and blood, or from a lack of balance in the complementary states of yin and yang.

PREPARATIONS

Mugwort leaf is available in bulk at Chinese pharmacies, Asian markets, and some Western health food stores. The herb is also available in pills. The dried, aged, powdered herb can be rolled into a cigarlike cylinder, using tissue paper; one end is burned near the site of an injury to increase blood circulation and relieve pain. Acupuncturists sometimes use this technique instead of or in addition to inserting needles.

COMBINATIONS: A mixture with gelatin is prescribed for vaginal bleeding and pain during pregnancy, or spotting between periods. Combining mugwort with dried ginger targets menstrual pain. And a preparation of mugwort leaf and kochia fruit is applied to itchy lesions on the skin.

For information on dosages and other preparations, check with a herbal practitioner.

TARGET AILMENTS
Take internally for:
Excessive menstrual bleeding
Menstrual cramps
Uterine bleeding
Vaginal pain and bleeding during pregnancy
Threatened miscarriage
Apply externally for:
Pain relief
Itchy lesions

SIDE EFFECTS

NONE EXPECTED

M

MULLEIN

LATIN NAME
Verbascum thapsus

VITAL STATISTICS

GENERAL DESCRIPTION
Mullein, a common roadside wildflower, has large velvety leaves and small, dense yellow flowers. Owing to its astringent or binding action on tissue, it is useful in treating diarrhea and hemorrhoids. As an expectorant, it helps the body remove excess mucus from the lungs and is used to treat bronchitis and coughs. The dried leaves, flowers, and roots are all used as remedies. Because it burns easily when dried, mullein was used to make candlewicks before the introduction of cotton; hence its name "candlewick plant." For visual characteristics of mullein, see the Color Guide to Prescription Drugs and Herbs.

PREPARATIONS
Over the counter:
Mullein is available as a tincture and as dried leaves, flowers, or roots.

At home:
TEA: Steep covered 1 to 2 tsp dried leaves, flowers, or roots per cup of boiling water for 10 to 15 minutes. Drink as many as 3 cups a day.
COMPRESS: Make a tea using vinegar, allow to cool; soak dry bandages in the tea, and apply to ulcers, tumors, or hemorrhoids.
INHALANT: Boil fresh leaves in water and inhale the steam to relieve coughs and congestion.
COMBINATIONS: Used with elder and red clover to ease painful coughing. Mixed with gumweed for asthma. Used as an extract in olive oil to apply to external ulcers, hemorrhoids, and tumors, and for ear problems. It also combines well with white horehound, coltsfoot, and lobelia for treating bronchitis.
Consult a qualified practitioner for the dosage appropriate for your specific condition.

PRECAUTIONS

WARNING
If you have a history of cancer, consult your doctor before taking this herb internally, since the tannin found in mullein is thought to have cancer-causing actions.

Although the leaves, flowers, and roots seem to be harmless, mullein seeds are toxic.

Do not take mullein if you are pregnant or are nursing a baby.

POSSIBLE INTERACTIONS
Combining mullein with other herbs may necessitate a lower dosage.

TARGET AILMENTS

Take internally for:

Respiratory ailments such as bronchitis, coughs, flu, asthma

Gastrointestinal ailments such as stomach cramps, diarrhea

Apply externally for:

External ulcers; tumors; hemorrhoids

Ear problems

SIDE EFFECTS

NOT SERIOUS
- Mild stomach upset; diarrhea

USE LESS OR DISCONTINUE. CONSULT A DOCTOR WHEN CONVENIENT.

M

MUPIROCIN

VITAL STATISTICS

DRUG CLASS
Antibiotics [Topical Antibiotics]

BRAND NAME
Bactroban

OTHER DRUGS IN THIS SUBCLASS
Rx: chlorhexidine (for gums); combination of neomycin, polymyxin B, and hydrocortisone (antibiotic-corticosteroid for ears)
OTC: bacitracin, neomycin, polymyxin B

GENERAL DESCRIPTION
Mupirocin is a topical antibiotic used to treat impetigo, a skin infection caused by certain strains of *Staphylococcus* and *Streptococcus* bacteria. Topical antibiotics are used to prevent or clear up bacterial infections of the skin, ears, or gums. Each drug is effective against a specific group of bacteria. They should never be used interchangeably; drugs for the skin, for example, should not be applied to the ears or mouth. Mupirocin should not be applied to the eyes or mucous membranes. However, there is a form of mupirocin (mupirocin calcium, or the brand-name drug Bactroban Nasal) specifically designed for use in the nose to treat bacterial nasal infections.

For more information on this and related medications, see Topical Antibiotics.

PRECAUTIONS

SPECIAL INFORMATION
- Check with your doctor if you notice no improvement after using this medication for two or three days.
- Prolonged use of a prescription topical antibiotic may result in fungal superinfection.
- The use of topical antibiotics increases the risk of kidney damage or hearing loss in people with impaired kidney function who are already taking nephrotoxic medicines.
- If you are pregnant or nursing, check with your doctor before using.

TARGET AILMENTS
Impetigo

SIDE EFFECTS

SERIOUS
- Allergic reaction such as itching, stinging, rash, redness, or swelling at the application site

CALL YOUR DOCTOR IMMEDIATELY.

Rx MUSCLE RELAXANTS

VITAL STATISTICS

GENERIC NAMES
carisoprodol, cyclobenzaprine

GENERAL DESCRIPTION
Muscle relaxants are a class of drugs that block messages from skeletal muscles to the brain. These messages may include pain or information related to muscle contraction and other movements. Some of these medications act at the site of the muscle, while others act at the brain or brainstem. They usually work by interfering with the body's response to various chemicals that transmit electrical impulses from the muscles to the brain.

There are two major therapeutic groups of skeletal muscle relaxants. One group includes neuromuscular blockers that are used for relaxing muscles in preparation for surgery; these drugs are not active in the central nervous system. The other group, called spasmolytics, are used to relieve spasticity in a number of neurological conditions, and they are active in the central nervous system. The generic drugs listed above belong to this second group. For more information, see the entries Carisoprodol and Cyclobenzaprine; for information on another drug that is used for this purpose, see Diazepam.

TARGET AILMENTS

Muscle spasms and strains

PRECAUTIONS

WARNING
An overdose of some types of muscle relaxants can be dangerous, resulting in breathing problems, stupor, or even coma. Contact a poison control center or seek emergency care if you have taken more than the amount prescribed.

SPECIAL INFORMATION
- Women who are pregnant or nursing should take muscle relaxants only under a doctor's supervision.
- Muscle relaxants may cause drowsiness. Use caution while taking these medications if you must drive or perform other tasks requiring alertness.

SIDE EFFECTS

NOT SERIOUS
- Dizziness; lightheadedness
- Drowsiness
- Headache

CALL YOUR DOCTOR IF THESE SYMPTOMS BECOME TROUBLESOME.

SERIOUS
- Skin rash, hives, or itching
- Confusion; visual hallucinations
- Breathing difficulties

CALL YOUR DOCTOR IF YOU EXPERIENCE THESE EFFECTS.

MYRRH

LATIN NAME
Commiphora molmol
(or C. myrrha)

VITAL STATISTICS

GENERAL DESCRIPTION

Myrrh is a resin produced by a knobby shrub that is native to the Middle East and found especially in the Red Sea area. Its flowers are white and its leaves are covered with fluff. The stems and shoots exude the resin, which hardens and drops to the ground.

In ancient times, myrrh was an important ingredient in perfumes, embalming, and incense. It was once used to facilitate the birthing process. Today myrrh is used as a flavoring in many foods and beverages and in toothpaste and mouthwash. In aromatherapy, it is valued for its wound-healing, antifungal, and antiseptic properties. It is also effective in treating respiratory illness, throat and gum problems, and mouth ulcers. For visual characteristics, see the Color Guide to Prescription Drugs and Herbs.

PREPARATIONS

Myrrh is available as an oil, a tincture, or in powdered form.

FOR A GARGLE AND RINSE, add 1 drop myrrh and 1 drop peppermint (for flavor) to half a glass of water. Do not swallow after use.

TO USE THE OIL FOR SKIN CONDITIONS AND AS A CHEST RUB, dilute 10 to 15 drops in 2 tbsp vegetable or nut oil.

FOR VAGINAL THRUSH, saturate a tampon with 2 to 4 drops myrrh oil mixed into 2 tsp vegetable or nut oil.

PRECAUTIONS

☠ *WARNING*

Avoid myrrh during pregnancy.

Do not ingest myrrh; it can irritate the kidneys.

SPECIAL INFORMATION

Buy only from a reputable source. Myrrh is sometimes adulterated with ammonia.

TARGET AILMENTS
Eczema and other skin conditions
Stretch marks
Ringworm
Athlete's foot
Wounds
Arthritis
Bronchitis
Mouth ulcers and gum problems
Sore throat
Colds and cough
Diarrhea
Candidiasis
Vaginal thrush

SIDE EFFECTS

MYRRH IS NONIRRITATING AND NONSENSITIZING. HOWEVER, IT MAY BE TOXIC IN HIGH CONCENTRATIONS.

M

MYRRH

LATIN NAME
Commiphora molmol
(or C. myrrha)

VITAL STATISTICS

GENERAL DESCRIPTION
Myrrh comes from an oil found in the bark of several species of shrubs native to northeast Africa and Arabia. The oil hardens into nuggets, called gum resin, which is powdered to make the healing herb. Myrrh fights infection by stimulating the production of white blood cells and by a direct antibacterial action. For visual characteristics of myrrh, see the Color Guide to Prescription Drugs and Herbs.

PREPARATIONS
Over the counter:
Available as powdered resin, tinctures, and as an ingredient in commercial toothpastes.

At home:
MOUTHWASH: Steep covered 1 tsp powdered herb and 1 tsp boric acid in 1 pt boiling water. Let stand 30 minutes and strain; use when cool.
TEA: Steep covered 1 to 2 tsp powdered herb per cup of boiling water for 10 to 15 minutes. Drink three times a day.
COMBINATIONS: With distilled witch hazel, applied externally. With garlic oil in ear drops.
Consult a qualified practitioner for the dosage appropriate for your specific condition.

PRECAUTIONS

WARNING
Any resin tends to be hard to eliminate and can cause minor kidney damage if taken internally for extended periods. Consult your physician or herbalist before using myrrh if you are pregnant or nursing, or have kidney disease. Do not exceed recommended doses.

Use of this herb by children for more than seven to 10 days should be done in conjunction with a healthcare practitioner. Do not give internally at all to children under two.

POSSIBLE INTERACTIONS
Combining myrrh with other herbs may necessitate a lower dosage.

TARGET AILMENTS

Take internally or use as a gargle for:

Mouth and throat infections

Gum disease; pharyngitis

Sinusitis; colds

Asthma; boils

Chest congestion; coughs

Apply externally for:

Wounds; abrasions

SIDE EFFECTS

NOT SERIOUS
- Stomach upset; diarrhea

REDUCE DOSE OR DISCONTINUE.

SERIOUS
- Severe diarrhea; sweating
- Vomiting; rapid heartbeat
- Kidney problems

LARGE AMOUNTS MAY CAUSE THESE EFFECTS. DISCONTINUE USE AND CALL YOUR DOCTOR.

M

Rx NABUMETONE

VITAL STATISTICS

DRUG CLASS
Analgesics [Nonsteroidal Anti-Inflammatory Drugs (NSAIDs)]

BRAND NAME
Relafen

OTHER DRUGS IN THIS SUBCLASS
diclofenac, etodolac, flurbiprofen, ibuprofen, ketoprofen, ketorolac, naproxen, oxaprozin

GENERAL DESCRIPTION
Introduced in 1984, nabumetone is an NSAID, a type of pain reliever acting at the site of pain. Because it reduces inflammation, it is used to treat rheumatoid and osteoarthritis. It may be prescribed when aspirin or acetaminophen is not effective. Since nabumetone is a prodrug, meaning it exhibits pharmaceutical action only after the body changes it to another form, it must first be metabolized by the liver. See also Nonsteroidal Anti-Inflammatory Drugs (NSAIDs).

PRECAUTIONS

SPECIAL INFORMATION
- Do not use if you are allergic to NSAIDs or to aspirin. It may cause bronchoconstriction or anaphylaxis.
- Consult your doctor before using if you have asthma, peptic ulcer, enteritis, high blood pressure, bleeding problems, or impaired liver or kidney function.

POSSIBLE INTERACTIONS
Antipsychotic drugs (e.g., chlorpromazine and clozapine): decreased effects of these drugs.
Benzodiazepines (such as chlordiazepoxide, diazepam, and oxazepam): decreased effects of these drugs.
Tricyclic antidepressants (such as amitriptyline): decreased effects of these drugs.

TARGET AILMENTS

Inflammation, especially of arthritis (osteo- and rheumatoid)

SIDE EFFECTS

NOT SERIOUS
- Dizziness; drowsiness; headache; abdominal pain or cramps; constipation; diarrhea; heartburn; nausea

CALL A DOCTOR IF THESE PERSIST.

SERIOUS
- Anaphylactic reaction (hives, rash, intense itching, and trouble breathing)

SEEK EMERGENCY HELP.

- Chest pain or irregular heartbeat; trouble breathing
- Diminished hearing; tinnitus
- Fluid retention
- Black or tarry stools; blood in urine
- Photosensitivity
- Jaundice

DISCONTINUE USE AND CALL YOUR DOCTOR IMMEDIATELY.

Rx NADOLOL

VITAL STATISTICS

DRUG CLASS
Beta-Adrenergic Blockers

BRAND NAME
Corgard

OTHER DRUGS IN THIS CLASS
atenolol, bisoprolol, metoprolol, propranolol, timolol

GENERAL DESCRIPTION
Introduced in 1976, nadolol is a nonselective beta-blocking drug commonly prescribed in the management of hypertension (high blood pressure) and angina. By blocking the action of certain parts of the nervous system, the drug reduces the oxygen requirements and contraction force of the heart while also relaxing blood vessels, thereby lowering blood pressure and easing the work load of the heart. For more information, including side effects and possible drug interactions, see Beta-Adrenergic Blockers.

PRECAUTIONS

SPECIAL INFORMATION
- Nadolol can make you drowsy, dizzy, and lightheaded. Avoid activities that require alertness, such as driving, until you know how you react to these drugs.
- Tell your doctor if you are planning surgery or have any of the following conditions, which nadolol may complicate: allergies, bronchial asthma, or emphysema; congestive heart failure; diabetes mellitus; hyperthyroidism; impaired liver or kidneys; mental depression; myasthenia gravis; poor circulation or circulatory disease.
- Do not use nadolol if you have a bronchospastic disease, bronchial asthma, or a severe chronic obstructive pulmonary disease.
- Beta-adrenergic blockers can both mask the symptoms of low blood sugar and cause a severe rise in blood sugar in people with diabetes mellitus.
- Beta-adrenergic blockers can increase the severity of allergic reactions to drugs, food, or insect stings. Contact your doctor immediately if a severe allergic reaction occurs.
- Suddenly stopping this drug may cause or increase heart problems. Dosage must be reduced gradually under your doctor's supervision.
- Before taking nadolol, let your doctor know if you are pregnant or breast-feeding.

TARGET AILMENTS

- Hypertension (high blood pressure)
- Heart disease
- Angina (chest pain)
- Heart attack
- Abnormal heart rhythms

SIDE EFFECTS
SEE BETA-ADRENERGIC BLOCKERS.

N

NAPROXEN

VITAL STATISTICS

DRUG CLASS
Analgesics [Nonsteroidal Anti-Inflammatory Drugs (NSAIDs)]

BRAND NAMES
Rx: Anaprox, Anaprox DS, Naprosyn
OTC: Aleve

OTHER DRUGS IN THIS CLASS
diclofenac, etodolac, flurbiprofen, ibuprofen, ketoprofen, ketorolac, nabumetone, oxaprozin

GENERAL DESCRIPTION
Made available in the 1990s, naproxen is a nonsteroidal anti-inflammatory drug, or NSAID, used to treat rheumatoid arthritis and osteoarthritis. Like other NSAIDs, naproxen not only reduces inflammation but also relieves muscle, joint, and menstrual pain and reduces fever. For more information, see Nonsteroidal Anti-Inflammatory Drugs (NSAIDs). For visual characteristics of naproxen and the brand-name drugs Anaprox and Naprosyn, see the Color Guide to Prescription Drugs and Herbs.

PRECAUTIONS

SPECIAL INFORMATION
- Do not use naproxen if you are allergic to NSAIDs or to aspirin. It may cause bronchoconstriction or anaphylaxis in aspirin-sensitive asthmatics.
- Avoid this drug or consult your doctor before using it if you have asthma, peptic ulcer, enteritis (intestinal inflammation), high blood pressure, bleeding problems, or impaired liver or kidney function.

TARGET AILMENTS

Inflammation, especially related to osteoarthritis and rheumatoid arthritis

Pain, especially from inflammation, dental and other surgeries, menstruation, and migraines

Fever

SIDE EFFECTS

NOT SERIOUS
- Dizziness, drowsiness, or headache
- Abdominal pain or cramps
- Constipation or diarrhea
- Heartburn; nausea

CONSULT YOUR DOCTOR IF THESE SYMPTOMS PERSIST.

SERIOUS
- Anaphylactic reaction (hives, rash, intense itching, and trouble breathing)
- Gastrointestinal bleeding; ulceration; stomach perforation (black or tarry stools)
- Chest pain; irregular heartbeat
- Diminished hearing or ringing in the ears
- Trouble breathing
- Fluid retention
- Jaundice; blood in urine
- Photosensitivity

CALL YOUR DOCTOR IMMEDIATELY.

Natrum muriaticum

LATIN NAME
Natrum muriaticum

Vital Statistics

GENERAL DESCRIPTION

Natrum muriaticum is simply salt, or sodium chloride, a substance present in the natural world in quantities greater than any other except water. Essential to life and health, salt has been valued in human commerce throughout history. Roman soldiers were given a stipend, called a salarium, which they used to buy salt; from this we get the word *salary.* Homeopaths prescribe dilute solutions of *Nat mur,* as they call it, for conditions that are coupled with symptoms of extreme thirst, emotional sensitivity, and a strong desire for salt.

Nat mur is prepared by adding pure sodium chloride to boiling water. Once the salt has dissolved, the solution is filtered and crystallized by evaporation. The final product is diluted in water to the desired potency. For more information on homeopathic medicine, see page 14.

PREPARATIONS

Nat mur is available over the counter in various potencies in both liquid and tablet form. Consult a homeopathic physician for more information.

Precautions

SPECIAL INFORMATION

- When a remedy is administered, no one but the patient should touch the pills. If tablets are spilled, throw them away.
- The mouth should be clear of flavors 15 minutes before and after taking a remedy, and strong flavors and aromas, such as coffee and heavy perfume, should be avoided for the duration of treatment.

TARGET AILMENTS

Anemia

Backaches that are relieved by firm pressure

Cold sores, especially in the corners of the mouth

Colds with sneezing, watery eyes, and runny nose

Constipation

Depression caused by grief, with a desire to be alone

Eczema

Fevers accompanied by weakness and chills

Genital herpes

Hay fever

Indigestion

Menstrual irregularity

Migraine headaches

SIDE EFFECTS

None expected

NEOMYCIN

VITAL STATISTICS

DRUG CLASS
Antibiotics [Topical Antibiotics]

BRAND NAME
Neosporin

OTHER DRUGS IN THIS SUBCLASS
Rx: chlorhexidine (for gums); mupirocin (for skin); combination of neomycin, polymyxin B, and hydrocortisone (antibiotic-corticosteroid for ears or eyes)
OTC: bacitracin, polymyxin B

GENERAL DESCRIPTION
Neomycin is an aminoglycoside, an antibiotic with a broad spectrum of activity and effectiveness. In oral forms the drug can be used to treat gastrointestinal infections, although it is rarely given orally because of the high risk of kidney and hearing damage. Neomycin is available over the counter as a topical ointment by itself, or in combination with polymyxin B and bacitracin. This combination is used on the skin to prevent infections in minor cuts, scrapes, and burns.

By prescription, neomycin comes in combination with polymyxin B and hydrocortisone for a combined antibiotic and corticosteroid treatment for external ear infections. Other forms of these three drugs are used to treat bacterial infections of the eye and skin. For more information, see Topical Antibiotics.

PRECAUTIONS

SPECIAL INFORMATION
- Check with your doctor if you notice no improvement after using these medications for two or three days.
- The use of topical antibiotics increases the risk of kidney damage or hearing loss in people with impaired kidney function who are already taking nephrotoxic medicines.
- If you are pregnant or nursing, check with your doctor before using.

POSSIBLE INTERACTIONS
Other aminoglycosides: possible hypersensitivity reaction and toxicity leading to permanent deafness.

TARGET AILMENTS

Minor cuts, scrapes, and burns (neomycin alone, or in combination with bacitracin and polymyxin B, to prevent bacterial infection)

External ear canal infections (neomycin, polymyxin B, and hydrocortisone in combination)

SIDE EFFECTS

SERIOUS
- Allergic reaction such as itching, stinging, rash, redness, or swelling at the application site
- Kidney damage or hearing loss (due to extensive systemic absorption of neomycin via application over large areas of the body or through prolonged use)

CALL YOUR DOCTOR IMMEDIATELY.

Rx NEOMYCIN, POLYMYXIN B, AND HYDROCORTISONE

VITAL STATISTICS

DRUG CLASS
Antibiotics [Topical Antibiotics]

BRAND NAMES
Cortisporin, Lazersporin-C, Otocort

OTHER DRUGS IN THIS SUBCLASS
Rx: chlorhexidine (for gums); mupirocin (for skin)
OTC: bacitracin, neomycin, polymyxin B

GENERAL DESCRIPTION
This steroid-antibiotic combination is used to treat bacterial infections of the external ear canal. Other forms of this combination of drugs are used to treat inflammation of the skin or eyes where bacterial infection exists or is likely to occur. You should never use these ear, skin, or eye preparations interchangeably; use each form only for its intended purpose. Don't use this drug in your ears if your eardrum is ruptured, and don't use it at all if you are sensitive to any of the ingredients. For more information about neomycin and bacitracin, see Topical Antibiotics. For information about the corticosteroid ingredient, see Hydrocortisone.

PRECAUTIONS

SPECIAL INFORMATION
- Do not use this combination if you are allergic to any of the component drugs, or if you have a fungal, viral, or herpes infection.
- Check with your doctor if you notice no improvement after using these medications for two or three days.
- Prolonged use of a prescription topical antibiotic may result in fungal superinfection.
- The use of topical antibiotics increases the risk of kidney damage or hearing loss in people with impaired kidney function who are already taking nephrotoxic medicines.
- If you are pregnant or nursing, check with your doctor before using.

POSSIBLE INTERACTIONS
Aminoglycosides: possible hypersensitivity reaction and toxicity, leading to permanent deafness if combined with neomycin, which is also an aminoglycoside.

TARGET AILMENTS

External ear canal infection

Inflammation and infection or possible infection of the eyes

Some skin infections

SIDE EFFECTS

SERIOUS
- Allergic reaction (itching, rash, redness, or swelling)
- Kidney damage or hearing loss (may result if extensive systemic absorption of neomycin occurs via application over large areas of the body or through prolonged use)

CALL YOUR DOCTOR IMMEDIATELY. SEE ALSO HYDROCORTISONE.

N

NEROLI

LATIN NAME
Citrus aurantium

VITAL STATISTICS

GENERAL DESCRIPTION

Neroli oil is distilled from freshly picked flowers of the bitter orange, also known as the Seville orange. The plant is native to the Far East. Neroli oil was discovered in the late 17th century and was used by the Venetians to counter the plague and other fevers. The oil is very expensive to produce.

Neroli oil is yellowish in color and has a strong scent. When exposed to light and air, it turns reddish brown. Once this reaction has taken place, neroli oil is useless for healing.

Neroli has a sedative, antispasmodic, and tranquilizing effect. It also has a slightly hypnotic action. Some women find neroli oil to be especially helpful as a relaxant during pregnancy and labor.

PREPARATIONS

For almost all neroli's target ailments, the oil can be used in baths, inhalations, and skin applications.

BATH: Add 5 drops to the bathwater.

INHALATION: Use a diffuser, or place a few drops of neroli on a handkerchief, hold to your nose and breathe.

SKIN APPLICATION OR BODY MASSAGE: Blend 4 drops in 1 tbsp of a carrier oil such as vegetable or nut oil or aloe gel. For scars, stretch marks, and wrinkles, it is even more effective to use vitamin E oil or rosa mosqueta oil as the carrier oil.

PRECAUTIONS

SPECIAL INFORMATION

Buy only from a reputable source. Because of its price, neroli oil is often adulterated with other oils.

TARGET AILMENTS
Anxiety and stress
Depression
Insomnia
Poor circulation
Menstrual symptoms
Broken capillaries
Scars, stretch marks, and wrinkles

SIDE EFFECTS

NONE EXPECTED

Nettle

LATIN NAME
Urtica dioica

Vital Statistics

GENERAL DESCRIPTION
Notorious for the stinging needles along its leaves, nettle can be safely ingested when the irritant is tamed by boiling or drying. A tonic made from the leaves and stems is said to strengthen the body. Herbalists consider nettle a diuretic capable of removing toxins, and its iron and vitamin C may help prevent anemia. Nettle has an erect stem and serrated, dark green, heart-shaped leaves. For visual characteristics of nettle, see the Color Guide to Prescription Drugs and Herbs.

PREPARATIONS
Over the counter:
Nettle is available as tincture, capsules, and dried leaves and stems.

At home:
Tea: Steep covered 1 to 3 tsp dried herb in 1 cup boiling water for 10 minutes. Drink up to 3 cups a day.
Juice: Add 2 tsp juice squeezed from nettle to a fresh vegetable or fruit drink.
Combinations: Nettle combines well with figwort and burdock to treat eczema; take orally as juice or tea.
Consult a qualified practitioner for the dosage appropriate for your specific condition.

Precautions

WARNING
Do not use uncooked nettle; it may cause kidney damage and other symptoms of poisoning. As a diuretic, nettle may remove potassium from the body. If you use it frequently, eat foods high in potassium, such as bananas and fresh vegetables.

Do not give nettle to children younger than two years old.

POSSIBLE INTERACTIONS
Combining nettle with other herbs may necessitate a lower dosage.

TARGET AILMENTS
Take internally for:
Arthritis; gout
Hay fever; eczema
Vaginal yeast infections
Hemorrhoids; diarrhea; chronic cystitis
Use internally only under the supervision of a physician for:
High blood pressure
Congestive heart failure

SIDE EFFECTS

NOT SERIOUS
- Stomach irritation
- Constipation
- Burning skin
- Urinary suppression

THESE SYMPTOMS MAY BE CAUSED BY LARGE DOSES OF NETTLE TEA. DISCONTINUE USE AND CALL YOUR DOCTOR.

N

Rx NIACIN

VITAL STATISTICS

DRUG CLASS
Cholesterol-Reducing Drugs

BRAND NAMES
Rx: Niacor, Nicolar
OTC: Niacin-Time, Nicobid, Slo-Niacin

OTHER DRUGS IN THIS CLASS
cholestyramine, colestipol, fluvastatin, gemfibrozil, lovastatin, pravastatin, simvastatin

GENERAL DESCRIPTION
Since 1937, large doses of niacin have been used to treat high blood levels of cholesterol and triglycerides in people at risk for coronary artery disease. For more information, see Cholesterol-Reducing Drugs.

PRECAUTIONS

SPECIAL INFORMATION
- Do not take niacin if you have low blood pressure or liver disease.
- Do not use niacin without telling your physician if you have or have had peptic ulcers, bleeding disorders, allergies, gout, or diabetes.
- Taking niacin with meals or milk reduces the likelihood of stomach upset.

POSSIBLE INTERACTIONS
Antidiabetic drugs: niacin may decrease the effect of insulin by raising the level of blood sugar.
Antihypertensive drugs: niacin may increase their effects and cause low blood pressure.
Lovastatin, pravastatin, simvastatin: the combination could potentially cause kidney failure or rhabdomyolysis (a fatal muscle disease). Your doctor will monitor you carefully.

TARGET AILMENTS

The major types of cholesterol disorders, particularly those in which high levels of blood fats have been linked to an increased risk of heart disease

SIDE EFFECTS

NOT SERIOUS
- Flushing
- Headache
- Nausea or vomiting
- A feeling of warmth on the face and neck

CALL YOUR DOCTOR IF SYMPTOMS CONTINUE OR ARE BOTHERSOME.

SERIOUS
- Light gray stools
- Darkening of urine
- Yellow skin or eyes
- Loss of appetite
- Dizziness or fainting
- Worsening of gout or diabetes

CALL YOUR DOCTOR RIGHT AWAY.

NIACIN (VITAMIN B3)

VITAL STATISTICS

OTHER NAME
vitamin B_3

GENERAL DESCRIPTION
Niacin contributes to more than 50 vital bodily processes. Among other things, it helps convert food into energy; build red blood cells; synthesize hormones, fatty acids, and steroids; maintain skin, nerves, and blood vessels; support the gastrointestinal tract; stabilize mental health; and detoxify certain drugs and chemicals in the body. In addition, it helps insulin regulate blood sugar levels. Niacin is also a powerful drug, capable of lowering blood cholesterol and triglycerides, dilating blood vessels to improve circulation, and alleviating depression, insomnia, and hyperactivity.

Extreme deficiency of niacin results in pellagra, characterized by diarrhea, dermatitis, and mental illness. Pellagra was common until the discovery that niacin was a cure; the disease is now virtually nonexistent in the United States thanks to niacin-enriched flour and other foods. Multivitamin supplements can raise niacin levels safely.

RDA
Men: 19 mg
Women: 15 mg
Pregnant women: 17 mg

NATURAL SOURCES
Niacin-rich foods include liver, poultry, lean meats, fish, nuts, peanut butter, and enriched flour. If you get enough protein, you are probably receiving adequate niacin as well. If adequate vitamin B_6 is present, the body can also produce niacin from the amino acid tryptophan, found in milk, eggs, and cheese.

PRECAUTIONS

WARNING
Niacin is toxic in high amounts, so large doses should be taken only under a doctor's supervision. Nausea is the first symptom, which often prevents further intake; continued overuse may cause a rash, itchy skin, and liver damage.

SPECIAL INFORMATION
- Signs of niacin deficiency include indigestion; diarrhea; muscle weakness; loss of appetite; dermatitis that is worsened by exposure to sunlight; mouth sores; a red, inflamed tongue; headaches; irritability; anxiety; and depression.
- Pregnant or breast-feeding women, the elderly, alcoholics, and people with hyperthyroidism are the most likely to be niacin deficient.

TARGET AILMENTS

Depression

High cholesterol

SIDE EFFECTS

NONE EXPECTED

NIAOULI

LATIN NAME
Melaleuca viridiflora

VITAL STATISTICS

GENERAL DESCRIPTION

Principally from Australia, this evergreen has a spongy bark and yellow or white flowers. The yellow or greenish oil has a camphorous odor and is found in health aids such as toothpaste, gargles, and cough drops.

The oil is distilled from the leaves and young twigs. Niaouli has antiseptic, analgesic, and antiallergenic properties. It is effective in reducing fever and diarrhea. It also stimulates tissue regeneration, making it helpful for healing.

PREPARATIONS

Niaouli can be misted in a room to eliminate airborne infections and aid in respiratory complaints. Add 1 tsp of oil to a cup of warm water and store in a spray bottle. It also makes an effective inhalation: Combine 2 to 4 drops of niaouli with 1 drop each of eucalyptus and myrtle. Add to a large bowl of hot water. Drape a towel around the bowl and over your head, and inhale.

FOR ALL NIAOULI'S TARGET AILMENTS, the oil can be diluted with a carrier oil and applied to the skin. To make a lotion, blend 15 drops of essential oil in 2 tbsp of a carrier oil such as vegetable oil or aloe gel.

FOR INSECT BITES, BOILS, MINOR WOUNDS, BURNS, AND TOOTHACHE, apply a single undiluted drop of niaouli oil to affected area.

FOR A BLADDER INFECTION, add 10 drops of niaouli to the bath. Apply the lotion to the lower abdomen and lower back.

TARGET AILMENTS

- Allergies
- Bronchitis
- Colds and flu
- Minor wounds and burns
- Acne
- Boils
- Insect bites
- Muscle aches and pains
- Toothache
- Bladder infection

SIDE EFFECTS

NIAOULI IS NONTOXIC AND NONIRRITATING.

Rx NICOTINE

VITAL STATISTICS

DRUG CLASS
Smoking Cessation Drugs

BRAND NAMES
Rx: Nicotrol NS (nasal spray)
OTC: NicoDerm CQ (transdermal); Nicorette (chewing gum); Nicotrol (transdermal)

GENERAL DESCRIPTION
Nicotine transdermal (skin) patches are designed to release a specific amount of nicotine through the skin and into the bloodstream every 24 hours; nicotine is also available in flavored chewing gum or in a prescription nasal spray. The drug allows gradual nicotine withdrawal for people who want to stop smoking but find abrupt cessation difficult and physically painful.

Nicotine acts on the peripheral and central nervous systems, producing stimulant and depressant effects. By slowly reducing nicotine intake, these products can lessen physical smoking-withdrawal effects, such as irritability, nervousness, drowsiness, fatigue, headache, and nicotine craving. There is no evidence that nicotine replacement drugs work unless the smoker also participates in a medically supervised stop-smoking program.

PRECAUTIONS

WARNING
Extremely high doses of nicotine can produce toxic symptoms; nicotine overdose can be fatal. Because of the risk of overdose, do not smoke when using a medicinal form of nicotine.

SPECIAL INFORMATION
- In order for nicotine replacement drugs to be safe and effective, stop smoking completely at the beginning of treatment. This is also essential because of the risk of nicotine overdose.
- Call your doctor immediately if you have any of the following symptoms of toxic overdose: nausea, vomiting, abdominal cramps, diarrhea, dizziness, sweating, hearing or vision problems, confusion, weakness.
- Nicotine replacement products should not be used by nonsmokers or others who are not addicted to the drug.
- Do not use this drug if you have had an allergic reaction to it before. Consult your doctor if you have angina or an abnormal heart rhythm; have had a recent heart attack; or are pregnant, planning a pregnancy, or nursing.

- Tell your doctor if you have diabetes, high blood pressure, skin disease, overactive thyroid, adrenaline-producing tumors, peptic ulcer, or liver or kidney disease, or if you get rashes from adhesive bandages or tape.
- Tell your doctor what other medications you take. Changes in nicotine levels may require dosage adjustments for other drugs, especially those affecting the nervous system.
- Nicotine can be very harmful to children and pets. Be sure to dispose of used patches carefully, and keep nasal sprays out of their reach at all times.
- Do not use nicotine replacement drugs for more than 12 to 20 weeks (depending on the system) if you have stopped smoking. Continued use can be harmful and addictive.

POSSIBLE INTERACTIONS

Bronchodilators, insulin, propoxyphene, and propranolol and other beta-adrenergic blockers: you may need decreased amounts of these drugs when you stop smoking.

Isoproterenol, phenylephrine: you may need increased amounts of these drugs when you stop smoking.

TARGET AILMENTS
Smoking cessation
Nicotine withdrawal

SIDE EFFECTS

NOT SERIOUS

- Mild, temporary irritation (redness, tingling, itchiness) at a patch site
- Fast heartbeat
- Coughing; dry mouth
- Muscle or joint pain
- Hot feeling at the back of the throat or nose; sneezing; watery eyes; runny nose (nasal spray)

CALL YOUR DOCTOR IF THESE SYMPTOMS PERSIST OR ARE BOTHERSOME.

- Increased appetite
- Mild headache, irritability, or nervousness
- Unusual dreams

THESE ARE SYMPTOMS OF SMOKING WITHDRAWAL.

SERIOUS

- Chest pain
- Irregular heartbeat
- Dizziness
- Allergic reactions (hives, rash, swelling)
- Tingling in the arms or legs
- Tingling, burning, numbness in the nose, throat, or mouth (nasal spray)

CHECK WITH YOUR DOCTOR. ALSO SEE SIGNS OF OVERDOSE UNDER SPECIAL INFORMATION.

NIFEDIPINE

VITAL STATISTICS

DRUG CLASS
Calcium Channel Blockers

BRAND NAMES
Adalat, Adalat CC, Procardia XL

OTHER DRUGS IN THIS CLASS
amlodipine, diltiazem, isradipine, verapamil

GENERAL DESCRIPTION
Used since 1972 to control high blood pressure, nifedipine inhibits the passage of calcium into heart muscle cells and muscle cells surrounding blood vessels, retarding electrical stimulation of the heart, dilating the arteries, slowing contraction of the heart, and preventing some spasms of the coronary arteries. Alone or in combination with other heart and blood pressure medications, nifedipine is used to treat mild to moderate high blood pressure (hypertension) and to prevent angina. It is sometimes used to treat Raynaud's syndrome. For information on possible drug interactions, see Calcium Channel Blockers.

PRECAUTIONS

SPECIAL INFORMATION
- Recent findings have prompted warnings from some healthcare professionals about the safety of nifedipine, particularly large doses of the short-acting form. Before using this drug, be sure to discuss the matter thoroughly with your doctor. If you are already taking it, do not stop the medication without first consulting your doctor.
- Pregnant and nursing women should use nifedipine only if clearly needed.
- Let your doctor know if you are suffering from low blood pressure (hypotension), heart or kidney disease, or pulmonary congestion.
- Drinking grapefruit juice may increase the effects of nifedipine.

TARGET AILMENTS
Angina
High blood pressure
Raynaud's syndrome

SIDE EFFECTS

NOT SERIOUS
- Nausea; constipation
- Tiredness; dizziness
- Headache; flushing

CALL YOUR DOCTOR IF THESE EFFECTS BECOME TROUBLESOME.

SERIOUS
- Heart problems, such as congestive heart failure, heart-rhythm irregularities, or increased angina
- Low blood pressure; fainting
- Edema (swelling of the ankles and feet)
- Allergic reactions, such as skin rash
- Bleeding or tender gums

CONTACT YOUR DOCTOR IMMEDIATELY.

NITRATES

VITAL STATISTICS

GENERIC NAMES
isosorbide dinitrate, isosorbide mononitrate, nitroglycerin

GENERAL DESCRIPTION
Nitrates are a class of drugs used for decades to relieve chest pain associated with angina. They work by relaxing and dilating the muscles of blood vessels. This dilation, which for the most part affects the veins, relieves pressure on the heart by reducing its work load and its need for oxygen. In most cases, the dilation also lowers blood pressure, especially systolic pressure.

Nitrates come in a variety of forms; your medical condition will determine which form is appropriate for you. For example, sublingual tablets (those that are dissolved under the tongue) and chewable tablets, both of which are fast acting, are prescribed for the treatment of acute angina. Standard pills and skin patches are commonly used to prevent angina attacks. Other uses of nitrates include the treatment of some kinds of congestive heart failure. For more information, see the entries for the generic drugs listed above.

PRECAUTIONS

SPECIAL INFORMATION
- The safety of nitrates has not been established for pregnant or nursing women or for children; consult your doctor before using these drugs.
- Standard oral dosages should be taken on an empty stomach (either one hour before or two hours after meals) and with a full glass of water. This will improve absorption of the drug.
- Tolerance to nitrates may occur, requiring an adjustment (increase) of dosage over time to achieve the same therapeutic result. If tolerance becomes a problem for you, your doctor may advise taking this drug intermittently, with a medication-free period each day. However, intermittent therapy can be done only so long as symptoms are under control and your doctor orders it.
- Discontinuation should be gradual, to prevent rebound symptoms of angina.
- Tell your doctor if you have severe anemia, recent head trauma, glaucoma, an overactive thyroid, or a digestive absorption problem. Your doctor may decide not to use nitrates or to give you a smaller dose.
- Nitrates may cause the Zlatkis-Zak cholesterol test to show a lower-than-actual cholesterol level.

CONTINUED

NITRATES

POSSIBLE INTERACTIONS

Alcohol: increased risk of orthostatic hypotension (lightheadedness upon standing); do not drink while using nitrates.

Cold, cough, and allergy remedies containing epinephrine-like drugs: may counteract effects of isosorbide mononitrate.

Marijuana: can increase angina and possibly reduce effects of isosorbide mononitrate.

Nicotine, sympathomimetics: can reduce effects of isosorbide mononitrate.

Norepinephrine: decreased action of this medication.

Opioid analgesics: increased orthostatic hypotension (lightheadedness upon standing).

Other cardiovascular medicines (including antihypertensives, beta blockers, vasodilators, and other nitrates): Use these drugs only under your doctor's direction; combining them with nitrates may cause a lowering of blood pressure and other side effects.

Stimulants (such as amphetamines, pseudoephedrine): decreased action of nitrates.

TARGET AILMENTS
Acute angina pectoris
Chronic angina pectoris
Hypertension (nitroglycerin)
Congestive heart failure
Heart attack (adjunct treatment)

SIDE EFFECTS

NOT SERIOUS

- Headaches and lightheadedness when changing position (orthostatic hypotension)
- Flushing of the face and neck
- Nausea or vomiting
- Restlessness
- Fast heartbeat

CALL YOUR DOCTOR IF THESE PROBLEMS PERSIST.

SERIOUS

- Blurred vision
- Severe or prolonged headache
- Feelings of pressure in the head
- Fever
- Convulsions
- Dizziness or fainting
- Weakness or change in heartbeat
- Bluish tinge to lips, fingernails, or palms of hands
- A skin rash not from an ointment or patch

THESE PROBLEMS ARE RARE. IF YOU EXPERIENCE ANY OF THEM, CONTACT YOUR DOCTOR IMMEDIATELY.

Rx NITROFURANTOIN

VITAL STATISTICS

DRUG CLASS
Antibiotics

BRAND NAMES
Macrobid, Macrodantin

GENERAL DESCRIPTION
Used since 1953 to treat urinary tract infections, nitrofurantoin is a synthetic, broad-spectrum antibacterial agent. Its mode of action, unique among antibacterials, is to react chemically with bacterial enzymes, producing new substances that inactivate or alter vital proteins in the organism. Depending on the concentration of nitrofurantoin used, these changes either kill the organism outright or retard its growth. Because of its mode of action, bacterial resistance to this drug is rare.

Use of nitrofurantoin is limited to the prevention and treatment of urinary tract infections caused by susceptible bacteria, including *E. coli* and some species of *Enterococci* and *Staphylococci.* Nitrofurantoin does have potentially serious side effects that may require discontinuation of the drug.

For visual characteristics of the brand-name drug Macrobid, see the Color Guide to Prescription Drugs and Herbs.

PRECAUTIONS

SPECIAL INFORMATION

- Take this medication with food or milk to reduce possible gastrointestinal effects.
- Nitrofurantoin should not be used by women who are pregnant and near term or at delivery, or by women who are nursing. The drug can cross the placenta and affect the fetus. It can also enter breast milk in small amounts, possibly causing anemia in breast-feeding infants. Caution is advised for use during early pregnancy. Consult your doctor.
- Do not give nitrofurantoin to infants less than one month old; the drug may cause anemia.
- Nitrofurantoin may exacerbate peripheral neuropathy (a tingling sensation caused by a nervous system disorder), especially if you have G6PD deficiency (glucose enzyme), lung disease, or kidney problems.
- Antibiotics kill not only harmful bacteria but also "good" bacteria that keep unwanted fungi and intestinal organisms in check. Eating yogurt containing *Lactobacillus acidophilus* culture (or taking acidophilus tablets) may help restore normal bacteria.
- Prolonged use of any antibiotic can lead to fungal infections, including candidiasis, or to bacterial infections such as pseudomembranous colitis.

TARGET AILMENTS

Urinary tract infections (prevention and treatment)

CONTINUED

NITROFURANTOIN

POSSIBLE INTERACTIONS

Nitrofurantoin may interact with a number of drugs that affect the blood, liver, or nervous system. Consult your doctor before taking any medication along with nitrofurantoin.

Anticholinergic (atropine-like) drugs: increased nitrofurantoin effect.

Magnesium trisilicate antacids: reduced nitrofurantoin effect.

Nalidixic acid and quinolones: nitrofurantoin interferes with the action of these drugs.

Probenecid and sulfinpyrazone (antigout): increased levels and effectiveness of nitrofurantoin; risk of nitrofurantoin toxicity.

SIDE EFFECTS

NOT SERIOUS

- Stomach pain, diarrhea, or nausea

LET YOUR DOCTOR KNOW IF THESE SYMPTOMS BECOME TROUBLESOME.

- A rusty or brownish color in the urine

THIS SIDE EFFECT DOES NOT REQUIRE A DOCTOR'S ATTENTION.

SERIOUS

- Pneumonitis (pneumonia symptoms, such as fever, cough, chest pain, difficulty in breathing)
- Blood problems, such as reduced white cell count (manifested as sore throat and fever)
- Tiredness or weakness
- Dizziness, drowsiness, or headache
- Nerve problems (numbness, tingling, a burning sensation in the face or mouth)
- Unusual muscle weakness
- Allergic reactions, such as skin rash
- Pale skin; unusual tiredness or weakness
- Jaundice (yellow skin or eyes)

CALL YOUR DOCTOR IMMEDIATELY IF YOU EXPERIENCE ANY OF THESE SYMPTOMS. PNEUMONITIS IS THE MOST COMMON OF THESE EFFECTS.

NITROGLYCERIN

VITAL STATISTICS

DRUG CLASS
Nitrates

OTHER DRUGS IN THIS CLASS
isosorbide dinitrate, isosorbide mononitrate

BRAND NAMES
Nitro-Dur, Nitrostat, Transderm-Nitro

GENERAL DESCRIPTION
Since 1847, nitroglycerin has been prescribed for cardiovascular disease. The drug is most commonly used to provide effective relief of acute angina (chest pain) from coronary artery disease. It is also offered as a preventive treatment for angina attacks and as a complementary treatment for heart attack, and is sometimes used to treat hypertensive emergencies.

Nitroglycerin comes in several forms, each prescribed according to its therapeutic use. For fast action, sublingual tablets (those that are dissolved under the tongue) or a spray form may be used. For long-term therapy, your doctor may prescribe standard tablets, ointment, or skin patches.

See Nitrates for more information, including side effects and possible food and drug interactions. For visual characteristics of the brand-name drug Nitrostat, see the Color Guide to Prescription Drugs and Herbs.

PRECAUTIONS

SPECIAL INFORMATION
- The safety of nitroglycerin has not been established for pregnant or nursing women or for children; consult your doctor before using this drug.
- Tolerance to nitroglycerin may occur, requiring an adjustment (increase) of dosage over time to achieve the same therapeutic result. If tolerance becomes a problem for you, your doctor may advise taking this drug intermittently, with a medication-free period each day. However, intermittent therapy can be done only so long as symptoms are under control and your doctor orders it.
- Discontinuation should be gradual to prevent rebound symptoms of angina.
- Tell your doctor if you have severe anemia, recent head trauma, glaucoma, an overactive thyroid, or a digestive absorption problem. Your doctor may decide not to use nitroglycerin or to give you a smaller dose.
- Keep sublingual tablets in the original container. After each use, replace the cap tightly to prevent loss of the drug's potency.
- Nitroglycerin may cause the Zlatkis-Zak cholesterol test to show a lower-than-actual cholesterol level.
- Nitroglycerin ointment or transdermal patches may irritate the skin at the application site.

TARGET AILMENTS

Angina pectoris

Hypertensive crises

Myocardial infarction (heart attack)

SIDE EFFECTS

SEE NITRATES.

NIZATIDINE

VITAL STATISTICS

DRUG CLASS
Antiulcer Drugs [Histamine H_2 Blockers]

BRAND NAMES
Rx: Axid
OTC: Axid AR

OTHER DRUGS IN THIS SUBCLASS
lansoprazole, omeprazole, sucralfate
Histamine H_2 Blockers: cimetidine, famotidine, ranitidine

GENERAL DESCRIPTION
Nizatidine is used primarily to treat ulcers of the stomach and duodenum (upper intestine). It is also prescribed for Zollinger-Ellison syndrome, gastroesophageal reflux (in which stomach acid flows backward into the esophagus), and other conditions involving the overproduction of stomach acid. In some cases, nizatidine is used to prevent upper gastrointestinal bleeding.

In the over-the-counter form, nizatidine is used not for ulcers but to relieve acid indigestion and heartburn. Although the OTC version is a lower dose of nizatidine than the prescription form, essentially the same interactions apply, although the side effects are milder.

Belonging to the subclass of antiulcer drugs known as histamine H_2 blockers, nizatidine works by blocking the effects of the chemical compound histamine in the stomach, thereby reducing the secretion of the digestive juice hydrochloric acid. For more information on side effects and possible drug interactions, see Antiulcer Drugs. For visual characteristics of the brand-name drug Axid, see the Color Guide to Prescription Drugs and Herbs.

PRECAUTIONS

SPECIAL INFORMATION
- Nizatidine may affect some medical tests, including blood platelet counts and liver function tests. Inform the person giving you the test that you are taking this medication.
- Avoid this drug if you are pregnant or nursing.
- Inform your doctor if you have a history of kidney or liver disease or are taking large doses of aspirin.
- If you are also using antacids for relief from ulcer pain, take the antacid at least two hours before or after taking nizatidine.
- If this drug causes dizziness or drowsiness, restrict your driving or your involvement in other potentially hazardous activities.

POSSIBLE INTERACTIONS
Alcohol, tobacco (smoking): increased stomach acidity, leading to decreased effectiveness of nizatidine.
Antacids containing aluminum and magnesium hydroxide: reduced effects of nizatidine; avoid taking antacids within two hours of taking nizatidine.
Aspirin: increased effect of aspirin if large doses of aspirin are being taken.
Enteric-coated tablets: changes in stomach acidity, causing these medications to dissolve prematurely in the stomach; avoid taking enteric-coated drugs with nizatidine.

NIZATIDINE

TARGET AILMENTS

Duodenal ulcer

Gastric ulcer

Upper gastrointestinal bleeding associated with gastric ulcer or duodenal ulcer, or with gastritis

Zollinger-Ellison syndrome

Multiple endocrine neoplasia

Other conditions characterized by an overproduction of stomach acid

Gastroesophageal reflux

Acid indigestion and heartburn (OTC)

SIDE EFFECTS

NOT SERIOUS

- Drowsiness and increased sweating (more common)
- Dizziness
- Headache
- Nausea
- Vomiting
- Skin rash
- Constipation
- Decreased libido or sexual ability
- Swelling or soreness of breasts (in women or men)

MOST OF THESE SIDE EFFECTS ARE RARE. CALL YOUR DOCTOR IF THESE SYMPTOMS PERSIST OR BECOME BOTHERSOME.

SERIOUS

- Allergic reaction (redness or swelling of the skin)
- Confusion
- Unusual bleeding or bruising
- Abdominal pain; yellow skin

THESE SIDE EFFECTS ARE RARE. IF THEY OCCUR, CALL YOUR DOCTOR IMMEDIATELY.

Nonsteroidal Anti-Inflammatory Drugs (NSAIDs)

Vital Statistics

GENERIC NAMES

Rx: diclofenac, etodolac, flurbiprofen, ibuprofen, ketoprofen, ketorolac, nabumetone, naproxen, oxaprozin

OTC: ibuprofen, ketoprofen, naproxen

GENERAL DESCRIPTION

NSAIDs are nonnarcotic analgesic drugs that reduce inflammation, especially from arthritis. These drugs are used by people who cannot tolerate aspirin, or when aspirin or acetaminophen is not effective. In addition to reducing inflammation, NSAIDs relieve pain. Some are indicated for reducing fever. For more information, see the entries for the generic drugs listed above.

TARGET AILMENTS
Inflammation, especially related to osteoarthritis and rheumatoid arthritis
Pain, especially from inflammation, dental and other surgeries, menstruation, or migraines
Fever

Precautions

SPECIAL INFORMATION

- If NSAIDs upset your stomach, take them with food or milk.
- Do not use NSAIDs if you are allergic to them or to aspirin. NSAIDs may cause bronchoconstriction or anaphylaxis in aspirin-sensitive asthmatics.
- Avoid these drugs or consult your doctor before using them if you have asthma, peptic ulcer, enteritis (intestinal inflammation), high blood pressure, bleeding problems, epilepsy, Parkinson's disease, or impaired liver or kidney function.
- Do not take more than the recommended dose and seek emergency help in case of overdose. Possible symptoms of overdose include drowsiness, increased sweating, rapid heartbeat, abdominal pain, vomiting, nausea, gastrointestinal bleeding, and disorientation.
- NSAIDs are not recommended for pregnant women, especially during the last trimester, or for nursing mothers.

POSSIBLE INTERACTIONS

Because NSAIDs interact with many substances, check with your doctor or pharmacist before taking in combination with other drugs. NSAIDs can affect liver and kidney function, thereby increasing the toxicity of other drugs. Some or all NSAIDs can interact with the following drugs:

Acetaminophen: increased risk of adverse liver or kidney effect.

Alcohol: possible bleeding and ulcers.

Antacids: decreased NSAID effect.

Anticoagulant drugs: increased anticoagulant effect, possible bleeding.

NONSTEROIDAL ANTI-INFLAMMATORY DRUGS (NSAIDs)

Anticonvulsant drugs (phenytoin): increased action of phenytoin.

Antidiabetic drugs and insulin: increased hypoglycemic effect; with diclofenac, either increased or decreased hypoglycemic effect.

Antipsychotic drugs (such as chlorpromazine and clozapine): with nabumetone, decreased effects of these drugs.

Aspirin: increased risk of stomach problems.

Benzodiazepines (such as chlordiazepoxide, diazepam, and oxazepam): with nabumetone, decreased effects of these drugs.

Beta-adrenergic blockers: decreased antihypertensive effect.

Cimetidine: may increase or decrease the effect of the NSAID.

Colchicine: possibility of bleeding and ulcers when combined with certain NSAIDs.

Corticosteroids: possible bleeding and ulcers. Don't combine unless directed to do so by your doctor.

Cyclosporine: increased risk of kidney damage.

Diuretics: reduced diuretic effect.

Methotrexate: increased toxicity of methotrexate; possibly fatal poisoning.

Probenecid: increased NSAID effect, possible NSAID toxicity.

Sulfonamides: possible sulfonamide toxicity.

Tricyclic antidepressants (such as amitriptyline): with nabumetone, decreased effects of these drugs.

Verapamil: increased toxicity.

SIDE EFFECTS

NOT SERIOUS

- Dizziness
- Drowsiness
- Headache
- Abdominal pain or cramps
- Constipation
- Diarrhea; heartburn
- Nausea

CONSULT YOUR DOCTOR IF THESE SYMPTOMS PERSIST.

SERIOUS

- Hives, rash, intense itching, and trouble breathing (anaphylactic reaction)

SEEK EMERGENCY HELP.

- Chest pain or irregular heartbeat
- Diminished hearing or ringing in the ears
- Trouble breathing
- Fluid retention
- Black or tarry stools
- Blood in urine
- Photosensitivity
- Jaundice (indicated by bleeding, bruising, tiredness, tenderness in upper abdomen, and yellow eyes or skin)
- Gastrointestinal ulceration, bleeding, and perforation of stomach

DISCONTINUE USE AND CALL YOUR DOCTOR IMMEDIATELY IF YOU NOTICE ANY OF THESE SYMPTOMS.

Rx NORTRIPTYLINE

VITAL STATISTICS

DRUG CLASS
Antidepressants [Tricyclic Antidepressants (TCAs)]

BRAND NAME
Pamelor

OTHER DRUGS IN THIS SUBCLASS
amitriptyline, doxepin

GENERAL DESCRIPTION
In use for three decades, nortriptyline is prescribed for treatment of primary depression and panic attacks. It is also used in combination with other drugs to manage chronic pain. Like other tricyclic antidepressants, nortriptyline acts to restore normal levels of important brain chemicals such as serotonin and norepinephrine. For visual characteristics, see the Color Guide to Prescription Drugs and Herbs. See Antidepressants for information about side effects and possible drug interactions.

TARGET AILMENTS

Primary depression

Panic attacks

SIDE EFFECTS

SEE ANTIDEPRESSANTS.

PRECAUTIONS

SPECIAL INFORMATION

- Before taking nortriptyline, let your doctor know if you are suffering from glaucoma, urinary retention, epilepsy, or hyperthyroidism.
- This drug may cause drowsiness. When taking nortriptyline, use care while driving, operating machinery, or performing tasks that require mental alertness.
- Nortriptyline can trigger manic attacks in individuals with manic-depression. Be sure to tell your doctor if you have manic-depression.
- Nortriptyline can affect blood sugar (glucose tolerance) tests by causing fluctuations in blood sugar levels.
- The full effects of this drug may not occur for several weeks.
- If you are pregnant, nursing, or planning a pregnancy, check with your doctor before taking nortriptyline.

POSSIBLE INTERACTIONS

Anticoagulant drugs (such as warfarin): TCAs may increase the anticlotting activity.

Barbiturates: decreased effectiveness of TCAs.

Cimetidine (antiulcer): increased TCA effects.

Clonidine (blood pressure medication): may cause a dangerous increase in blood pressure.

Haloperidol (antipsychotic), oral contraceptives, phenothiazines (antipsychotic), levodopa (anti-Parkinsonism): increased levels of TCAs.

Thyroid medications: combining TCAs with thyroid drugs may increase the effects, including side effects, of both medications.

Tobacco (smoking): increased elimination of TCAs from the body, lessening their effectiveness.

Rx NORVASC

VITAL STATISTICS

DRUG CLASS
Calcium Channel Blockers

GENERIC NAME
amlodipine

OTHER DRUGS IN THIS CLASS
diltiazem, isradipine, nifedipine, verapamil

GENERAL DESCRIPTION
Norvasc is a brand name for the generic drug amlodipine, a calcium channel blocker used to treat hypertension and angina (chest pain). Like other drugs in its class, Norvasc inhibits the passage of calcium into vascular smooth muscle cells, thus dilating the arteries and lowering blood pressure. These actions also reduce the strain on the heart and open the coronary arteries—blocking spasms of the coronary arteries and thus lessening angina. Norvasc is used alone or in carefully selected combinations with other heart and blood pressure medications. For visual characteristics of Norvasc, see the Color Guide to Prescription Drugs and Herbs. For information on possible drug interactions, see Calcium Channel Blockers.

PRECAUTIONS

WARNING
Rarely, people with advanced coronary artery disease experience increased angina or myocardial infarction (heart attack) on beginning treatment with a calcium channel blocker. Contact your doctor immediately if this occurs.

SPECIAL INFORMATION
- Recent findings have prompted warnings about the safety of calcium channel blockers. Before using Norvasc, be sure to discuss this matter thoroughly with your doctor. If you are already taking this drug, do not stop the medication without first consulting your doctor.
- Let your doctor know if you are suffering from low blood pressure, heart or liver disease, congestive heart failure, or severe obstruction of the coronary arteries.

TARGET AILMENTS

Angina (chest pain)

High blood pressure

SIDE EFFECTS

NOT SERIOUS
- Gastrointestinal upset
- Drowsiness; fatigue
- Lightheadedness; dizziness
- Headache; flushing
- Weight gain; increased appetite; muscle cramps (rare)

CALL YOUR DOCTOR IF THESE EFFECTS BECOME TROUBLESOME.

SERIOUS
- Edema (swelling)
- Heart problems, such as congestive heart failure, heart-rhythm irregularities, or increased angina (rare)
- Shortness of breath (rare)
- Allergic reactions, such as skin rash (rare)

CONTACT YOUR DOCTOR AT ONCE.

Notoginseng Root

LATIN NAME
Panax notoginseng

Vital Statistics

GENERAL DESCRIPTION

Notoginseng root is used to stop bleeding, reduce swelling, and alleviate pain from injuries. Unlike Western medications, the root seems to halt the bleeding without making the blood clot, and to stop the clotting or hematoma without causing bleeding. Western practitioners of sports medicine frequently use this herb as a tonic to improve stamina. Powdered notoginseng has been used to treat individuals with coronary artery disease who complained primarily of chest pain. Many seemed to improve, and some also experienced reductions in blood pressure. Notoginseng is sometimes used to treat acute attacks of Crohn's disease.

The best variety of notoginseng root is large, solid, and dark brown, with thin skin. Also known as pseudoginseng root *(Panax pseudoginseng),* it is grown in several Chinese provinces and harvested in the fall or winter of the plant's third or seventh year, after the fruit is ripe. Chinese herbalists classify it as sweet, bitter, and warm.

Chinese medicine takes a holistic approach to healthcare, fashioning remedies to treat the entire being as well as the specific parts or areas. Single herbs may be used alone or in combination with other herbs to prevent and combat disease, which is thought to arise from disturbances in the flow of a bodily energy called chi (pronounced "chee") and blood, or from a lack of balance in the complementary states of yin and yang.

PREPARATIONS

Notoginseng root is available in bulk from Chinese pharmacies, Asian markets, and Western health food stores, where it is sold as loose, dried roots or in the form of tablets.

Combinations: Notoginseng can be made into a liniment for swelling and pain and is included in many injury tonics. It is also taken internally to heal injuries, cuts, and even gunshot wounds. A preparation containing notoginseng root and bletilla root is prescribed for vomiting, for coughing up blood, for nosebleeds, and for blood in the urine. A mixture with dragon bone and gallnut from the Chinese sumac makes a poultice for bleeding caused by trauma. For information on appropriate preparations and doses, check with a herbal practitioner.

Precautions

SPECIAL INFORMATION

Pregnant women should avoid this herb; notoginseng may cause a miscarriage in at-risk pregnancies.

TARGET AILMENTS

Take internally for:

Internal bleeding such as nosebleeds and blood in the stool and urine, coughing up blood

Take both internally and externally for:

Bleeding from injuries; swelling and pain of fractures, falls, contusions and sprains, cuts, gunshot wounds

SIDE EFFECTS

None expected

NUTMEG

LATIN NAME
Myristica fragrans

VITAL STATISTICS

GENERAL DESCRIPTION

As early as the seventh century, Arabs used nutmeg for digestive disorders, kidney problems, and lymphatic ailments. Today it is used principally as a spice in cooking and by herbalists as a treatment for diarrhea, insomnia, indigestion, and flatulence. It relaxes muscles, sedates the body, and helps remove gas from the digestive tract. Early reports describe hallucinogenic reactions to ingesting whole seeds, but these have not been substantiated. Nutmeg is native to a province of Indonesia once known as the Spice Islands, where it is still used as a culinary seasoning and medicinal herb. It comes from an evergreen tree that produces a fruit called the nutmeg apple. Nutmeg comes from the nut, which is removed and dried.

It is reported that in some Middle Eastern cultures, nutmeg is used in love potions as an aphrodisiac.

PREPARATIONS

Nutmeg is available as a powder and tincture. Consult a qualified practitioner for the dosage appropriate for you and the specific condition being treated.

PRECAUTIONS

☠ *WARNING*

Women have suffered toxic reactions when attempting to use nutmeg to induce abortions. It is no longer thought to precipitate abortion.

Use of this herb by children for more than seven to 10 days should be done in conjunction with a healthcare practitioner.

POSSIBLE INTERACTIONS

Combining nutmeg with other herbs may necessitate a lower dosage.

TARGET AILMENTS
Diarrhea; indigestion
Loss of appetite
Colic
Flatulence
Insomnia

SIDE EFFECTS

SERIOUS

MYRISTICIN, A COMPONENT OF NUTMEG, HAS NARCOTIC PROPERTIES. AS LITTLE AS A TEASPOON OF THIS SUBSTANCE CAN CAUSE TOXIC SYMPTOMS IN HUMANS. INGESTION OF 6 TO 12 TSP (OR 1 TO 2 OZ) OF GROUND NUTMEG CAN CAUSE PROLONGED DELIRIUM, DISORIENTATION, AND DRUNKENNESS.

N

NUX VOMICA

LATIN NAME
Nux vomica

VITAL STATISTICS

GENERAL DESCRIPTION

Nux vomica, also known as poison nut, is a remedy made from seeds of an evergreen tree indigenous to parts of India, Thailand, China, and Australia. The seeds contain strychnine and have a bitter, unpleasant taste. Small doses of the seed stimulate the appetite, while somewhat larger doses decrease the appetite and cause motor dysfunction, including stiffness in the arms and legs and a staggered walk. Toxic doses can cause convulsions and death. *Nux vomica* is prescribed by homeopaths for ailments that occur from overindulgence in food, coffee, or alcohol, usually accompanied by irritability. To prepare the homeopathic remedy, poison-nut seeds are ground to a powder and then diluted with milk sugar to the desired potency. For more information on homeopathic medicine, see page 14.

PREPARATIONS

Nux vomica is available over the counter in various potencies, in both liquid and tablet form. Consult a homeopathic practitioner for more precise information.

PRECAUTIONS

SPECIAL INFORMATION

- When a remedy is administered, no one but the patient should touch the pills. If tablets are spilled, throw them away.
- The mouth should be clear of flavors 15 minutes before and after taking a remedy, and strong flavors and aromas, such as coffee, camphor, and heavily scented perfumes, should be avoided for the duration of treatment.

TARGET AILMENTS

Colds with sneezing and a stuffy nose

Colic and stomach cramps from overeating; indigestion

Constipation resulting from physical inactivity

Cystitis

Fever with chills

Gas and gas pains

Hangovers

Headache with dizziness

Insomnia

Irritable bowel syndrome

Menstrual cramps with heavy flow

Nausea (especially morning sickness)

Sinusitis

Stomach flu

Vomiting brought on by overeating or eating rich foods

SIDE EFFECTS

NONE EXPECTED

OATS

LATIN NAME
Avena sativa

VITAL STATISTICS

GENERAL DESCRIPTION

Oats, of proved nutritional value, also alleviate such ailments as depression and nervous anxiety, high cholesterol, insomnia, and indigestion. With their vitamins, minerals, and alkaloids providing both relaxing and stimulating effects, oats can improve the overall condition of the nerves and relieve general feelings of weakness and fatigue. Oatmeal applied externally can relieve discomfort from poison ivy, hives or other allergic reactions, shingles, and similar skin conditions.

PREPARATIONS

Over the counter:

Available as raw rolled oats, oat straw, and oat bran, or as tincture. Commercial preparations for external use are also available.

At home:

TEA: For nerves, pour 1 cup boiling water over 2 to 3 tsp dried oat straw; steep covered 10 to 15 minutes. Drink three times a day.

TINCTURE: Drink 1/4 to 1/2 tsp three times a day.

NUTRITION AND DIET: Include 2 to 3 oz oat fiber per day in a low-fat diet to help reduce cholesterol. Oatmeal, porridge, or oat bran is suggested.

BATH: To relieve hives, place up to 1 cup raw rolled oats directly into bathwater. For neuralgia or skin irritation, put 1 to 3 cups raw oats into a muslin bag, then place bag in bathwater or hang the bag under the tap, letting water run over it into the bath. Or boil 1 pound shredded oat straw in 2 quarts of water for 30 minutes; strain liquid and add to bathwater. Oat straw may also be used for soothing footbaths.

COMBINATIONS: May be combined with damiana, kola, skullcap, mugwort, and lady's-slipper *(Cypripedium pubescens)* to treat depression and anxiety. Consult a qualified practitioner for the dosage appropriate for your specific condition.

PRECAUTIONS

SPECIAL INFORMATION

- If adding oat bran to the diet, increase your intake gradually. Increasing it too fast can cause cramps and gas.
- If using a bath preparation, be careful not to stay in the bath too long; lengthy immersion can strip sensitive skin of essential oils.

POSSIBLE INTERACTIONS

Combining oats with other herbs may necessitate a lower dosage.

TARGET AILMENTS
Take internally for:
Depression; anxiety; insomnia
High cholesterol; indigestion
Use externally for:
Eczema and allergy-related skin conditions; dry skin

SIDE EFFECTS

NOT SERIOUS

- Headaches

VERY LARGE DOSES CAN CAUSE THESE. DISCONTINUE USE.

O

Rx OFLOXACIN

VITAL STATISTICS

DRUG CLASS
Antibiotics [Fluoroquinolones]

BRAND NAMES
Floxin, Ocuflox

GENERAL DESCRIPTION
Introduced in 1984, ofloxacin is a synthetic fluoroquinolone that shares a wide range of uses with other drugs of its type. Besides the ailments typically targeted by fluoroquinolones, ofloxacin is used to fight infections caused by *Chlamydia trachomatis* bacteria. It has also been approved for use in treating corneal ulcers caused by bacteria. See Fluoroquinolones for more information about uses and side effects. For visual characteristics of the brand-name drug Floxin, see the Color Guide to Prescription Drugs and Herbs.

TARGET AILMENTS
Bronchitis (bacterial exacerbations); pneumonia (bacterial)

Chlamydia and other sexually transmitted diseases

Corneal ulcers (bacterial)

Otitis media; sinusitis

Prostatitis (bacterial)

Infections of the skin and soft tissue

Urinary tract infections; diarrhea

O

PRECAUTIONS

SPECIAL INFORMATION
A rare condition known as pseudomembranous colitis may occur during or after the use of fluoroquinolones. Call your doctor at once if you experience abdominal or stomach cramps, severe pain and bloating, watery and severe diarrhea (may be bloody); fever, increased thirst; nausea or vomiting; tiredness or weakness; unusual weight loss. These symptoms may occur at any time while you are using fluoroquinolones, or they may strike weeks after you have stopped taking the drug.

POSSIBLE INTERACTIONS
Antacids; didanosine (antiviral); ferrous sulfate, laxatives containing magnesium; sucralfate (antiulcer); zinc: reduced fluoroquinolone effect. Take ofloxacin at least two hours before or two hours after taking antacids and similar drugs.

Cimetidine (antiulcer) and probenecid (antigout): decreased elimination of fluoroquinolones, heightening risk of adverse effects and toxicity.

Theophyllines (asthma drugs): ofloxacin may inhibit metabolism of these drugs, increasing the risk of adverse effects and theophylline toxicity. (Generally, ofloxacin has less effect on theophylline metabolism than does ciprofloxacin, another fluoroquinolone drug.)

Warfarin (anticoagulant): increased anticoagulant effect.

SIDE EFFECTS
SEE FLUOROQUINOLONES.

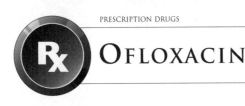

OMEGA-3 FATTY ACIDS

VITAL STATISTICS

GENERAL DESCRIPTION

Omega-3 fatty acids have earned a wide reputation for preventing heart disease. They are linked to low incidences of heart disease in world populations that eat large amounts of fatty fish. These fatty acids help lower blood levels of LDL, the harmful type of cholesterol that can lead to atherosclerosis. Omega-3 fatty acids also contribute to functions in the body that help thin the blood and decrease plaque along artery walls, improving blood circulation.

Omega-3 fatty acids may relieve inflammation associated with colitis or arthritis, and skin problems such as skin cancer or psoriasis. Purported to have overall health benefits, omega-3 fatty acids are sometimes recommended to treat kidney problems, multiple sclerosis, and cancer, among other ailments.

NATURAL SOURCES

cold-water fish, including tuna, salmon, mackerel, and sardines; walnuts; flaxseed oil; canola oil

PREPARATIONS

Available in flaxseed, flaxseed oil, and gel capsules.

TARGET AILMENTS

Heart disease; high cholesterol; arthritis; colitis; psoriasis; atopic dermatitis (eczema); lupus; multiple sclerosis; cancer

PRECAUTIONS

WARNING

Avoid concentrated supplements unless recommended by your doctor.

Omega-3 fatty acids may slow blood clotting. Do not take these supplements if you have a blood-clotting disorder.

SPECIAL INFORMATION

- No standard recommended dosage has been determined. Consult your doctor for advice on adding omega-3 fatty acids to your diet. Most doctors recommend eating fish rather than taking supplements.
- If you are pregnant or breast-feeding, consult your doctor before taking supplements.
- With excessive amounts, unusual bleeding may result.
- Omega-3 fatty acid supplements may raise blood levels of HDL, the good kind of cholesterol, causing an increase in overall blood cholesterol levels.

POSSIBLE INTERACTIONS

Anticoagulant medications, including aspirin: may increase anticoagulant effect. Consult your doctor before taking omega-3 fatty acid supplements.

SIDE EFFECTS

NOT SERIOUS

- Unusual tiredness (anemia)

CALL YOUR DOCTOR.

Omeprazole

Vital Statistics

DRUG CLASS
Antiulcer Drugs

BRAND NAME
Prilosec

OTHER DRUGS IN THIS CLASS
lansoprazole, sucralfate
Histamine H_2 Blockers: cimetidine, famotidine, nizatidine, ranitidine

GENERAL DESCRIPTION
Omeprazole is used to treat several conditions associated with excessive production of stomach acid, such as ulcers of the stomach and duodenum (first portion of the small intestine), Zollinger-Ellison syndrome, multiple endocrine neoplasia, systemic mastocytosis, gastritis, gastroesophageal reflux (in which stomach acid flows backward into the esophagus), and gastrointestinal symptoms associated with the use of nonsteroidal anti-inflammatory drugs (NSAIDs) and aspirin. The drug works by inhibiting the action of enzymes in the acid-producing cells of the stomach lining. For more information on possible drug interactions, see Antiulcer Drugs. For visual characteristics of the brand-name drug Prilosec, see the Color Guide to Prescription Drugs and Herbs.

Precautions

SPECIAL INFORMATION
- Avoid this drug if you are breast-feeding.
- Check with your doctor before taking omeprazole with antacids.

Target Ailments

Duodenal ulcer; gastric ulcer; upper gastrointestinal bleeding associated with gastric ulcer or duodenal ulcer, or with gastritis

Zollinger-Ellison syndrome; multiple endocrine neoplasia; other conditions characterized by an overproduction of stomach acid

Gastroesophageal reflux

Gastrointestinal symptoms associated with the use of nonsteroidal anti-inflammatory drugs (NSAIDs) and aspirin

Side Effects

Not Serious

- Abdominal pain; dizziness or headache; drowsiness; chest pain; heartburn; constipation, gas, or diarrhea; nausea and vomiting; rash or itching

Call your doctor if these symptoms become bothersome.

Serious

- Anemia (unusual tiredness); combined sore throat and fever; mouth sores; bloody urine; urinary tract infection (pain or burning when urinating); unusual bleeding or bruising

Call your doctor right away.

O

Ophthalmic Antibiotics

Vital Statistics

GENERIC NAMES
erythromycin, tobramycin

GENERAL DESCRIPTION
Ophthalmic antibiotics, available as ointments or eye drops, fight eye infections caused by bacteria. The generic drugs used in these eye medications may also come in the form of tablets, skin creams, or injectables for treating other, nonocular infections. However, you should never use these forms interchangeably; use each form only for its intended purpose. For more information, see the entries for the generic drugs listed above.

Precautions

SPECIAL INFORMATION
- Tell your doctor if you have ever had an allergic reaction to these drugs. You may need a different treatment.
- Prolonged use of ophthalmic antibiotics may result in a superinfection in the eye, with symptoms of a worsening infection. Discontinue the antibiotic and call your doctor.
- Unless they are clearly needed, do not use these drugs if you are pregnant or breast-feeding.
- Tobramycin may slow the healing of corneal wounds.

POSSIBLE INTERACTIONS
None expected for ophthalmic forms. However, since systemic absorption through the eyes can occur, you should tell your doctor about any other medicine you are using.

TARGET AILMENTS

Eye infections due to strains of strep, staph, *Hemophilus influenzae,* and other bacteria (also used to prevent conjunctivitis in newborns who have been exposed in the birth canal to chlamydia or gonorrhea)

SIDE EFFECTS

NOT SERIOUS
- Blurred vision, slight burning, or stinging that occurs momentarily upon each application

SERIOUS
- Eye irritation that develops and persists after using these drugs
- Itching, redness, or swelling

THESE MAY INDICATE AN ALLERGY OR A SUPERINFECTION. DISCONTINUE USE AND CALL YOUR DOCTOR RIGHT AWAY.

Opioid Analgesics

Vital Statistics

GENERIC NAMES
codeine, hydrocodone, oxycodone, propoxyphene, tramadol

GENERAL DESCRIPTION
Opioid analgesics are narcotic drugs that act on the central nervous system (the spinal cord and brain) to alter the perception of pain. They are used to treat temporary moderate to severe pain and are often combined with nonnarcotic analgesics such as aspirin or acetaminophen. As narcotics, opioid analgesics may cause physical and psychological dependence, especially if used for long periods of time. For more information, see entries for the generic drugs listed above.

Precautions

SPECIAL INFORMATION

- Opioid analgesics can lead to addiction, both physical and psychological.
- Tell your doctor if you notice the following withdrawal symptoms after you stop taking an opioid drug: fever, runny nose, or sneezing; diarrhea; goose flesh; unusually large pupils; nervousness or irritability; fast heartbeat.
- Seek emergency medical care if you overdose on opioid analgesics. Symptoms of overdose include pinpoint pupils; slow, shallow, or troubled breathing; slow heartbeat; extreme dizziness or weakness; confusion; convulsions.
- These drugs are not recommended if you are pregnant or breast-feeding.
- Before taking these drugs, tell your physician if you have kidney or liver impairment, asthma, breathing problems, glaucoma, a stomach ulcer, a history of convulsions or drug abuse, inflammatory bowel disease, gallbladder disease, hypothyroidism, a bladder obstruction, or prostate problems.
- Do not drive or operate machinery until you know how the drug you are taking affects you.
- Do not drink alcoholic beverages while you are taking these drugs.
- Combining propoxyphene with alcohol, tranquilizers, sedatives, muscle relaxants, or antidepressants can lead to death. Do not combine without your doctor's knowledge.
- Rarely, propoxyphene can cause jaundice and reduced liver function, which may include such symptoms as weakness, loss of appetite, and nausea.
- Some opioid analgesic drugs also contain a nonnarcotic analgesic, such as aspirin or acetaminophen. Before taking any other medication, read the label carefully to avoid accidental overdose.

TARGET AILMENTS

Moderate to severe pain, especially short-term pain from acute trauma or surgery

Moderate to severe tension headaches

Nonproductive cough in bronchial disorders (codeine, hydrocodone)

Opioid Analgesics

POSSIBLE INTERACTIONS

Amphetamines: risk of convulsions if a patient taking amphetamines takes an overdose of propoxyphene.

Anticholinergic drugs: opioid drugs may increase the effects of these drugs; risk of severe constipation and urinary retention (difficulty in urination, with frequent urge to urinate).

Anticoagulants: propoxyphene may increase the effects of some anticoagulants.

Antidepressants [especially monoamine oxidase (MAO) inhibitors]: increased sedative effect and serious toxicity.

Antidiarrheal drugs: risk of severe constipation.

Antihypertensives, diuretics: may lower blood pressure, causing orthostatic hypotension (dizziness related to change in body position).

Carbamazepine: propoxyphene may increase the effects of carbamazepine, leading to an increased risk of toxicity.

Central nervous system depressants and drugs with sedative effects (such as alcohol, antihistamines, benzodiazepines, and other opioid drugs): increased sedative effects; risk of coma.

Cimetidine: with propoxyphene, possible central nervous system toxicity.

Metoclopramide: opioids render this drug less effective.

Smoking cessation drugs, such as nicotine patches or chewing gum: may increase the effects of propoxyphene.

SIDE EFFECTS

NOT SERIOUS

- Dry mouth
- Dizziness
- Fatigue
- Drowsiness
- Headache
- Nervousness
- Difficulty in urination; frequent urge to urinate
- Mild nausea
- Mild constipation

CONSULT YOUR DOCTOR IF SYMPTOMS CONTINUE OR ARE BOTHERSOME.

SERIOUS

- Slow or shallow breathing
- Somnolence
- Skin rash, hives or itching, or facial swelling
- Decrease in blood pressure or heart rate
- Fast heartbeat with increased sweating and shortness of breath
- Severe constipation, nausea, stomach pain, or vomiting
- Propoxyphene only: reduced liver function (brownish urine or whitish stool) or jaundice

DISCONTINUE USE AND CALL YOUR DOCTOR.

Rx ORAL HYPOGLYCEMICS

VITAL STATISTICS

DRUG CLASS
Antidiabetic Drugs

GENERIC NAMES
glipizide, glyburide

GENERAL DESCRIPTION
A subclass of antidiabetic drugs, oral hypoglycemics (also known as sulfonylureas) are used to treat a form of non-insulin-dependent (Type 2) diabetes that cannot be controlled by diet and exercise alone. Oral hypoglycemic drugs stimulate the release of existing insulin in people whose bodies are capable of producing insulin. These drugs do not lower blood sugar on their own but can work effectively when used in conjunction with a prescribed diet and exercise program. For information on specific oral hypoglycemics, see entries for the generic drugs listed above. For information about other medications used to treat diabetes (including other oral medications classified as "antihyperglycemics," which work by a different mechanism from hypoglycemics), see the entries for Acarbose, Metformin, Troglitazone, Antidiabetic Drugs, and Insulin.

PRECAUTIONS

SPECIAL INFORMATION
- An overdose of these drugs can result in hypoglycemia (abnormally small concentrations of sugar in the blood). Signs of hypoglycemia include excessive hunger, cold sweats, shakiness, nervousness or anxiety, rapid pulse, headache, drowsiness, confusion, nausea, and cool, pale skin. Keep hard candy or fruit juice handy to raise your blood sugar level and counteract hypoglycemia. Call your doctor.
- Tell your doctor if you are allergic to sulfa drugs; you may also be allergic to oral hypoglycemics.
- Avoid oral antidiabetic drugs if you are pregnant or nursing; abnormal blood sugar levels have been associated with birth defects in laboratory animals. Injectable insulin is more effective than oral medications at maintaining close-to-normal blood sugar concentrations in women who are pregnant or nursing.
- People who are elderly, debilitated, or malnourished, as well as those with adrenal, thyroid, pituitary, kidney, or liver problems, have an increased susceptibility to the hypoglycemic action of antidiabetic drugs and should use them with caution.
- Do not stop taking this medication without your doctor's approval.
- Mild stress may reduce the effectiveness of oral hypoglycemics.

Oral Hypoglycemics

- Some studies have shown that the use of oral hypoglycemic drugs to control diabetes is more likely to lead to fatal heart problems than the use of diet alone or diet in conjunction with insulin. Your doctor can help determine the best course of treatment.
- These drugs may cause photosensitivity; avoid prolonged exposure to the sun and sunlamps.
- It is important to self-monitor your glucose level when taking these drugs.
- Strict adherence to your prescribed regimen of diet and exercise is required for these medications to be effective.

POSSIBLE INTERACTIONS

Oral hypoglycemics may interact with a number of other drugs. Check with your doctor or pharmacist before taking any medication, and be sure to read all labels for sugar content.

Alcohol, aspirin, and other salicylates: avoid these substances while taking oral hypoglycemics.

Beta-adrenergic blockers, bumetanide, diazoxide, estrogens, ethacrynic acid, oral contraceptives, phenytoin, rifampin: decreased effects of oral hypoglycemics.

Cimetidine, clofibrate, fenfluramine, monoamine oxidase (MAO) inhibitors, phenylbutazone, ranitidine: increased effects of oral hypoglycemics.

TARGET AILMENTS

Non-insulin-dependent (Type 2) diabetes

SIDE EFFECTS

NOT SERIOUS

- Constipation or diarrhea
- Nausea, vomiting, or stomach pain
- Dizziness; mild drowsiness
- Headache
- Heartburn
- Change in appetite
- Skin allergies
- Weakness
- Tingling of hands and feet

CALL YOUR DOCTOR IF THESE SYMPTOMS CONTINUE OR BECOME BOTHERSOME.

SERIOUS

- Sore throat and unusual bleeding or bruising
- Water retention (edema)
- Weight gain
- Yellowing of the skin or eyes (jaundice)
- Abnormally light-colored stools
- Low-grade fever, fatigue, chills

CONTACT YOUR DOCTOR IMMEDIATELY. ALSO SEE THE OVERDOSE SYMPTOMS LISTED IN SPECIAL INFORMATION.

OREGON GRAPE

LATIN NAME
Berberis aquifolium

VITAL STATISTICS

GENERAL DESCRIPTION

Also known as mountain grape, this herb comes from the Pacific Northwest, where it was long used by Native Americans to treat arthritis, liver disease, and cancer. Like its British cousin, the herb barberry, Oregon grape is considered a blood purifier having a cleansing effect on the liver, gallbladder, and digestive system. Today the herb's most common use is in treating skin problems such as psoriasis, eczema, pimples, and boils, which can arise from systemic imbalances involving the liver and gallbladder. A tea or decoction can help stimulate the appetite and ease nausea, especially nausea related to gallbladder problems. The herb also serves as a mild tonic laxative and may help improve the body's absorption of minerals. Men may find this herb helpful in treating prostate infections.

PREPARATIONS

Over the counter:
Available in bulk.

At home:

DECOCTION: To help reduce symptoms of psoriasis, simmer covered 1 tbsp dried herbs in 1 cup boiling water for 10 minutes; strain and drink hot, up to 3 cups a day.

TINCTURE: Take 15 to 30 drops three times a day.

COMBINATIONS: For skin problems, combine with burdock and/or cleavers. To relieve constipation, combine with yellow dock or cascara sagrada. For hepatitis and jaundice, combine with dandelion root.

Consult a qualified practitioner for the dosage appropriate for you and the specific condition being treated.

PRECAUTIONS

WARNING

Do not use if pregnant.

SPECIAL INFORMATION

Use of this herb by children for more than seven to 10 days should be done in conjunction with a healthcare practitioner.

POSSIBLE INTERACTIONS

Combining Oregon grape with other herbs may necessitate a lower dosage.

TARGET AILMENTS
Skin diseases
Jaundice; other liver problems
Anemia
Constipation
Indigestion; nausea

SIDE EFFECTS

NOT SERIOUS

- Nausea; vomiting; upset stomach
- Allergic reaction

DISCONTINUE USE. IF PROBLEMS PERSIST, CALL YOUR DOCTOR.

SERIOUS

- Heart failure (very large doses)

SEEK EMERGENCY HELP.

Rx ORTHO-NOVUM

VITAL STATISTICS

DRUG CLASS

Estrogens and Progestins [Oral Contraceptives]

BRAND NAMES

Ortho-Novum 1/35:
1 mg norethindrone, 35 mcg ethinyl estradiol
Ortho-Novum 1/50:
1 mg norethindrone, 50 mcg mestranol
Ortho-Novum 10/11 (biphasic):
White tablet: 0.5 mg norethindrone, 35 mcg ethinyl estradiol
Peach tablet: 1 mg norethindrone, 35 mcg ethinyl estradiol
Ortho-Novum 7/7/7 (triphasic):
White tablet: 0.5 mg norethindrone, 35 mcg ethinyl estradiol
Light peach tablet: 0.75 mg norethindrone, 35 mcg ethinyl estradiol
Peach tablet: 1 mg norethindrone, 35 mcg ethinyl estradiol

OTHER DRUGS IN THIS SUBCLASS

Estrogens: conjugated estrogens, estradiol, estropipate, ethinyl estradiol, mestranol
Progestins: desogestrel, ethynodiol diacetate, levonorgestrel, medroxyprogesterone, norethindrone, norgestimate, norgestrel

GENERAL DESCRIPTION

Oral contraceptives such as the brand-name drug Ortho-Novum are used to prevent pregnancy. Ortho-Novum oral contraceptives combine the progestin drug norethindrone with an estrogen such as ethinyl estradiol or mestranol. They work mainly by preventing ovulation. Combination contraceptives also alter both the cervical mucus (making it more difficult for sperm to enter the uterus) and the uterine lining (preventing a fertilized egg from attaching to the uterus as it does in a normal pregnancy).

Ortho-Novum comes in monophasic, biphasic, and triphasic regimens. Monophasic formulas provide 21 pills with constant doses of estrogen and progestin. In general, biphasic and triphasic formulas provide lower overall doses of estrogen and/or progestin by using two (biphasic) or three (triphasic) different dose ratios. For example, in a biphasic regimen you take a lower-dose pill for the first 10 days and then switch to a pill that contains a higher dose for the next 11 days. The overall lower dosage helps lessen any side effects from these hormones. Your doctor will select an oral contraceptive based on the relative strength and proportion of each ingredient to best fit your menstrual cycle and medical history. For more information about these drugs, including possible interactions, see Estrogens and Progestins. For visual characteristics of the brand-name drugs Ortho-Novum 1/35 and Ortho-Novum 7/7/7, see the Color Guide to Prescription Drugs and Herbs.

O

PRECAUTIONS

WARNING

Do not use Ortho-Novum if you are pregnant or breast-feeding. If you suspect you are pregnant, discontinue use immediately to avoid severely harming the fetus.

Do not smoke if you are using oral contraceptives. The combination can increase the risk of heart-related side effects, including heart attack, stroke, and blood clots, especially in women over 35.

Get medical attention immediately if you experience any of the following: severe pain in leg, chest, or abdomen; sudden headaches; changes in speech, vision, or breathing; weak-

Ortho-Novum

ness or numbness in extremities. These symptoms may indicate blood clots.

SPECIAL INFORMATION

- Before taking Ortho-Novum, let your doctor know if you are a smoker or have liver disease, gallbladder disease, a history of depression, a history of breast cancer, fibrocystic breast changes, endometriosis, uterine fibroids, diabetes, asthma, epilepsy, heart disease, high cholesterol, blood-clotting disorders, or high blood pressure. Your doctor will use this information to determine whether or not you should use these drugs and what your dosage should be.
- Oral contraceptives increase your risk of blood clots. Do not use them if you have a history of heart attack, stroke, thrombophlebitis, or embolism.
- These drugs may cause fluid retention, which can aggravate asthma, epilepsy, migraines, and heart and kidney disease.
- Follow dosage instructions carefully. Consult your doctor for guidance if you forget to take a pill.
- Taking these drugs with or after meals can help reduce nausea.
- Oral contraceptives thin the cervical mucus, which in turn increases susceptibility to vaginal infections.
- Oral contraceptives do not protect against HIV infection (AIDS) or other sexually transmitted diseases.

POSSIBLE INTERACTIONS

See Estrogens and Progestins.

TARGET AILMENTS

Primarily for birth control

SIDE EFFECTS

NOT SERIOUS

- Acne
- Headache or migraine
- Mild nausea, diarrhea, or vomiting or abdominal pain
- Appetite or weight changes
- Fluid and sodium retention
- Breast tenderness
- Changes in sexual desire
- Blotches on skin; increased body hair; loss of hair on scalp; photosensitivity; intolerance to contact lenses; mild dizziness (less common)

LET YOUR DOCTOR KNOW IF THESE SYMPTOMS PERSIST OR BECOME BOTHERSOME.

SERIOUS

- Lumps in the breasts or breast enlargement
- Spotting or changes in menstrual bleeding (may indicate uterine cancer)
- Painful or frequent urination
- Fainting
- Cataracts
- Jaundice (yellow skin)
- Pain in the stomach or right side of the abdomen
- Increased blood pressure
- Rash; new or changed mole
- Vaginitis (itching, irritation, or thick whitish discharge)

CALL YOUR DOCTOR RIGHT AWAY IF YOU EXPERIENCE THESE SYMPTOMS OR THE BLOOD-CLOT SYMPTOMS LISTED UNDER WARNING.

OSTEOPOROSIS TREATMENT

VITAL STATISTICS

GENERIC NAMES
alendronate, calcitonin

GENERAL DESCRIPTION
Antiosteoporosis drugs slow the loss of bone tissue and help increase bone mass, and they can often be used to treat women for whom estrogen replacement therapy is inappropriate. Osteoporosis, which means "porous bones," is a condition that causes formerly strong bones to gradually thin and weaken, leaving them susceptible to fractures. Although all bones are affected by the disease, those of the spine, hip, and wrist are most likely to break. In elderly people, spine and hip fractures can be particularly dangerous, because the prolonged immobility required during the healing process often leads to blood clots or pneumonia.

Experts believe women are more susceptible to osteoporosis because their bones tend to be lighter and thinner, and because their bodies experience hormonal changes after menopause that appear to accelerate the loss of bone mass. This is primarily due to a loss of estrogen. Estrogen replacement therapy maintains bone mass and protects against fracture. In men osteoporosis is uncommon until after the age of 70.

In addition to medication, intake of adequate calcium and vitamin D and weight-bearing exercise are essential to preventing loss of bone. Calcium supplements have been shown to increase bone mass and to decrease the incidence of fracture. Your doctor may recommend supplements and a program of exercise. See the entries for the generic drugs listed above for more information.

PRECAUTIONS

WARNING
Do not take alendronate if you have hypocalcemia (low blood levels of calcium) or a serious kidney disease. (People with mild to moderate kidney disease can use alendronate. Consult your doctor.)

SPECIAL INFORMATION
- Consult with your doctor or pharmacist about the proper dosing schedule and what to do if you miss a dose.
- Swallow alendronate with six to eight ounces of water, and to avoid throat irritation, don't lie down for at least 30 minutes after you take it. Take alendronate with plain water only; wait at least 30 minutes before ingesting any other liquid, medicine, or food, any of which can interfere with the body's absorption of alendronate. Waiting longer than 30 minutes before ingesting any beverage or food will improve the absorption of alendronate.
- These drugs may affect medical tests; notify any doctor or dentist you consult that you are taking this medicine.
- Visit your doctor regularly to monitor bone loss, and consult your doctor before stopping the use of this medication.
- These drugs are not normally used or recommended for premenopausal women or for children. Do not use during pregnancy or while breast-feeding.
- An allergy skin test is recommended before beginning therapy with calcitonin, especially if you are allergic to any protein.

CONTINUED

Osteoporosis Treatment

POSSIBLE INTERACTIONS

Antacids: antacids can decrease the body's absorption of alendronate. Take antacids at least 30 minutes after taking a dose of alendronate.

Aspirin and other salicylates: taken with alendronate, these drugs can increase the risk of stomach irritation.

Calcium supplements: can interfere with the body's absorption of antiosteoporosis drugs and should be taken at least 30 minutes after taking alendronate and four hours after a dose of calcitonin.

Estrogen replacement therapy: the effect of combining alendronate with estrogen therapy is not known; their combination is not recommended.

Plicamycin: taken with calcitonin this drug will cause reduction in blood calcium levels (hypocalcemia).

Vitamin supplements: can interfere with the body's absorption of alendronate and should be taken at least 30 minutes after taking alendronate and four hours after taking calcitonin.

O

TARGET AILMENTS

Osteoporosis

SIDE EFFECTS

NOT SERIOUS

- Nausea, constipation or diarrhea, gas, bloated feeling

For alendronate:

- Headache

For calcitonin nasal spray:

- Nasal inflammation; dryness; crusting; sores; irritation; itching; redness
- Swollen, runny, or stuffy nose; slight nasal bleeding, discomfort, or tenderness
- Salty or metallic taste in the mouth

CALL YOUR DOCTOR IF THESE PROBLEMS PERSIST.

SERIOUS

For calcitonin:

- Swelling of hands, feet, face, mouth, or neck
- Skin rash or hives

SEEK EMERGENCY TREATMENT IF YOU NOTICE ANY OF THE ABOVE.

For calcitonin nasal spray:

- Ulceration of the nose

CONSULT YOUR DOCTOR AT ONCE.

For alendronate:

- Abdominal pain; heartburn
- Irritation, pain, or ulceration of the esophagus
- Difficulty swallowing
- Muscle pain; skin rash

CALL YOUR DOCTOR RIGHT AWAY.

Rx OXAPROZIN

VITAL STATISTICS

DRUG CLASS
Analgesics [Nonsteroidal Anti-Inflammatory Drugs (NSAIDs)]

BRAND NAME
Daypro

OTHER DRUGS IN THIS SUBCLASS
diclofenac, etodolac, flurbiprofen, ibuprofen, ketoprofen, ketorolac, nabumetone, naproxen

GENERAL DESCRIPTION
Introduced in 1992, oxaprozin is an NSAID, a type of pain reliever acting at the site of the pain. It may be used by people who cannot tolerate aspirin, or when aspirin or acetaminophen is not effective. Because it reduces inflammation, this drug is prescribed in the treatment of osteoarthritis and rheumatoid arthritis. For information on possible interactions, see Nonsteroidal Anti-Inflammatory Drugs (NSAIDs).

PRECAUTIONS

SPECIAL INFORMATION
- If oxaprozin upsets your stomach, take it with food or milk.
- Do not use oxaprozin if you are allergic to NSAIDs or to aspirin. It may cause bronchoconstriction or anaphylaxis in aspirin-sensitive asthmatics.
- Avoid this drug or consult your doctor before using it if you have asthma, peptic ulcer, enteritis, high blood pressure, bleeding problems, epilepsy, Parkinson's disease, or liver or kidney impairment.
- Seek emergency help in case of overdose. Possible symptoms include drowsiness, rapid heartbeat, abdominal pain, vomiting, nausea, gastrointestinal bleeding, and disorientation.
- Oxaprozin is not recommended during pregnancy, especially the last trimester, or for nursing mothers.

TARGET AILMENTS

Inflammation, especially related to osteoarthritis and rheumatoid arthritis

SIDE EFFECTS

NOT SERIOUS
- Drowsiness
- Rash
- Mild abdominal pain; constipation or diarrhea; nausea; indigestion

CONSULT YOUR DOCTOR IF THESE SYMPTOMS PERSIST.

SERIOUS
- Anaphylactic reaction (hives, rash, intense itching, and trouble breathing)
- Gastrointestinal bleeding, ulceration, stomach perforation (black or tarry stools)
- Angina; irregular heartbeat
- Diminished hearing or ringing in the ears
- Fluid retention
- Photosensitivity
- Jaundice; blood in urine

DISCONTINUE USE AND CALL YOUR DOCTOR IMMEDIATELY.

Oxycodone

Vital Statistics

DRUG CLASS
Analgesics [Opioid Analgesics]

BRAND NAMES
Percocet, Roxicet, Roxicodone

OTHER DRUGS IN THIS SUBCLASS
codeine, hydrocodone, propoxyphene, tramadol

GENERAL DESCRIPTION
A narcotic pain reliever, oxycodone acts on the central nervous system (the spinal cord and brain) to alter the perception of pain. It is prescribed for moderate to severe pain relief, often in combination with acetaminophen or aspirin. As a narcotic, this drug may cause physical and psychological dependence, especially if used for long periods of time. For more information, including possible drug interactions and additional precautions, see Opioid Analgesics. For visual characteristics of Roxicet, see the Color Guide to Prescription Drugs and Herbs.

Precautions

SPECIAL INFORMATION
- Tell your doctor if you notice the following withdrawal symptoms after you stop taking oxycodone: fever, runny nose, or sneezing; diarrhea; goose flesh; unusually large pupils; nervousness or irritability; fast heartbeat.
- Seek emergency medical care if you overdose on oxycodone. Symptoms include pinpoint pupils; slow, shallow, or troubled breathing; slow heartbeat; extreme dizziness or weakness; coma, cardiac arrest.
- Oxycodone can lead to addiction, both physical and psychological.
- Do not drive or operate machinery until you know how this drug affects you.
- Do not drink alcoholic beverages while you are taking this drug.

TARGET AILMENTS

Moderate to severe pain, especially short-term pain from acute trauma or surgery

SIDE EFFECTS

NOT SERIOUS
- Dry mouth
- Dizziness; headache
- Fatigue; nervousness
- Difficulty in urination
- Frequent urge to urinate
- Mild nausea or constipation

CONSULT YOUR DOCTOR IF SYMPTOMS CONTINUE OR ARE BOTHERSOME.

SERIOUS
- Slow or shallow breathing
- Rash, hives, itching, or facial swelling
- Decrease in blood pressure or heart rate
- Increased sweating and shortness of breath
- Severe constipation, nausea, stomach pain, or vomiting

CALL YOUR DOCTOR RIGHT AWAY.

OXYMETAZOLINE

VITAL STATISTICS

DRUG CLASS
Decongestants

BRAND NAMES
Afrin, Neo-Synephrine Maximum Strength

OTHER DRUGS IN THIS CLASS
Rx: phenylpropanolamine
OTC: phenylephrine, phenylpropanolamine, pseudoephedrine

GENERAL DESCRIPTION
Used as an active ingredient in over-the-counter nose sprays, oxymetazoline relieves nasal congestion caused by colds, allergies, or sinusitis by constricting blood vessels in nasal passages. Its best use is as a short-term (over several days) decongestant. While short-term use as directed on the label usually produces minimal side effects, long-term use or overuse may result in rebound congestion or absorption into the bloodstream, producing central nervous system effects similar to those of oral decongestants (dizziness, headache, insomnia, nervousness, high blood pressure, heart-rhythm problems). For more information, see Decongestants.

TARGET AILMENTS
Congestion of the nose and sinuses caused by allergy or upper respiratory infection

PRECAUTIONS

SPECIAL INFORMATION
Check with your doctor before taking this drug if you have cardiovascular disease (including angina, coronary artery disease, and hypertension), hyperthyroidism (overactive thyroid), diabetes, prostate enlargement, or glaucoma. Oxymetazoline may exacerbate these conditions.

POSSIBLE INTERACTIONS
Tricyclic antidepressants (such as amitriptyline): increased serious central nervous system side effects if oxymetazoline is absorbed into the bloodstream.

SIDE EFFECTS

NOT SERIOUS
- Sneezing
- Burning, stinging, or dryness of nose

CONSULT YOUR DOCTOR IF SYMPTOMS CONTINUE OR ARE BOTHERSOME.

SERIOUS
- Severe headache; trembling
- Nervousness or restlessness
- Insomnia
- Pounding or irregular heartbeat
- High blood pressure
- Rebound congestion

CALL YOUR DOCTOR RIGHT AWAY.

Palmarosa

LATIN NAME
Cymbopogon martinii

Vital Statistics

GENERAL DESCRIPTION

Native to India and Pakistan, this wild tropical grass has a long stem and aromatic leaves. Palmarosa is closely related to lemongrass and citronella. The oil is distilled from the leaves and flowers. It is pale yellow or olive in color, with a sweet floral scent.

Palmarosa has antiviral, antibacterial, and antiseptic properties, as well as an overall strengthening effect on the digestive system. When diluted, palmarosa is an effective treatment for a variety of skin conditions because it regulates sebum production and regenerates skin cells.

PREPARATIONS

For nearly all palmarosa's target ailments, the oil can be used in the bath or as a skin application. Inhalations are helpful for all but skin problems.

Bath: Add 10 drops to bathwater.

Skin applications: Apply the undiluted essential oil to small cuts and wounds. For other ailments, apply a more dilute formula: Blend 15 drops in 2 tbsp of a carrier oil such as almond oil or aloe gel.

Inhalation: Use a diffuser to scent the air or place a few drops of palmarosa on a handkerchief. Hold to your nose and breathe.

Precautions

SPECIAL INFORMATION

Buy from a reputable source. Palmarosa is easily adulterated with cedar and turpentine.

TARGET AILMENTS
Flu
Intestinal infections and digestive problems
Anxiety and stress
Anorexia
Minor cuts and wounds
Acne
Dermatitis
Oily or dry skin
Cold sores
Scarring

SIDE EFFECTS

PALMAROSA IS NONTOXIC AND NONIRRITATING.

PAPAIN

VITAL STATISTICS

DAILY DOSAGE
For celiac disease, 500 mg to 1,000 mg daily, with meals.

GENERAL DESCRIPTION
Papain is a protein-digesting enzyme found in the papaya fruit. In supplements it may be available by itself or combined with the enzyme bromelain. Papain is not universally accepted as a therapeutic substance. Its benefits have not been confirmed by rigorous study, and as a supplement the amounts used in the tablets or capsules are not standardized and therefore are unreliable. Some authorities advise against using the supplement at all.

Papain is recommended by some practitioners, however, especially in the treatment of celiac disease, a condition in which the body cannot digest gluten in grains such as wheat. Left untreated the disease can result in cancer of the small intestine. Some studies show that papain helps digest gluten and renders it harmless to the celiac patient. This would be a significant benefit for sufferers from the disease, as it is difficult to eliminate every trace of gluten from the diet. Taken regularly, papain may allow the patient to eat gluten products or serve as a preventive against small amounts of gluten that enter the diet.

Papain is a plant enzyme, a family of supplements that some nutritionists use for a variety of problems including food allergies, poor digestion, and constipation. Plant enzymes are also used to fight inflammation and to help clear the arteries in people with cardiovascular disease.

NATURAL SOURCES
papaya

PREPARATIONS
Available in tablets and capsules.

TARGET AILMENTS
Celiac disease
Poor digestion
Constipation
Food allergies

SIDE EFFECTS
NONE EXPECTED

PRECAUTIONS

WARNING
Consult your doctor for guidance before taking papain supplements. The natural source may be safer.

SPECIAL INFORMATION
Papain's benefits are still considered to be speculative.

PAROXETINE

VITAL STATISTICS

DRUG CLASS

Antidepressants [Selective Serotonin Reuptake Inhibitors (SSRIs)]

BRAND NAME

Paxil

OTHER DRUGS IN THIS SUBCLASS

fluoxetine, sertraline, venlafaxine

GENERAL DESCRIPTION

Paroxetine belongs to a subclass of antidepressants known as selective serotonin reuptake inhibitors (SSRIs), but it is chemically unrelated to other similar-acting drugs used to treat depressive illness. Although this drug has not been shown to be habit forming, long-term studies have not been completed on its addictive potential. See Antidepressants for more information on possible drug interactions.

TARGET AILMENTS

Major depressive disorders

Obsessive-compulsive disorder

SIDE EFFECTS

SEE ANTIDEPRESSANTS.

PRECAUTIONS

SPECIAL INFORMATION

- Paroxetine may cause drowsiness. When taking this drug, use care while driving, operating machinery, or performing tasks that require mental alertness.
- Paroxetine can trigger manic attacks in individuals with manic-depression. Be sure to tell your doctor if you have manic-depression.
- Paroxetine can affect blood sugar (glucose tolerance) tests by causing fluctuations in blood sugar levels.
- The full effects of this drug may not occur for several weeks.
- The severity of any side effects may decrease with time (after two weeks) or with lowered dosages. If you have any questions about potential side effects, ask your doctor.
- If you are pregnant, nursing, or planning a pregnancy, check with your doctor before taking paroxetine.

POSSIBLE INTERACTIONS

Alcohol and other drugs that depress the central nervous system: increased paroxetine effects, leading to problems such as respiratory depression or very low blood pressure.

Anticonvulsants: decreased effectiveness of anticonvulsants, making seizures more likely.

Antihistamines: increased antihistamine action, including any side effects; antihistamines may also increase the action of paroxetine, including any side effects.

Monoamine oxidase (MAO) inhibitors: WARNING: severe, possibly fatal reactions such as seizures, tremor, and coma because of additive effects of the drugs.

Other antidepressants: combining antidepressants will likely increase the action of one or both drugs, leading to increased side effects.

PARSLEY

LATIN NAME
Petroselinum crispum

VITAL STATISTICS

GENERAL DESCRIPTION
The feathery leaves of parsley, added to salads and cooked foods or used as a decorative garnish, are also a source of chlorophyll and vitamins C and A, as well as a versatile herbal remedy. Because of its ability to ease muscle spasms or cramps, parsley is used as a digestive aid. Considered an expectorant, it is prescribed for coughs and asthma, and it is also prescribed as a diuretic and mild laxative. Native to the eastern Mediterranean area, parsley is now cultivated around the world. One of the first herbs to appear in the spring, the plant develops tiny chartreuse flowers on an umbrella-shaped canopy. For visual characteristics of parsley, see the Color Guide to Prescription Drugs and Herbs.

PREPARATIONS
Over the counter:
Available as tincture and as fresh or dried leaves, seeds, stems, and roots.

At home:
TEA: Steep covered 1 to 2 tsp dried leaves or roots per cup of boiling water for 5 to 10 minutes in a closed container. Drink up to 3 cups a day. Or steep, covered, chopped fresh leaves and stems in hot water.
NUTRITION AND DIET: Eat raw green leaves as a breath freshener.
Consult a qualified practitioner for the dosage appropriate for you and the specific condition being treated.

SIDE EFFECTS
NONE EXPECTED

PRECAUTIONS

WARNING
Pregnant and nursing women should not take parsley juice or oil in medicinal doses, because it may stimulate uterine contractions. Eating a few sprigs served as garnish will probably not cause any harm.

If you use this herb frequently as a medicine, you should increase your intake of foods high in potassium, such as bananas and fresh vegetables, because diuretics deplete the body of potassium.

SPECIAL INFORMATION
- Do not give medicinal doses to children younger than two years old.
- Use of this herb by older children for more than seven to 10 days should be done in conjunction with a healthcare practitioner.
- Only experienced field botanists should pick wild parsley, because of its resemblance to toxic plants.

POSSIBLE INTERACTIONS
Combining parsley with other herbs may necessitate a lower dosage.

TARGET AILMENTS
Take internally for:
- Indigestion
- Urinary tract infections
- Irregular menstruation
- Premenstrual syndrome

PASSIONFLOWER

LATIN NAME
Passiflora incarnata

VITAL STATISTICS

GENERAL DESCRIPTION

Passionflower was named by Spanish explorers who saw in its flowers' ornate design elements of the "passion," or suffering, of Jesus. Native Americans in the southeastern United States, particularly the Cherokee, used the pleasant-tasting herb in healing; it soon became popular in Europe. Today, passionflower is thought to have a calming effect on the central nervous system. Herbalists recommend it as a sedative, a digestive aid, and a pain reliever. Because it dilates blood vessels, it is also being tested as a heart disease preventive. For visual characteristics, see the Color Guide to Prescription Drugs and Herbs.

PREPARATIONS

Over the counter:

Available in commercial herbal remedies and as dried or fresh leaves, capsules, or tincture.

At home:

Tea: Steep covered 1 to 2 tsp dried herb per cup of boiling water for 15 minutes. For insomnia, drink 1 cup in the evening.

Tincture: 1 dropperful in warm water, up to four times a day, for anxiety.

Combinations: For insomnia, use with valerian, hops, Jamaican dogwood, or chamomile.

Consult a practitioner for the dosage appropriate for you and your specific condition.

PRECAUTIONS

☠ *WARNING*

Because passionflower can cause sleepiness, do not take this herb during the day if you operate heavy machinery or drive.

Always use under medical supervision. Many herbalists recommend only professionally prepared remedies; another species, *Passiflora caerulea,* contains cyanide, and there is some fear that this might be used instead.

Pregnant women should avoid passionflower; it may stimulate the uterine muscles.

SPECIAL INFORMATION

Do not use with children unless it is specifically prescribed by a healthcare practitioner who is knowledgeable about herbs; use low-strength preparations for adults over 65.

POSSIBLE INTERACTIONS

Use caution when taking passionflower with prescription sedatives and antianxiety medications to avoid overmedication.

TARGET AILMENTS

Insomnia; anxiety; tension; neuralgia; shingles; menstrual cramps; seizures of Parkinson's disease, epilepsy; asthma; addictive disorders (to aid withdrawal)

SIDE EFFECTS

NOT SERIOUS

- Upset stomach
- Nausea
- Vomiting
- Diarrhea
- Sleepiness (do not operate heavy machinery)

DISCONTINUE AND CALL YOUR DOCTOR.

P

PATCHOULI

LATIN NAME
Pogostemon patchouli

VITAL STATISTICS

GENERAL DESCRIPTION

This bushy herb has a sturdy stem and large, fragrant leaves. Its white flowers are tinged with purple. Patchouli is native to Indonesia and the Philippines. It is cultivated in India, China, Malaysia, and South America. Patchouli oil has had a role in traditional Japanese, Chinese, and Malay medicine and was at one time the principal remedy against venomous snake and insect bites.

The oil has bactericidal and fungicidal properties, making it an excellent treatment for skin disorders such as athlete's foot and impetigo. It is also used as an antidepressant, anti-inflammatory, astringent, and antiseptic.

PREPARATIONS

Patchouli oil is distilled from the dried leaves of the plant. The oil has a sweet, earthy scent that improves as the oil ages. Patchouli oil is amber to dark orange in color.

For skin problems, mix 10 to 15 drops in vegetable or nut oil or aloe gel and apply wherever needed. Skin application is also good for relieving allergies, anxiety, stress, and sexual problems. For these problems it is helpful to inhale the oil by diffusing it into the air or by smelling drops placed on a tissue.

For most conditions, 10 drops of the oil can be added to the bath.

PRECAUTIONS

SPECIAL INFORMATION

Buy patchouli from a reputable source. The oil is sometimes adulterated with cedar or other oils.

TARGET AILMENTS

- Acne
- Athlete's foot
- Impetigo
- Cracked, chapped skin
- Cellulite and mature skin
- Dandruff
- Anxiety and stress
- Sexual problems
- Allergies
- Hemorrhoids

SIDE EFFECTS

PATCHOULI IS NONTOXIC, NONIRRITATING, AND NONSENSITIZING.

Pau d'Arco

LATIN NAME
Tabebuia impetiginosa

Vital Statistics

GENERAL DESCRIPTION

Pau d'arco is the name of both a tree and a medicinal extract from the tree's bark or heartwood. The extract is believed to be effective against bacterial, fungal, viral, and parasitic infections, and is also considered an anti-inflammatory agent. It is thought to destroy microorganisms by increasing the supply of oxygen to cells. For centuries before modern science isolated some 20 of its chemical ingredients, pau d'arco was used as a folk remedy. The pau d'arco tree, also called the trumpet tree, is native to Central and South America and the West Indies; it can reach a height of 125 feet.

PREPARATIONS

Over the counter:

Pau d'arco is available as capsules, tinctures, and dried bark.

At home:

Decoction: Boil covered 1 tbsp bark in 2 to 3 cups water for 10 to 15 minutes. Drink 2 to 4 cups a day.

Consult a qualified practitioner for the dosage appropriate for you and the specific condition being treated.

Precautions

SPECIAL INFORMATION

Use of this herb by children for more than seven to 10 days should be done in conjunction with a healthcare practitioner.

POSSIBLE INTERACTIONS

Combining pau d'arco with other herbs may necessitate a lower dosage.

TARGET AILMENTS

Take internally for:

Bacterial, fungal, viral, and parasitic infections

Indigestion

SIDE EFFECTS

None expected

Paxil

Vital Statistics

DRUG CLASS
Antidepressants [Selective Serotonin Reuptake Inhibitors (SSRIs)]

GENERIC NAME
paroxetine

OTHER DRUGS IN THIS SUBCLASS
fluoxetine, sertraline

GENERAL DESCRIPTION
Paxil is the brand-name form of the generic drug paroxetine, which belongs to a subclass of antidepressants known as selective serotonin reuptake inhibitors (SSRIs). Paxil is chemically unrelated to other similar-acting drugs used to treat depressive illness. Although this drug has not been shown to be habit forming, long-term studies have not been completed on its addictive potential. See Antidepressants for more information on possible drug interactions. For visual characteristics of Paxil, see the Color Guide to Prescription Drugs and Herbs.

Precautions

SPECIAL INFORMATION
- Paxil may cause drowsiness. When taking this drug, use care while driving, operating machinery, or performing tasks that require mental alertness.
- Paxil can trigger manic attacks in individuals with manic-depression. Be sure to tell your doctor if you have manic-depression.
- Paxil can affect blood sugar (glucose tolerance) tests by causing fluctuation in blood sugar levels.
- The full effects of this drug may not occur for several weeks.
- The severity of any side effects may decrease with time (after two weeks) or with lowered dosages. If you have any questions about potential side effects, discuss them with your doctor.
- If you are pregnant, nursing, or planning a pregnancy, check with your doctor before taking Paxil.

POSSIBLE INTERACTIONS
Alcohol and other drugs that depress the central nervous system: increased paroxetine effects, leading to problems such as respiratory depression or very low blood pressure.
Anticonvulsants: decreased effectiveness of anticonvulsants, making seizures more likely.
Antihistamines: increased antihistamine action, including any side effects; antihistamines may also increase the action of paroxetine, including any side effects.
MAO inhibitors: severe, possibly fatal reactions such as seizures, tremor, and coma because of additive effects of the drugs.
Other antidepressants: combining antidepressants is likely to increase the action of one or both drugs, leading to increased side effects.

TARGET AILMENTS

Major depressive disorders

Obsessive-compulsive disorders

SIDE EFFECTS

See Special Information.

PECTIN

VITAL STATISTICS

BRAND NAMES

Kaopectate, Luden's Cough Drops

GENERAL DESCRIPTION

Pectin, a fruit extract, has been used for centuries to help jell fruit preserves and as an ingredient in numerous other foods and medicines. It is generally believed to be a safe ingredient for medications, although experts disagree over its effectiveness in some products.

Pectin is recognized as a safe and effective demulcent, or soother, for the membranes of the mouth and throat. It also has been shown to form a protective coating over sore or ulcerated areas in the mouth and throat, helping to relieve pain by preventing further stimulation of nerve endings in these areas. Pectin is sometimes used in cough drops, lozenges, mouth rinses, gargles, and sprays. (It has not been shown to be effective against cold sores.) To work, pectin must be applied in sufficient quantities and thickness to form a solid or semisolid coating over the affected area.

Because of its protectant action and its ability to absorb liquids, pectin also serves as a safe and effective antidiarrheal agent.

PRECAUTIONS

SPECIAL INFORMATION

When taken in an antidiarrheal medication, pectin may interfere with the absorption of other drugs. For this reason, you should exercise caution in combining it with other oral medicines. Take pectin at least two hours before or after taking other drugs.

POSSIBLE INTERACTIONS

Digitalis preparations, such as digoxin: pectin may interfere with the absorption of digitalis preparations, decreasing their effectiveness. Make sure that you take the different medications at least two hours apart.

TARGET AILMENTS

Mouth and throat irritations

Diarrhea and intestinal cramps

SIDE EFFECTS

NOT SERIOUS

- Constipation (when taken in an antidiarrheal medication)

SERIOUS

NONE EXPECTED, ALTHOUGH AN OVERDOSE OF THIS MEDICATION MAY LEAD TO AN INABILITY TO DEFECATE.

Rx PENICILLINS

VITAL STATISTICS

GENERIC NAMES
amoxicillin, amoxicillin and clavulanate, ampicillin, penicillin V

GENERAL DESCRIPTION
A subclass of antibiotic drugs, penicillins act by killing sensitive strains of growing bacteria. Penicillins are ineffective against fungi, viruses, and parasites.

When discovered in 1928, "penicillin" referred to a single drug. Today, more than 20 penicillins—some derived from molds or bacteria, others produced synthetically—are used to treat a wide range of bacterial infections. Penicillins work by attacking a bacterium's cell wall. Because body cells have a membrane but no cell wall, the drugs can selectively destroy invading bacteria without harming body tissues. See the entries for the generic drugs listed above for more information.

PRECAUTIONS

SPECIAL INFORMATION
- Take the full course of your prescription, even if you feel better before finishing the medicine; otherwise, the infection may return.
- Most penicillins are better absorbed if taken on an empty stomach. However, amoxicillin, amoxicillin and clavulanate, and penicillin V work equally well whether taken on a full or on an empty stomach.
- Tell your doctor if you are allergic to cephalosporins; you may also be allergic to penicillins.

TARGET AILMENTS

Otitis media

Sinusitis

Infections of the skin and soft tissues

Pharyngitis

Pneumonia

Genitourinary tract infections

Each generic drug in this subclass targets a different spectrum of disease organisms, including *Escherichia coli, Hemophilus influenzae,* as well as the streptococcal, staphylococcal, and gonorrheal bacteria. These organisms are responsible for a number of disorders in addition to the ones listed here.

P

CONTINUED

PENICILLINS

- Let your doctor know if you have impaired kidneys, gastrointestinal disease, or a history of bleeding disorders. Your doctor may need to adjust your dosage, monitor you more closely, or prescribe a different drug.
- Penicillins also kill "good" intestinal bacteria that keep harmful fungi and intestinal bacteria in check. Eating yogurt containing *Lactobacillus acidophilus* culture or taking acidophilus tablets may help restore the body's normal bacteria.
- Prolonged use of any antibiotic drug can lead to fungal infections, including candidiasis, or to bacterial infections such as pseudomembranous colitis.
- Taking amoxicillin when you have mononucleosis may produce a skin rash.
- Penicillin may cause false-positive results in tests for glucose and protein in urine.
- If possible, avoid taking penicillins if you are pregnant or breast-feeding.

POSSIBLE INTERACTIONS

Allopurinol: may cause a skin rash.

Bacteriostatic drugs (chloramphenicol, erythromycins, sulfonamides, tetracyclines): these medicines can interfere with the bacteria-killing action of all penicillins.

Disulfiram: do not combine with amoxicillin and clavulanate.

Estrogen (oral contraceptives): decreased efficacy of contraceptives when taken with penicillin V.

Probenecid: decreases the kidneys' ability to excrete penicillins. Possible penicillin toxicity. However, probenecid is sometimes prescribed in combination with penicillin when the treatment of severe infections requires that high levels of penicillin remain in the body.

SIDE EFFECTS

NOT SERIOUS

- Mild nausea
- Mild diarrhea
- Oral candidiasis (sore mouth or tongue)
- Vaginal candidiasis

TELL YOUR DOCTOR WHEN CONVENIENT.

SERIOUS

- Allergic reaction (skin rash, hives, intense itching, or difficulty breathing)
- Severe allergic reactions (anaphylactic shock) can be life threatening; call your doctor, 911, or your emergency number immediately.
- Unusual bruising or bleeding
- Sore throat with fever
- Severe abdominal pain with diarrhea
- Seizures

CALL YOUR DOCTOR IMMEDIATELY.

Penicillin V

Vital Statistics

DRUG CLASS
Antibiotics [Penicillins]

BRAND NAMES
Betapen-VK, Penicillin VK, Veetids

OTHER DRUGS IN THIS SUBCLASS
amoxicillin, amoxicillin and clavulanate, ampicillin

GENERAL DESCRIPTION
Introduced in 1953, penicillin V is commonly used to treat otitis media and infections of the respiratory tract, and skin infections. It may be prescribed to prevent endocarditis and rheumatic fever. This type of penicillin is not used to treat severe infections. For more information, see Penicillins.

Precautions

SPECIAL INFORMATION
- Most penicillins are better absorbed if taken on an empty stomach. However, penicillin V works equally well whether taken on a full or an empty stomach.
- If possible, avoid taking penicillin V if you are pregnant or breast-feeding.

POSSIBLE INTERACTIONS
Allopurinol: may cause a skin rash.
Bacteriostatic drugs (chloramphenicol, erythromycins, sulfonamides, tetracyclines): these medicines can interfere with the bacteria-killing action of all penicillins.
Estrogen (oral contraceptives): decreased effectiveness in preventing pregnancy.

Target Ailments

Otitis media

Skin infections

Respiratory tract infections

Endocarditis

Rheumatic fever

Side Effects

Not Serious
- Mild nausea
- Mild diarrhea
- Oral candidiasis (sore mouth or tongue)
- Vaginal candidiasis

Tell your doctor when convenient.

Serious
- Allergic reaction (skin rash, hives, intense itching, or difficulty breathing)
- Severe allergic reactions (anaphylactic shock) can be life threatening; call your doctor, 911, or your emergency number immediately.
- Unusual bruising or bleeding
- Sore throat with fever
- Severe abdominal pain with diarrhea
- Seizures

Call your doctor immediately.

PENNYROYAL

LATIN NAME
Mentha pulegium

VITAL STATISTICS

GENERAL DESCRIPTION

Pennyroyal, a plant with smooth oval leaves, has been used since ancient times as a cough remedy and digestive aid and as a flea repellent. The strong aroma of its infusion acts as a decongestant and possibly as an expectorant, helping to remove excess mucus from the lungs; it is therefore useful for coughs. While the dried herb is safe in recommended doses, the oil of the pennyroyal plant should not be ingested, since even small amounts of it are toxic.

PREPARATIONS

Over the counter:

Pennyroyal is available as tinctures and as dried leaves and flowers.

At home:

TEA: Steep covered 1 to 2 tsp dried leaves in 1 cup boiling water for 10 to 15 minutes. Drink up to 2 cups a day.

Consult a qualified practitioner for the dosage appropriate for you and the specific condition being treated.

PRECAUTIONS

WARNING

Present-day practitioners advise against taking pennyroyal oil in any amount because of its toxicity.

Pennyroyal stimulates uterine contractions and should not be used during pregnancy.

SPECIAL INFORMATION

- Do not exceed the recommended dose of the herb and do not take for longer than a week at a time.
- In the past pennyroyal has been used to induce abortion because of its ability to stimulate menstruation and strengthen uterine contractions; but it should never be used for that purpose, since it may cause serious complications, such as hemorrhage or convulsions. The amount needed to abort a fetus is close to a lethal dose.
- This herb should not be used with children unless it is specifically prescribed by a healthcare practitioner who is knowledgeable about herbs. Do not give to children younger than two.

POSSIBLE INTERACTIONS

Combining pennyroyal with other herbs may necessitate a lower dosage.

TARGET AILMENTS
Use internally for:
Colds; coughs
Premenstrual syndrome; menstrual cramps
Gas; indigestion
Anxiety
Apply externally for:
Fleas on pets (use as you would commercial flea powder)

SIDE EFFECTS

NONE EXPECTED IF USED PRECISELY AS DIRECTED.

PENTOXIFYLLINE

VITAL STATISTICS

DRUG CLASS
Blood Viscosity-Reducing Agents

BRAND NAME
Trental

GENERAL DESCRIPTION
Since 1972, pentoxifylline (also known as oxypentifylline) has been used to relieve painful leg cramps and intermittent claudication (blood vessel spasms) associated with peripheral vascular disease, a chronic blood vessel disorder that primarily affects the legs. The cramping, which usually occurs during walking, is the result of oxygen deprivation in leg muscles. Pentoxifylline eases the pain by improving blood flow to the small vessels in the legs, thus increasing the supply of oxygen to the leg muscles.

As the first real "blood thinner," pentoxifylline works by reducing blood viscosity (thickness), increasing the flexibility of oxygen-carrying red blood cells, and preventing the formation of red blood cells and platelets. When taken at the recommended dosages, the drug usually produces no side effects.

For visual characteristics of the brand Trental, see the Color Guide to Prescription Drugs and Herbs.

PRECAUTIONS

SPECIAL INFORMATION

- In managing peripheral vascular disease, pentoxifylline should be part of an overall treatment that includes physical exercise and a low-fat diet.
- Do not take pentoxifylline if you have had an allergic reaction to this drug in the past.
- Before taking pentoxifylline, tell your doctor if you smoke tobacco, are taking any antihypertensive drugs, or are allergic to caffeine, theobromine, theophylline, or other xanthine drugs.
- Before taking this drug, tell your physician if you have angina or cerebral atherosclerosis, kidney or liver disease, low blood pressure, or any condition (such as a stroke) in which there is a risk of bleeding.
- Do not use pentoxifylline during the first three months of pregnancy or while nursing.
- Do not stop using this drug on your own: It takes several weeks for pentoxifylline to work, and at least three months to assess its full effectiveness in preventing or easing leg pains.
- Pentoxifylline should be taken with meals or with antacids to lessen the chance of stomach upset. Tablets should be swallowed whole.
- Do not smoke tobacco. Nicotine constricts blood vessels and may make your condition worse.

CONTINUED

PENTOXIFYLLINE

POSSIBLE INTERACTIONS

Alcohol and antihypertensive drugs: may increase blood-pressure-lowering effects of both medications.

Anticoagulants: pentoxifylline also inhibits blood clotting; concurrent use may increase the risk of unwanted bleeding.

Caffeine and nicotine: may decrease the effectiveness of pentoxifylline.

TARGET AILMENTS

Intermittent claudication (blocked blood vessels in the legs, causing spasms) associated with peripheral vascular disease

SIDE EFFECTS

NOT SERIOUS

- Headache
- Dizziness
- Tremors
- Indigestion
- Nausea
- Vomiting

CALL YOUR DOCTOR IF THESE EFFECTS PERSIST OR BECOME BOTHERSOME.

SERIOUS

- Chest pains
- Irregular heart rhythms

CALL YOUR DOCTOR IMMEDIATELY.

PEONY

LATIN NAME
Paeonia lactiflora

VITAL STATISTICS

GENERAL DESCRIPTION
The root of the white peony flower is a commonly used herb in Chinese medicine. Chinese herbalists believe that this herb nourishes the blood; it is thus often used for menstrual problems. White peony root helps relieve spasms and cramping pain and helps alleviate irritability. If a person is profusely sweating or losing vital fluids, this herb can help protect against dehydration and weakness. Good-quality roots are thick, firm, straight, and not cracked.

Chinese medicine takes a holistic approach to healthcare, fashioning remedies to treat the entire being as well as the specific parts or areas. Single herbs may be used alone or in combination with other herbs to prevent and combat disease, which is thought to arise from disturbances in the flow of a bodily energy called chi (pronounced "chee") and blood, or from a lack of balance in the complementary states of yin and yang.

PREPARATIONS
Over the counter:
White peony root is available in dried form in Chinese pharmacies and in combinations in pills and capsules in Chinese pharmacies and Oriental grocery stores.

At home:
DECOCTION: Cook peony root in water at a high simmer, covered, with other herbs for 20 to 30 minutes.
COMBINATIONS: With cyperus and corydalis, peony is used to treat abdominal pain with menstruation. With licorice root, peony is used to treat cramps in the calf. Peony combined with bupleurum is used to treat flank and breast pain.

PRECAUTIONS

WARNING
Use peony with caution if you have diarrhea with undigested food, or if you are cold and have a very pale colored tongue.

POSSIBLE INTERACTIONS
Some sources suggest that you should not take peony with dendrobium, mirabilite, tortoiseshell, cephalanoplos, or veratrum root and rhizome.

TARGET AILMENTS
Menstrual pain; irregular periods; premenstrual syndrome
Irritability
Cramping pain in limbs or abdomen
Cramps with diarrhea
Weakness with excessive sweating or loss of fluids

SIDE EFFECTS
NONE EXPECTED

Pepcid

Vital Statistics

DRUG CLASS
Antiulcer Drugs [Histamine H_2 Blockers]

GENERIC NAME
famotidine

GENERAL DESCRIPTION
Pepcid is a brand name for the generic drug famotidine. This drug is used mainly to treat ulcers of the stomach and duodenum. It is also prescribed for Zollinger-Ellison syndrome, gastroesophageal reflux (in which stomach acid flows back into the esophagus), and other conditions involving the overproduction of stomach acid. In some cases the drug is used to prevent upper gastrointestinal bleeding.

Pepcid works by blocking the effects of the chemical histamine in the stomach, thereby reducing the secretion of the digestive juice hydrochloric acid. For information on additional drug interactions, see Antiulcer Drugs. For visual characteristics, see the Color Guide to Prescription Drugs and Herbs.

Precautions

SPECIAL INFORMATION
- Avoid this drug while pregnant or nursing.
- Inform your doctor if you have a history of liver or kidney disease.
- This drug can interfere with skin allergy tests and cause false-negative results.
- You may need to avoid driving or other potentially hazardous activities while taking this drug.
- Antacids can be taken with Pepcid.

POSSIBLE INTERACTIONS
Alcohol, tobacco: may cause decreased effectiveness of famotidine.
Enteric-coated tablets: changes in stomach acidity may cause these medications to dissolve prematurely in the stomach; avoid taking them with famotidine.
Itraconazole, ketoconazole: decreased absorption of these drugs into the body.

Target Ailments

Duodenal ulcer; gastric ulcer; upper gastrointestinal bleeding associated with gastric ulcer or duodenal ulcer, or with gastritis

Zollinger-Ellison syndrome; multiple endocrine neoplasia; other conditions characterized by an overproduction of stomach acid

Gastroesophageal reflux

Side Effects

SEE FAMOTIDINE AND ANTIULCER DRUGS.

Peppermint

LATIN NAME
Mentha x piperita

Vital Statistics

GENERAL DESCRIPTION
Peppermint, native to Europe and western Asia, is cultivated around the world. This perennial herb promotes an overall sense of well-being. It can be used to loosen mucus and stimulate the liver, and can also be used as an antiseptic, antiviral, and antibacterial agent. It is also helpful in relieving pain, stomach discomfort, and nausea. Preceded by an initial cooling action, peppermint produces a warming effect.

Peppermint oil is colorless, pale yellow, or green and is a popular flavoring agent—as well as an effective insect repellent. The oil darkens and thickens as it ages. The United States is the largest producer of peppermint essential oil.

PREPARATIONS
The flowering tops and leaves are distilled to produce the essential oil. The oil glands are easily accessible on the outside of the leaves.

Peppermint oil must be diluted before it is applied to the skin: Mix 8 to 20 drops peppermint oil with 2 tbsp vegetable or nut oil or aloe gel. Use fewer drops for sensitive skin; more drops for tough skin.

For inhalation, either scent the air with a diffuser or sniff drops placed on a tissue. Keep eyes closed when inhaling the vapor.

Precautions

WARNING
Avoid peppermint if you have epilepsy or other neural disorders.

SPECIAL INFORMATION
- Do not use peppermint if you are pregnant.
- Do not give to children under 30 months of age.
- Do not use if you also are undergoing homeopathic treatment. Mint acts as an antagonist to many homeopathic remedies.
- Use in moderation; peppermint may cause skin irritation if it is too concentrated.
- Do not use peppermint at bedtime; it may keep you awake at night.

TARGET AILMENTS
Indigestion; nausea
Headaches
Neuralgia
Muscle and joint pain; menstrual pain
Bronchitis
Sinus problems
Colds and flu
Motion sickness
Shock
Sore feet
Mental fatigue

SIDE EFFECTS
None expected if used as directed.

P

PEPPERMINT

LATIN NAME
Mentha x piperita

VITAL STATISTICS

GENERAL DESCRIPTION

Peppermint plants have long, serrated leaves and a familiar, minty aroma. This pleasant-tasting herb has been used as a remedy for indigestion since the era of ancient Egypt. Menthol, the principal active ingredient of peppermint, stimulates the stomach lining, thereby reducing the amount of time food spends in the stomach. It also relaxes the muscles of the digestive system. Peppermint can be grown easily from root cuttings; but if it is not confined, it tends to spread rapidly. For visual characteristics of peppermint, see the Color Guide to Prescription Drugs and Herbs.

PREPARATIONS

Over the counter:

Peppermint is available as commercial tea, tinctures, and fresh or dried leaves and flowers.

At home:

Tea: Drink commercial brands, or steep covered 1 to 2 heaping tsp dried herb per cup of boiling water for 10 minutes. Drink up to 3 cups a day.

Bath: Fill a cloth bag with several handfuls of dried or fresh herb and let hot water run over it.

Combinations: For colds and flu, peppermint may be used as a tea or tincture with boneset, elder flower, and yarrow.

Consult a qualified practitioner for the dosage appropriate for you and the specific condition being treated.

SIDE EFFECTS

None expected

PRECAUTIONS

WARNING

Do not ingest pure menthol or pure peppermint oil; these substances are extremely toxic. Pure peppermint oil may cause cardiac arrhythmias, and pure menthol can be fatal in a dose as small as a teaspoon.

Give only very dilute preparations to children younger than two years old and only under the supervision of a doctor or herbalist.

Pregnant women with morning sickness should use a dilute tea rather than a more potent infusion. Peppermint should not be used by women who have a history of miscarriage.

POSSIBLE INTERACTIONS

Combining peppermint with other herbs may necessitate a lower dosage.

TARGET AILMENTS

Take internally for:

Cramps (including menstrual); stomach pain

Gas; nausea associated with migraine headaches

Morning sickness; travel sickness

Insomnia; anxiety

Fever; colds; flu

Apply tea externally for:

Itching; inflammation

PERMETHRIN

VITAL STATISTICS

DRUG CLASS
Antilouse Drugs

BRAND NAMES
Nix Creme Rinse, Elimite

GENERAL DESCRIPTION
Permethrin is the active component in most over-the-counter preparations for the topical treatment of head lice. This drug kills both living insects, by attacking their nervous systems and paralyzing them, and their tiny white eggs (nits) attached to human hairs. Permethrin does not have the potent side effects of other, more toxic antilouse drugs.

Permethrin is found in medicated shampoos and hair-rinse products, and also in a 5 percent cream formula for treating scabies (caused by mites). Most preparations work well with a single application, but a second application five to seven days after the first may sometimes be necessary. Protective residues of the product remain in the hair for 10 to 14 days.

Most permethrin preparations can effectively treat three different kinds of lice infestations—head, pubic, and body lice. However, a 1 percent permethrin creme-rinse product that protects the head from head lice reinfestation for a full 14 days is not approved by the FDA as safe and effective for treating pubic lice or body lice.

PRECAUTIONS

WARNING
Susceptible individuals may experience breathing difficulty or an asthmatic reaction when using any form of this product.

SPECIAL INFORMATION
- Individuals sensitive to ragweed, chrysanthemums, pyrethrins, or veterinary insecticides containing permethrin are likely to be sensitive to all permethrin products.
- This is a topical medication. It should not be taken orally or internally. If swallowed, immediately call your doctor and/or a poison control center.
- Avoid getting this medication near or in the eyes. If you accidentally get permethrin in your eyes, flush them thoroughly with water.
- Permethrin is not recommended for children under two years of age.
- A second application is necessary if live lice are observed seven days after the first application.

CONTINUED

PERMETHRIN

- Nursing mothers should either not use permethrin or consider temporarily discontinuing breast-feeding while using it.
- Directions for the use of these products must be followed carefully to ensure total disinfection. Careful attention must be paid to the disinfection of all clothing, headgear, bedding, and personal belongings where insects can hide.

TARGET AILMENTS

Head, pubic, and body lice

Scabies (caused by mites)

SIDE EFFECTS

NOT SERIOUS

- Itching, burning, stinging, tingling skin
- Swelling; rash
- Numbness; discomfort
- Possible asthmatic reactions
- Temporary increased itching, redness, stinging, or swelling of the scalp (accompanies lice infestations)

CALL YOUR DOCTOR IF THESE EFFECTS PERSIST OR BECOME BOTHERSOME.

P

PETROLEUM

LATIN NAME
Oleum petrae

VITAL STATISTICS

GENERAL DESCRIPTION

The oil we use to produce gasoline, heating fuel, and materials such as plastics originates beneath the earth's surface and is formed from the decomposition of plants and animals over millions of years. Its name—petroleum—is derived from the Latin words for rock *(petra)* and oil *(oleum).* Petroleum generally has not been used medicinally, but it was employed as a caulking substance in shipbuilding and as a source of light in ancient times, sometimes going under the name of burning water. As a homeopathic remedy, *Petroleum* is used today principally for motion sickness, especially of the type made worse by fresh air, and for cracked, dry skin. It is prepared from unrefined oil.

Like most homeopathic prescriptions, *Petroleum* was developed as a remedy by observation of the reactions of healthy individuals to doses of various strengths. When a patient exhibits a set of symptoms that matches the cataloged symptoms brought on by *Petroleum,* the homeopathic practitioner then prescribes the substance in an extremely dilute form. For more information on homeopathic medicine, see page 14.

PREPARATIONS

Petroleum is available over the counter in various potencies, in both liquid and tablet form, at selected stores and pharmacies. Consult your homeopath for further information.

SIDE EFFECTS

NONE EXPECTED

PRECAUTIONS

SPECIAL INFORMATION

- Only the patient should touch the pills. If tablets are spilled, throw them away.
- The mouth should be clear of flavors 15 minutes before and after taking a remedy, and strong flavors and aromas, such as coffee, camphor, and heavily scented perfumes, should be avoided for the duration of treatment.

TARGET AILMENTS
Motion sickness consisting of dizziness and nausea accompanied by faintness, pallor, and cold sweats as well as by hunger, increased salivation, giddiness worsened by loud noise and by sitting up, and pain in back of head and neck
Confusion when in fresh air
Forgetfulness; irritability
Pain and itching on feet, hands, and toes, occurring in moist, cold weather
Diarrhea during the day, with strong appetite
Headache in back of head
Nausea with dizziness and headache

Rx PHENELZINE

VITAL STATISTICS

DRUG CLASS
Antidepressants [Monoamine Oxidase (MAO) Inhibitors]

BRAND NAME
Nardil

OTHER DRUGS IN THIS SUBCLASS
isocarboxazid, tranylcypromine

GENERAL DESCRIPTION
Introduced in 1961, phenelzine—like other medications in the subclass of antidepressants known as MAO inhibitors—is used to treat depression, anxiety, and phobias when other antidepressant drugs have failed. See Monoamine Oxidase (MAO) Inhibitors for information about side effects and possible drug interactions.

TARGET AILMENTS

Major depression, especially if the condition has not responded to other drugs

Panic disorder

Prevention of vascular headache (including migraine) or tension headache

SIDE EFFECTS
SEE MONOAMINE OXIDASE (MAO) INHIBITORS.

PRECAUTIONS

WARNING
Phenelzine reacts with many drugs and foods. Following are some of the substances you should avoid when taking this drug: high-protein foods that are aged, fermented, or pickled, including (but not limited to) aged or processed cheeses; sour cream; alcohol, especially wine and beer (including alcohol-free wine and beer); pickled fish; dry sausages (salami); soy sauce; bean curd; yogurt; liver; figs; raisins; bananas; avocados; chocolate; papaya; meat tenderizers; and fava beans. Also avoid caffeine. But beware: This is only a partial list. Talk to your doctor and pharmacist about other drugs and foods you should avoid.

SPECIAL INFORMATION
- Let your doctor know if you have diabetes, epilepsy, hyperthyroidism, or manic or suicidal tendencies, or if you have had a stroke.
- Phenelzine may suppress heart pain, thereby masking heart problems. Let your doctor know if you have any history of angina or other heart disease.
- The full effects of phenelzine may not be felt until after several weeks of therapy.
- Use this drug during pregnancy or breast-feeding only if your doctor says that the benefits outweigh the risks.

Phenol

Vital Statistics

DRUG CLASS
Antiseptics

BRAND NAMES
Anbesol, Chloraseptic

GENERAL DESCRIPTION
Phenol was discovered in 1834 as a component of coal tar (hence its other name, carbolic acid). Used alone, phenol is extremely toxic and potentially fatal, so this antiseptic is used only in small amounts and in combination with other chemicals. These preparations are used to inhibit the growth of bacteria and to reduce the chance of infection in minor scrapes, cuts, and burns. Sometimes phenol is included in preparations used to treat poison ivy rashes and insect bites, or to relieve the pain associated with toothaches, teething, fever blisters, and other soreness of the gums, mouth, and throat. Combined with certain other drugs, such as benzocaine, phenol has an analgesic or local anesthetic effect, which makes it useful in temporarily reducing pain and itching when applied directly on the skin.

TARGET AILMENTS

Minor cuts, scrapes, and burns

Local infections

Pain and soreness of gums and mouth

Pain and itching due to insect bites or poison ivy

SIDE EFFECTS

NOT SERIOUS

When used according to package label instructions, products containing phenol are considered safe and effective and very rarely produce side effects.

SERIOUS

- Irritation
- Pain
- Redness
- Rash
- Swelling
- Fever

Discontinue use and contact your doctor immediately.

P

CONTINUED

PHENOL

PRECAUTIONS

☠ ***WARNING***

Overuse or overapplication of this drug can lead to serious, potentially life-threatening side effects.

SPECIAL INFORMATION

- Although some preparations containing phenol are specially formulated for use in the mouth or throat, this drug is potentially fatal if swallowed in large enough amounts. Keep this drug away from children.
- Do not use phenol if you are allergic to local anesthetics containing benzocaine.
- Do not use this drug near the eyes.
- Do not use on children under age two or for diaper rash, as this medication is easily absorbed into the skin.
- Do not apply topical preparations over large areas of skin, and never cover the treated area with a bandage or dressing.
- Do not use for longer than seven days; if the irritation has not improved within that period, see your doctor or dentist.
- If you are pregnant or nursing, check with your doctor before using this drug.
- To treat a teething baby, use only the recommended amount. Do not overdose.
- If you have an infection or many sores in your mouth, check with your doctor or dentist before using oral preparations containing phenol.

POSSIBLE INTERACTIONS

Phenol preparations have not been shown to interact with any specific drugs. However, before using these medications, be sure to inform your doctor, dentist, or pharmacist of any other prescription or nonprescription drug you are taking.

PHENOLPHTHALEIN

VITAL STATISTICS

DRUG CLASS
Laxatives

BRAND NAMES
Correctol, some types of Ex-Lax

OTHER DRUGS IN THIS CLASS
sennosides (stimulant); calcium polycarbophil, methylcellulose, psyllium hydrophilic mucilloid (bulk); docusate (stool softener)

GENERAL DESCRIPTION
Phenolphthalein is a stimulant type of laxative used to relieve constipation. Stimulant laxatives are believed to promote evacuation by increasing peristalsis (waves of contractions) in the intestinal muscles. For additional special information and possible interactions, see Laxatives.

PRECAUTIONS

SPECIAL INFORMATION
- Overdose or prolonged use or misuse of this drug may result in an electrolyte imbalance. Symptoms include irregular heartbeat, confusion, unusual fatigue or weakness, and muscle cramps.
- Do not use phenolphthalein or any other stimulant type of laxative if you think you may have an intestinal obstruction.

TARGET AILMENTS

Constipation

Straining during bowel movements following rectal surgery, heart attacks, or childbirth, or when hemorrhoids are present

SIDE EFFECTS

NOT SERIOUS
- Rectal irritation; pink or red urine or feces; belching; cramps; nausea; diarrhea

CALL YOUR DOCTOR IF THESE PROBLEMS PERSIST.

SERIOUS
- An allergic reaction, most often displayed on the skin in the form of increased pigmentation, eruptions, rashes, burning, and itching (rare)
- Irritability, confusion, skin rash, breathing difficulty, burning sensation when urinating, kidney problems, respiratory problems, and heart-rhythm problems that could lead to cardiac arrest (rare)

DISCONTINUE USE AND CALL YOUR DOCTOR IMMEDIATELY.

PHENTERMINE

VITAL STATISTICS

DRUG CLASS
Appetite Suppressants

OTHER DRUGS IN THIS CLASS
fenfluramine

GENERAL DESCRIPTION
An appetite suppressant, phentermine is used to reduce weight in obese patients who have no physiological basis for their disorder. Its appetite-suppressing effects are thought to result at least partially from stimulation of the hypothalamus, the part of the brain that controls appetite. Phentermine also causes increased levels of the neurochemical norepinephrine in the brain. This drug is intended to be used for a few weeks only, and within a program of weight reduction based on calorie restriction, behavior modification, and exercise.

Phentermine is related chemically and pharmacologically to amphetamines, drugs that can produce severe psychological dependence and antisocial behavior. Phentermine causes less harm from stimulation of the central nervous system than do the amphetamines and is not as strongly addictive. This drug, though, can cause tolerance and psychological dependence. Because of these problems, phentermine has limited usefulness; the possible benefits must be weighed against the risks, as described below. For visual characteristics, see the Color Guide to Prescription Drugs and Herbs. For more information about this class of drugs, see Appetite Suppressants.

PRECAUTIONS

WARNING
Do not take phentermine if you have glaucoma, advanced hardening of the arteries, symptoms of cardiovascular disease, moderate to severe high blood pressure, hyperthyroid disease, or allergy or sensitivity to drugs that stimulate the nervous system. Tell your doctor about any drug reactions you have had in the past.

Do not take this drug if you are agitated, have a history of drug abuse, or have taken an MAO inhibitor within the past 14 days. These antidepressant drugs, used with phentermine, can cause a hypertensive crisis.

To avoid an overdose, take only the recommended doses of phentermine for the recommended length of time. Overdosage may cause rapid respiration, confusion, assaultive behavior, hallucinations, and panic states, as well as other symptoms. Extreme overdoses can cause convulsions, coma, and death.

SPECIAL INFORMATION
- Talk with your doctor before taking this drug if you have mildly elevated blood pressure.
- This drug may cause drowsiness. When taking phentermine, use care while driving, operating machinery, or performing tasks that require mental alertness.
- When the appetite-suppressing effect of this drug subsides, meaning that tolerance has developed, consult your doctor about gradually stopping the drug. Do not exceed the recommended dose in an attempt to achieve additional appetite suppression.
- To avoid withdrawal symptoms such as depression or insomnia, do not stop taking this drug abruptly, especially after taking high doses for a long time.

PHENTERMINE

- If you are pregnant, nursing, or planning a pregnancy, check with your doctor before taking phentermine.
- This drug is not recommended for children under the age of 12 years.
- Do not take this drug late in the evening; it may cause insomnia.
- Do not drink alcoholic beverages while taking this drug.
- If you miss a dose of this medication, skip it completely, and take the next dose at the scheduled time.

POSSIBLE INTERACTIONS

Alcohol: intensified effects of alcohol.

Antacids, acetazolamide, and sodium bicarbonate: prolonged action of phentermine.

Antihypertensive drugs such as guanethidine: decreased antihypertensive effects.

Caffeine: may overstimulate the nervous system.

Insulin or oral diabetic agent: may change dosage requirements for the diabetic drug.

Monoamine oxidase (MAO) inhibitors: possible hypertensive crisis, with symptoms such as severe headache and heart palpitations. Do not take with phentermine.

General anesthetics: may cause cardiac arrhythmias.

Phenothiazines and haloperidol: decreased phentermine effect.

Thyroid hormones: may increase stimulating effects of the hormones, with symptoms such as rapid heart rate, increased appetite, insomnia, and anxiety.

TARGET AILMENTS

Obesity with no physiological basis

SIDE EFFECTS

NOT SERIOUS

- Constipation; diarrhea; nausea
- Dry mouth; unpleasant taste
- Nervousness; dizziness; fainting
- Insomnia
- Overstimulation; restlessness
- Chills; fever; sweating
- Headache

CALL YOUR DOCTOR IF THESE EFFECTS PERSIST OR BECOME BOTHERSOME.

SERIOUS

- Elevated blood pressure
- Euphoria; depression
- Hives; skin rash
- Hair loss
- Palpitations; rapid or uneven heartbeat
- Changes in sex drive; impotence
- Increased urination; menstrual problems
- Shortness of breath
- Blurred vision
- Breast development in males
- Psychotic episodes (rare)

CALL YOUR DOCTOR IMMEDIATELY.

PHENYLEPHRINE

VITAL STATISTICS

DRUG CLASS
Decongestants

OTHER DRUGS IN THIS CLASS
oxymetazoline, phenylpropanolamine, pseudoephedrine

GENERAL DESCRIPTION
A drug with several distinct uses, phenylephrine is available over the counter as a decongestant for the nose, sinuses, or Eustachian tubes. It is also an ingredient in many combination products intended to treat coughs, colds, and allergies. For more information, including additional special information, see Decongestants.

SIDE EFFECTS

NOT SERIOUS

- Rebound nasal congestion
- Nasal burning or dryness
- Headache; weakness, dizziness, or lightheadedness

CALL YOUR DOCTOR IF THESE PROBLEMS PERSIST.

SERIOUS

- Unusual sweating
- Blurred vision or increased sensitivity to light
- Nervousness; restlessness; insomnia; anxiety
- Rapid or pounding heartbeat
- Vomiting

CONTACT YOUR DOCTOR IMMEDIATELY.

PRECAUTIONS

WARNING
Do not take phenylephrine if you have severe heart or blood vessel disease, seriously high blood pressure, or ventricular tachycardia.

SPECIAL INFORMATION

- Check with your doctor before taking this drug if you are elderly or ill or have hepatitis or acute pancreatitis.
- Use the weakest effective dose to prevent rebound congestion.
- Take only the recommended dose.

POSSIBLE INTERACTIONS

Antihypertensive drugs, including diuretics: may inhibit their effect.

Caffeine: may increase stimulant effect.

Diet pills containing amphetamines or phenylpropanolamine: severe rise in blood pressure. Do not take with these drugs.

Epinephrine, levodopa, digitalis: may increase risk of an irregular heart rhythm.

Guanadrel or guanethidine: may cause heart or blood pressure problems.

MAO inhibitors: severe rise in blood pressure. Do not take phenylephrine with these drugs or use within two weeks of each other.

Nitrates: may reduce the effect of nitrates.

Thyroid hormones: may increase effects of either medication.

Tricyclic antidepressants: increased phenylephrine effect. Use with caution.

TARGET AILMENTS

Nasal congestion; mild to moderate hypotension; severe hypotension (adjunct); various eye conditions

PHENYLPROPANOLAMINE

VITAL STATISTICS

DRUG CLASS
Decongestants

BRAND NAMES
Rx: Entex LA
OTC: Alka-Seltzer Plus, Comtrex Liqui-Gel, Dexatrim (diet aid), Dimetapp (for adults and children), Naldecon-DX, Robitussin-CF, Tavist-D, Triaminic DM Syrup, Triaminic Expectorant, Triaminicol Multi-Symptom Relief, Triaminic Syrup, Tylenol Cold (effervescent formula)

OTHER DRUGS IN THIS CLASS
OTC: oxymetazoline, phenylephrine, pseudoephedrine

GENERAL DESCRIPTION
A nasal decongestant sometimes used as an appetite suppressant, phenylpropanolamine is widely used in over-the-counter cold and allergy products. This medication is banned for use during athletic competitions. For the visual characteristics of phenylpropanolamine-guaifenesin combination drug and the prescription brand-name drug Entex LA, see the Color Guide to Prescription Drugs and Herbs. For more information, see Decongestants.

PRECAUTIONS

SPECIAL INFORMATION
- In rare cases, phenylpropanolamine has been associated with serious cardiovascular, central nervous system, and psychological effects such as stroke, irregular heart rhythms, high blood pressure, hallucinations, and seizures. These effects may be more likely in individuals who take high dosages or who have an underlying cardiovascular or psychological illness.
- Check with your doctor before taking this drug if you have cardiovascular disease (including angina, coronary artery disease, and hypertension), hyperthyroidism (overactive thyroid), diabetes, or glaucoma. Phenylpropanolamine may exacerbate these conditions.

TARGET AILMENTS
Congestion of the nose and sinuses
Bronchial asthma
Obesity (used as an appetite suppressant)
Urinary incontinence

CONTINUED

PHENYLPROPANOLAMINE

POSSIBLE INTERACTIONS

Anticoagulant (blood-thinning) drugs: decreased anticoagulant effect.

Beta blockers: phenylpropanolamine can lessen the effectiveness of beta blockers, causing hypertension.

Digitalis preparations: possible heart-rhythm problems.

High blood pressure drugs containing rauwolfia: decreased effectiveness of phenylpropanolamine.

Monoamine oxidase (MAO) inhibitors: increased stimulant action of phenylpropanolamine, causing effects such as hypertension and heart-rhythm problems.

Stimulants (such as other decongestants, amphetamines, caffeine): increased stimulant effects, leading to excessive nervousness, insomnia, irregular heart rhythm, or seizures.

Tricyclic antidepressants (such as amitriptyline): increased action of phenylpropanolamine, making serious central nervous system side effects more likely.

SIDE EFFECTS

NOT SERIOUS

- Mild nervousness
- Restlessness
- Insomnia
- Dizziness
- Lightheadedness
- Nausea
- Dryness of mouth or nose
- Rebound congestion

CALL YOUR DOCTOR IF THESE EFFECTS PERSIST OR BECOME BOTHERSOME.

SERIOUS

- Stroke
- Irregular heart rhythms
- High blood pressure
- Hallucinations
- Seizures

CALL YOUR DOCTOR IMMEDIATELY.

Phenytoin

Vital Statistics

DRUG CLASS
Anticonvulsant Drugs

BRAND NAMES
Dilantin, Diphenylan

OTHER DRUGS IN THIS CLASS
carbamazepine, valproic acid

GENERAL DESCRIPTION
Introduced in 1938, phenytoin is one of several hydantoin anticonvulsant drugs used primarily in the suppression and control of epileptic seizures. Although the exact mechanisms by which these drugs work are unknown, anticonvulsants appear to inhibit the sudden spread of excessive or abnormal electrical impulses in the brain, thereby limiting or preventing epileptic convulsions. Phenytoin, formerly known as diphenylhydantoin, is used to treat all types of epilepsy except absence (petit mal) seizures. It may be used alone or in combination with other anticonvulsants. For more information, see Anticonvulsant Drugs.

TARGET AILMENTS
Epileptic seizures, except absence (petit mal) type
Prevention and treatment of seizures during and following neurosurgery
Relief of pain in trigeminal neuralgia (tic douloureux). May be used alone or with carbamazepine

Precautions

WARNING
Seek immediate medical help for overdose. Overdose signs include double or blurred vision; jerky or rolling eye movements; slurred speech or stuttering; severe clumsiness, unsteadiness, confusion, and trembling; and staggering walk.

SPECIAL INFORMATION
- Do not use phenytoin if you have had an allergic reaction to this drug or to any of the hydantoin drugs in the past.
- Tell your doctor if you are taking any other drugs (prescription or over the counter); have diabetes, heart disease, or low blood pressure; have a history of impaired liver function or liver disease; or may soon have surgery under general anesthesia.
- Using phenytoin during pregnancy increases the risk of birth defects (fetal hydantoin syndrome). Be sure to tell your doctor if you are pregnant or planning to become pregnant soon.
- Since phenytoin may cause folic acid deficiency, talk with your doctor about taking a daily multivitamin supplement.
- Since phenytoin can cause gum problems (bleeding, tenderness, abnormal growth), good oral hygiene is essential: Be sure to brush and floss your teeth and massage your gums regularly and carefully. You should also see your dentist every three months to have your teeth cleaned.
- Phenytoin may affect complete blood cell counts; blood cholesterol, calcium, glucose, thyroid hormone, and other levels; and liver function tests.
- Do not abruptly discontinue this drug or switch to another brand or generic unless advised by your physician.

PHENYTOIN

POSSIBLE INTERACTIONS

Phenytoin interacts with a vast number of drugs, only a few of which are described here. Be sure to check with your physician before taking any other medication.

Alcohol, antacids, antidepressants (tricyclic), antihistamines, central nervous system depressants, diazoxide, and rifampin: decreased effectiveness of phenytoin in controlling epileptic seizures.

Anticoagulants, drugs for high blood pressure, sedatives, propranolol and other beta-adrenergic blockers, caffeine, corticosteroids, cyclosporine, doxycycline, and oral contraceptives: phenytoin may increase or decrease the effects of these drugs.

Cimetidine, sulfonamides, and valproic acid: increased effects of phenytoin and increased risk of severe side effects.

SIDE EFFECTS

NOT SERIOUS

- Mild sluggishness and fatigue; diarrhea
- Excessive growth of facial and body hair; enlargement of jaw; widening of nose tip; thickening of lips
- Swollen breasts (in males)
- Muscle twitching
- Nausea and vomiting
- Headache; dizziness
- Insomnia

CONSULT YOUR DOCTOR IF THESE EFFECTS PERSIST OR ARE BOTHERSOME.

SERIOUS

- Gum overgrowth
- Bleeding or tender gums
- Fever
- Enlarged glands in underarms or neck
- Mood changes
- Increase in seizures
- Muscle pain or weakness
- Excitability or nervousness
- Severe skin rash
- Joint pain and swelling
- Blurred or double vision
- Elevated blood sugar
- Sore throat; weakness; fever; abnormal bruising or bleeding (bone marrow depression)
- Discolored urine; drug-induced hepatitis or nephritis

CONTACT YOUR DOCTOR IMMEDIATELY.

PHOSPHORUS

LATIN NAME
Phosphorus

VITAL STATISTICS

GENERAL DESCRIPTION

The chemical element phosphorus can be found in the cellular fluid of all living tissue. Phosphorus plays a vital role in the activity of the body's cells, most importantly in the transfer of genetic information. Many phosphorus compounds are used commercially in toothpaste, fertilizer, and laundry detergent. Phosphorus poisoning causes irritation of the mucous membranes and inflammation of tissue; over time, it can destroy bone. As a homeopathic remedy, minute doses are prescribed by practitioners for conditions accompanied by symptoms of fatigue and nervousness, with a tendency to bleed easily and an unquenchable thirst for cold water. To prepare the homeopathic remedy, pure phosphorus is diluted in large quantities of milk sugar. For more information on homeopathic medicine, see page 14.

PREPARATIONS

Phosphorus is available over the counter in various potencies, in both liquid and tablet form, at selected stores and pharmacies. Consult your homeopathic practitioner for further information.

PRECAUTIONS

SPECIAL INFORMATION

- When a remedy is administered, no one but the patient should touch the pills. If tablets are spilled, throw them away.
- The mouth should be clear of flavors 15 minutes before and after taking a remedy, and strong flavors and aromas, such as coffee and heavy perfume, should be avoided for the duration of treatment.

TARGET AILMENTS

- Bronchitis
- Pneumonia
- Coughs with congestion and burning pains in the chest
- Visual problems resulting from eyestrain
- Gastritis
- Nosebleeds
- Indigestion accompanied by vomiting or pain
- Stomach ulcers
- Kidney infections
- Nasal polyps
- Hepatitis
- Anemia
- Hemorrhages
- Diarrhea
- Menstrual problems

SIDE EFFECTS

NONE EXPECTED

PHOSPHORUS

VITAL STATISTICS

GENERAL DESCRIPTION

Phosphorus is the second most plentiful mineral in the body and is found in every cell. Like calcium, phosphorus is essential for bone formation and maintenance; more than 75 percent of the body's phosphorus is contained in bones and teeth. Phosphorus stimulates muscle contraction and contributes to tissue growth and repair, energy production, nerve-impulse transmission, and heart and kidney function.

RDA

Adults over 25 years old: 800 mg
Young adults and pregnant women: 1,200 mg

NATURAL SOURCES

Phosphorus exists to some degree in nearly all foods, especially meats, poultry, eggs, fish, nuts, dairy products, whole grains, and soft drinks.

PRECAUTIONS

SPECIAL INFORMATION

- Deficiency is rare—most people take in far more phosphorus than they need through preserved foods—but may be induced by long-term use of antacids or anticonvulsant drugs that contain aluminum hydroxide. Symptoms of phosphorus deficiency include general weakness, loss of appetite, bone pain, and increased susceptibility to bone fracture.
- Do not try to self-administer phosphorus. Supplementation, if necessary, must be done as part of a balanced formula developed by a qualified practitioner.
- Excess phosphorus in the bloodstream promotes calcium loss, which may weaken bones. Extreme phosphorus toxicity is rare, except in the event of kidney disease.

TARGET AILMENTS

Fatigue

Fractures (prevention)

SIDE EFFECTS

NONE EXPECTED

PHYTOLACCA

LATIN NAME
Phytolacca decandra

VITAL STATISTICS

GENERAL DESCRIPTION

Phytolacca, sometimes called pokeweed or pokeroot, is a perennial bush that grows in wet areas in various parts of the world. The herb is quite high in potassium, and its active ingredient affects several parts of the body, including muscles and joints, the nervous and digestive systems, the throat, and bone. It has been used as a folk remedy to make a salve for ulcers and cancerous growths and by Native American tribes as a purgative and to treat rheumatism. Homeopathic practitioners use the remedy *Phytolacca* to relieve painful conditions of several types. It may be prepared from the ripe berries or fresh leaves of the plant; alternatively, especially in the winter, the fresh root may be used after being pounded to a pulp. For more information on homeopathic medicine, see page 14.

PREPARATIONS

Phytolacca is available over the counter in various potencies, in both liquid and tablet form, at selected stores and pharmacies. Consult your homeopathic practitioner for further information.

PRECAUTIONS

SPECIAL INFORMATION

- When a remedy is administered, no one but the patient should touch the pills. If tablets are spilled, throw them away.
- The mouth should be clear of flavors 15 minutes before and after taking a remedy, and strong flavors and aromas, such as coffee and heavy perfume, should be avoided for the duration of treatment.

TARGET AILMENTS

Breast abscess and infection, and cracked nipples in nursing mothers

Nipple pain that radiates throughout the body

Mumps with pressure around the glands, possibly with pains that shoot into the ear on swallowing

Painful sore throat and swollen tonsils, with difficulty swallowing

Sore throat with aching, fever, and swollen glands that worsens with warm drinks and is relieved by cold drinks, possibly with pains that shoot into the ear on swallowing

Painful teething

Shooting pains that feel like electric shocks

Pains where tendons attach to bones

Hip pain relieved by rubbing

SIDE EFFECTS

NONE EXPECTED

Pill Curing

Vital Statistics

CHINESE NAME
Kang Ning Wan

ALSO SOLD AS
Po Chai Pills (almost identical form)

GENERAL DESCRIPTION
Pill Curing and *Po Chai* Pills are well-known remedies for nausea, vomiting, and diarrhea caused by overeating or by contaminated food or water. Historically, these remedies have been used to treat summertime stomach and intestinal symptoms, such as those mentioned above, with headache and low-grade fever. The formulas are also used to prevent and treat motion sickness. A number of herbs contained in the formulas are good for treating headaches and for strengthening and clearing the digestive tract.

Chinese medicine takes a holistic approach to healthcare, fashioning remedies to treat the entire being as well as the specific parts or areas. Precise combinations of herbs are used to prevent and combat disease, which is thought to arise from disturbances in the flow of a bodily energy called chi (pronounced "chee") and blood, or from a lack of balance in the complementary states of yin and yang. A patent formula, Pill Curing is made by using a standardized combination of herbs and method of preparation.

INGREDIENTS
gastrodia, angelica root, chrysanthemum, mint, kudzu, trichosanthes root, gray atractylodes, Job's-tears, poria, saussurea, magnolia bark, red citrus peel, agastache, mixture with fermented grain sprouts, rice sprouts

PREPARATIONS
Pill Curing and a very similar formula known as *Po Chai* Pills are available in pill form at many Chinese pharmacies and Oriental grocery stores.

TARGET AILMENTS
Nausea
Vomiting
Abdominal pain and distention
Diarrhea; motion sickness
Gastroenteritis with fever and headache

SIDE EFFECTS
None expected

PINE

LATIN NAME
Pinus sylvestris

VITAL STATISTICS

GENERAL DESCRIPTION

The needles of the fragrant Scotch pine are used to produce pine oil, a safe, useful, and therapeutic oil said to have expectorant and decongestant properties. The oil is colorless to pale yellow, with a strong balsamic and camphoric aroma. It is used to treat pulmonary problems and the flu as well as other viral infections.

The Scotch pine is native to Eurasia and is most widespread in western and northern Europe and in Russia. The trees can grow up to 120 feet high. In earlier seafaring days, the trunks were prized as masts for sailing ships. Native Americans stuffed mattresses with the needles to repel fleas and lice. Today the Scotch pine, with its long, stiff needle pairs, is a favorite for decorating at Christmas.

PREPARATIONS

The oil can either be applied externally or inhaled to relieve respiratory problems or calm the mind. For a steam inhalation, place 6 drops in a bowl of boiling water. Lean over the bowl, drape a towel over your head and the bowl, and inhale for up to 5 minutes.

Add 10 to 15 drops to a warm bath to ease circulatory problems, swelling from arthritis and rheumatism, premenstrual syndrome, and anxious or depressed states of mind. Pine oil is also effective at countering urinary tract problems by using it in a sitz bath or applying it to the skin. For a massage oil, mix 10 to 15 drops in vegetable or nut oil or aloe gel. (Skin applications can be used for all target ailments.)

If the quality of the oil is suspect, a tea made from steeping pine needles in boiling water may substitute for pine oil.

PRECAUTIONS

SPECIAL INFORMATION

Buy only from a reputable source. Pine oil is easily adulterated with turpentine, which compromises its effectiveness.

TARGET AILMENTS
Anxiety; depression
Nervous tension
Skin disorders
Arthritis; rheumatism
Cystitis and other urinary problems
Bronchitis; sinus problems
Coughs; viral infections, including the flu
Pneumonia

SIDE EFFECTS

NOT SERIOUS

PINE CAN IRRITATE THE SKIN. AVOID USING THIS OIL IF YOU HAVE SENSITIVE SKIN.

PINELLIA

LATIN NAME
Pinellia ternata

VITAL STATISTICS

GENERAL DESCRIPTION

Pinellia is used in Chinese medicine for a variety of disorders that are said to have phlegm. These include cough, runny nose, and sinus congestion. Practitioners also use this rhizome to treat phlegmlike nodules, such as fatty cysts and swollen nodes in the neck or armpits, and for certain types of nausea and vomiting that are believed to be caused by phlegm. In Chinese medicine, phlegm also refers to the sensation that one's thinking and feeling capacity are clouded and thick.

Chinese medicine takes a holistic approach to healthcare, fashioning remedies to treat the entire being as well as the specific parts or areas. Single herbs may be used alone or in combination with other herbs to prevent and combat disease, which is thought to arise from disturbances in the flow of a bodily energy called chi (pronounced "chee") and blood, or from a lack of balance in the complementary states of yin and yang.

PREPARATIONS

Over the counter:

The raw form of pinellia is toxic and is generally not available. Chinese pharmacies usually sell the dried herb that has been cooked with ginger, vinegar, or alum so that it is not toxic. It can also be found as a pill or in capsules in combinations with other herbs in Oriental groceries and some Western health food stores.

At home:

The treated form is cooked with other herbs at a high simmer for 20 to 30 minutes.

COMBINATIONS: Pinellia is used with aged citrus peel for abdominal distention, nausea, and vomiting, and also for cough and heaviness in the chest. Fritillaria and pinellia are used for cough and also to treat phlegm nodules, especially in the neck.

PRECAUTIONS

WARNING

Do not use raw pinellia internally. Do not use in the case of bleeding, dry cough, or general dryness.

POSSIBLE INTERACTIONS

According to some sources, pinellia is incompatible with aconite *(wu tou).*

SPECIAL INFORMATION

In one report, four people who ate the raw herb in large amounts experienced burning and numbness in the throat and lips, nausea, and heaviness in the chest. One recovered without help; the others were cured by eating ginger.

TARGET AILMENTS

Cough with mucus and congestion; phlegmlike nodules (such as swollen lymph glands, goiter, sebaceous cysts)

Certain types of nausea and vomiting, including morning sickness

Cloudy, phlegmlike thinking, feeling, or perceiving

SIDE EFFECTS

NONE EXPECTED WHEN THE HERB HAS BEEN PROPERLY PREPARED.

Ping Chuan Wan

Vital Statistics

ENGLISH NAME
Dyspnea-Calming Pills

GENERAL DESCRIPTION
Ping Chuan Wan is used to treat chronic coughing or shortness of breath. It is often prescribed for people who have a cough in the evening or after exertion. *Ping Chuan Wan* strengthens the lungs and helps resolve the cough, making this formula particularly helpful for people who have had bronchitis and cannot quite get back to normal.

Chinese medicine takes a holistic approach to healthcare, fashioning remedies to treat the entire being as well as the specific parts or areas. Precise combinations of herbs are used to prevent and combat disease, which is thought to arise from disturbances in the flow of a bodily energy called chi (pronounced "chee") and blood, or from a lack of balance in the complementary states of yin and yang. A patent formula, *Ping Chuan Wan* is made by using a standardized combination of herbs and method of preparation.

INGREDIENTS
codonopsis, gecko, cordyceps, bitter almond, aged orange peel, licorice root, mulberry root bark, cynanchum, phlogopitum, ficus, elaeagnus

PREPARATIONS
Ping Chuan Wan is available in pill form at many Chinese pharmacies and Oriental grocery stores.

Precautions

WARNING
Do not use this formula if you have a full, productive (phlegm-producing) cough.

TARGET AILMENTS

- Chronic bronchitis
- Emphysema
- Cough from lung weakness
- Shortness of breath from weakness

SIDE EFFECTS
None expected

P

PLANTAIN

LATIN NAME
Plantago major

VITAL STATISTICS

GENERAL DESCRIPTION
A perennial weed, plantain bears leaves that grow low to the ground and a spiked stalk with inconspicuous flowers. It is as useful to the herbalist as it is annoying to the homeowner trying to grow an attractive lawn. Because of its astringent or binding properties, it can aid in the treatment of diarrhea and hemorrhoids. Plantain also helps the body remove excess mucus from the lungs and soothes inflamed and sore membranes, making it useful for treating coughs and mild bronchitis. And its antimicrobial and anti-inflammatory actions help in healing skin wounds.

PREPARATIONS
Over the counter:
Plantain is available as tinctures, powdered seeds, dried leaves, seeds, and aboveground parts.

At home:
TEA: Steep covered 2 tsp dried herb per cup of boiling water for 10 minutes. Drink 3 cups a day.
DECOCTION: Simmer partly covered 1 oz dried leaves in $1\frac{1}{2}$ pt water until reduced to 1 pt. Sweeten with honey. Take 1 tbsp three to four times a day.
DRESSING: Use the tincture as a dressing for cuts, wounds, bruises, and bites.
COMBINATIONS: A liniment made from plantain juice (or tea) and rose oil can be used externally for gout.
Consult a qualified practitioner for the dosage appropriate for you and the specific condition being treated.

PRECAUTIONS

SPECIAL INFORMATION
A piece of cotton may be soaked with plantain juice or tincture and applied to a tooth to control toothache until you get to a dentist.

POSSIBLE INTERACTIONS
Combining plantain with other herbs may necessitate a lower dosage.

TARGET AILMENTS
Take internally for:
Diarrhea
Cough
Bronchitis
Kidney and bladder infection
Urinary incontinence
Hemorrhoids
Apply externally for treatment of:
External tumors and ulcers
Itchy, burning, or inflamed skin; cuts
Snake and insect bites

SIDE EFFECTS
NONE EXPECTED

PLATYCODON

LATIN NAME
Platycodon grandiflorum

VITAL STATISTICS

GENERAL DESCRIPTION

The Chinese herb platycodon is the root of the common garden flower known as balloonflower. (It is worth noting that one of the herb's uses in Chinese medicine is to direct upward the action of the herbs combined with it.) Good-quality herbs are thick, firm, large, and white.

Platycodon is most commonly used to treat all kinds of coughs, as well as sore throat and loss of voice. It even helps clear up the pus in a bad sore throat. In laboratory experiments, preparations of platycodon lowered blood sugar levels in rabbits, especially those with artificially induced diabetes. In another study, platycodon showed a beneficial reduction of cholesterol in the livers of rats.

Chinese medicine takes a holistic approach to healthcare, fashioning remedies to treat the entire being as well as the specific parts or areas. Single herbs may be used alone or in combination with other herbs to prevent and combat disease, which is thought to arise from disturbances in the flow of a bodily energy called chi (pronounced "chee") and blood, or from a lack of balance in the complementary states of yin and yang.

PREPARATIONS

Over the counter:

Platycodon is available in dried form at Chinese pharmacies. The herb is also sold as pills and cough syrups in Chinese pharmacies and Oriental grocery stores.

At home:

Platycodon is cooked with other herbs at a high simmer for 20 to 30 minutes.

COMBINATIONS: Mixed with licorice root, platycodon is used for hoarseness, pain, and swelling in the throat from a cold or flu. It can also be combined with perilla leaves and bitter almond to treat cough with phlegm.

PRECAUTIONS

WARNING

Do not use this herb if you are coughing up blood.

POSSIBLE INTERACTIONS

Some sources say platycodon counteracts gentiana and longan.

TARGET AILMENTS
Cough
Abscess of the throat or lung
Sore throat or hoarseness

SIDE EFFECTS

NONE EXPECTED

Pleurisy Root

LATIN NAME
Asclepias tuberosa

Vital Statistics

GENERAL DESCRIPTION
As its name suggests, pleurisy root has proved valuable in the treatment of pleurisy, a painful lung disease; it helps clear excess mucus from the lungs and reduces inflammation in lung tissues. The herb is also considered excellent for people with colds and helpful for those recovering from pneumonia.

In addition to its use in respiratory ailments, pleurisy root is valued as a digestive aid; as a mild laxative, it can bring relief in some cases of indigestion. The herb was used extensively by North American Indians for its expectorant and diaphoretic properties.

PREPARATIONS
Over the counter:
Pleurisy root is available in dried bulk and as tincture.

At home:
Decoction: To help fight pneumonia, simmer covered 1 tbsp pleurisy root in 1 cup water for 10 minutes; steep 5 minutes and strain. Drink three or four times daily.
Tincture: Take 1/8 to 1/2 tsp three times a day.
Combinations: Mix with cayenne, lobelia, and grindelia for treatment of respiratory congestion.
Consult a qualified practitioner for the dosage appropriate for you and the specific condition being treated.

Precautions

WARNING
The fresh root can cause nausea and vomiting. Use commercial preparations of pleurisy root only.

Use of this herb by children for more than seven to 10 days should be done in conjunction with a healthcare practitioner.

POSSIBLE INTERACTIONS
Combining pleurisy root with other herbs may necessitate a lower dosage.

TARGET AILMENTS
Cold
Flu
Bronchitis
Indigestion

SIDE EFFECTS
None expected

PODOPHYLLUM

LATIN NAME
Podophyllum peltatum

VITAL STATISTICS

GENERAL DESCRIPTION

Called American mandrake or May apple, *Podophyllum* grows in wet meadows and woods in North America. A malodorous white flower blooms in May and is followed by the fruit, which resembles the rose hip. The shape of the leaves gives the plant another of its common names: duck's foot. The resin from *Podophyllum,* called podophyllin, is used medicinally as a caustic. Resins from this plant have also been said to contain substances that have antitumor activity, a property that may have been recognized by the Chinese 2,000 years ago.

North American Indians used the herb to kill parasites, and as an emetic and purgative. Early Americans also used it in cathartic preparations to clean out the intestines. Although large doses of the herb are poisonous, smaller doses have been employed as a liver and bowel stimulant. Homeopathic practitioners today use *Podophyllum* to treat diarrhea and flatulence. To prepare the remedy, the fresh root is gathered before the fruit ripens. It is then chopped and pounded and left to sit in an alcohol solution. For more information on homeopathic medicine, see page 14.

PREPARATIONS

Podophyllum is available over the counter in various potencies, in both liquid and tablet form, at selected stores and pharmacies. Consult your homeopathic practitioner for further information.

PRECAUTIONS

SPECIAL INFORMATION

- Only the patient should touch the pills. If tablets are spilled, throw them away.
- The mouth should be clear of flavors 15 minutes before and after taking a remedy, and strong flavors and aromas, such as coffee, camphor, and heavily scented perfumes, should be avoided for the duration of treatment.

TARGET AILMENTS

Diarrhea with these characteristics:

Frequent profuse and offensive liquid stools the color of pea soup

Gurgling and rumbling in the abdomen

Alternating with constipation and headache

Faintness after passing stool

Worsening after drinking water and eating

Driving a patient out of bed at 4 or 5 a.m.

Flatulence with gurgling before a stool; loud wind during stool

SIDE EFFECTS

NONE EXPECTED

P

Polygonum

LATIN NAME
Polygonum multiflorum (root)

Vital Statistics

GENERAL DESCRIPTION

Polygonum, also known as fleeceflower root, is frequently called fo-ti by sellers, users, and practitioners. It is prescribed for a wide variety of disorders that includes such disparate conditions as signs of premature aging and symptoms of malaria. In test-tube studies, polygonum root seems to have an antibiotic effect. The herb usually appears heavy, solid, and reddish brown. In traditional Chinese medicine it is classified as bitter, sweet, astringent, and slightly warm.

PREPARATIONS

Polygonum is available at Chinese pharmacies, Asian markets, and some Western health food stores. You can also find it in pill form.

Combinations: With lycium fruit, psoralea fruit, and cuscuta it is prescribed for sore knees and back, dizziness, and premature aging. A preparation containing polygonum, scrophularia, and forsythia fruit is prescribed for scrofula, abscesses, and other swellings. A combination with Asian ginseng, dong quai, and tangerine peel is recommended for chronic malarial symptoms.

Precautions

SPECIAL INFORMATION

Practitioners do not prescribe the herb for patients with phlegm or diarrhea.

POSSIBLE INTERACTIONS

Some traditional sources suggest that you should avoid taking this herb with onions, chives, or garlic.

TARGET AILMENTS

Take internally for:

- Dizziness and blurred vision; chronic fatigue
- Insomnia
- Prematurely gray hair
- Nocturnal emission
- Vaginal discharge
- Carbuncles, sores, abscesses, scrofula (a form of tuberculosis in the neck), goiter, and neck lumps
- Constipation
- Sore knees and back

SIDE EFFECTS

NOT SERIOUS

- Flushing of the face
- Increased frequency of bowel movements
- Diarrhea
- Mild abdominal pain

CALL YOUR DOCTOR IF THESE EFFECTS PERSIST OR BECOME BOTHERSOME.

POLYMYXIN B

VITAL STATISTICS

DRUG CLASS
Antibiotics [Topical Antibiotics]

BRAND NAME
Neosporin

OTHER DRUGS IN THIS SUBCLASS
Rx: chlorhexidine (for gums); mupirocin (for skin); combination of neomycin, polymyxin B, and hydrocortisone (antibiotic-corticosteroid for ears)
OTC: bacitracin, neomycin

GENERAL DESCRIPTION
Over-the-counter forms of polymyxin B, combined with bacitracin and neomycin, are used topically to prevent infections in minor cuts, scrapes, and burns. Polymyxin B also comes in a prescription medication in combination with neomycin and hydrocortisone for a combined antibiotic and corticosteroid treatment for external ear infections. For more information, see Topical Antibiotics.

PRECAUTIONS

SPECIAL INFORMATION
- Check with your doctor if you notice no improvement after using this medication for two or three days.
- Prolonged use of a prescription topical antibiotic may result in fungal superinfection.
- The use of topical antibiotics increases the risk of kidney damage or hearing loss in people with impaired kidney function who are already taking nephrotoxic medicines.
- If you are pregnant or nursing, check with your doctor before using.

POSSIBLE INTERACTIONS
Aminoglycosides: possible hypersensitivity reaction and toxicity, leading to permanent deafness if combined with neomycin, which is also an aminoglycoside and is found in a prescription combination drug along with polymyxin B and hydrocortisone.

TARGET AILMENTS
Minor cuts, scrapes, and burns

External ear canal infection (in combination with neomycin and hydrocortisone)

SIDE EFFECTS

SERIOUS
- Allergic reaction such as itching, stinging, rash, redness, or swelling at the application site
- Kidney damage or hearing loss (may result if extensive systemic absorption of neomycin occurs via application over large areas of the body or through prolonged use)

CALL YOUR DOCTOR IMMEDIATELY. ALSO SEE HYDROCORTISONE.

P

PONDIMIN

VITAL STATISTICS

DRUG CLASS
Appetite Suppressants

GENERIC NAME
fenfluramine

OTHER DRUGS IN THIS CLASS
phentermine

GENERAL DESCRIPTION
Pondimin, a brand name of the generic drug fenfluramine, is used for short-term treatment of obesity when the disorder has no physiological basis; it is not intended for long-term or intermittent use. The drug is used to control appetite and is administered in conjunction with a low-calorie diet, exercise, and behavior-modification techniques.

Fenfluramine is believed to work by stimulating the hypothalamus, the part of the brain thought to control appetite. Because it may improve glucose tolerance, fenfluramine is especially useful in patients with non-insulin-dependent (Type 2) diabetes.

Fenfluramine is related chemically to amphetamines, which can cause severe psychological dependence and produce harmful physical and mental effects. Although amphetamines and other appetite-suppressant drugs stimulate the central nervous system and raise blood pressure, fenfluramine is more likely to depress the central nervous system, and it may reduce blood pressure. It therefore can be useful for patients with anxiety or who need to avoid stimulation for any reason. For more information, see Appetite Suppressants, keeping in mind that fenfluramine differs in some ways from the other drugs in its class. For visual characteristics of Pondimin, see the Color Guide to Prescription Drugs and Herbs.

PRECAUTIONS

WARNING
Do not take Pondimin if you have glaucoma, a history of drug abuse, severe hypertension, symptomatic cardiovascular disease, mental depression, or a history of psychotic illness.

Do not take this drug within 14 days of taking a monoamine oxidase (MAO) inhibitor. Combining these drugs poses the risk of a hypertensive crisis, causing symptoms such as severe headache and heart palpitations.

Avoid anesthesia, if possible, while taking Pondimin. If surgery with anesthesia is unavoidable, intensive cardiac monitoring is required to prevent serious or even fatal cardiac arrhythmias.

Taking an anorexiant such as fenfluramine for longer than three months within a one-year period has been associated with an increased risk of primary pulmonary hypertension, a serious and often fatal cardiopulmonary disease. Tell your doctor immediately if you notice reduced tolerance for exercise, including shortness of breath or chest pain; faintness; or swelling of your feet or ankles.

Overdoses of fenfluramine may produce a variety of symptoms, including drowsiness, confusion, flushing, tremor, fever, and sweating. Extreme overdoses can cause convulsions, coma, and even death. In case of overdose or ingestion by a child, seek emergency help immediately.

Pondimin

SPECIAL INFORMATION

- Alcoholics and people with mental illness should check with a doctor before using this drug. Pondimin can increase the risk of paranoia, depression, delusions, or agitation in susceptible people. Severe depression may also result if fenfluramine is stopped abruptly.
- Avoid this drug if you are pregnant. It's also best to avoid Pondimin when nursing a baby, although it is not known whether fenfluramine passes into human breast milk.
- The safety and efficacy of Pondimin in children younger than age 12 is unknown.
- People with mild or moderate hypertension should have their blood pressure monitored when taking this drug.
- Avoid alcohol while taking Pondimin.
- Refrain from driving or engaging in other potentially hazardous activities until you know how this drug will affect you.

POSSIBLE INTERACTIONS

Antihypertensive drugs (such as guanethidine, reserpine, methyldopa): increased effects of these drugs.

Central nervous system depressants: increased depressant effects.

Insulin: the combination may reduce the requirement for insulin. Glucose levels should be monitored.

Monoamine oxidase (MAO) inhibitors: may cause hypertensive crisis.

TARGET AILMENTS

Obesity without physiological basis

SIDE EFFECTS

NOT SERIOUS

- Drowsiness
- Diarrhea
- Dry mouth; bad taste in mouth
- Sweating; fever; chills
- Dizziness
- Weakness; fatigue; insomnia
- Increased or decreased libido
- Constipation; abdominal pain; nausea
- Painful or frequent urination
- Muscle pain
- Rash
- Burning sensation

CALL YOUR DOCTOR IF THESE PROBLEMS PERSIST.

SERIOUS

- Blurred vision
- Palpitations
- Incoordination; confusion
- Elevated mood; depression; anxiety
- Nervousness; tension; agitation
- Difficulty articulating
- Eye irritation
- Chest pain
- Hives
- Shortness of breath
- Increased or decreased blood pressure

CONTACT YOUR DOCTOR IMMEDIATELY.

Po Sum On Medicated Oil

Vital Statistics

ENGLISH NAME
Maintain Peaceful Heart Oil

PINYIN NAME
Bao Xin An You

GENERAL DESCRIPTION
Po Sum On Medicated Oil is a liniment used for treating general aches in the joints when they are not hot to the touch and for pain resulting from injury. It is also used for toothache pain and as a chest rub to relieve coughing.

Chinese medicine takes a holistic approach to healthcare, fashioning remedies to treat the entire being as well as the specific parts or areas. Precise combinations of herbs are used to prevent and combat disease, which is thought to arise from disturbances in the flow of a bodily energy called chi (pronounced "chee") and blood, or from a lack of balance in the complementary states of yin and yang. A patent formula, *Po Sum On* Medicated Oil is made by using a standardized combination of herbs and method of preparation.

INGREDIENTS
mint oil, camellia, dragon blood resin, scutellaria, cinnamon oil, licorice root, alcohol

PREPARATIONS
This formula is sold in bottles at many Chinese pharmacies and Oriental grocery stores.

Precautions

☠ ***WARNING***
Wash hands after use to avoid getting the oil in the eyes. Keep away from flames. Do not use on open wounds.

TARGET AILMENTS

Use externally for:

Joint pain (when joint is not red)

Pain from injury

Toothache (apply to gum)

Cough (chest rub)

SIDE EFFECTS

No medical side effects are expected, but the formula can stain clothes.

POTASSIUM

VITAL STATISTICS

GENERAL DESCRIPTION
Potassium is the third most abundant mineral in the body, after calcium and phosphorus. It works closely with sodium and chloride to maintain fluid distribution and pH balance and to augment nerve-impulse transmission, muscle contraction, and regulation of heartbeat and blood pressure. Potassium is also required for protein synthesis, carbohydrate metabolism, and insulin secretion by the pancreas. Studies suggest that people who regularly eat potassium-rich foods are less likely to develop atherosclerosis, heart disease, and high blood pressure, or to die of a stroke.

Many Americans may get only marginal amounts of potassium, but supplements, such as potassium aspartate, are best taken only under a doctor's guidance.

Marginal potassium deficiency causes no symptoms but may increase the risk of developing high blood pressure or aggravate existing heart disease. More severe deficiency can result in constipation, muscle cramps and muscle weakness, poor reflexes, poor concentration, heart arrhythmias, and, rarely, death due to heart failure. Acute potassium toxicity may have similar effects, including possible heart failure. However, acute toxicity is rarely linked to diet and tends to occur only in the event of kidney failure.

EMDR
Adults: 2,000 mg

NATURAL SOURCES
Dietary sources include lean meats, raw vegetables, fruits (especially citrus fruits, bananas, and avocados), potatoes, and dandelion greens.

PRECAUTIONS

WARNING
Consult a doctor before taking potassium supplements.

People with kidney disease should never take potassium supplements.

TARGET AILMENTS

Heart disease

High blood pressure

SIDE EFFECTS
NONE EXPECTED

P

Potassium Chloride

Vital Statistics

DRUG CLASS
Diuretics [Adjunct Therapy]

BRAND NAMES
K-Dur, Klor-Con 10, Micro-K 10, Slow-K

GENERAL DESCRIPTION
Potassium chloride is a mineral supplement prescribed for the prevention and treatment of potassium depletion. Such depletion usually results from the use of drugs known as non-potassium-sparing diuretics, which promote the excretion of minerals through increased urine flow. For more information, see Diuretics. For visual characteristics of potassium chloride and the brand-name drug K-Dur, see the Color Guide to Prescription Drugs and Herbs.

Precautions

SPECIAL INFORMATION
- Inform your doctor if you have stomach ulcers; potassium chloride can cause stomach irritation.
- Do not use this drug if you are taking potassium-sparing diuretics or salt substitutes.

POSSIBLE INTERACTIONS
Angiotensin-converting enzyme (ACE) inhibitors: increased potassium chloride levels.
Digoxin: increased digoxin levels.
Potassium-sparing diuretics (such as amiloride or triamterene): increased potassium chloride levels.

Target Ailments

Potassium depletion

Side Effects

Not Serious
- Gastrointestinal upset (take the medication with meals to alleviate this discomfort)
- Muscle cramps

Serious
- Black stools (a symptom of gastrointestinal bleeding)
- Severe vomiting
- Heart-rhythm problems
- Mental confusion

If you experience an irregular heartbeat or feel confused, call your doctor immediately. Elevated potassium levels in the blood can also cause muscle cramps, a less serious side effect but one that also warrants consultation with your doctor.

PRAMOXINE

VITAL STATISTICS

DRUG CLASS
Anesthetics

BRAND NAMES
Caladryl, Fleet Hemorrhoidal Preparation, Anusol

OTHER DRUGS IN THIS CLASS
benzocaine, dyclonine

GENERAL DESCRIPTION
Pramoxine is a local anesthetic used topically for the temporary relief of pain, itching, and inflammation associated with minor skin disorders. It works by blocking nerve impulses to the brain. The drug is considered safe and effective for use by adults and children over the age of two, although it is not recommended for treatment of diaper rash. Pramoxine is chemically unrelated to other anesthetics, reducing the likelihood of cross-sensitivity reactions in people who are allergic to other local anesthetics. Drug interactions are uncommon, and it seldom causes serious side effects. See Anesthetics for additional information.

PRECAUTIONS

SPECIAL INFORMATION
- Pramoxine is for external use only. Avoid applying it over large areas, to open wounds, where there may be a risk of infection, or to broken skin. Keep this product away from the eyes, ears, or mouth.
- If the condition worsens, the problem area becomes infected, bleeding occurs, or symptoms persist for more than seven days, discontinue use and consult a physician.
- Before using this drug, seek the advice of your doctor if you are pregnant or nursing or if you have heart disease, high blood pressure, thyroid disease, or diabetes.

TARGET AILMENTS
Minor skin disorders
Cold sores
Uncomplicated hemorrhoidal itching and pain

SIDE EFFECTS

NOT SERIOUS
- Irritation of some mucous membranes; a burning sensation in the eyes

CALL YOUR DOCTOR IF THESE EFFECTS BECOME BOTHERSOME.

SERIOUS
- Allergic skin reactions, including large swellings, burning, or stinging
- Cardiovascular depression, indicated by low blood pressure, irregular heartbeat, paleness, or sweating (rare)
- Central nervous system toxicity (breathing difficulties, blurred vision, convulsions, dizziness, anxiety, ringing in the ears) caused by absorption of pramoxine through damaged skin (rare)

CALL YOUR DOCTOR RIGHT AWAY.

PRAVASTATIN

VITAL STATISTICS

DRUG CLASS
Cholesterol-Reducing Drugs

BRAND NAME
Pravachol

OTHER DRUGS IN THIS CLASS
cholestyramine, colestipol, fluvastatin, gemfibrozil, lovastatin, niacin, simvastatin

GENERAL DESCRIPTION
Introduced in 1986, pravastatin is an HMG-CoA reductase inhibitor, a type of drug that alters blood levels of cholesterol and other fats. It works by blocking a liver enzyme needed in the production of cholesterol. Pravastatin may also increase the blood level of high-density lipoproteins (HDLs), the so-called good cholesterol that seems to protect against heart disease. Recently this drug was found to reduce the risk of first heart attack in patients with high cholesterol. For more information, see Cholesterol-Reducing Drugs.

PRECAUTIONS

SPECIAL INFORMATION
- Do not take pravastatin if you are pregnant or nursing. If you become pregnant while taking this drug, stop using it immediately and inform your doctor.
- Do not use this drug if you have had an allergic reaction to it in the past, or if you have active liver disease.
- Because pravastatin can cause liver damage, liver function must be monitored during therapy.

POSSIBLE INTERACTIONS
Erythromycin, immunosuppressants, niacin: may cause severe muscle pain or kidney failure if used with pravastatin.
Gemfibrozil: may affect the absorption and excretion of pravastatin; do not take concurrently.

TARGET AILMENTS
The major types of cholesterol disorders

SIDE EFFECTS

NOT SERIOUS
- Constipation
- Gas

CALL YOUR DOCTOR IF THESE EFFECTS BECOME TROUBLESOME.

SERIOUS
- Fever
- Muscle aches
- Cramps
- Blurred vision

CALL YOUR DOCTOR RIGHT AWAY.

Precose

Vital Statistics

DRUG CLASS
Antidiabetic Drugs

GENERIC NAME
acarbose

OTHER DRUGS IN THIS CLASS
glipizide, glyburide, insulin, metformin, troglitazone

GENERAL DESCRIPTION
Precose is a brand name for the generic drug acarbose, which is used to treat excess blood sugar in people with non-insulin-dependent (Type 2) diabetes when diet, weight loss, and exercise do not produce sufficient control but insulin is not required. This drug helps to lower blood sugar but does not cure diabetes.

Introduced in 1996, acarbose is different from other diabetes medications in that it doesn't enhance insulin production or the body's sensitivity to insulin. Rather, it acts by inhibiting the digestion and absorption of dietary sugars (carbohydrates). Precose can be combined with a sulfonylurea drug for more effective blood sugar control. For more information, including possible drug interactions and other important facts about this drug, see Acarbose. See also Antidiabetic Drugs.

Precautions

WARNING
Precose, when used in combination with other antidiabetes agents, can cause symptoms of hypoglycemia, or low blood sugar (unusual weakness, shakiness, stomach pain, nausea or excessive hunger, cold sweats or chills, confusion, rapid heartbeat, anxiety, convulsions, or unconsciousness). For mild symptoms of hypoglycemia, consume something that contains dextrose—not sucrose (table sugar), because of the way the drug acts on it—as soon as possible. For more severe symptoms, contact a poison control center or seek emergency care immediately.

Make sure that you can recognize the symptoms of hypoglycemia before you begin to take a combination of Precose and any other antidiabetes drug.

Avoid driving and other dangerous activities until you see how the drug affects you. Use caution if you participate in heavy exercise, since your blood sugar levels may be insufficient for the effort.

TARGET AILMENTS

Diabetes

SIDE EFFECTS

NOT SERIOUS

- Gas
- Bloating
- Diarrhea
- Nausea
- Stomach cramps
- Skin rash or itching

CALL YOUR DOCTOR IF THESE EFFECTS PERSIST OR BECOME TROUBLESOME.

SERIOUS

- Yellow eyes or skin (jaundice)

DISCONTINUE USE AND CALL YOUR DOCTOR IMMEDIATELY.

P

PREDNISONE

VITAL STATISTICS

DRUG CLASS
Corticosteroids

BRAND NAME
Deltasone

OTHER DRUGS IN THIS CLASS
Rx: beclomethasone, betamethasone, fluticasone, methylprednisolone, mometasone furoate, triamcinolone
OTC: hydrocortisone

GENERAL DESCRIPTION
Introduced in 1955, prednisone is a powerful medication used to treat a wide variety of disorders, including ulcerative colitis, Crohn's disease, serious skin problems, severe allergies, and rheumatic disorders (including bursitis, tendinitis, and arthritis). Prednisone is also used to speed recovery from acute attacks of multiple sclerosis; to prevent rejection of transplanted organs; as replacement therapy in adrenocortical deficiency; and is used in some cancer cases. For more information, see Corticosteroids. For visual characteristics of the brand-name drug Deltasone and the generic drug Prednisone Oral, see the Color Guide to Prescription Drugs and Herbs.

PRECAUTIONS

SPECIAL INFORMATION

- Ask your doctor about the risks and benefits of corticosteroid treatment if you have or have had any of the following conditions: HIV infection or AIDS, heart disease, hypertension, ulcerative colitis, diabetes, diverticulitis, gastritis or peptic ulcers, recent chickenpox or measles, candidiasis or other fungal infections, glaucoma, herpes simplex, liver or kidney disease, myasthenia gravis, osteoporosis, anastomoses, lupus, tuberculosis, recent intestinal problems, or any infection, such as a cold or flu.
- Prolonged use of prednisone can cause birth defects. Pregnant and nursing women should avoid this drug.
- Prolonged use of prednisone increases the risk of osteoporosis, cataracts, glaucoma, Cushing's syndrome (moon face), and diabetes. It can also reactivate tuberculosis.
- Check with your doctor before you stop using this drug. It may be necessary to reduce the dosage gradually to avoid serious consequences.

Prednisone

POSSIBLE INTERACTIONS

Aminoglutethimide, antacids, barbiturates, phenytoin, and rifampin: decreased effectiveness of prednisone.

Diuretics: decreased effectiveness of both combined drugs.

Growth hormones, isoniazid, potassium supplements, and salicylates: prednisone may decrease the effectiveness of these drugs.

Oral anticoagulants: prednisone may increase or decrease the effectiveness of oral anticoagulants.

Vaccines (live virus, other immunizations): prednisone may make you more susceptible to the injected virus.

TARGET AILMENTS
Arthritis
Bursitis
Tendinitis
Ulcerative colitis
Crohn's disease

SIDE EFFECTS

NOT SERIOUS

- Stomach upset
- Increased or decreased appetite
- Restlessness
- Dizziness
- Sleeplessness
- Change in skin color
- Unusual hair growth on face or body

SERIOUS

- Eye pain
- Loss of or blurred vision
- Stomach pain or burning feeling in stomach
- Black, tarry stools
- Severe and lasting skin rash, hives, or burning, itching, or painful skin
- Blisters, acne, or other skin problems
- Nausea or vomiting
- High blood pressure
- Foot or leg swelling
- Rapid weight gain
- Fluid retention (edema)
- Unusual bruising
- Menstrual irregularities
- Prolonged sore throat, fever, cold, or other sign of infection

CONTACT YOUR DOCTOR IMMEDIATELY.

PREMARIN

VITAL STATISTICS

DRUG CLASS
Estrogens and Progestins [Hormone Replacement]

GENERIC NAME
conjugated estrogens

OTHER DRUGS IN THIS SUBCLASS
Estrogens: estradiol, estropipate
Progestin: medroxyprogesterone

GENERAL DESCRIPTION
Premarin is the brand name for the generic drug known as conjugated estrogens. Premarin tablets replace the body's estrogen at natural menopause or after surgical removal of the ovaries or uterus. Replacement therapy lessens any resulting symptoms such as hot flashes and vaginal dryness and, at the same time, helps prevent osteoporosis and atherosclerosis. Premarin is also prescribed for young women whose ovaries do not produce sufficient quantities of estrogen. As a vaginal cream, Premarin is used short term to treat the degeneration of genital tissues and vulvar itching associated with estrogen deficiencies. In injection form, Premarin treats abnormal uterine bleeding caused by a hormonal imbalance. See Estrogens and Progestins for more information, including side effects and possible drug interactions. For visual characteristics of Premarin tablets, see the Color Guide to Prescription Drugs and Herbs.

SIDE EFFECTS
SEE ESTROGENS AND PROGESTINS.

PRECAUTIONS

WARNING
Do not use Premarin if you are pregnant or breast-feeding. If you suspect you are pregnant, discontinue use immediately to avoid severely harming the fetus.

Estrogens increase the risk of uterine cancer in menopausal and postmenopausal women. Abnormal vaginal bleeding is a possible symptom. If you have had menopause and experience unusual vaginal bleeding, call your doctor right away.

Get medical attention immediately if you experience any of the following: severe pain in leg, chest, or abdomen; sudden headaches; changes in speech, vision, or breathing; weakness or numbness in extremities. These symptoms may indicate a blood clot.

TARGET AILMENTS

Hot flashes, vaginal dryness, and other symptoms occurring at natural menopause or after removal of the ovaries or uterus

Osteoporosis and heart disease in postmenopausal women (preventive treatment)

Genital itching and degeneration of genital tissues

Abnormal uterine bleeding (injection form only)

Palliative treatment of advanced inoperable cancers: breast cancer in women and prostate cancer in men

Prempro

Vital Statistics

DRUG CLASS
Estrogens and Progestins [Hormone Replacement]

GENERIC NAMES
conjugated estrogens, medroxyprogesterone

OTHER DRUGS IN THIS SUBCLASS
estradiol, estropipate

GENERAL DESCRIPTION
The brand-name drug Prempro is used to replace the hormones in a woman's body that decline at menopause. Drug therapy lessens any resulting symptoms such as hot flashes and vaginal dryness and, at the same time, helps prevent osteoporosis. Prempro is also prescribed for young women whose ovaries do not produce enough estrogen, and to treat the degeneration of vulvar and vaginal tissues associated with estrogen deficiencies. Prempro, unlike the brand-name drug Premarin, is prescribed only for women with an intact uterus. The addition of a small dose of the progestin drug medroxyprogesterone in Prempro helps alleviate the side effects of estrogen therapy and also reduces the risk of endometrial hyperplasia (a precancerous uterine condition associated with long-term estrogen use). See Estrogens and Progestins for more information, including side effects and possible drug interactions. For visual characteristics of Prempro, see the Color Guide to Prescription Drugs and Herbs.

SIDE EFFECTS
See Estrogens and Progestins.

Precautions

WARNING
Do not use Prempro if you are pregnant or breast-feeding. If you suspect you are pregnant, discontinue use immediately to avoid severely harming the fetus.

Estrogens increase the risk of uterine cancer in menopausal and postmenopausal women. Abnormal vaginal bleeding is a possible symptom. If you have had menopause and experience unusual vaginal bleeding, call your doctor right away.

Get medical attention immediately if you experience any of the following: severe pain in leg, chest, or abdomen; sudden headaches; changes in speech, vision, or breathing; weakness or numbness in extremities. These symptoms may indicate a blood clot.

SPECIAL INFORMATION
Before taking Prempro, let your doctor know if you are a smoker, have ever had a stroke, or have liver disease, gallbladder disease, a history of breast cancer, fibrocystic breast changes, endometriosis, uterine fibroids, diabetes, asthma, epilepsy, migraine, heart disease, a blood-clotting disorder, or high blood pressure.

TARGET AILMENTS

Hot flashes, vaginal dryness, and other symptoms occurring at natural menopause or after surgical removal of the ovaries

Osteoporosis in postmenopausal women (preventive treatment)

Vulvar and vaginal atrophy

PRILOSEC

VITAL STATISTICS

DRUG CLASS
Antiulcer Drugs

GENERIC NAME
omeprazole

OTHER DRUGS IN THIS CLASS
lansoprazole, sucralfate
Histamine H_2 Blockers: cimetidine, famotidine, nizatidine, ranitidine

GENERAL DESCRIPTION
Prilosec is a brand name for the generic drug omeprazole. It is used to treat several conditions associated with excessive production of stomach acid, such as ulcers of the stomach and duodenum (upper portion of the small intestine), Zollinger-Ellison syndrome, multiple endocrine neoplasia, systemic mastocytosis, gastritis, gastroesophageal reflux (in which stomach acid flows backward into the esophagus), and gastrointestinal symptoms associated with the use of nonsteroidal anti-inflammatory drugs (NSAIDs) and aspirin. Prilosec works by inhibiting the action of enzymes in the acid-producing cells of the stomach lining.

For information on possible drug interactions, see Antiulcer Drugs. For visual characteristics of Prilosec, see the Color Guide to Prescription Drugs and Herbs.

PRECAUTIONS

SPECIAL INFORMATION
- Avoid this drug if you are breast-feeding.
- Prilosec may be taken with antacids.

TARGET AILMENTS

Duodenal ulcer; gastric ulcer; upper gastrointestinal bleeding associated with gastric ulcer or duodenal ulcer, or with gastritis

Zollinger-Ellison syndrome; multiple endocrine neoplasia; other conditions characterized by an overproduction of stomach acid

Gastroesophageal reflux

Gastrointestinal symptoms associated with the use of nonsteroidal anti-inflammatory drugs (NSAIDs) and aspirin

SIDE EFFECTS

NOT SERIOUS

- Abdominal pain; dizziness or headache; drowsiness; chest pain; heartburn; constipation, gas, or diarrhea; nausea and vomiting; rash or itching

CALL YOUR DOCTOR IF THESE SYMPTOMS BECOME BOTHERSOME.

SERIOUS

- Anemia (unusual fatigue); combined sore throat and fever; mouth sores; bloody urine; urinary tract infection (pain or burning when urinating); unusual bleeding or bruising

CALL YOUR DOCTOR RIGHT AWAY.

PRINIVIL

VITAL STATISTICS

DRUG CLASS
Angiotensin-Converting Enzyme (ACE) Inhibitors

GENERIC NAME
lisinopril

OTHER DRUGS IN THIS CLASS
benazepril, captopril, enalapril, fosinopril, quinapril, ramipril

GENERAL DESCRIPTION
Prinivil is a brand name for the generic ACE inhibitor lisinopril. Introduced in 1988, lisinopril relaxes arterial walls, thereby lowering blood pressure. It is used in the management of hypertension (high blood pressure) and congestive heart failure. For increased blood-pressure-lowering action, this drug may be combined with hydrochlorothiazide, a diuretic. For further information, see Angiotensin-Converting Enzyme (ACE) Inhibitors. For visual characteristics of Prinivil, see the Color Guide to Prescription Drugs and Herbs.

TARGET AILMENTS
High blood pressure
Congestive heart failure (in conjunction with digitalis preparations and diuretics)
Heart attacks (used within 24 hours to improve survival)

PRECAUTIONS

WARNING
Get medical attention immediately if you notice swelling of your face, tongue, or vocal cords or have difficulty swallowing or breathing; this reaction can be life threatening.

This drug should not be taken during pregnancy; it has been associated with death of the fetus and newborn.

SPECIAL INFORMATION
- Prinivil increases blood potassium levels. Do not use potassium-rich products without first consulting your doctor. The potassium in your blood could rise to dangerous levels, leading to heart-rhythm problems.
- Do not abruptly stop taking this drug. Your doctor must reduce the dosage gradually.

SIDE EFFECTS

NOT SERIOUS
- Dry, persistent cough
- Headache; fatigue
- Nausea; mild diarrhea
- Loss of sense of taste
- Temporary skin rash

CALL YOUR DOCTOR IF THESE EFFECTS BECOME BOTHERSOME.

SERIOUS
- Fainting or dizziness
- Persistent skin rash
- Fever or chills; joint pain
- Numbness and tingling
- Abdominal pain; vomiting
- Chest pain or palpitations

CALL YOUR DOCTOR IMMEDIATELY.

PROANTHOCYANIDIN

VITAL STATISTICS

OTHER NAMES
oligomeric procyanidolic complexes (OPC); procyanidolic oligomers (PCO)

GENERAL DESCRIPTION
Proanthocyanidin is among a group of naturally occurring plant compounds, called bioflavonoids, that have been found to protect and strengthen living tissue. A number of fruits—including blueberries, raspberries, cranberries, and cherries—contain proanthocyanidin. The substance is also found in pine bark, a fact that French explorer Jacques Cartier and his crew reportedly discovered in the 1500s while on expedition in Canada. With nothing to eat but biscuits and dried pork, the men began experiencing weakness, muscle aches, joint pains, and bruising. An Indian showed them how to make tea from pine bark. The explorers drank it, and their symptoms disappeared.

But by far the highest concentrations of proanthocyanidin are found in the seeds and skin of grapes. Recent research suggests that drinking red wine can help reduce the risk of cardiovascular disease, and many experts attribute these benefits to high levels of proanthocyanidin in the grapes.

Because it acts as an antioxidant, neutralizing "free radicals" that can harm the body, proanthocyanidin has been used in France for years as a treatment for blood vessel disorders. Considered an effective antihistamine and anti-inflammatory agent, the substance is also thought to protect and heal connective tissue, reduce inflammation, and stabilize collagen and elastin, thereby improving and preserving the elasticity of the skin.

PREPARATIONS
Proanthocyanidin is available in tablet and capsule form as a dietary supplement.

TARGET AILMENTS

- Allergies that respond to antihistamines
- Arthritis
- Bruises
- Gum disease
- Phlebitis
- Ulcers
- Varicose veins and other vascular problems

SIDE EFFECTS

NONE EXPECTED

PROCARDIA

VITAL STATISTICS

DRUG CLASS
Calcium Channel Blockers

GENERIC NAME
nifedipine

OTHER DRUGS IN THIS CLASS
amlodipine, diltiazem, isradipine, verapamil

GENERAL DESCRIPTION
Procardia is a brand name for the generic drug nifedipine. Used since 1972 to control high blood pressure, nifedipine inhibits the passage of calcium into heart muscle cells and muscle cells surrounding blood vessels, retarding electrical stimulation of the heart, dilating the arteries, slowing contraction of the heart, and preventing some spasms of the coronary arteries. Alone or in combination with other heart and blood pressure medications, nifedipine is used to treat mild to moderate high blood pressure (hypertension) and to prevent angina. It is sometimes used to treat Raynaud's syndrome. Procardia is available in short-acting and extended-release tablets. For more information, including possible drug interactions, see Calcium Channel Blockers. For visual characteristics of Procardia XL, see the Color Guide to Prescription Drugs and Herbs.

TARGET AILMENTS
Angina; high blood pressure
Raynaud's syndrome

PRECAUTIONS

SPECIAL INFORMATION
- Recent findings have prompted warnings from some healthcare professionals about the safety of nifedipine, particularly large doses of the short-acting form. Before using this drug, be sure to discuss the matter thoroughly with your doctor. If you are already taking it, do not stop the medication without first consulting your doctor.
- Pregnant and nursing women should use Procardia only if clearly needed.
- Drinking grapefruit juice may increase the effects of this drug.

SIDE EFFECTS

NOT SERIOUS
- Nausea; constipation
- Fatigue; dizziness
- Headache; flushing

CALL YOUR DOCTOR IF THESE EFFECTS BECOME TROUBLESOME.

SERIOUS
- Heart problems, such as congestive heart failure, heart-rhythm irregularities, or increased angina
- Low blood pressure; fainting
- Edema (swelling of the ankles and feet)
- Allergic reactions, such as skin rash
- Bleeding or tender gums

CONTACT YOUR DOCTOR IMMEDIATELY.

P

Rx PROCHLORPERAZINE

VITAL STATISTICS

DRUG CLASS
Antinausea Drugs

BRAND NAME
Compazine

OTHER DRUGS IN THIS CLASS
scopolamine

GENERAL DESCRIPTION
Prochlorperazine, introduced in 1956, controls nausea and vomiting by blocking stimulation of the area of the brain that controls vomiting. This drug is sometimes prescribed for short bouts of flulike nausea but is usually used to control severe nausea induced by surgery, radiation therapy, chemotherapy, and other drugs. Prochlorperazine must be used with care, as its antiemetic action can mask signs of overdosage of other drugs and obscure symptoms of other diseases, such as intestinal obstructions, Reye's syndrome, and brain tumor. For more information, including possible interactions, see Antinausea Drugs.

P

PRECAUTIONS

SPECIAL INFORMATION
- Prochlorperazine interacts with many OTC cold, cough, and allergy medicines and with many prescription drugs.
- Do not take prochlorperazine if you have had an allergic reaction to it in the past or if you have a blood or bone marrow disease, Parkinson's disease, breast cancer, or any liver or kidney disease.
- If you are too nauseated to swallow tablets, capsules, or syrup, you can ask for this drug in suppository or injection form.
- This drug may cause unusual sensitivity to the sun or to sunlamps.
- Prochlorperazine can cause a decrease in white blood cell count, an increase in liver enzymes and bilirubin, and false-positive pregnancy test results.
- Prochlorperazine should not be given to children under age two or to those who weigh less than 20 pounds. Children with acute illnesses, such as measles, chickenpox, or flulike infections, are very susceptible to adverse reactions to this drug.

TARGET AILMENTS

Nausea and vomiting

SIDE EFFECTS

NOT SERIOUS

- Drowsiness; dizziness; blurred vision; dry mouth; nasal congestion
- Constipation; impaired urination; pink- or purple-colored urine
- Decreased sex drive; menstrual irregularities; swollen breasts

SEE YOUR DOCTOR IF THESE SYMPTOMS PERSIST.

SERIOUS

- Jaundice; muscle spasms of the face and neck
- Extreme restlessness or agitation; fainting; skin rashes

CALL YOUR DOCTOR RIGHT AWAY.

Promethazine

Vital Statistics

DRUG CLASS
Antihistamines

BRAND NAME
Phenergan

OTHER DRUGS IN THIS CLASS
Rx: astemizole, cetirizine, diphenhydramine, fexofenadine, loratadine, terfenadine
OTC: brompheniramine, chlorpheniramine, clemastine, dexbrompheniramine, diphenhydramine, doxylamine, triprolidine

GENERAL DESCRIPTION
Promethazine is a sedating antihistamine prescribed for allergies, motion sickness, nausea related to anesthesia, and pain control following surgery. See Antihistamines for more information. For visual characteristics of the brand-name drug Phenergan, see the Color Guide to Prescription Drugs and Herbs.

Precautions

SPECIAL INFORMATION
- Promethazine causes drowsiness in varying degrees: Avoid driving or operating dangerous machinery until you know how the drug affects you.
- If you have sleep apnea, avoid this drug.
- Check with your doctor before using promethazine if you have a seizure disorder, glaucoma, high blood pressure, an enlarged prostate, stomach ulcer, bladder obstruction, liver disease, or heart disease; this drug may exacerbate these conditions.

POSSIBLE INTERACTIONS
Alcohol, antianxiety drugs, barbiturates, or other sedatives: do not take with promethazine, since the combination may result in excessive sedation.
Epinephrine: may cause hypotension. Do not combine with promethazine.
Levodopa: reduced levodopa effect.
Monoamine oxidase (MAO) inhibitors: hypotension and dryness of the respiratory passages. Do not combine with promethazine.

TARGET AILMENTS

Nasal and respiratory allergies; motion sickness; insomnia

Nausea related to anesthesia; anxiety before surgery; pain after surgery (adjunct therapy)

SIDE EFFECTS

NOT SERIOUS
- Drowsiness; dryness of the mouth, nose, or throat
- Dizziness, weakness, and slower reaction time, especially in the elderly
- Nervousness and insomnia, especially in children

CALL YOUR DOCTOR IF THESE SYMPTOMS PERSIST.

SERIOUS
- Confusion; disorientation
- Uncontrolled movements

CALL YOUR DOCTOR RIGHT AWAY.

PROPOXYPHENE

VITAL STATISTICS

DRUG CLASS
Analgesics [Opioid Analgesics]

BRAND NAMES
Darvocet-N 100, Propacet 100

OTHER DRUGS IN THIS SUBCLASS
codeine, hydrocodone, oxycodone, tramadol

GENERAL DESCRIPTION
Propoxyphene is an opioid analgesic that acts on the central nervous system (the spinal cord and brain) to alter the perception of pain. Prescribed for mild to moderate pain relief, it is often combined with acetaminophen. This drug is less likely than other opiates to cause psychological or physical dependence and severe withdrawal symptoms, but it should be used with caution. See Opioid Analgesics for additional information on drug interactions and side effects. For visual characteristics of the brand-name drug Darvocet-N 100 and of the generic combination drugs propoxyphene napsylate and acetaminophen and propoxyphene hydrochloride [HCL] and acetaminophen, see the Color Guide to Prescription Drugs and Herbs.

TARGET AILMENTS

Mild to moderate pain, especially from acute trauma or surgery

SIDE EFFECTS

See Opioid Analgesics.

PRECAUTIONS

SPECIAL INFORMATION
- Combining propoxyphene with alcohol, tranquilizers, sedatives, muscle relaxants, or antidepressants can lead to death. Do not combine without your doctor's knowledge.
- Tell your doctor if you notice these symptoms after you stop taking propoxyphene: fever, runny nose, or sneezing; diarrhea; goose flesh; unusually large pupils; nervousness or irritability; fast heartbeat.
- Seek emergency medical care if you overdose on propoxyphene. Symptoms include pinpoint pupils; slow, shallow, or troubled breathing, and slow heartbeat; extreme dizziness or weakness; confusion; convulsions.
- Do not drive or operate machinery until you know how this drug affects you.

POSSIBLE INTERACTIONS
Amphetamines: risk of convulsions if a patient taking amphetamines takes an overdose of propoxyphene.
Anticoagulants: may increase the effects of some anticoagulants.
Carbamazepine: may increase the effects of carbamazepine, leading to an increased risk of toxicity.
Cimetidine: possible central nervous system toxicity.
Smoking cessation drugs, such as nicotine patches or chewing gum: may increase the effects of propoxyphene.
Tobacco (smoking): may decrease the effects of propoxyphene.
See also Opioid Analgesics.

PROPRANOLOL

VITAL STATISTICS

DRUG CLASS
Beta-Adrenergic Blockers

BRAND NAMES
Inderal, Inderal LA

OTHER DRUGS IN THIS CLASS
atenolol, bisoprolol, metoprolol, nadolol, timolol

GENERAL DESCRIPTION
A nonselective beta-blocking drug, propranolol is prescribed to help manage high blood pressure (hypertension), heart-rhythm disorders, angina, tremors, and myocardial infarction (heart attack). Other uses include the prevention of migraine headaches.

By blocking the action of certain parts of the nervous system, propranolol reduces the oxygen requirements and contraction force of the heart while also relaxing blood vessels, thereby lowering blood pressure and easing the heart's work load. The drug also affects the movement of nerve impulses in the heart, helping to control some heart-rhythm problems. Since propranolol has a stronger effect on the central nervous system than other beta-adrenergic blockers, it is more likely to cause fatigue or dizziness. For more information, including side effects, contraindications, and possible drug interactions, see Beta-Adrenergic Blockers.

PRECAUTIONS

SPECIAL INFORMATION
- Propranolol can make you drowsy, dizzy, and lightheaded. Avoid activities that require alertness, such as driving, until you know how you react to this drug.
- Do not use propranolol if you have a bronchospastic disease, bronchial asthma, or a severe chronic obstructive pulmonary disease.
- Suddenly stopping this drug may cause or increase heart problems. Dosage must be reduced gradually by your doctor.

TARGET AILMENTS

Heart disease, especially angina (chest pain), myocardial infarction (heart attack), and abnormal heart rhythms

High blood pressure (hypertension)

Migraine headaches

Tremors

Anxiety

Alcohol withdrawal

SIDE EFFECTS
SEE BETA-ADRENERGIC BLOCKERS.

P

PROSTATE GLAND PILLS

VITAL STATISTICS

CHINESE NAME
Qian Lie Xian Wan

GENERAL DESCRIPTION
Prostate Gland Pills are used generally for symptoms of dribbling and painful urination and painful or swollen testicles. The herbs in the formula help clear pus and inflammation and increase the circulation of fluids and blood in the area.

Chinese medicine takes a holistic approach to healthcare, fashioning remedies to treat the entire being as well as the specific parts or areas. Precise combinations of herbs are used to prevent and combat disease, which is thought to arise from disturbances in the flow of a bodily energy called chi (pronounced "chee") and blood, or from a lack of balance in the complementary states of yin and yang. A patent formula, Prostate Gland Pills are made by using a standardized combination of herbs and method of preparation.

INGREDIENTS
vaccaria seeds, tree peony root, red peony root, astragalus, patrinia, hogfennel, licorice, saussurea, akebia stem

PREPARATIONS
This formula can be found in pill form in many Chinese pharmacies and Oriental grocery stores.

TARGET AILMENTS

- Prostate infection or swelling
- Dribbling urine (in men)
- Painful urination (in men)
- Painful testicles
- Urinary tract infection

SIDE EFFECTS

NONE EXPECTED

Rx PROVENTIL

VITAL STATISTICS

DRUG CLASS
Bronchodilators

GENERIC NAME
albuterol

OTHER DRUGS IN THIS CLASS
Rx: epinephrine, ipratropium, salmeterol, terbutaline, theophylline
OTC: ephedrine, epinephrine, theophylline

GENERAL DESCRIPTION
Proventil is a brand name for albuterol, an antiasthmatic drug that acts by relaxing the muscles surrounding the bronchial tubes in the lungs. Proventil is commonly prescribed for symptoms of acute bronchial asthma. The drug is also used to reduce the frequency and severity of recurrent asthma attacks and exercise-induced bronchospasms. Proventil is available as an inhalation aerosol, an inhalation solution, and in syrup and tablet form. For more information, see Bronchodilators.

PRECAUTIONS

☠ ***WARNING***
Your body can build up tolerance to bronchodilator inhalants, causing them to become less effective. If this happens, discontinue the drug and tell your doctor. Do not increase the dose. Increasing the dose can lead to serious, perhaps fatal bronchial constriction. It may also cause heart-rhythm irregularities.

SPECIAL INFORMATION
- Before you use Proventil, tell your doctor if you have cardiovascular disease, narrow-angle glaucoma, prostatic hypertrophy, or difficulty urinating.
- Women who are pregnant or breast-feeding should consult a doctor before using a bronchodilator.

POSSIBLE INTERACTIONS
Beta blockers: decreased effects of both the beta blockers and Proventil.
See Bronchodilators for more interactions.

TARGET AILMENTS

Bronchial asthma

Bronchospasms induced by exercise

SIDE EFFECTS

NOT SERIOUS
- Mild nausea or weakness
- Insomnia
- Nervousness; restlessness

CALL YOUR DOCTOR IF THESE EFFECTS BECOME BOTHERSOME.

SERIOUS
- Change in blood pressure; change in heartbeat (irregular or pounding)
- Trembling; anxiety
- Breathing problems
- Dizziness; lightheadedness
- Muscle cramps
- Nausea or vomiting
- Chest pain or discomfort

CALL YOUR DOCTOR RIGHT AWAY.

Provera

Vital Statistics

DRUG CLASS
Estrogens and Progestins [Hormone Replacement]

GENERIC NAME
medroxyprogesterone

OTHER DRUGS IN THIS CLASS
Estrogens: conjugated estrogens, estradiol, estropipate, ethinyl estradiol, mestranol
Progestins: desogestrel, ethynodiol diacetate, levonorgestrel, norethindrone, norgestimate, norgestrel

GENERAL DESCRIPTION
Provera is a brand-name drug prescribed for abnormal uterine bleeding (heavy or prolonged menstruation) and amenorrhea (absence of menstruation). Medroxyprogesterone, the active ingredient in Provera, is the progestin drug most often used to treat menstrual problems that are caused by hormonal imbalance. See Estrogens and Progestins for more information, including side effects, possible drug interactions, and additional precautions. For visual characteristics, see the Color Guide to Prescription Drugs and Herbs.

TARGET AILMENTS

Lack of menstruation

Abnormal uterine bleeding due to hormonal imbalance

SIDE EFFECTS

SEE ESTROGENS AND PROGESTINS.

Precautions

WARNING
Do not use Provera during the first four months of pregnancy or if you are breastfeeding. If you suspect you are pregnant, discontinue use immediately to avoid harming the fetus.

Get medical attention immediately if you experience any of the following: severe pain in leg, chest, or abdomen; sudden headaches; changes in speech, vision, or breathing; weakness or numbness in extremities. These symptoms may indicate blood clots.

SPECIAL INFORMATION
- Before taking Provera, let your doctor know if you are a smoker or have kidney disease, liver disease, gallbladder disease, a history of breast cancer, fibrocystic breast changes, endometriosis, uterine fibroids, diabetes, asthma, epilepsy, migraine, stroke, heart disease, blood-clotting disorders, or high blood pressure. Your doctor will use this information to determine whether or not you should use Provera and what your dosage should be.
- Provera may increase blood glucose levels; if you are diabetic, your doctor may have to adjust your dosage of insulin or other antidiabetic drug.
- Taking Provera with or after meals can help reduce nausea.
- Provera may cause mental depression, especially in women who have a history of depression. Consult with your doctor if you notice this side effect.
- Treatment with Provera may mask the onset of menopause because you may continue to experience regular menstrual bleeding.

Rx PROZAC

VITAL STATISTICS

DRUG CLASS
Antidepressants [Selective Serotonin Reuptake Inhibitors (SSRIs)]

GENERIC NAME
fluoxetine

OTHER DRUGS IN THIS SUBCLASS
paroxetine, sertraline, venlafaxine

GENERAL DESCRIPTION
Prozac is a brand name for the well-known antidepressant drug fluoxetine, which is prescribed for control of a wide range of depressive illnesses. It is also used to treat alcohol dependence and obsessive-compulsive disorder.

Fluoxetine belongs to a subclass of antidepressants known as selective serotonin reuptake inhibitors (SSRIs). It works by enhancing the action of the neurotransmitter serotonin in the brain. See Antidepressants for information on side effects and possible drug interactions.

TARGET AILMENTS

Major depression

Obsessive-compulsive disorder

SIDE EFFECTS

SEE ANTIDEPRESSANTS.

PRECAUTIONS

SPECIAL INFORMATION
- Although Prozac benefits many of those who take it, a greater percentage of people experience side effects with this drug than with other antidepressants. If you have any questions about possible side effects, discuss them with your doctor.
- Rarely, Prozac can trigger manic attacks; this side effect may be more common in individuals with manic-depressive (bipolar) disorder. Be sure to tell your doctor if you have a history of manic-depression.
- Fluoxetine may exacerbate suicidal tendencies in some individuals. Be sure to tell your healthcare provider if you have experienced thoughts of suicide or believe you may be susceptible to such thoughts.
- This drug may cause drowsiness. When taking fluoxetine, use care while driving, operating machinery, or performing tasks that require mental alertness.
- Prozac can affect blood sugar levels; dosage adjustment in oral antidiabetic medication or insulin may be required.
- If you are pregnant, nursing, or planning a pregnancy, check with your doctor before taking Prozac.
- The full effects of this drug may not be felt for several weeks.
- The severity of any side effects may decrease with time (after two weeks) or with lowered dosages. If you have any questions about potential side effects, discuss them with your doctor.

PSEUDOEPHEDRINE

VITAL STATISTICS

DRUG CLASS
Decongestants

BRAND NAMES
Actifed, Advil Cold and Sinus, Claritin-D, Comtrex Multi-Symptom Cold Reliever Tablets or Liquid, Contac, Drixoral, NyQuil, PediaCare (various forms), Sudafed, TheraFlu, Triaminic Nite Light, Triaminic Sore Throat Formula, Tylenol Allergy Sinus, Tylenol Cold (adults and children), Tylenol Sinus

OTHER DRUGS IN THIS CLASS
Rx: phenylpropanolamine
OTC: oxymetazoline, phenylephrine, phenylpropanolamine

GENERAL DESCRIPTION
Pseudoephedrine is a synthetic decongestant drug modeled on the ephedrine found in plants of the *Ephedra* genus. The drug is used to treat congestion of the nasal, sinus, and Eustachian passages caused by colds, allergies, or related respiratory problems. It is often available in combination with analgesics, antihistamines, and expectorants. Pseudoephedrine is banned for use during athletic competitions. For more information, see Decongestants.

PRECAUTIONS

SPECIAL INFORMATION
- Some preparations that contain pseudoephedrine also contain antihistamines, which can cause other side effects, including drowsiness. See Antihistamines for further information.
- Check with your doctor before taking pseudoephedrine if you have cardiovascular disease (including angina, coronary artery disease, and hypertension), hyperthyroidism (overactive thyroid), prostate enlargement, diabetes, or glaucoma. The drug may exacerbate these conditions.

PSEUDOEPHEDRINE

POSSIBLE INTERACTIONS

Beta blockers: Pseudoephedrine can lessen the effectiveness of beta blockers, causing hypertension.

Digoxin: possible heart-rhythm problems.

High blood pressure drugs: decreased antihypertensive effect.

Levodopa (anti-Parkinsonism drug): increased risk of heart-rhythm problems.

Monoamine oxidase (MAO) inhibitors: increased stimulant action of pseudoephedrine, causing effects such as hypertension and heart-rhythm problems.

Rauwolfia: decreased effectiveness of pseudoephedrine.

Stimulants (such as other decongestants, amphetamines, caffeine): increased stimulant effects, leading to excessive nervousness, insomnia, irregular heart rhythm, or seizures.

Thyroid hormones: increased effects of both combined drugs. Your doctor may have to adjust the dosage of both medications.

Tricyclic antidepressants (such as amitriptyline): increased action of pseudoephedrine, making serious central nervous system side effects more likely.

TARGET AILMENTS

Nasal and sinus congestion

Congestion of Eustachian tubes, which join the ear with the nose and throat

SIDE EFFECTS

NOT SERIOUS

- Mild nervousness
- Mild restlessness
- Insomnia
- Dizziness
- Lightheadedness
- Nausea
- Dryness of mouth or nose
- Rebound congestion

CALL YOUR DOCTOR IF THESE EFFECTS CONTINUE OR BECOME BOTHERSOME.

SERIOUS

- Severe headache
- Nervousness
- Restlessness
- Pounding or irregular heartbeat
- High blood pressure
- Trouble breathing

CONTACT YOUR DOCTOR IMMEDIATELY.

PSYLLIUM

LATIN NAME
Plantago psyllium

VITAL STATISTICS

GENERAL DESCRIPTION

For centuries, traditional Chinese and Ayurvedic (Hindu) physicians have used psyllium to treat diarrhea, constipation, hemorrhoids, and urinary problems. The ground-up seeds, rich in fiber, make a safe, gentle, bulk-forming laxative and are the active ingredient in many commercial laxative products. Both diarrhea and constipation may be treated, because the herb absorbs excess fluid in the intestinal tract and increases stool volume. Recently it has been suggested that psyllium may help prevent heart disease by clearing excess cholesterol from the body. This 18-inch-tall herb produces white flowers and abundant small brown seed pods.

PREPARATIONS

Over the counter:

Psyllium is available as whole seeds, ground or powdered seeds, and in various commercial bulk-forming laxative preparations.

At home:

DRINK: Mix 1 tsp ground seeds or powder in 1 cup cool liquid. Drink 2 to 3 cups a day.

SEEDS: Take 1 tsp seeds with water at mealtimes.

Consult a qualified practitioner for the dosage appropriate for you and the specific condition being treated.

TARGET AILMENTS

Take internally for:

Ulcers; colitis

Constipation, diarrhea, or hemorrhoidal irritation

PRECAUTIONS

☠ *WARNING*

You must drink eight to 10 glasses of water throughout the day when taking psyllium as a laxative, to prevent blockage of the intestines.

SPECIAL INFORMATION

- Start using this herb gradually, so your body can adjust to the increase in fiber.
- Do not use psyllium to treat ulcers or colitis without consulting your doctor.
- Do not give this herb to children younger than two years of age. Consult your pediatrician if your infant or child is constipated.
- Use of this herb by children for more than seven to 10 days should be done in conjunction with a healthcare practitioner.
- Pregnant women should avoid psyllium and all laxatives, because they stimulate the lower pelvis near the uterus.

POSSIBLE INTERACTIONS

Combining psyllium with other herbs may necessitate a lower dosage.

SIDE EFFECTS

NOT SERIOUS

Psyllium can cause allergic reactions in people who have allergies to dust or grasses. Call your doctor if bothersome.

SERIOUS

Severe allergic reactions are rare; if you have difficulty breathing, seek emergency help.

Psyllium Hydrophilic Mucilloid

Vital Statistics

DRUG CLASS
Laxatives

BRAND NAME
Metamucil

OTHER DRUGS IN THIS CLASS
Bulk: calcium polycarbophil, methylcellulose
Stimulant: phenolphthalein, sennosides
Stool softener: docusate

GENERAL DESCRIPTION
Psyllium hydrophilic mucilloid is a bulk-forming laxative used to relieve chronic constipation. It also helps relieve chronic, watery diarrhea. This type of laxative may be especially beneficial to people on low-fiber diets and to those with irritable bowel syndrome (spastic colon), diverticulitis, or hemorrhoids. For more information, including additional precautions, see Laxatives.

TARGET AILMENTS

Constipation

Diarrhea

Irritable bowel syndrome, or spastic colon

Straining during bowel movements following rectal surgery, heart attacks, or childbirth, or when hemorrhoids are present

Precautions

SPECIAL INFORMATION
- When taking this laxative, be sure to drink plenty of water or other fluid to avoid obstruction of the throat and esophagus. Taking this medication without enough liquid may cause choking.
- This laxative is slow acting; you may not experience its effects for 12 to 72 hours after taking it.
- Bulk-forming laxatives are best for geriatric patients with poorly functioning colons.
- If you are diabetic, avoid psyllium-type laxatives that contain large amounts of sugar; instead, use sugar-free types that contain the artificial sweetener aspartame.
- If you have difficulty swallowing—as with dysphagia—do not take bulk-forming laxatives, which can cause an esophageal obstruction.
- Call your doctor if the laxative fails to have the desired effect after one week of use.

POSSIBLE INTERACTIONS
Oral anticoagulants, digoxin, salicylate, tetracycline: these drugs may be less effective when taken concurrently with bulk-forming laxatives. After taking any of these medications, wait two hours before taking a laxative.

SIDE EFFECTS

SERIOUS

In rare cases, people with respiratory problems may have adverse reactions to inhaled particles from powder preparations.

PULSATILLA

LATIN NAME
Pulsatilla nigricans

VITAL STATISTICS

GENERAL DESCRIPTION

Common in meadowlands in northern and central Europe, *Pulsatilla,* or windflower, contains a caustic substance that may cause mouth or throat blisters if the plant is chewed. Homeopathic physicians prescribe *Pulsatilla* for patients with conditions accompanied by a thick yellow or white discharge. For homeopathic use, *Pulsatilla* is collected in full bloom and pounded to a pulp. The pulp is steeped in an alcohol-and-water solution, then strained and diluted. For more information on homeopathic medicine, see page 14.

PREPARATIONS

Pulsatilla is available over the counter in various potencies, both in liquid and in tablet form, at selected stores and pharmacies. Consult your homeopathic physician for more precise information.

PRECAUTIONS

SPECIAL INFORMATION

- When a remedy is administered, no one but the patient should touch the pills. If tablets are spilled, throw them away.
- The mouth should be clear of flavors 15 minutes before and after taking a remedy, and strong flavors and aromas, such as coffee, camphor, and heavily scented perfumes, should be avoided for the duration of treatment.

SIDE EFFECTS

NONE EXPECTED

TARGET AILMENTS

- Bedwetting
- Breast infections
- Chickenpox
- Conjunctivitis
- Coughs causing a rattle in the chest and interfering with sleep
- Headaches in the forehead
- Eye inflammation, with aching eyes and a thick discharge
- Fever with chills
- Hay fever
- Incontinence
- Indigestion from rich foods
- Aching joints that improve with movement and cold compresses
- Urethritis in men
- Late menstrual periods
- Otitis media (middle ear infection)
- Sciatica
- Sinusitis
- Varicose veins
- Depression with excessive crying

Rx QUINAPRIL

VITAL STATISTICS

DRUG CLASS
Angiotensin-Converting Enzyme (ACE) Inhibitors

BRAND NAME
Accupril

OTHER DRUGS IN THIS CLASS
benazepril, captopril, enalapril, fosinopril, lisinopril, ramipril

GENERAL DESCRIPTION
Quinapril is prescribed for mild-to-moderate high blood pressure and for congestive heart failure. Like other ACE inhibitors, this drug blocks a body enzyme needed for the production of a substance that causes blood vessels to constrict. As a result, it relaxes the artery walls, thereby lowering blood pressure. For further information, see Angiotensin-Converting Enzyme (ACE) Inhibitors.

PRECAUTIONS

WARNING
This drug should not be taken during pregnancy; it has been associated with death of the fetus and newborn.

SPECIAL INFORMATION
- Quinapril causes an increase in blood levels of potassium. Do not use potassium-rich products, including salt substitutes and low-salt milk, without consulting your doctor. Potassium levels could rise dangerously, leading to heart-rhythm problems.
- Do not stop taking this medication abruptly. Your doctor may tell you to reduce the dosage gradually.
- Quinapril's high magnesium content may reduce the body's absorption of drugs interacting with magnesium.

TARGET AILMENTS

High blood pressure

Sometimes congestive heart failure (in conjunction with digitalis preparations and diuretics)

SIDE EFFECTS

NOT SERIOUS
- Dry, persistent cough; fatigue; nausea; diarrhea; temporary skin rash; low blood pressure; dizziness on suddenly rising or changing position

CALL YOUR DOCTOR IF THESE EFFECTS BECOME BOTHERSOME.

SERIOUS
- Fainting; persistent skin rash; joint pain; drowsiness; numbness and tingling; abdominal pain; vomiting; diarrhea; signs of infection; chest pain; heart palpitation; jaundice (yellowing of skin or eyes)

CALL YOUR DOCTOR RIGHT AWAY. GET MEDICAL ATTENTION IMMEDIATELY IF YOU NOTICE SWELLING OF YOUR FACE, TONGUE, OR VOCAL CORDS OR HAVE DIFFICULTY SWALLOWING OR BREATHING; THIS REACTION CAN BE LIFE THREATENING.

Rx RAMIPRIL

VITAL STATISTICS

DRUG CLASS
Angiotensin-Converting Enzyme (ACE) Inhibitors

BRAND NAME
Altace

OTHER DRUGS IN THIS CLASS
benazepril, captopril, enalapril, fosinopril, lisinopril, quinapril

GENERAL DESCRIPTION
The ACE inhibitor ramipril blocks an enzyme in the body that is essential for the production of a substance that causes blood vessels to constrict. Because it relaxes arterial walls, thereby lowering blood pressure and putting less stress on the heart, ramipril is prescribed for mild-to-severe high blood pressure (hypertension). For further information, see Angiotensin-Converting Enzyme (ACE) Inhibitors.

PRECAUTIONS

WARNING
Get medical attention immediately if you notice swelling of your face, tongue, or vocal cords or have difficulty swallowing or breathing; this reaction can be life threatening.

This drug should not be taken during pregnancy because it has been associated with death of the fetus and newborn baby.

SPECIAL INFORMATION
- Ramipril causes an increase in blood levels of potassium. Do not use potassium-rich products, including salt substitutes and low-salt milk, without first consulting your doctor. Potassium levels could rise dangerously, which could lead to heart-rhythm problems.
- Do not abruptly stop taking this drug. Your doctor may tell you to reduce the dosage gradually.

TARGET AILMENTS

High blood pressure

Congestive heart failure following heart attack

SIDE EFFECTS

NOT SERIOUS
- Dry, persistent cough; headache; fatigue; nausea; diarrhea; loss of sense of taste; temporary skin rash; low blood pressure or dizziness on suddenly rising or changing position

CALL YOUR DOCTOR IF THESE EFFECTS BECOME BOTHERSOME.

SERIOUS
- Fainting; persistent skin rash; joint pain; drowsiness; numbness and tingling; abdominal pain; vomiting; diarrhea; chest pain; heart palpitation; jaundice (yellowing of skin or eyes)

CALL YOUR DOCTOR RIGHT AWAY.

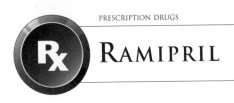

Rx RANITIDINE

VITAL STATISTICS

DRUG CLASS
Antiulcer Drugs [Histamine H_2 Blockers]

BRAND NAMES
Rx: Zantac 150, Zantac 300, Tritec
OTC: Zantac 75

OTHER DRUGS IN THIS CLASS
lansoprazole, omeprazole, sucralfate
Histamine H_2 Blockers: cimetidine, famotidine, nizatidine

GENERAL DESCRIPTION
Ranitidine is used primarily to treat ulcers of the stomach and duodenum (upper intestine). It is also prescribed for Zollinger-Ellison syndrome, gastroesophageal reflux (in which stomach acid flows backward into the esophagus), and other conditions involving the overproduction of stomach acid. In some cases, ranitidine is used to prevent upper gastrointestinal bleeding.

In the over-the-counter form, ranitidine is used not for ulcers but to relieve acid indigestion and heartburn. Although the OTC version is a lower dose of ranitidine than the prescription form, essentially the same interactions apply, though the side effects are milder.

Belonging to the subclass of antiulcer drugs known as histamine H_2 blockers, ranitidine works by blocking the effects of the chemical compound histamine in the stomach, thereby reducing the secretion of the digestive juice hydrochloric acid. For more information on side effects and possible drug interactions, see Antiulcer Drugs.

PRECAUTIONS

SPECIAL INFORMATION
- You may need to take this drug for several days before experiencing any relief from stomach pain.
- Tell your doctor if you have a history of kidney or liver disease.
- If you are also using antacids for relief from ulcer pain, take the antacid at least two hours before or after taking ranitidine.
- Because this drug may cause dizziness or drowsiness, you may need to restrict your driving or involvement in potentially hazardous activities.
- Avoid this drug if pregnant or nursing.
- Ranitidine may cause a false-positive result in urine protein tests.

TARGET AILMENTS
Duodenal ulcer
Gastric ulcer
Upper gastrointestinal bleeding associated with gastric ulcer or duodenal ulcer, or with gastritis
Zollinger-Ellison syndrome
Multiple endocrine neoplasia
Other conditions characterized by an overproduction of stomach acid
Gastroesophageal reflux
Acid indigestion and heartburn (OTC)

CONTINUED

RANITIDINE

POSSIBLE INTERACTIONS

Alcohol: significantly increased concentration of alcohol in the blood.

Antacids: decreased absorption of ranitidine into the body; avoid taking antacids within two hours of taking ranitidine.

Anticoagulants, including warfarin: decreased elimination of warfarin from the body, possibly resulting in bleeding complications.

Diazepam: inhibited absorption of diazepam into the body.

Glipizide, glyburide, theophylline: increased effects of these drugs.

Itraconazole, ketoconazole: decreased absorption of these drugs.

Sucralfate: decreased absorption of ranitidine.

SIDE EFFECTS

NOT SERIOUS

- Constipation or diarrhea
- Dizziness
- Drowsiness
- Headache
- Nausea or vomiting
- Skin rash
- Blurred vision (less common)
- Joint or muscle pain (less common)
- Hair loss (less common)
- Decreased libido or sexual ability (less common)
- Swelling of breasts or breast soreness in women or men (less common)

CALL YOUR DOCTOR IF THESE SYMPTOMS PERSIST OR BECOME BOTHERSOME.

SERIOUS

- Allergic reaction (burning, redness, or swelling of the skin)
- Irregular heartbeat (rare)
- Tightness in the chest (rare)
- Confusion (rare)
- Combined weakness, fever, and sore throat (rare)
- Unusual bleeding or bruising (rare)
- Unusual fatigue or weakness (rare)

CALL YOUR DOCTOR IMMEDIATELY IF YOU EXPERIENCE THESE SYMPTOMS.

Red Clover

LATIN NAME
Trifolium pratense

Vital Statistics

GENERAL DESCRIPTION

The medicinal parts of the perennial plant red clover are the red or purple ball-shaped flowers, which are gathered between May and September. Red clover has been used medicinally in many parts of the world. It was prescribed as an expectorant in China and as a cure for asthma in Russia. Other cultures have used it to treat skin sores and eye irritations, and as a diuretic. Herbalists today prescribe red clover for skin ailments, indigestion, and coughs. It is an anti-inflammatory agent and also, as an expectorant, helps remove excess mucus from the lungs. In addition, the herb appears to act like the hormone estrogen and may help women with menopausal symptoms. For visual characteristics of red clover, see the Color Guide to Prescription Drugs and Herbs.

PREPARATIONS

Over the counter:

Available in dried bulk and tincture.

At home:

Infusion: Steep covered 1 to 3 tsp dried flower tops in 1 cup boiling water for 10 to 15 minutes. Drink up to 3 cups a day.

Compress: Soak a clean cloth in the infusion and apply to the skin.

Consult a practitioner for the dosage appropriate for you and your specific condition.

Precautions

WARNING

Do not use red clover if you are pregnant, because of its estrogen-like behavior.

Avoid red clover if you have estrogen-dependent cancer or if you have a history of heart disease, stroke, or thrombophlebitis.

If you are taking birth-control pills, consult your doctor before using red clover.

Do not give to children under the age of two. Older children and people over 65 should start with a low dose and increase as needed.

SPECIAL INFORMATION

Red clover contains four antitumor compounds among its chemical components, and some herbalists believe it may find a use in combination with more powerful drugs to treat cancers that are not aggravated by estrogen.

POSSIBLE INTERACTIONS

Combining red clover with other herbs may necessitate a lower dosage.

TARGET AILMENTS

Take internally for:

Coughs; bronchitis; whooping cough; indigestion; menopausal symptoms

Use internally and externally for:

Skin problems such as eczema and psoriasis

SIDE EFFECTS

SERIOUS

- Stomachaches
- Diarrhea

Overdoses may produce these symptoms. Discontinue if you experience them.

RED RASPBERRY

LATIN NAME
Rubus idaeus

VITAL STATISTICS

GENERAL DESCRIPTION

The berry of this biennial bush is commonly used in gourmet desserts, but herbalists value the leaves. These have high concentrations of tannin, a chemical that herbalists believe is effective in treating diarrhea, nausea, vomiting, and morning sickness in pregnancy. It is also thought that tannin, an astringent substance, helps prevent miscarriages and, during labor, strengthens contractions, checks hemorrhaging, and reduces labor pains; you should not, however, use red raspberry for this purpose at home. Red raspberry leaves are included in several herbal pregnancy formulas sold in the United States. The herb is also used as a gargle for sore throats. For visual characteristics of red raspberry, see the Color Guide to Prescription Drugs and Herbs.

PREPARATIONS

Over the counter:

Red raspberry is available as dried leaves or berries, and as a tincture.

At home:

INFUSION: Use 1 to 2 tsp dried leaves or berries per cup of boiling water. Steep covered for 10 to 15 minutes. Drink cold and as desired. During pregnancy, steep ½ oz dried leaves with 1 pt boiling water for 3 to 5 minutes and drink warm, 1 pt per day. For children, dilute the infusion with more water.

Consult a qualified practitioner for the dosage appropriate for you and the specific condition being treated.

PRECAUTIONS

SPECIAL INFORMATION

- Pregnant women should take red raspberry only with the consent and under the supervision of a physician.
- Animal tests suggest that red raspberry may reduce levels of glucose (blood sugar) in animals and hence may help in the management of diabetes.

POSSIBLE INTERACTIONS

Combining red raspberry with other herbs may necessitate a lower dosage.

TARGET AILMENTS
Morning sickness; threatened miscarriage; problems arising during labor
Diarrhea
Mouth ulcers; bleeding gums

SIDE EFFECTS

NOT SERIOUS

MAY CAUSE STOMACH UPSET OR DIARRHEA IF THE RECOMMENDED DOSE IS EXCEEDED.

R

RELAFEN

VITAL STATISTICS

DRUG CLASS

Analgesics [Nonsteroidal Anti-Inflammatory Drugs (NSAIDs)]

GENERIC NAME

nabumetone

GENERAL DESCRIPTION

Relafen is the brand-name form of nabumetone, which is an NSAID—a type of pain reliever acting at the site of pain. Because it reduces inflammation, it is used to treat rheumatoid arthritis and osteoarthritis. It may be prescribed when aspirin or acetaminophen is not effective. Since Relafen is a prodrug, meaning it exhibits pharmaceutical action only after the body changes it to another form, it must first be metabolized by the liver. See also Nonsteroidal Anti-Inflammatory Drugs (NSAIDs). For visual characteristics, see the Color Guide to Prescription Drugs and Herbs.

PRECAUTIONS

SPECIAL INFORMATION

- Do not use if you are allergic to NSAIDs or to aspirin. It may cause bronchoconstriction or anaphylaxis.
- Consult your doctor before using if you have asthma, peptic ulcer, enteritis, high blood pressure, bleeding problems, or impaired liver or kidney function.

TARGET AILMENTS

Inflammation, especially if related to osteoarthritis and rheumatoid arthritis

POSSIBLE INTERACTIONS

Antipsychotic drugs (chlorpromazine and clozapine): decreased effects of these drugs.

Benzodiazepines (such as chlordiazepoxide, diazepam, and oxazepam): decreased effects of these drugs.

Tricyclic antidepressants (such as amitriptyline): decreased effects of these drugs.

SIDE EFFECTS

NOT SERIOUS

- Dizziness; drowsiness; headache; abdominal pain or cramps; constipation; diarrhea; heartburn; nausea

CONSULT YOUR DOCTOR IF THESE SYMPTOMS PERSIST.

SERIOUS

- Anaphylactic reaction (hives, rash, intense itching, and trouble breathing). Seek emergency help.
- Chest pain or irregular heartbeat; trouble breathing
- Diminished hearing or ringing in the ears
- Fluid retention
- Black or tarry stools; blood in urine
- Photosensitivity
- Jaundice

DISCONTINUE USE AND CALL YOUR DOCTOR IMMEDIATELY.

R

Rhus toxicodendron

LATIN NAME
Rhus toxicodendron

Vital Statistics

GENERAL DESCRIPTION

This vinelike shrub, also known as poison ivy, grows throughout North America and is well known for the itchy red rash its oil can cause on the skin. The medicinal history of its leaves and stalk began in the late 18th century, when it was used to treat conditions such as paralysis and rheumatism. The effects of its undilute form can range from a rash to nausea, fever, delirium, swollen glands, and ulcers in the oral cavity. For this reason, homeopathic practitioners use *Rhus toxicodendron,* or *Rhus tox,* as it is also called, to treat conditions that may be accompanied by a fever, restlessness, and swollen glands.

Rhus tox is prepared from plants gathered at night, when the oil is said to be at its most potent. The leaves and stalks are pounded to a pulp and mixed with alcohol, then strained and diluted. For more information on homeopathic medicine, see page 14.

PREPARATIONS

Rhus tox is available over the counter in various potencies, both in liquid and in tablet form, at selected stores and pharmacies. Consult your homeopathic physician for more precise information.

Precautions

SPECIAL INFORMATION

- Only the patient should touch the pills. If tablets are spilled, throw them away.
- The mouth should be clear of flavors 15 minutes before and after taking a remedy, and strong flavors and aromas, such as coffee and heavy perfume, should be avoided for the duration of treatment.

TARGET AILMENTS

- Arthritis with stiffness that is worse in the morning and is lessened by movement
- Backache with stiffness along the spine
- Bursitis
- Carpal tunnel syndrome
- Eye inflammation with swelling and itching, and with sticky matter between the eyelids
- Genital herpes
- Hamstring injury
- Influenza with painful joints
- Headaches
- Hives that itch, sting, and intensify after they are scratched
- Joint, back pains from overexertion
- Impetigo
- Poison ivy
- Sprains with stiffness
- Toothaches

SIDE EFFECTS

None expected

R

RISPERIDONE

VITAL STATISTICS

DRUG CLASS
Antipsychotic Drugs

BRAND NAME
Risperidal

GENERAL DESCRIPTION
Risperidone, introduced in 1994, is used to treat the symptoms of severe psychotic disorders, including chronic schizophrenia. The drug apparently acts by blocking specific receptors to the neurotransmitters dopamine and serotonin, thereby restoring a more normal mood and more normal thought processes.

Risperidone affects a wider range of symptoms than other medications that have been used to treat schizophrenia. Symptoms that risperidone has been shown to improve include hallucinations, delusions, apathy, withdrawal, and poor impulse control. This drug also has less potential for harmful or bothersome side effects such as movement disorders, apparently because of its more narrowly targeted effect on electrochemical receptors in the nervous system. For visual characteristics, see the Color Guide to Prescription Drugs and Herbs.

TARGET AILMENTS

Psychotic disorders

PRECAUTIONS

WARNING
An overdose of risperidone can be dangerous, causing effects such as low blood pressure, rapid heartbeat, difficulty breathing, and seizure. Contact a poison control center or seek emergency care if you've taken more than the amount prescribed. Risperidone can cause drowsiness and can significantly lower your ability to concentrate; restrict your activities as necessary, and do not drive or operate dangerous machinery until you know how the medicine affects you.

This drug can cause permanent tardive dyskinesia (involuntary muscle movements), although it is less likely to do so than previously available antischizophrenia drugs. If you notice any involuntary movement, contact your doctor immediately.

Another possible side effect of risperidone is neuroleptic malignant syndrome, with symptoms including high fever, stiff muscles, increased sweating, high or low blood pressure, and fast or irregular heartbeat.

Risperidone increases production of the hormone prolactin in the body. Because some cancers need prolactin for growth, this drug should be used with caution by anyone with a history of breast cancer.

Contact your doctor if you notice any abnormal bleeding, tendency to bruise, or increased infections while taking risperidone.

SPECIAL INFORMATION
- Before taking risperidone, inform your doctor if you have any decreased liver or kidney function, are allergic to risperidone or any major tranquilizers, or have a history of heart disease, seizures, breast cancer, thyroid disorders, pituitary tumors, tardive dyskinesia, neuroleptic malignant syndrome,

R

CONTINUED

RISPERIDONE

or Parkinson's disease.
- Older people are more susceptible to the adverse effects of risperidone and must be monitored closely.
- Dosages vary; consult your doctor about any concerns you may have in order to achieve the best results.
- Risperidone tablets can be crushed and taken with or without food.
- This drug can affect some laboratory tests. Make sure any doctor you consult knows you are taking it.
- Risperidone may cause heightened sensitivity to the sun and sunlamps. Avoid overexposure, and use a sunblocking agent when you go outside.
- Consult your doctor before you decide to stop taking this drug.
- The safety and effectiveness of this drug have not been established for people under the age of 18.
- Risperidone has not been proved safe for pregnant women, and it should not be used while you are breast-feeding. Consult your doctor if you are pregnant or trying to become pregnant.

POSSIBLE INTERACTIONS

Alcohol and other central nervous system depressants (tranquilizers, sedatives, narcotics): increased sedative effect; combination should be avoided.

Antihypertensive drugs: increased antihypertensive effect.

Carbamazepine: decreased effects of risperidone.

Clozapine: increased effects of risperidone.

Levodopa, dopamine agonists: decreased effects of these drugs.

SIDE EFFECTS

NOT SERIOUS

- Anxiety; drowsiness; fatigue; headache; difficulty concentrating
- Joint pain; muscle stiffness or weakness; trembling; dizziness (temporary); weight gain; sore throat; runny nose; cough; fever
- Breast tenderness (male and female); rash, dry skin, or darkening of skin
- Heartburn, nausea, constipation, or diarrhea; lightheadedness, fast heartbeat, or fainting upon standing; increased sweating
- Reduced sexual functioning; excessive sleep; increased or decreased salivation

CONTACT YOUR DOCTOR IF THESE EFFECTS PERSIST.

SERIOUS

- Insomnia; restlessness, anxiety, or nervousness; difficulty breathing
- Severe rash; seborrhea
- Seizures; chest pain; difficulty speaking or swallowing; fainting; vision problems; menstrual changes
- Increased urination, problems in urinating
- Problems balancing or walking; aggressiveness

CALL YOUR DOCTOR RIGHT AWAY.

Ritalin

Vital Statistics

DRUG CLASS
Central Nervous System Stimulants

GENERIC NAME
methylphenidate

GENERAL DESCRIPTION
Ritalin is a brand name for the generic drug methylphenidate, a mild central nervous system (CNS) stimulant that seems to work by activating the brainstem arousal system and cerebral cortex.

For some children with an attention deficit disorder, CNS stimulation decreases motor restlessness, increases attention span, and improves concentration. In adults, it can lead to increased motor activity and mental alertness, decreased fatigue, a cheerier outlook, and mild euphoria.

Because Ritalin is an amphetamine-like drug, it can be habit forming, leading to marked tolerance and serious physical and psychological dependence. Dosages must be prescribed on an individual basis, and physician supervision is essential.

Drugs in the central nervous system stimulant class are used to treat various organic, psychological, and behavioral disorders, such as attention deficit disorders, narcolepsy, depression, and obesity. Amphetamines and cocaine are major drugs in this class. Minor drugs include appetite suppressants, bronchodilators, caffeine, and the sympathomimetics. For visual characteristics of Ritalin, see the Color Guide to Prescription Drugs and Herbs.

Precautions

SPECIAL INFORMATION
- Seek immediate medical help for overdose. Signs of overdose include rapid, pounding, or irregular heartbeat; fever and sweating; confusion, convulsions, hallucinations, agitation, delirium, vomiting, dry mouth, trembling, muscle twitching, increased blood pressure, and loss of consciousness.
- Do not take if you have had an allergic reaction to this drug; have glaucoma or motor tics; or are suffering from severe tension, agitation, anxiety, or emotional depression.
- Before taking this drug, tell your doctor if you have high blood pressure, epilepsy, angina, liver problems, or a history of alcoholism or drug dependence.
- Sleeping problems may be avoided if you take the last dose before 6 p.m.
- Although Ritalin may be the primary agent in treating attention deficit disorders, its long-term effects are unknown. Your doctor may recommend occasional drug-free periods during treatment and discontinuance of the drug after puberty.

CONTINUED

RITALIN

POSSIBLE INTERACTIONS

Anticholinergics, anticoagulants, anticonvulsants, and antidepressants (tricyclic): Ritalin may increase the effects of these drugs.

Antihypertensives, guanethidine, minoxidil, and terazosin: Ritalin may decrease the effects of these drugs.

Monoamine oxidase (MAO) inhibitors: Ritalin should not be taken within two weeks of using MAO inhibitors. Concurrent use of the two drugs could cause dangerously high blood pressure and severe convulsions.

TARGET AILMENTS

Attention deficit disorders in children

Narcolepsy (uncontrollable spells of drowsiness or sleep)

Mild to moderate depression

In the elderly, apathy and withdrawal

Chronic pain (used with other drugs)

SIDE EFFECTS

NOT SERIOUS

- Nervousness
- Trouble sleeping
- Loss of appetite
- Headache
- Dizziness
- Nausea
- Stomach pains
- Mild skin rash
- Unusual fatigue

SEE YOUR DOCTOR IF THESE SYMPTOMS PERSIST.

SERIOUS

- Severe skin rash or hives
- Irregular or fast heartbeat
- Chest pain
- Unusual bruising
- Blurred vision
- Joint pain
- Sore throat and fever
- Weight loss
- Mood or mental changes
- Abnormal behavior patterns
- Psychotic reactions

CALL YOUR DOCTOR RIGHT AWAY.

Rose

LATIN NAME
Rosa damascena

Vital Statistics

GENERAL DESCRIPTION

Rose oil, one of the most highly valued oils, is used both in aromatherapy and in making perfume. Much of the rose oil used in aromatherapy is produced from the damask rose, which originated in Syria and has been prized throughout the world for its sweet, soothing scent and the color and shape of its blooms, as well as for its therapeutic properties.

The petals and stamens are used to produce the oil, which is a pale yellow-green, oily in texture, and strongly scented. Rose water, also believed to have medicinal properties, is a by-product of this distillation process.

Rose oil is used externally to treat a wide variety of disorders, including respiratory infections, liver congestion, sensitive skin, broken capillaries, nausea, and stress. It is said to have antidepressant, antiseptic, astringent, and sedative properties and is considered a tonic for the heart, liver, stomach, and uterus.

PREPARATIONS

Rose water can be used as a gargle and rinse for sore throat and mouth ulcers. Cotton balls can be soaked in rose water and placed over the eyes to relieve fatigue and irritation.

Body oil: Combine 10 drops rose oil with 2 oz almond oil or aloe gel. Rub on the stomach, solar plexus, back of neck, temples, and other areas twice a day to relieve premenstrual or menopausal symptoms, to aid the liver, stomach, and circulatory system, or to help with skin problems.

Rose oil can be used in a diffuser to scent a room, sprinkled on a tissue and inhaled, or worn like perfume. For use in the bath, add 3 to 5 drops rose oil to the bathwater.

Precautions

SPECIAL INFORMATION

Buy rose oil only from a reputable source. Because the oil is so expensive to produce, its purity may be compromised.

TARGET AILMENTS
Insomnia
Anxiety; depression
Nervous tension
Diminished sex drive
Loss of appetite
Nausea
Menstrual pain
Cough; hay fever
Sore throat
Mouth ulcers
Skin problems
Eye and eyelid complaints (rose water only)

SIDE EFFECTS

None expected

R

Rose Hip

LATIN NAME
Rosa spp.

Vital Statistics

GENERAL DESCRIPTION

In the 1930s, herbalists discovered vitamin C in fresh rose hips—the cherry-sized bright red fruits that remain after the rose petals have fallen off. Since then, scientists have found that rose hips also contain flavonoids, which increase the body's utilization of the vitamin. For these reasons, herbalists prescribe rose hips for colds and flu. Between 45 and 90 percent of the vitamin is lost, however, when the herb is dried. Beware when buying prepackaged rose hip teas, jams, extracts, purées, and soups: While often consumed for their natural vitamin C, they may actually contain very small amounts of it. For visual characteristics of rose hip, see the Color Guide to Prescription Drugs and Herbs.

PREPARATIONS

Over the counter:

Rose hips are available as dried bulk and in tincture.

At home:

Infusion: Use 2 to 3 tsp dried, chopped hips per cup of boiling water. Steep covered for 10 minutes. Drink hot or warm, as desired.

Jam: Collect the hips after the first frost (do not use any that have been sprayed with insecticide). Place in a heavy stainless steel pan and simmer until tender, using 1 cup water to 1 lb rose hips. Rub through a fine sieve. Weigh the pulp and add 1 lb heated sugar for each lb pulp. Simmer until thick.

Consult a qualified practitioner for the dosage appropriate for you and the specific condition being treated.

Precautions

SPECIAL INFORMATION

If you have a kidney infection, consult your doctor before taking large quantities of rose hip.

POSSIBLE INTERACTIONS

Combining rose hip with other herbs may necessitate a lower dosage.

TARGET AILMENTS

Take internally for:

Colds and flu

SIDE EFFECTS

NOT SERIOUS

High doses of vitamin C may cause diarrhea and may slightly strain the kidneys.

R

ROSEMARY

LATIN NAME
Rosmarinus officinalis

VITAL STATISTICS

GENERAL DESCRIPTION

This Mediterranean evergreen shrub has silvery green leaves and pale blue flowers. Its name in Latin means "dew of the sea." Rosemary had many symbolic associations in ancient times: love, death, and loyalty, for example. Today, it is one of the best known and most used of the aromatic herbs. Planted in the garden, rosemary discourages pests. The oil is colorless to pale yellow-green, and its scent is minty in oils of good quality.

A stimulant, rosemary is thought to invigorate the whole body and help eliminate toxins. Rosemary is said to have antiseptic and diuretic properties, and as an antispasmodic agent it is considered useful in relieving the pain of premenstrual tension and cramping, asthma, and rheumatic aches and pains.

PREPARATIONS

The best-quality oil is distilled from the flowering tops. It can also be distilled from the leaves and stems before the plant flowers, but the oil will be of an inferior quality.

For nearly all uses, rosemary can be applied to the skin: Add 15 drops of oil to 2 tbsp of vegetable or nut oil, or aloe gel. To add it to the bath, use 5 to 10 drops of oil. For treating hair loss and dandruff, add 20 drops of rosemary oil to 1 oz of shampoo, or add 7 to 10 drops of oil to 2 tbsp of aloe gel, then apply to scalp and leave on overnight.

To inhale, use a room diffuser or sprinkle a few drops of oil on a tissue or handkerchief and inhale the fragrance.

PRECAUTIONS

SPECIAL INFORMATION

- Avoid using rosemary during pregnancy.
- Do not use rosemary if you have epilepsy or high blood pressure.

TARGET AILMENTS
Indigestion and gas; constipation
Liver problems; fluid retention
Asthma and bronchitis; colds and flu
Depression
Rheumatism and arthritis
Mental fatigue; poor memory
Headache (apply diluted or undiluted to areas of pain)
Hair loss; dandruff
Low blood pressure
Varicose veins (skin application)
Irregular menstrual periods and menstrual pain

SIDE EFFECTS

NONE EXPECTED

ROSEMARY

LATIN NAME
Rosmarinus officinalis

VITAL STATISTICS

GENERAL DESCRIPTION

The evergreen perennial known as rosemary has a variety of uses that go beyond its popularity as a culinary spice. Herbalists believe that rosemary leaves stimulate the circulatory and nervous systems and therefore serve as an antidepressant. The leaves are also used to treat muscle pain and are thought to contain antispasmodic chemicals that relax the smooth muscle lining of the digestive tract. In recent years, rosemary has shown promise for its antibacterial and antifungal action, and herbalists recommend that the leaves be used externally for skin infections. It is even prescribed as a gargle for bad breath.

Before the advent of refrigeration, crushed rosemary leaves were wrapped around meats to help prevent spoilage and to add flavor. Today, some herbalists suggest putting rosemary leaves in the bath for relaxation and rubbing them on the head to treat premature baldness. Recent studies indicate that rosemary may contain antioxidant chemicals that help prevent food poisoning and fight tumors.

PREPARATIONS

Over the counter:

Rosemary is available as dried bulk, in tincture, and as two types of oil, one for internal use and the other for external application.

At home:

Infusion: Use 1 tsp crushed leaves per cup of boiling water. Steep covered 10 to 15 minutes. To settle the stomach or clear a stuffy nose, drink 3 cups a day. For children younger than two years, dilute the infusion with more water.

Consult a qualified practitioner for the dosage appropriate for your specific condition.

PRECAUTIONS

☠ *WARNING*

Do not confuse rosemary oil for internal use with that intended for external application. Never ingest the external variety.

Avoid rosemary if you are pregnant.

POSSIBLE INTERACTIONS

Combining rosemary with other herbs may necessitate a lower dosage.

TARGET AILMENTS

Take internally for:

Indigestion; upper respiratory infections that require a decongestant; tension; muscle pain; sprains; rheumatism; neuralgia

Apply externally, as an antiseptic, for:

Skin infections

SIDE EFFECTS

NOT SERIOUS

Rosemary oil for internal use may cause mild stomach, kidney, and intestinal irritation, even in small doses. If you experience any of these discomforts, consult your physician.

SERIOUS

Rosemary oil, taken internally in large amounts, can be poisonous. Keep to the prescribed dosage.

RUMEX

LATIN NAME
Rumex crispus

VITAL STATISTICS

GENERAL DESCRIPTION

Also called yellow dock or curly dock, *Rumex* comes from a bitter-tasting weed with yellow roots and curled leaves that grows abundantly worldwide. Historically, people have used the root as a tonic and laxative, to cleanse the blood, and as therapy for a variety of conditions including ulcers, rheumatism, and cancer. Present-day herbalists use yellow dock for skin complaints and constipation, whereas homeopathic practitioners find *Rumex* successful in treating a specific type of dry cough. The root is gathered in late fall, pounded to a pulp, mixed with alcohol and water, then strained, diluted, and shaken in the usual manner of such remedies.

Like most homeopathic prescriptions, *Rumex* was developed as a remedy by studying the reactions of healthy individuals to doses of various strengths. The mental, emotional, and physical changes induced by *Rumex* were then cataloged. When a patient exhibits a set of symptoms that matches the cataloged symptoms brought on by *Rumex,* the homeopathic practitioner then prescribes it in an extremely dilute form. It is presumed that in this highly dilute dosage, *Rumex* can counter the symptoms that are similar to the ones it induces when it is at full strength. For more information on homeopathic medicine, see page 14.

PREPARATIONS

Rumex is available over the counter in various potencies, in both liquid and tablet form, at selected stores and pharmacies. Consult your homeopathic practitioner for more precise information.

PRECAUTIONS

SPECIAL INFORMATION

When a remedy is administered, no one but the patient should touch the pills. If tablets are spilled, throw them away.

TARGET AILMENTS

Cough with these characteristics:

- Irritation, rawness, and tickling in back of throat and larynx
- Worsening with talking, breathing cold air, and at night
- Production of mucus from back of mouth
- Burning chest pain, usually on left side, that worsens on breathing cold air
- Worsening on lying down and when uncovered in bed or when undressing
- Sore throat with irritated air passages and laryngitis that worsens when breathing cold air
- Cough provoked by any change in temperature, including cold to warm

SIDE EFFECTS

NONE EXPECTED

R

RUTA

LATIN NAME
Ruta graveolens

VITAL STATISTICS

GENERAL DESCRIPTION

Native to southern Europe, *Ruta* spread across the Continent in the wake of the Romans, who valued it for its medicinal properties. *Ruta* comes from the Greek *reuo,* meaning "to set free," an allusion to its historical popularity as a cure for numerous complaints, including headaches, coughs, and croup. Through centuries of use, this small shrub, sometimes called rue or rue bitterwort, has spread to herb gardens worldwide.

In large doses, *Ruta* has toxic properties, but homeopathic practitioners prescribe minute doses to treat conditions or injuries that may be accompanied by symptoms of weakness or a bruised sensation. The plant is collected for homeopathic use just before blossoming; it is pounded to a pulp and pressed for its juice, which is then diluted in a water-and-alcohol base.

Like most homeopathic prescriptions, *Ruta* was developed as a remedy by observation of the reactions of healthy individuals to doses of various strengths. The mental, emotional, and physical changes induced by *Ruta* were then cataloged. When a patient exhibits a set of symptoms that matches the cataloged symptoms brought on by *Ruta,* the homeopathic practitioner then prescribes it in an extremely dilute form. It is presumed that in this highly dilute dosage, *Ruta* can counter symptoms that are similar to the ones it induces when it is at full strength. For more information on homeopathic medicine, see page 14.

SIDE EFFECTS

NONE EXPECTED

PREPARATIONS

Ruta is available over the counter in various potencies, in both liquid and tablet form, at selected stores and pharmacies. Consult your homeopathic practitioner for more precise information.

PRECAUTIONS

SPECIAL INFORMATION

- When a remedy is administered, no one but the patient should touch the pills. If tablets are spilled, throw them away.
- The mouth should be clear of flavors 15 minutes before and after taking a remedy, and strong flavors and aromas, such as coffee, camphor, and heavily scented perfumes, should be avoided for the duration of treatment.

TARGET AILMENTS
Carpal tunnel syndrome
Eyestrain caused by overwork and accompanied by heat and pain
Sciatica
Groin strain
Sprains with pain and a bruised sensation
Tennis elbow
Injuries to tendons and cartilage

SAFFLOWER FLOWER

LATIN NAME
Carthamus tinctorius

VITAL STATISTICS

GENERAL DESCRIPTION

Herbalists prescribe safflower flower, whose Chinese name means "red flower," for several conditions related to the flow of blood through the body. In a clinical trial, the herb seemed effective in treating the swelling and bruising that result from acute sprains.

Safflower flower is harvested in several Chinese provinces throughout June and July, when the color of the blossoms changes from yellow to red; traditionalists prefer picking safflower flower on the morning of a cloudy day, before the dew has dried. In addition to having a fresh red color, the best safflower flowers feel soft and have long petals. Practitioners characterize this herb as acrid and warm.

Chinese medicine takes a holistic approach to healthcare, fashioning remedies to treat the entire being as well as the specific parts or areas. Single herbs may be used alone or in combination with other herbs to prevent and combat disease, which is thought to arise from disturbances in the flow of a bodily energy called chi (pronounced "chee") and blood, or from a lack of balance in the complementary states of yin and yang.

PREPARATIONS

Dried safflower flower is available in bulk at Chinese pharmacies, Asian markets, and some Western health food stores. You can also obtain it in tablet form. The herb is frequently sold in liniments for treating bruises and injuries.

COMBINATIONS: Safflower flower is mixed with cnidium root for chest pain. It is combined with dong quai and sappan wood to make a preparation for treating the pain and swelling associated with trauma. A mixture with Chinese foxglove root, red peony root, and forsythia fruit is prescribed for pain, redness, and swelling of the eyes. Safflower flower and groomwell root are combined into a decoction and taken internally or used externally to treat boils, carbuncles, and childhood measles.

PRECAUTIONS

WARNING

Do not use safflower flower if you are pregnant, because there is evidence that the herb stimulates the uterus.

TARGET AILMENTS

Take internally for:

Delayed menstruation; poor blood circulation; blood clots; stabbing chest pain

Apply externally for:

Burns, bruises, and other injuries to the skin

Use both internally and externally for:

Sores and carbuncles; measles in its early stages

SIDE EFFECTS

NONE EXPECTED

S

SAFFRON

LATIN NAME
Crocus sativus

VITAL STATISTICS

GENERAL DESCRIPTION

Saffron is one of the most expensive herbs, with prices ranging from $55 to $250 an ounce. The price is high because the valuable components are not the leaves or the violet petals but the three tiny, orange, antenna-like stigmas inside the flower of this member of the crocus family. An ingredient of the stigmas known as crocetin is the active agent. To produce one ounce of saffron, you would need to harvest almost 5,000 flowers. Even if you have the energy, you should never try to harvest your own saffron; you might use the wrong kind of crocus.

Herbalists prescribe saffron primarily in conjunction with the conventional treatment for high blood pressure and heart disease. Laboratory studies have indicated that injections of crocetin may decrease cholesterol levels in animals. Some herbalists believe that saffron may increase the amount of oxygen in the blood; the oxygen, in turn, may slow the growth of artery-clogging plaque deposits. Because crocetin is also thought to stimulate the uterus and the digestive process, practitioners also recommend saffron for digestion and to promote menstruation.

S

PREPARATIONS

Over the counter:

Saffron is available as dried powder and dried stigmas.

At home:

INFUSION: Place 12 to 15 stigmas in 1 cup boiling water. Steep covered 10 minutes. Drink up to 1 cup a day.

Consult a qualified practitioner for the dosage appropriate for you and the specific condition being treated.

PRECAUTIONS

WARNING

In large amounts, saffron is highly toxic. Take the herb only in the recommended dosage, in consultation with your practitioner.

Do not use saffron to induce an abortion. Women have died as a result of overdose in an attempt to end their pregnancies.

Do not give saffron to children under two years of age. For older children and adults over 65, begin with low-strength preparations and increase gradually.

Do not attempt to harvest your own saffron; one species is toxic.

SPECIAL INFORMATION

Use of this herb by children for more than seven to 10 days should be done in conjunction with a healthcare practitioner.

POSSIBLE INTERACTIONS

Combining saffron with other herbs may necessitate a lower dosage.

TARGET AILMENTS
Take internally for:
High cholesterol; high blood pressure
Atherosclerosis
Indigestion; delayed menstruation

SIDE EFFECTS

NONE EXPECTED

SAGE

LATIN NAME
Salvia officinalis

VITAL STATISTICS

GENERAL DESCRIPTION

The scientific name of sage, *Salvia*, derives from the Latin for "to save," underscoring the herb's early reputation as a cure-all. Modern herbalists believe that sage contains an aromatic oil that reduces excessive perspiration and the night sweats associated with such diseases as tuberculosis. In addition, the oil, which is antiseptic, combines with another component, the astringent tannin, to relieve sore throats or gums. For visual characteristics of sage, see the Color Guide to Prescription Drugs and Herbs.

PREPARATIONS

Over the counter:
Sage is available as tincture, prepared tea, or dried or fresh leaves.

At home:

INFUSION: Steep covered 2 to 3 tsp leaves per cup of boiling water for 10 minutes. Drink 3 cups a day, hot or cold, or use as a wash for bacterial infections in wounds.

COMPRESS: Soak a clean cloth in the infusion and apply to insect bites.

TINCTURE: Take 1 to 1½ tsp three times daily with water or juice.

MOUTHWASH: Add 3 tsp leaves to 1 pt water, boil, and let stand covered for 15 minutes. Gargle the warm liquid three times daily.

FRESH: Apply fresh sage leaves to minor cuts or scrapes before washing and bandaging.

PRECAUTIONS

WARNING

Sage can cause convulsions in high doses. However, the heat of cooking or preparing an infusion reduces toxicity.

SPECIAL INFORMATION

- Do not use if you are pregnant or nursing.
- Sage oil should not be ingested.
- Use dilute preparations for children under 12 and adults over 65. Use of this herb by children for more than seven to 10 days should be done in conjunction with a healthcare practitioner.

POSSIBLE INTERACTIONS

Combining sage with other herbs may necessitate a lower dosage.

TARGET AILMENTS

Take internally for:

Indigestion; gas; nausea; to stem lactation or reduce the night sweats of menopause

Use as a mouthwash or gargle for:

Mouth and throat infections

Apply externally for:

Bacterial infections in wounds; insect bites

SIDE EFFECTS

NOT SERIOUS

- Drinking the tea may inflame the lips and mouth lining

DISCONTINUE USE IF THESE EFFECTS ARE BOTHERSOME.

Salmeterol

Vital Statistics

DRUG CLASS
Bronchodilators

BRAND NAME
Serevent

GENERAL DESCRIPTION
Used principally as a treatment for chronic asthma, salmeterol opens the airways and causes the bronchial smooth muscle to relax, thereby increasing the capacity of the lungs and relieving spasm. This drug is also helpful for preventing bronchospasm caused either by asthma or by exercise. It is not recommended for acute asthma, since its onset of action is longer than that of other bronchodilators.

Salmeterol is available as an oral inhalant by prescription only and exerts its action locally in the lungs. It is sometimes used in conjunction with short-acting inhaled bronchodilators such as albuterol. For more information, including possible drug interactions and other important facts about this class of medications, see Bronchodilators.

Precautions

WARNING
Do not take salmeterol if your asthma is getting worse or you have acute symptoms; people with worsening asthma should be treated with short-acting inhaled bronchodilators, possibly with oral steroids. You should also avoid using this drug if you have had an allergic reaction to it in any form or dosage before, if you have an irregular heart rhythm, or if you have taken an MAO inhibitor within the past two weeks.

SPECIAL INFORMATION
Tell your doctor before starting this drug if you have very high blood pressure, diabetes, a history of a heart disorder, or a history of convulsions.

TARGET AILMENTS

Asthma

Exercise-induced bronchospasm (prevention)

SIDE EFFECTS

NOT SERIOUS

- Headache; dizziness; abdominal pain; nausea; diarrhea; dryness or irritation of the mouth or throat; muscle cramps; nervousness; trembling

CALL YOUR DOCTOR IF THESE PROBLEMS PERSIST.

SERIOUS

- Bronchospasm (shortness of breath, tightness in chest, wheezing)
- Swelling of face, lips, or eyelids; hives; fast or pounding heartbeat
- Respiratory arrest (rare)

CONTACT YOUR DOCTOR IMMEDIATELY.

Sang Ju Yin Pian

Vital Statistics

ENGLISH NAME
Mulberry Chrysanthemum Medicine Pills

ALSO SOLD AS
Sang Chu Yin Pien, Sang Ju Gan Mao Pian

GENERAL DESCRIPTION
Sang Ju Yin Pian is used in the early stages of disease to treat a cold or flu with stuffy head or chest, watery eyes, fever, sore throat, and headache. If taken soon enough it can sometimes ward off the cold or flu, but the remedy is less effective once the patient has entered the fever and achy stage.

Chinese medicine takes a holistic approach to healthcare, fashioning remedies to treat the entire being as well as the specific parts or areas. Precise combinations of herbs are used to prevent and combat disease, which is thought to arise from disturbances in the flow of a bodily energy called chi (pronounced "chee") and blood, or from a lack of balance in the complementary states of yin and yang. A patent formula, *Sang Ju Yin Pian* is made by using a standardized combination of herbs and method of preparation.

INGREDIENTS
mulberry leaf, chrysanthemum, forsythia, bitter almond, balloonflower, phragmitis, licorice, mint

PREPARATIONS
This formula is available under the various names mentioned above at many Chinese pharmacies and Oriental grocery stores.

Target Ailments

Early stage of cold or flu with symptoms such as headache, chest or nose congestion, sneezing, watery eyes, sore throat, and fever

Side Effects

None expected

SAN SHE DAN CHUAN BEI YE

VITAL STATISTICS

ENGLISH NAME
Three Snake Gallbladder Fritillaria Liquid

GENERAL DESCRIPTION
San She Dan Chuan Bei Ye is used to treat phlegm or mucus conditions that are quite stubborn. This formula is appropriate for all sorts of coughs, including those associated with asthma, and for emphysema. Because of its greater strength, *San She Dan Chuan Bei Ye* is generally used only after other remedies have failed.

Chinese medicine takes a holistic approach to healthcare, fashioning remedies to treat the entire being as well as the specific parts or areas. Precise combinations of herbs are used to prevent and combat disease, which is thought to arise from disturbances in the flow of a bodily energy called chi (pronounced "chee") and blood, or from a lack of balance in the complementary states of yin and yang. A patent formula, *San She Dan Chuan Bei Ye* is made by using a standardized combination of herbs and method of preparation.

INGREDIENTS
fritillaria, bitter almond, snake gallbladder, honey

PREPARATIONS
This formula is available at many Chinese pharmacies and Oriental grocery stores. It is sold in small vials of liquid that are drunk through a tiny straw.

TARGET AILMENTS

Cough with phlegm

Bronchitis

Emphysema

Asthma with lots of phlegm

SIDE EFFECTS

NONE EXPECTED

SARGASSUM SEAWEED

LATIN NAME
Sargassum pallidum

VITAL STATISTICS

GENERAL DESCRIPTION

More commonly known as seaweed, sargassum is collected from the coastal provinces of China and from other coastlines around the world. Its high content of the element iodine makes it effective in treating a variety of ailments related to the thyroid gland. It also promotes urination and is traditionally prescribed for the pain of hernia. In laboratory trials, the cholesterol levels of rats fell when they were given sargassum, and large doses of sargassum have lowered blood pressure in dogs and rabbits. In other tests, extracts of the herb inhibited the growth of fungi. Practitioners of Chinese medicine characterize sargassum as a cold, salty herb.

Chinese medicine takes a holistic approach to healthcare, fashioning remedies to treat the entire being as well as the specific parts or areas. Single herbs may be used alone or in combination with other herbs to prevent and combat disease, which is thought to arise from disturbances in the flow of a bodily energy called chi (pronounced "chee") and blood, or from a lack of balance in the complementary states of yin and yang.

PREPARATIONS

Sargassum is available in bulk at Chinese pharmacies, Asian markets, and Western health food stores.

COMBINATIONS: A mixture of sargassum, silkworm, prunella, and scrophularia is used for goiter and scrofula. The same symptoms can also be treated with a preparation of sargassum and licorice; some traditional texts suggest that these two herbs are incompatible, although animal experiments have shown no adverse reactions. A combination of sargassum and water chestnut is prescribed for the lung disease silicosis. For information on dosages and other preparations, consult a qualified practitioner.

PRECAUTIONS

SPECIAL INFORMATION

Sargassum's ability to stimulate the excretion of fluids from the body makes it useful for individuals trying to lose weight. The herb is not appropriate for all weight-loss patients, however, because its impact on the thyroid gland affects the metabolism rate. Consult a practitioner of Chinese medicine before using this herb.

TARGET AILMENTS

Take internally for:

- Nodules in the neck, including goiter and other thyroid disorders
- Scrofula (a form of tuberculosis)
- Inadequate urination
- Edema (retention of body fluids)
- Pain from hernia
- Swollen, painful testes

SIDE EFFECTS

NONE EXPECTED

S

SASSAFRAS

LATIN NAME
Sassafras albidum

VITAL STATISTICS

GENERAL DESCRIPTION

The root bark of this native American tree yields a tea with not only a pleasant taste but also a wide reputation as a tonic. It contains a volatile oil once prized as a flavoring for root beer and other beverages. Laboratory tests in the 1960s, however, revealed that the main component of the oil, safrole, is carcinogenic in rats and mice, and the U.S. Food and Drug Administration has prohibited the internal use of sassafras containing safrole. Until the ban, the herb was widely used for a variety of ailments, including colic, rheumatism, and poison ivy. The essential oil of the root bark has recently been found to have mild antiseptic action and is still used to combat external infections.

PREPARATIONS

Over the counter:
Sassafras is available as an essential oil and tincture and as fresh or dried root bark, although internal use is prohibited.

At home:
LINIMENT: Mix 1 oz each of the tinctures of sassafras, prickly ash, cayenne, myrrh, and camphor with 3 oz water; shake well and apply to areas afflicted by rheumatism.
Consult a qualified practitioner for the dosage appropriate for you and the specific condition being treated.

PRECAUTIONS

SPECIAL INFORMATION

This herb should not be used with children unless it is specifically prescribed by a health-care practitioner who is knowledgeable about herbs.

POSSIBLE INTERACTIONS

Combining sassafras with other herbs may necessitate a lower dosage.

TARGET AILMENTS

The only approved applications are external. Use as liniment for:

Rheumatism

Use a compress for:

Skin irritations such as acne, boils, poison ivy, and poison oak

SIDE EFFECTS

NONE EXPECTED IF USED EXTERNALLY.

SAW PALMETTO

LATIN NAME
Serenoa repens

VITAL STATISTICS

GENERAL DESCRIPTION

An extract made from the berries of this shrub is used to strengthen and treat problems with the male reproductive system. It is particularly recommended for benign enlargement of the prostate gland, which is indicated by urination difficulties and can lead to bladder infections and kidney problems. Common among men over 50, the condition is thought to be caused by an accumulation of a testosterone derivative called dihydrotestosterone; saw palmetto appears to block the production of this chemical.

Saw palmetto has also been used as an expectorant, diuretic, tonic, antiseptic, sedative, and digestive aid. It is native to the sandy coast of the southeastern United States, where the plant reaches a height of about 10 feet. For visual characteristics of saw palmetto, see the Color Guide to Prescription Drugs and Herbs.

PREPARATIONS

Over the counter:

Available as fresh or dried berries and in powder or capsule form. Gel capsules are preferable to tea or tincture, because the active ingredients of the herb are fat soluble and do not dissolve well in water.

At home:

INFUSION: If you have fresh berries, prepare by steeping covered ½ to 1 tsp berries per cup of boiling water for 10 minutes. Drink 6 oz, two or three times a day.

DECOCTION: Add ½ to 1 tsp dried berries to 1 cup water, bring to a boil, and simmer covered for 5 minutes. Drink three times daily.

TINCTURE: Drink ¼ to ½ tsp in water two or three times daily.

Consult a practitioner for the dosage appropriate for you and your condition.

PRECAUTIONS

WARNING

Do not substitute saw palmetto for medical treatment. Although this herb is thought to be effective for treating an enlarged prostate, it has no known effect against prostate cancer. Because the symptoms of prostate enlargement and prostate cancer are similar, men should see a doctor when they have urological symptoms such as urine retention, dribbling, and passage of blood in the urine.

SPECIAL INFORMATION

This herb should not be used with children unless it is prescribed by a healthcare practitioner who is knowledgeable about herbs.

POSSIBLE INTERACTIONS

Combining saw palmetto with other herbs may necessitate a lower dosage.

TARGET AILMENTS

Use internally for treatment of:

- Benign prostatic hyperplasia (enlargement of the prostate gland)
- Nasal congestion
- Bronchitis
- Coughs due to colds

SIDE EFFECTS

NONE EXPECTED

SCALLION

LATIN NAME
Allium fistulosum

VITAL STATISTICS

GENERAL DESCRIPTION

The white bulb and green parts of scallions, or spring onions, are prescribed to improve digestion and help regulate the metabolism rate. They affect the body in a manner similar to garlic but are often preferred because of their less powerful odor. In a clinical trial, a combination of scallions, pinellia root, and ginger juice, given as an enema, seemed useful in treating acute mastitis (breast inflammation). The essential oils of scallions seemed to inhibit the spread of staphylococcus, streptococcus, and other types of bacteria in trials with diseased persons. Traditional Chinese medicine characterizes the herb as acrid and warm.

Chinese medicine takes a holistic approach to healthcare, fashioning remedies to treat the entire being as well as the specific parts or areas. Single herbs may be used alone or in combination with other herbs to prevent and combat disease, which is thought to arise from disturbances in the flow of a bodily energy called chi (pronounced "chee") and blood, or from a lack of balance in the complementary states of yin and yang.

PREPARATIONS

Over the counter:

Scallions are available at Chinese pharmacies as well as at Asian and Western food markets. You can also obtain tablets containing the herb.

At home:

Tea: Chop two to five scallions and steep in a cup of boiling water. Top the brew with honey and drink at the first signs of chills and fever.

Poultice: Mix chopped scallions with honey, wrap in a cloth; apply to relieve sores and abscesses.

Combinations: The herb is prepared with soybeans for chills, fever, and nasal congestion. For more information on appropriate preparations and doses, check with a Chinese medicine practitioner.

PRECAUTIONS

WARNING

Do not use scallions if you are sweating profusely, since the herb promotes sweating.

Some traditional Chinese authorities warn against ingesting mixtures of honey and scallions, but others recommend the use of such preparations.

TARGET AILMENTS

Take internally for:

Chills and fevers

Nasal congestion

Abdominal pain and distention

Apply externally for:

Sores and abscesses

SIDE EFFECTS

None expected

S

SCHISANDRA

LATIN NAME
Schisandra chinensis

VITAL STATISTICS

GENERAL DESCRIPTION

The fruit of schisandra, a member of the magnolia family, is valued for its medicinal properties. Look for shiny, purplish red fruit that is thick, fleshy, and oily. Chinese medicine practitioners prescribe it for a variety of disorders as varied as allergic skin reactions, insomnia, and hepatitis. Western herbalists often use it as a tonic to help the body resist physical, biological, and environmental stresses. Traditional Chinese medicine characterizes the fruit as sour and slightly warm.

Chinese medicine takes a holistic approach to healthcare, fashioning remedies to treat the entire being as well as the specific parts or areas. Single herbs may be used alone or in combination with other herbs to prevent and combat disease, which is thought to arise from disturbances in the flow of a bodily energy called chi (pronounced "chee") and blood, or from a lack of balance in the complementary states of yin and yang.

PREPARATIONS

Dried schisandra fruit is available at Chinese pharmacies, Asian markets, and some Western health food stores. The fruit also comes in tablet form. It is sometimes prepared in wine as a tonic.

COMBINATIONS: Schisandra is mixed with zizyphus and Chinese foxglove root to treat insomnia, irritability, and forgetfulness. When combined with Asian ginseng and ophiopogon tuber, it is prescribed for shortness of breath accompanied by coughing and thirst, and for irregular heartbeat or palpitations.

For additional information, consult a Chinese medicine practitioner.

PRECAUTIONS

SPECIAL INFORMATION

- The herb is not recommended for use in the early stages of coughs or rashes.
- Overdose symptoms include restlessness, insomnia, or difficulties in breathing.

TARGET AILMENTS

Take internally for:

Chronic coughs and wheezing; asthma

Allergic skin reactions; irritated skin

Excessive sweating

Insomnia; irritability; forgetfulness; dream-disturbed sleep; general lethargy

Irregular heartbeat with coughing and thirst, palpitations, shortness of breath

Nocturnal emission; vaginal discharge; frequent urination

SIDE EFFECTS

NOT SERIOUS

- Heartburn

DISCONTINUE USE AND CALL YOUR PRACTITIONER.

Rx SCOPOLAMINE

VITAL STATISTICS

DRUG CLASS
Antinausea Drugs

BRAND NAME
Transderm-Scōp

GENERAL DESCRIPTION
Scopolamine is well known for its ability to prevent the nausea, dizziness, and vomiting of motion sickness. In eye drop form it is used to aid in eye examinations and to prevent eye inflammation. The motion-sickness medication comes in the form of a transdermal patch that releases a controlled therapeutic dose of scopolamine.

PRECAUTIONS

☠ ***WARNING***
Do not use scopolamine if you have myasthenia gravis, narrow-angle glaucoma, cardiovascular disease, intestinal obstruction, stomach bloating, or difficulty urinating.

Remove the patch or stop taking the drug and contact your doctor immediately if you have pain and reddening of the eyes with dilated pupils and blurry vision. These may be symptoms of narrow-angle glaucoma.

SPECIAL INFORMATION
- Use of the patch for longer than 72 hours may cause withdrawal symptoms such as nausea, vomiting, and headache.
- Wash your hands after handling the patch to avoid contact with the eyes, which can cause pupil dilation and blurred vision.
- If you are pregnant or nursing, consult your doctor before using scopolamine.
- Scopolamine may cause drowsiness and disorientation. Do not drive until you learn how this medicine affects you.

POSSIBLE INTERACTIONS
This is a partial listing. Consult your doctor about other drugs you are taking.
Alcohol, tricyclic antidepressants, antihistamines, sedatives and hypnotics: increased depressant effects.
Digoxin: increased digoxin effect.
Ketoconazole, levodopa: decreased effects of ketoconazole and levodopa.
Opioid analgesics: risk of severe constipation.
Potassium supplements: risk of ulcers.

TARGET AILMENTS

Motion sickness (skin patch)

Irritable bowel syndrome (oral)

Iritis; uveitis (eye drops)

SIDE EFFECTS

NOT SERIOUS
- Dry eyes, nose, or mouth
- Drowsiness

CALL YOUR DOCTOR IF THESE PROBLEMS PERSIST.

SERIOUS
- Hives; rash; severe itching
- Confusion; dizziness; hallucinations; rapid heartbeat
- Eye pain; blurred vision
- Severe constipation

REMOVE THE PATCH OR STOP TAKING THE DRUG AND CONTACT YOUR DOCTOR IMMEDIATELY.

Selective Serotonin Reuptake Inhibitors (SSRIs)

Vital Statistics

DRUG CLASS
Antidepressants

GENERIC NAMES
fluoxetine, paroxetine, sertraline, venlafaxine

GENERAL DESCRIPTION
Drugs in this subclass of antidepressant medications work by altering the level of the neurotransmitter serotonin in the brain. This group includes the widely used drug fluoxetine, which is better known by the brand name Prozac. See Antidepressants for additional special information as well as information about possible drug interactions.

Precautions

SPECIAL INFORMATION
The severity of any side effects may decrease with time (after two weeks) or with lowered dosages. If you have any questions about potential side effects, discuss them with your doctor.

TARGET AILMENTS
Major depressive disorders
Obsessive-compulsive disorder

SIDE EFFECTS

NOT SERIOUS

- Dizziness, drowsiness, or weakness
- Dry mouth; headache
- Increased appetite or food cravings; weight gain
- Nausea or diarrhea
- Increased sweating
- Insomnia
- Photosensitivity

LET YOUR DOCTOR KNOW IF THESE SYMPTOMS PERSIST OR BECOME TROUBLESOME.

SERIOUS

- Blurred vision, confusion, delirium, or hallucinations
- Paralytic ileus (blockage of intestines, possibly indicated by abdominal pain or swelling, difficulty in breathing, and severe constipation)
- Difficulty in urination
- Eye pain from aggravated glaucoma
- Tremors; changes in heartbeat; nervousness
- Parkinson's-like symptoms (shuffling walk, stiffness in the extremities)
- Allergic reaction; skin rash or spots; bruising or bleeding; jaundice; sore throat; fever (rare)

CALL YOUR DOCTOR IMMEDIATELY. YOU MAY BE REACTING TO THE DRUG OR TAKING TOO MUCH.

SELENIUM

VITAL STATISTICS

GENERAL DESCRIPTION
An antioxidant, selenium protects cells and tissues from damage wrought by free radicals. Because its antioxidant effects complement those of vitamin E, the two are said to potentiate, or reinforce, each other. Selenium also supports immune function and neutralizes certain poisonous substances, such as cadmium, mercury, and arsenic, that may be ingested or inhaled. Although its full therapeutic value is unknown, adequate selenium levels may help combat arthritis, deter heart disease, and prevent cancer.

Very little selenium is required to maintain good health, and most people get adequate amounts through diet alone. Some multinutrients contain selenium, but always in small, safe amounts.

RDA
Men: 70 mcg
Women: 55 mcg
Pregnant women: 65 mcg

NATURAL SOURCES
Whole grains, asparagus, garlic, eggs, and mushrooms are typically good sources, as are lean meats and seafood.

PRECAUTIONS

WARNING
Selenium can be toxic in extremely high doses, causing hair loss, nail problems, accelerated tooth decay, and swelling of the fingers, among other symptoms.

SPECIAL INFORMATION
High-dose supplements such as selenium citrate and selenium picolinate should be taken only if prescribed by a doctor.

TARGET AILMENTS
Arthritis
Cancer
Heart disease
Immune problems

SIDE EFFECTS
NONE EXPECTED

SENNA

LATIN NAME
Cassia senna

VITAL STATISTICS

GENERAL DESCRIPTION

Senna is a powerful laxative that should not be taken casually. This woody shrub contains colon-stimulating chemicals known as anthraquinones, which in high doses act as cathartics, or extremely strong laxatives. Both the leaves and the seed pods are used medicinally, although the pods are milder. Anthraquinones, derived from senna and other herbs, are among the ingredients of many commercial laxatives. The medicinal use of senna dates to ancient civilizations; it was introduced into European medicine by Arab healers in the ninth century. The herb grows primarily in India and Egypt.

PREPARATIONS

Over the counter:

Available in prepared tea bags, tinctures, and tablets, and as dried leaves and seed pods.

At home:

INFUSION: Steep three to six pods per cup of cold water and let sit overnight. Drink cold, ½ cup a day, in the morning or at night for a maximum of three days. If desired, offset the bitter taste by adding anise, peppermint, fennel, lemon, or a sweetener.

DECOCTION: Simmer covered four chopped pods in 1 cup warm water for 5 to 10 minutes; drink as above.

TINCTURE: Take ½ to 1 tsp in juice or water once a day in the morning or at night for no more than three days.

This herb should not be used with children unless it is specifically prescribed by a healthcare practitioner who is knowledgeable about herbs.

Consult a qualified practitioner for the dosage appropriate for you and the specific condition being treated.

PRECAUTIONS

☠ *WARNING*

Avoid senna if you are pregnant, nursing, or have gastrointestinal ailments such as ulcers, colitis, or hemorrhoids.

SPECIAL INFORMATION

- Because senna is so strong, try milder laxatives first, or fiber-rich foods.
- Overdependence on senna can result in lazy bowel syndrome; use this herb for no more than three days.
- Because senna has an unpleasant taste, herbalists recommend using over-the-counter preparations instead of teas.

POSSIBLE INTERACTIONS

Digoxin: increased digoxin effect, causing stress on the heart.

Combining senna with other herbs may necessitate a lower dosage.

TARGET AILMENTS

Constipation

SIDE EFFECTS

NOT SERIOUS

- Mild gastrointestinal cramps; skin rash

SERIOUS

- Diarrhea; nausea; severe stomach cramps
- Dehydration

LARGE DOSES MAY CAUSE THESE EFFECTS. DISCONTINUE USE AND CALL YOUR DOCTOR IMMEDIATELY.

S

SENNOSIDES

VITAL STATISTICS

DRUG CLASS
Laxatives

BRAND NAME
Ex-Lax Gentle Natural Laxative Pills

OTHER DRUGS IN THIS CLASS
calcium polycarbophil, docusate, methylcellulose, phenolphthalein, psyllium hydrophilic mucilloid

GENERAL DESCRIPTION
A stimulant type of laxative, sennosides is used to relieve constipation. Stimulant laxatives are believed to promote evacuation by increasing peristalsis (waves of contractions) in the intestinal muscles. See Laxatives for information about other drugs in this class.

TARGET AILMENTS

Constipation

Straining during bowel movements following rectal surgery, heart attacks, or childbirth, or when hemorrhoids are present

SIDE EFFECTS

NOT SERIOUS
- Temporary discoloration of urine
- Diarrhea

PRECAUTIONS

SPECIAL INFORMATION
- Laxatives can be habit forming. Use them infrequently, at the lowest effective dosage, and for no longer than a week. Long-term use, particularly of stimulant laxatives, can cause physical dependence, resulting in loss of normal bowel function and chronic constipation.
- An overdose or prolonged use of this drug may result in an electrolyte imbalance. Symptoms can include irregular heartbeat, confusion, unusual tiredness or weakness, and muscle cramps.
- Do not use laxatives if you have nausea, abdominal pain, or vomiting.
- Do not use stimulant laxatives if you think you may have an intestinal obstruction.
- If you have congestive heart failure or rectal bleeding of unknown cause, consult your physician before using laxatives.
- If you are diabetic, avoid laxative brands that contain large amounts of sugar; instead, use sugar-free types.
- Call your doctor if the laxative fails to have the desired effect after one week of use.

For more information, see Laxatives.

SEPIA

LATIN NAME
Sepia

VITAL STATISTICS

GENERAL DESCRIPTION

The cuttlefish is a soft-bodied mollusk with eight arms that is closely related to the squid and octopus; it propels itself by squirting jets of water from special organs in its body. When threatened, it releases spurts of dark ink called sepia that cloud the water and camouflage its retreat. Sepia has been used for artistic purposes, although its ingestion, such as occurs when a painter licks the brush, can bring about unpleasant side effects.

Homeopathic practitioners prescribe *Sepia* for patients with conditions whose symptoms include apathy, moodiness, and weakness. For the homeopathic preparation, cuttlefish ink is collected and diluted with large quantities of milk sugar for final use.

Like most homeopathic prescriptions, *Sepia* was developed as a remedy by observation of the reactions of healthy individuals to doses of various strengths. The mental, emotional, and physical changes induced by *Sepia* were then cataloged. When a patient exhibits a set of symptoms that matches the cataloged symptoms brought on by *Sepia,* the homeopathic practitioner then prescribes it in an extremely dilute form. For more information on homeopathic medicine, see page 14.

PREPARATIONS

Sepia is available over the counter in various potencies, in both liquid and tablet form, at selected stores and pharmacies. Consult your homeopathic practitioner for more information.

SIDE EFFECTS

NONE EXPECTED

PRECAUTIONS

SPECIAL INFORMATION

- Only the patient should touch the pills. If tablets are spilled, throw them away.
- The mouth should be clear of flavors 15 minutes before and after taking a remedy, and strong flavors and aromas should be avoided for the duration of treatment.

TARGET AILMENTS
Backaches and weakness in the small of the back
Violent fits of coughing
Cold sores and fever blisters around the mouth; genital herpes
Exhaustion
Hair loss
Gas
Headache with throbbing pain
Sinusitis
Urinary incontinence
Menopausal hot flashes
Menstrual cramps with intense, bearing-down pain
Nausea resulting from motion sickness or during pregnancy
Brown spots on the skin

S

SERTRALINE

VITAL STATISTICS

DRUG CLASS
Antidepressants [Selective Serotonin Reuptake Inhibitors (SSRIs)]

BRAND NAME
Zoloft

OTHER DRUGS IN THIS SUBCLASS
fluoxetine, paroxetine, venlafaxine

GENERAL DESCRIPTION
Introduced in 1986, sertraline belongs to a subclass of antidepressants known as selective serotonin reuptake inhibitors (SSRIs) and works by altering levels of serotonin, an important brain chemical. This medication is prescribed for treatment of depression and obsessive-compulsive disorder. See Antidepressants for side effects and additional precautions.

TARGET AILMENTS
Major depressive disorders
Obsessive-compulsive disorder

SIDE EFFECTS
SEE ANTIDEPRESSANTS.

PRECAUTIONS

SPECIAL INFORMATION
- The severity of any side effects may decrease with time (after two weeks) or with lowered dosages. If you have any questions about potential side effects, discuss them with your doctor.
- If you are pregnant, nursing, or planning a pregnancy, check with your doctor before taking sertraline.

POSSIBLE INTERACTIONS
Alcohol and other drugs that depress the central nervous system: increased sertraline effects, leading to problems such as respiratory depression or very low blood pressure.
Anticonvulsants: decreased effectiveness of anticonvulsants, making seizures more likely.
Antihistamines: increased antihistamine action, including any side effects; antihistamines may also increase the action of sertraline, including any side effects.
Digitalis preparations: using sertraline with heart medications may increase blood levels of both the antidepressant and the heart drugs, increasing the risk of side effects.
Lithium: taking sertraline with lithium could increase blood levels of lithium, leading to toxicity.
Monoamine oxidase (MAO) inhibitors: WARNING: severe, possibly fatal reactions such as seizures, tremor, and coma because of additive effects of the drugs.
Other antidepressants: combining antidepressants will likely increase the action of one or both drugs, leading to increased side effects.

S

SESAME OIL

LATIN NAME
Sesamum indicum

VITAL STATISTICS

GENERAL DESCRIPTION

Sesame oil is prepared from large, round, black sesame seeds, which have a sweet taste. Chinese medicine practitioners often prescribe the oil, sometimes called *hu ma you,* for constipation. They also use the sesame seeds as a laxative. Traditional Chinese medicine characterizes sesame oil as sweet and neutral.

Chinese medicine takes a holistic approach to healthcare, fashioning remedies to treat the entire being as well as the specific parts or areas. Single herbs may be used alone or in combination with other herbs to prevent and combat disease, which is thought to arise from disturbances in the flow of a bodily energy called chi (pronounced "chee") and blood, or from a lack of balance in the complementary states of yin and yang.

PREPARATIONS

Sesame seeds or oil is available at Chinese pharmacies, Asian markets, and Western health food stores. The seeds are also available in tablet form. A tablespoonful of the oil by itself in the evening is considered effective for constipation.

COMBINATIONS: Sesame oil is also mixed with therapeutic oils that contain other medicinally useful herbs. One remedy for constipation combines the seeds with chicken eggs; another formula mixes sesame seeds, dong quai, and biota seeds. Chinese medicine practitioners prescribe a combination of sesame seeds and white mulberry leaf for dizziness, blurred vision, tinnitus (ringing in the ears), and headaches.

For information on dosages and other preparations, ask a Chinese medicine practitioner.

PRECAUTIONS

WARNING

Do not use this herb if you have diarrhea.

TARGET AILMENTS

Take internally for:

- Constipation
- Certain types of blurred vision
- Tinnitus (ringing in the ears)
- Dizziness
- Recuperation after severe illness—to help restore the vitality that serious illness depletes

SIDE EFFECTS

NONE EXPECTED

S

SHARK CARTILAGE

VITAL STATISTICS

GENERAL DESCRIPTION

Shark cartilage is a nutritional supplement that has generated considerable controversy. Proponents say the substance has numerous potential uses, from stimulating the immune system to treating cancer. Some claim it is an effective anti-inflammatory that can relieve joint swelling, pain, and stiffness. Critics, on the other hand, say there is no scientific evidence of its effectiveness. Even manufacturers of the supplement acknowledge that, although studies are encouraging, the usefulness of shark cartilage as a cancer treatment has not been scientifically proved.

Shark cartilage is thought to have medicinal value largely because of two characteristics of the creatures themselves: Sharks have no bones, only cartilage, and they rarely get cancer. One theory is that something in the cartilage blocks the formation of new blood vessels, which tumors need in order to grow.

PREPARATIONS

Shark cartilage is sold in the United States in tablet form as a dietary supplement.

PRECAUTIONS

WARNING

This supplement should never be substituted for conventional cancer treatment. Because little is known about the potential effects of shark cartilage, do not take this supplement if you are pregnant.

SPECIAL INFORMATION

Taken at therapeutic levels, shark cartilage provides extremely high doses of calcium. Have your blood calcium level monitored if you are taking large amounts of this supplement.

TARGET AILMENTS
Joint pain
Stiffness
Swelling

SIDE EFFECTS

NONE EXPECTED

SHARK LIVER OIL

VITAL STATISTICS

DRUG CLASS
Antihemorrhoid Drugs

BRAND NAME
Preparation H

GENERAL DESCRIPTION
A brown fatty oil, rich in vitamin A, shark liver oil is a skin protectant, a chemically inactive substance that provides a physical barrier between the skin and the environment. Shark liver oil is used only in combination with other skin protectants, such as cocoa butter, lanolin, petrolatum, and glycerin. Shark liver oil is sometimes used to treat diaper rash, although its safety and effectiveness have not been established.

In hemorrhoid medications, shark liver oil coats the skin in the anorectal area, protecting it against rough, chafing bowel movements. Like other skin protectants, this oil helps prevent loss of moisture for temporary relief of skin irritation and burning associated with hemorrhoids.

PRECAUTIONS

SPECIAL INFORMATION
- In case of rectal bleeding or persistent itching, see your physician.
- Check with your doctor before using shark liver oil to treat diaper rash in children under the age of two.

TARGET AILMENTS

Burning and itching of the anorectal surface due to hemorrhoids

Diaper rash

SIDE EFFECTS

NONE EXPECTED

S

SHEEP SORREL

LATIN NAME
Rumex acetosella

VITAL STATISTICS

GENERAL DESCRIPTION
Herbalists use the leaves, roots, stems, and flowers of sheep sorrel, a common native European weed, for its purported astringent properties to treat mild ulcerative conditions, such as mouth and throat ulcers. A topical wash of sheep sorrel is also recommended for itchy skin rashes. The juice of the fresh plant is said to help urinary conditions. Recently sheep sorrel has been used in treating the side effects of chemotherapy. Its mechanism of action is not well understood.

PREPARATIONS
Over the counter:
Available as tinctures, capsules, and prepared tea, or as fresh or dried plant parts (leaves, root, flowers, stems) in combination with other herbs.

At home:
INFUSION: Steep leaves or stems covered for 5 minutes, or roots for 10 minutes, in hot (not boiling) water and drink two or three times a day.
TINCTURE: Stir 30 drops into a glass of water and drink 4 glasses (120 drops) daily.
Consult a qualified practitioner for the dosage appropriate for your specific condition.

PRECAUTIONS

WARNING
Large doses of this herb can be toxic. Sheep sorrel contains high levels of oxalic acid, which can cause kidney stones, worsen existing kidney ailments, and otherwise irritate the kidneys. If you have kidney problems, do not take sheep sorrel.

This herb should not be used with children unless it is prescribed by a healthcare practitioner who is knowledgeable about herbs.

POSSIBLE INTERACTIONS
Combining sheep sorrel with other herbs may necessitate a lower dosage.

TARGET AILMENTS

Take internally for:

Constipation; diarrhea

Mouth, throat, and stomach ulcers; excessive menstruation

Apply externally for:

Itchy skin rashes, such as hives and poison ivy; mild abrasions

SIDE EFFECTS

NOT SERIOUS
- Nausea
- Tingling tongue
- Severe headache

CALL YOUR DOCTOR IF THESE EFFECTS PERSIST.

SERIOUS
- Kidney problems, including kidney stones

DO NOT TAKE SHEEP SORREL IF YOU HAVE KIDNEY PROBLEMS.

SHIITAKE

LATIN NAME
Lentinus edodes

VITAL STATISTICS

GENERAL DESCRIPTION

A tasty, meaty-flavored fungus that grows on the trunks of dead trees, the shiitake mushroom has long been a staple of Chinese cuisine. In both China and Japan, shiitake mushrooms have been used for hundreds of years as cancer-fighting agents.

Today, Chinese herbalists also use the mushroom to lower blood cholesterol. The fungus contains cortinelin, a strong antibacterial agent that kills many disease-causing germs. A sulfide component of shiitake mushrooms also has antibiotic properties. Moreover, these mushrooms contain a polysaccharide complex called lentinan, which may be effective in stimulating the immune system. Herbalists think that this chemical may eventually prove useful in shrinking cancerous tumors; they base this hope on the fact that lentinan has slowed the growth of malignancies in several animal studies.

PREPARATIONS

Over the counter:
Available in dried form in Asian food markets or in capsules at health food stores.

At home:

Tea: Cover a handful of dried shiitakes with boiling water; soak 10 to 30 minutes. Strain the liquid and drink the tea; you can use the mushrooms in cooking.

Food: After soaking mushrooms in boiling water, eat one a day (many recipes are available) to maintain good health. Chinese medicine practitioners recommend eating 2 to 4 oz of shiitake mushrooms two or three times a week for general health benefits.

Consult a qualified practitioner for the dosage appropriate for you and the specific condition being treated.

PRECAUTIONS

SPECIAL INFORMATION

Shiitake mushrooms are rich in protein, in vitamins B_1, B_2, and B_{12}, in niacin, and in pantothenic acid.

POSSIBLE INTERACTIONS

Combining shiitake with other herbs may necessitate a lower dosage.

TARGET AILMENTS

Take internally for:

High blood cholesterol

Depressed immune system disorders

Chronic fatigue syndrome

Possibly, some forms of cancer (use only in consultation with a doctor)

SIDE EFFECTS

NONE EXPECTED

Shi Lin Tong Pian

Vital Statistics

ENGLISH NAME
Stone Strangury Tablets

GENERAL DESCRIPTION
Shi Lin Tong Pian is used to relieve blockages that inhibit the flow of urine. (The word *lin* in the name refers to the sensation of passing wood.) Practitioners usually prescribe this remedy when urination is frequent, scanty, and painful. The herb in this pill is said to help small stones pass more easily. Some people, in fact, have used *Shi Lin Tong Pian* to treat small gallstones as well as kidney stones.

Chinese medicine takes a holistic approach to healthcare, fashioning remedies to treat the entire being as well as the specific parts or areas. Precise combinations of herbs are used to prevent and combat disease, which is thought to arise from disturbances in the flow of a bodily energy called chi (pronounced "chee") and blood, or from a lack of balance in the complementary states of yin and yang. A patent formula, *Shi Lin Tong Pian* is made by using a standardized combination of herbs and method of preparation.

INGREDIENTS
gold money grass

PREPARATIONS
Shi Lin Tong Pian is available in pill form at many Chinese pharmacies and Oriental grocery stores.

Target Ailments

Frequent and scanty urination

Kidney stones or gallstones (if small)

Urinary tract infection (with or without bleeding)

Liver disease with swelling

Kidney disease with edema (swelling)

Side Effects

None expected

Shi Quan Da Bu Wan

Vital Statistics

ENGLISH NAME
All-Inclusive Great Tonifying Pills

ALSO SOLD AS
Shih Chuan Ta Bu Wan

GENERAL DESCRIPTION
Shi Quan Da Bu Wan is a tonic for a condition known in Chinese medicine as depletion of the basic substances of chi and blood when the person is also cold. Such depletion can come after a long illness or may result simply from the stresses of everyday living. A person with this condition is fatigued and has a pale complexion as well as a pale tongue. Other symptoms can include weakness, palpitations, and slight dizziness.

Chinese medicine takes a holistic approach to healthcare, fashioning remedies to treat the entire being as well as the specific parts or areas. Precise combinations of herbs are used to prevent and combat disease, which is thought to arise from disturbances in the flow of a bodily energy called chi (pronounced "chee") and blood, or from a lack of balance in the complementary states of yin and yang. A patent formula, *Shi Quan Da Bu Wan* is made by using a standardized combination of herbs and method of preparation.

INGREDIENTS
codonopsis, astragalus, white peony root, atractylodes, poria, cooked rehmannia, dang gui, cinnamon bark, ligusticum, licorice

PREPARATIONS
This formula is available in pill form at many Chinese pharmacies and Oriental grocery stores.

Precautions

WARNING
Discontinue taking this remedy if signs of heat or fever occur.

TARGET AILMENTS
Fatigue with coldness
Pale tongue; pale complexion

SIDE EFFECTS
SEE WARNING.

SILICA

LATIN NAME
Silica

VITAL STATISTICS

GENERAL DESCRIPTION

Silica, also called flint, is a mineral that is present in the human body in only trace amounts but is vital to the development of bones, the flexibility of cartilage, and the health of the skin and connective tissues. Many industrial operations rely on it, including the manufacture of concrete, paper, glass, and enamelware. Silica's medicinal use is limited to homeopathy. Minute doses are prescribed for patients with conditions accompanied by excessive sweating, weakness, and extreme sensitivity to cold. For homeopathic use, silica powder is mixed with sodium carbonate through a pharmaceutical process of dry substance dilution.

Like most homeopathic prescriptions, *Silica* was developed as a remedy by observation of the reactions of healthy individuals to doses of various strengths. The mental, emotional, and physical changes induced by *Silica* were then cataloged. When a patient exhibits a set of symptoms that matches the cataloged symptoms brought on by *Silica,* the homeopathic practitioner then prescribes it in an extremely dilute form. For more information on homeopathic medicine, see page 14.

PREPARATIONS

Silica is available over the counter in various potencies, in both liquid and tablet form, at selected stores and pharmacies. Consult your homeopath for further information.

SIDE EFFECTS

NONE EXPECTED

S

PRECAUTIONS

SPECIAL INFORMATION

- Only the patient should touch the pills. If tablets are spilled, throw them away.
- The mouth should be clear of flavors 15 minutes before and after taking a remedy, and strong flavors and aromas, such as coffee and heavy perfume, should be avoided for the duration of treatment.

TARGET AILMENTS

- Athlete's foot
- Constipation resulting from large stools
- Wounds inflamed by foreign matter
- Earache with decreased hearing and a stopped-up sensation
- Fingernails that have white spots and split easily
- Headaches beginning in the back of the head and spreading forward to the eyes
- Abscesses
- Swollen glands in the neck
- Gum infections
- Hemorrhoids
- Breast cysts

SIMETHICONE

VITAL STATISTICS

DRUG CLASS
Antigas Drugs

BRAND NAMES
Tums Antigas/Antacid formula; some types of Mylanta; Mylanta Gas; some types of Maalox

GENERAL DESCRIPTION
Simethicone is an antigas drug used to relieve the pain, cramping, bloating, intestinal pressure, and "full" sensation that accompany flatulence, or gas. Gas can build up in the gastrointestinal tract as a result of excessive swallowing of air or from eating foods the body does not tolerate well.

The defoaming properties of simethicone act in the gastrointestinal tract to disperse gas bubbles and to prevent their formation. The drug changes the surface tension of small gas bubbles in the stomach, causing them to coalesce and form larger ones. These larger bubbles are more easily expelled through belching or passing flatus. Simethicone is often combined with antacids for the dual relief of gas and heartburn.

Simethicone tablets should be chewed thoroughly before swallowing.

PRECAUTIONS

WARNING
Do not take this drug if you have kidney disease.

SPECIAL INFORMATION
- Simethicone is nontoxic; when used as indicated, the drug produces no side effects. A possible adverse effect could include excessive expulsion of gas in belching or flatus.
- The adult dosages of this drug are not recommended for treating infant colic. Infant drops are available, but check with your pediatrician for guidance on their use.
- Do not take this medication for more than two weeks.
- Do not exceed the recommended dosage.

POSSIBLE INTERACTIONS
Although unlikely, this drug may interact with some medications. Check with your doctor before using a product containing simethicone if you are taking other drugs.

TARGET AILMENTS
Symptoms of gas (bloating, abdominal cramps, intestinal pressure, fullness)
Postoperative gaseous distention

SIDE EFFECTS
NONE EXPECTED

SIMVASTATIN

VITAL STATISTICS

DRUG CLASS
Cholesterol-Reducing Drugs

BRAND NAME
Zocor

OTHER DRUGS IN THIS CLASS
cholestyramine, colestipol, fluvastatin, gemfibrozil, lovastatin, niacin, pravastatin

GENERAL DESCRIPTION
Introduced in 1986, simvastatin is an HMG-CoA reductase inhibitor, a type of drug that alters the blood levels of cholesterol and other fats. These drugs work by blocking a liver enzyme needed in the production of cholesterol. Simvastatin may also increase the blood level of high-density lipoproteins (HDLs), the so-called good cholesterol that seems to protect against heart disease. For more information, see Cholesterol-Reducing Drugs.

PRECAUTIONS

SPECIAL INFORMATION
- If you become pregnant while taking this drug, stop using it immediately and inform your doctor.
- Do not use this drug if you have had an allergic reaction to it in the past.
- Do not stop taking simvastatin without first checking with your doctor; your blood cholesterol levels may increase again.
- Before undergoing emergency treatment or medical or dental surgery, be sure to tell your healthcare practitioner if you are taking this drug.

S

POSSIBLE INTERACTIONS
Erythromycin, immunosuppressants, niacin: severe muscle pain or kidney failure.
Gemfibrozil: may affect the absorption and excretion of simvastatin; do not take concurrently.

TARGET AILMENTS

The major types of cholesterol disorders

SIDE EFFECTS

NOT SERIOUS
- Constipation or gas

CALL YOUR DOCTOR IF THESE EFFECTS PERSIST.

SERIOUS
- Fever
- Muscle aches
- Cramps

TELL YOUR DOCTOR IF YOU EXPERIENCE ANY OF THESE EFFECTS.

SKULLCAP

LATIN NAME
Scutellaria baicalensis

VITAL STATISTICS

GENERAL DESCRIPTION

Chinese herbalists prescribe the long, thick, skinless yellow root of skullcap for a wide range of disorders. In laboratory tests, the root seemed to have a diuretic effect on healthy animals and humans; it was also found to have broad antimicrobial effects. In traditional Chinese medicine, skullcap is characterized as bitter and cold.

Chinese medicine takes a holistic approach to healthcare, fashioning remedies to treat the entire being as well as the specific parts or areas. Single herbs may be used alone or in combination with other herbs to prevent and combat disease, which is thought to arise from disturbances in the flow of a bodily energy called chi (pronounced "chee") and blood, or from a lack of balance in the complementary states of yin and yang.

PREPARATIONS

Skullcap root is available in bulk from Chinese pharmacies, Asian markets, and Western health food stores. You can also obtain the herb as pills.

The root is usually decocted, but it can be fried dry for use in pregnancy and to treat diarrhea and infections of the urinary tract, or cooked in wine for upper respiratory infections and redness of the face and eyes.

COMBINATIONS: A mixture with coptis is prescribed for high fever and irritability. Skullcap root mixed with anemarrhena is thought to alleviate chronic coughs.

For further information on preparations and doses, consult a Chinese medicine practitioner.

PRECAUTIONS

SPECIAL INFORMATION

Before using skullcap to treat diarrhea or problems of pregnancy, check with a Chinese medicine practitioner.

POSSIBLE INTERACTIONS

Some sources in traditional Chinese medicine suggest that skullcap counteracts the effects of moutan and veratrum.

TARGET AILMENTS

Take internally for:

Diarrhea; dysentery

Upper respiratory infections with fever; urinary tract infections; jaundice; hepatitis

Nervous tension; irritability; headache; insomnia

Epilepsy and other seizures; red face or eyes

Coughing up or vomiting blood; nosebleeds; blood in the stool

Abdominal pain and vaginal bleeding; threatened miscarriage during pregnancy; premenstrual stress

SIDE EFFECTS

NONE EXPECTED

SKULLCAP

LATIN NAME
Scutellaria lateriflora

VITAL STATISTICS

GENERAL DESCRIPTION

The leaves and blue flowers of this two-foot-tall perennial are used as an ingredient in many over-the-counter herbal sleep remedies. Some researchers, especially in Europe and Asia, report that skullcap contains chemicals that calm the nervous system. Practitioners of Chinese medicine believe that skullcap is effective for treating hepatitis, a serious liver disease. In the United States, however, skullcap is considered controversial and even useless by many medical authorities, at least partly because of its early—and unearned—reputation for curing rabies, for which it garnered the now archaic name of mad dog weed. Its current name comes from an elongated, caplike appendage on the upper lip of the flower. Two Japanese animal studies showed that skullcap increases levels of the "good" kind of cholesterol, raising the possibility that skullcap may one day be useful in preventing heart disease and strokes.

For visual characteristics of skullcap, see the Color Guide to Prescription Drugs and Herbs.

PREPARATIONS

Over the counter:

Available as prepared tea, tinctures, dried leaves, and capsules.

At home:

TEA: Pour a cup of boiling water over 2 tsp dried leaves and steep covered for 10 to 15 minutes; drink this amount up to three times daily.

TINCTURE: Take ½ to 1 tsp in warm water one to two times per day.

Consult a qualified practitioner for the appropriate dosage.

PRECAUTIONS

☠ ***WARNING***

Skullcap may cause drowsiness. Do not operate a car or heavy machinery after taking it.

Large amounts of the tincture may cause confusion, giddiness, twitching, and possibly convulsions.

This herb should not be used with children unless it is prescribed by a healthcare practitioner who is knowledgeable about herbs.

POSSIBLE INTERACTIONS

Combining skullcap with other herbs may necessitate a lower dosage.

TARGET AILMENTS

Take internally for:

Nervous tension; tension-caused headaches and muscle aches

Insomnia; convulsions

Drug or alcohol withdrawal

Symptoms of premenstrual syndrome aggravated or caused by stress

SIDE EFFECTS

NOT SERIOUS

- Stomach upset; diarrhea

REDUCE INTAKE OR STOP USING SKULLCAP.

SEE WARNING.

S

Slippery Elm

LATIN NAME
Ulmus fulva

Vital Statistics

GENERAL DESCRIPTION

The U.S. Food and Drug Administration calls slippery elm a good demulcent, or soothing agent. Herbalists recommend its use externally to ease wounds and skin problems, and internally to soothe sore throats, coughing, and diarrhea and other gastrointestinal disorders. Slippery elm's active ingredient is found in the white inner bark, whose mucilaginous cells expand into a spongy mass when mixed with water. Elm trees were prized in the 18th and 19th centuries by American settlers, for whom slippery elm was a valuable cure. They soaked it in water and applied it to wounds, where it dried into a natural bandage. Mixed with water, it made a soothing gruel for children and sick people. Lozenges, powder, and other elm products are still available in health food stores, but the great elm forests once common throughout the East Coast of the United States have been ravaged by Dutch elm disease.

PREPARATIONS

Over the counter:
Available as capsules, tea, and powder.

At home:

Poultice: For wounds that have been thoroughly cleaned with soap and water, moisten powdered bark with enough water to make a paste; apply to wound and allow to dry. This forms a natural bandage that delivers soothing agents to the wound.

Tea: Add 2 tsp powder to a cup of boiling water; simmer covered for 15 minutes. Drink up to 3 cups a day for throat, digestive, and gynecological problems.

Food: Mix slippery elm powder into applesauce or oatmeal, or make it into a thin porridge with water.

Precautions

SPECIAL INFORMATION

Consult your doctor if your symptoms do not improve significantly within two weeks.

POSSIBLE INTERACTIONS

Combining slippery elm with other herbs may necessitate a lower dosage.

TARGET AILMENTS

Apply externally for:

Wounds; cuts; abrasions

Take internally for:

Cough and sore throat

Digestive complaints

Ulcers

Colitis

SIDE EFFECTS

NOT SERIOUS

Some people may be allergic to the powdered bark. If you experience any problems, stop using it. Consult your doctor before taking doses that are larger than recommended.

S

SMOKING CESSATION DRUGS

VITAL STATISTICS

GENERIC NAME
nicotine

BRAND NAMES
Rx: Nicotrol NS (nasal spray)
OTC: NicoDerm CQ (transdermal), Nicorette (chewing gum); Nicotrol (transdermal)

GENERAL DESCRIPTION
Smoking cessation drugs, available in the form of flavored chewing gum, transdermal (skin) patches, and nasal spray, are used to reduce nicotine craving and withdrawal effects in people who want to stop smoking. These aids serve as temporary alternative sources of nicotine and are most useful to those smokers who have a strong physical dependence on the drug.

Nicotine acts on the peripheral and central nervous systems, producing stimulant and depressant effects. By slowly reducing nicotine intake, these products can lessen the physical effects of smoking withdrawal, such as irritability, nervousness, drowsiness, fatigue, headache, and nicotine craving. There is no evidence that nicotine replacement drugs work unless the smoker also participates in a medically supervised stop-smoking program.

S

PRECAUTIONS

WARNING
Extremely high doses of nicotine can produce toxic symptoms; nicotine overdose can be fatal. Because of the risk of overdose, do not smoke when using a medicinal form of nicotine.

SPECIAL INFORMATION
- In order for smoking cessation drugs to be safe and effective, stop smoking completely at the beginning of treatment. This is also essential because of the risk of nicotine overdose.
- Call your doctor immediately if you have any of the following symptoms of toxic nicotine overdose: nausea, vomiting, abdominal cramps, diarrhea, dizziness, sweating, hearing or vision problems, confusion, weakness.
- Nicotine replacement products should not be used by nonsmokers or others who are not addicted to the drug.
- Do not use smoking cessation drugs if you have had an allergic reaction to them before. Consult your doctor if you have angina or an abnormal heart rhythm; have had a recent heart attack; or are pregnant, planning a pregnancy, or nursing.

- Tell your doctor if you have diabetes, high blood pressure, skin disease, overactive thyroid, adrenaline-producing tumors, peptic ulcer, or liver or kidney disease, or if you get rashes from adhesive bandages or tape.
- Tell your doctor what other medications you are taking. Changes in nicotine levels may require dosage adjustments for other drugs, especially those affecting the nervous system.
- Nicotine can be very harmful to children and pets. Be sure to dispose of used patches carefully, and keep nasal sprays out of reach at all times.
- Do not use smoking cessation drugs for more than 12 to 20 weeks (depending on the system) if you have succeeded in stopping smoking. Continued use can be harmful and addictive.

POSSIBLE INTERACTIONS

Bronchodilators, insulin, propoxyphene, and propranolol and other beta-adrenergic blockers: you may need decreased amounts of these drugs when you stop smoking.

Isoproterenol, phenylephrine: you may need increased amounts of these drugs when you stop smoking.

TARGET AILMENTS
Smoking cessation
Nicotine withdrawal

SIDE EFFECTS

NOT SERIOUS

- Mild, temporary irritation (redness, tingling, itchiness) at a patch site
- Fast heartbeat
- Coughing; dry mouth
- Muscle or joint pain
- Hot feeling at the back of the throat or nose; sneezing; watery eyes; runny nose (nasal spray)

CALL YOUR DOCTOR IF THESE SYMPTOMS PERSIST OR ARE BOTHERSOME.

- Increased appetite
- Mild headache, irritability, or nervousness
- Unusual dreams

THESE ARE SYMPTOMS OF NICOTINE WITHDRAWAL.

SERIOUS

- Chest pain
- Irregular heartbeat
- Dizziness
- Allergic reactions (hives, rash, swelling)
- Tingling in the arms or legs
- Tingling, burning, numbness in the nose, throat, or mouth (nasal spray)

CHECK WITH YOUR DOCTOR. ALSO SEE SIGNS OF OVERDOSE UNDER SPECIAL INFORMATION.

SODIUM

VITAL STATISTICS

GENERAL DESCRIPTION

All bodily fluids—including blood, tears, and perspiration—contain sodium. Together with potassium and chloride, sodium maintains fluid distribution and pH balance; with potassium, sodium also helps control muscle contraction and nerve function.

Keeping sodium intake within reasonable limits is critical for long-term health. When sodium levels are persistently elevated, the body loses potassium and retains water, making blood pressure rise. Adopting a low-sodium diet can reduce high blood pressure and correct a potassium deficiency. Overexertion can induce temporary sodium deficiency, characterized by nausea, dehydration, muscle cramps, and other symptoms of heatstroke. Drinking several glasses of water with a pinch of salt added replaces the sodium and eases the symptoms.

EMDR

Adults: 500 mg

NATURAL SOURCES

Most of the sodium in American diets is from table salt. Among many other sources are processed foods, soft drinks, meats, shellfish, condiments, snack foods, food additives, and over-the-counter laxatives.

SPECIAL INFORMATION

Americans generally consume far too much sodium. A single teaspoon of salt contains 2,000 mg—four times the daily minimum—but average daily consumption in the United States ranges from 3,000 mg to 7,000 mg.

TARGET AILMENTS

High blood pressure (low-sodium diet)

SIDE EFFECTS

NONE EXPECTED

SODIUM BICARBONATE AND CITRIC ACID

VITAL STATISTICS

DRUG CLASS
Antacids

BRAND NAME
Alka-Seltzer

OTHER DRUGS IN THIS CLASS
aluminum hydroxide, calcium carbonate, magnesium carbonate, magnesium hydroxide

GENERAL DESCRIPTION
The combination of sodium bicarbonate and citric acid is used to relieve symptoms of upset and sour stomach, acid indigestion, and heartburn. Most effective when taken on an empty stomach, this drug is absorbed quickly and easily into the body. If taken by itself for a long time, sodium bicarbonate may cause systemic alkalosis, a condition in which the blood becomes less acidic than normal. This can adversely affect the blood and kidneys. Citric acid is added to sodium bicarbonate to add acidity to the stomach and help correct the imbalance. See Antacids for information about additional side effects, other special information, and possible drug interactions.

PRECAUTIONS

SPECIAL INFORMATION
- Do not take antacids containing sodium if you have high blood pressure, congestive heart failure, cirrhosis, renal failure, or edema, or if you are on a low-sodium diet; the high sodium content of the drugs may exacerbate these problems.
- Sodium bicarbonate antacids can cause milk-alkali syndrome, characterized by headache, nausea, irritability, and weakness. In time, milk-alkali syndrome can lead to kidney disease or failure.
- Notify your doctor if you develop black, tarry stools or vomit the consistency of coffee grounds. These are symptoms of bleeding in the stomach or intestines.

TARGET AILMENTS

Upset stomach; heartburn; acid indigestion; sour stomach

Ulcers

SIDE EFFECTS

NOT SERIOUS
- Mild constipation; diarrhea; stomach cramps, vomiting; belching; flatulence

CALL YOUR DOCTOR IF THESE PROBLEMS PERSIST.

SERIOUS
- Swelling of the wrist, foot, or lower leg
- Nervousness or restlessness
- Slow breathing
- Irregular heartbeat
- Pain upon urinating or frequent need to urinate
- Continuing loss of appetite
- Unusual tiredness or weakness; continuing headache

CONSULT YOUR DOCTOR AT ONCE.

SOYBEAN MILK

VITAL STATISTICS

GENERAL DESCRIPTION

As more people in the United States cut down on the amount of red meat in their diet, soy is rapidly gaining popularity. The main reason is that soy products, including soybean milk, are among the few plant foods that provide complete proteins, which are essential for a healthy diet and can be more difficult to obtain in a diet that includes little meat.

Not only is soy a good source of protein, it also contains chemical compounds that can play a role in fighting cancer. These compounds are plant-based hormones called phytoestrogens. High levels of a specific class of phytoestrogens known as isoflavones are found in soy products. Isoflavones play two roles in preventing cancer. They act as antioxidants, protecting body cells from the harmful effects of "free radicals," or unstable oxygen by-products that can damage cell DNA. Isoflavones also act as antimutagens, preventing cell mutations that can develop into cancerous tumors.

Some research also suggests isoflavones may prevent the negative effects of naturally occurring estrogen hormones that play a role in the development of breast, ovarian, and endometrial cancers. The rates of breast and prostate cancers are far lower in Asian countries, where soy-based diets are the norm. The phytoestrogens in soy may also help lessen the severity of symptoms for women going through menopause. Many experts suggest that women approaching menopause include soy in their daily diets.

In addition to these benefits, soy can help reduce blood cholesterol levels. Soy is also a good source of folate, iron, and magnesium as well as calcium, which can help prevent osteoporosis.

Soybean milk, or soya milk, is a particularly good choice for people who are lactose intolerant, since it contains no lactose, a difficult-to-digest milk sugar that some people must avoid. There's no cholesterol in soya milk, although it does contain fat. Regular formulas of soya milk have nearly as much fat as 2 percent milk; light versions contain about as much as 1 percent milk. The taste can be a little chalky.

PREPARATIONS

Soya milk is available in the United States at health food stores and in a number of grocery stores. The taste varies from brand to brand.

TARGET AILMENTS
High cholesterol
Lactose intolerance
Osteoporosis
Breast, ovarian, and endometrial cancers (risk reduction)

SIDE EFFECTS

NONE EXPECTED

SPEARMINT

LATIN NAME
Mentha spicata

VITAL STATISTICS

GENERAL DESCRIPTION

Spearmint has been used since ancient times to promote digestion, heal wounds, and relieve colds and congestion. When the lance-shaped, serrated leaves are crushed or boiled, they release carvone, a chemical similar to but milder than the menthol found in peppermint, a close relative. Modern herbalists suggest using spearmint externally for itching and inflammation, and internally for digestive ailments, colds, and insomnia.

This perennial, fast-spreading plant is praised in an Egyptian papyrus thought to be the world's oldest surviving medical text. Spearmint was used by the Greeks and Romans for ailments from hiccups to leprosy. Chinese and Ayurvedic (Hindu) physicians have used it for centuries to treat indigestion, colds, coughs, and fever. Many herbalists prescribe spearmint and peppermint interchangeably as medicines, although the latter is considered more potent.

PREPARATIONS

Over the counter:

Available as capsules, prepared tea, fresh or dried leaves, tinctures, and oil.

At home:

TEA: Boil 1 to 2 tsp dried herb or several fresh leaves per cup of water; steep covered 10 minutes. Drink up to 3 cups a day.

TINCTURE: Add ¼ to 1 tsp to an 8-oz glass of water and drink up to three glasses a day.

HERBAL BATH: Fill a cloth bag with a few handfuls of dried or fresh spearmint leaves and add to running bathwater.

Consult a qualified practitioner for the dosage appropriate for your specific condition.

PRECAUTIONS

SPECIAL INFORMATION

- Spearmint oil may cause stomach upset if ingested. Use externally only.
- For children under two, dilute spearmint tea or tincture with water.

POSSIBLE INTERACTIONS

Combining spearmint with other herbs may necessitate a lower dosage.

TARGET AILMENTS

Take internally for:

Upset stomach; stomach spasms or cramps; flatulence; heartburn

Morning sickness

Nasal, sinus, and chest congestion; colds; headache

Sore mouth or throat

Take internally and apply externally for:

Muscle pains

External infections

Chapped hands

SIDE EFFECTS

NONE EXPECTED

SPIRONOLACTONE

VITAL STATISTICS

DRUG CLASS
Diuretics

BRAND NAMES
Aldactazide (combination of spironolactone and hydrochlorothiazide); Aldactone

OTHER DRUGS IN THIS CLASS
amiloride, bumetanide, furosemide, hydrochlorothiazide, indapamide, potassium chloride (adjunct therapy), triamterene

GENERAL DESCRIPTION
Spironolactone is a potassium-sparing diuretic, which means that in addition to increasing the flow of urine from the body, it increases sodium excretion and decreases potassium excretion. An important use of the drug is in the treatment of high blood pressure, for which it is usually prescribed in conjunction with other medications. Spironolactone is also available in combination with another diuretic, hydrochlorothiazide. In this combination product, spironolactone helps to minimize the loss of potassium that may result from the use of hydrochlorothiazide.

Spironolactone is used to treat certain types of edema, or overaccumulation of fluid in body tissues. It is also helpful in treating hypokalemia (low blood levels of potassium), which can be caused by other types of diuretics. Additionally, the drug is used to treat primary hyperaldosteronism, a disease marked by oversecretion of the adrenal hormone aldosterone. For more information about this class of drugs, see Diuretics.

PRECAUTIONS

WARNING
Do not take spironolactone if you have severely impaired kidney function, difficulty urinating, or high blood levels of potassium.

While taking this drug, do not use potassium supplements or other diuretics that do not reduce blood potassium levels unless they are prescribed by your doctor. High blood levels of potassium can be life threatening.

Do not take the combination product containing spironolactone and hydrochlorothiazide if you have liver failure or liver disease, or if you are sensitive to sulfa drugs or either of these two medications. Tell your doctor of any drug reactions you have had in the past.

Spironolactone has been shown to cause tumors in laboratory rats; therefore, it should be used only when necessary and in conditions for which it is specifically indicated.

SPECIAL INFORMATION
- Take spironolactone with caution if you have liver disease.
- Use the spironolactone-hydrochlorothiazide combination with caution if you have lupus.
- Avoid excessive sweating while taking this drug. Dehydration, diarrhea, and vomiting can cause you to lose too much water and

TARGET AILMENTS

Edema in congestive heart failure, cirrhosis, and nephrotic syndrome, as well as edema of unknown cause

Hypertension (adjunct therapy)

Primary hyperaldosteronism

can severely reduce your blood pressure.

- Your dosage should be adjusted according to your response to the drug; however, the lowest effective dose must be used to minimize an imbalance of electrolytes.
- If you have been given a drug containing spironolactone to treat your high blood pressure, take it as directed, even if you are feeling well. Because blood pressure comes down gradually, it may take several weeks for the full benefit to be seen. Do not discontinue the drug abruptly.
- Your doctor will likely order a complete kidney assessment before starting you on this drug and continue to monitor your kidney function while you are taking it.
- Tell your doctor or dentist that you are taking this drug if you have a medical emergency or are going to have surgery or dental treatment. Spironolactone may alter the body's response to anesthetics.
- Spironolactone may have an effect on certain diagnostic tests. Be sure to tell any healthcare practitioner conducting tests that you are taking this drug.
- Use of spironolactone during pregnancy should be restricted to edema due to pathological causes.
- Do not use this drug while you are nursing a baby. If it is essential, stop breast-feeding.

POSSIBLE INTERACTIONS

Antihypertensive agents and diuretics: increased antihypertensive effects.

Aspirin: causes decreased effectiveness of spironolactone.

Digoxin: increased levels of digoxin; possible digitalis toxicity.

Other potassium-sparing diuretics, ACE inhibitors, potassium supplements: may cause excessively high potassium level. Do not combine with spironolactone.

SIDE EFFECTS

NOT SERIOUS

- Abdominal cramps; vomiting
- Dry mouth; excessive thirst
- Muscle pain or cramps; diarrhea; drowsiness; fever; headache
- Skin eruptions
- Anemia or decreased white blood cell count (spironolactone and hydrochlorothiazide combination)

CALL YOUR DOCTOR IF THESE PROBLEMS PERSIST.

SERIOUS

- Breast development in males
- Deepening of voice, excessive hairiness
- Irregular menstruation; breast soreness in females
- Postmenopausal bleeding
- Sexual dysfunction
- Hives; weak or irregular heartbeat
- Lack of coordination
- Lethargy; mental confusion
- Ulcers; stomach bleeding or inflammation

CONTACT YOUR DOCTOR IMMEDIATELY.

SPONGIA

LATIN NAME
Spongia tosta

VITAL STATISTICS

GENERAL DESCRIPTION

This remedy is derived from the sponge, a primitive form of marine animal life that lacks mobility (and therefore initially was believed to be a plant) and has the unusual capacity to regenerate from broken-off parts of itself. Although most household sponges today are made from cellulose, in ancient times mops and paintbrushes were made from these animals. In the Middle Ages sponges were used medicinally for various purposes.

The homeopathic form is used today for treating specific types of colds, coughs, and sore throat. The remedy is prepared by roasting or toasting the sponge and letting it stand in an alcohol solution. For more information on homeopathic medicine, see page 14.

PREPARATIONS

Spongia is available over the counter in various potencies, in both liquid and tablet form, at selected stores and pharmacies. Consult your homeopathic practitioner for further information.

PRECAUTIONS

SPECIAL INFORMATION

- When a remedy is administered, no one but the patient should touch the pills. If tablets are spilled, throw them away.
- The mouth should be clear of flavors 15 minutes before and after taking a remedy, and strong flavors and aromas, such as coffee and heavy perfume, should be avoided for the duration of treatment.

TARGET AILMENTS

Colds and coughs with these characteristics:

Tickly throat and hoarseness; sore, burning feeling in larynx

Sore throat worsened by coughing, swallowing, and eating sweets; dry mucous membranes

Croupy or harsh cough with raspy barking sound and constricted throat upon awakening

Cough worsened by excitement, talking, alcohol, lying down, and cold drinks; cough improved by warm drinks and eating; burning pains in chest; inflamed bronchial tubes

Asthma with these characteristics:

Difficult, noisy breathing and little phlegm; worsened by both lying down and motion

Improved with leaning head back and taking warm food or drink; feeling of heaviness and exhaustion in which blood rushes to chest, neck, and face

Anxiety, apprehension, fear of dying

SIDE EFFECTS

NONE EXPECTED

St.-John's-Wort

LATIN NAME
Hypericum perforatum

Vital Statistics

GENERAL DESCRIPTION

Herbalists now know that the flowers of the plant called St.-John's-wort, used for centuries to heal wounds, contain hypericin, a substance with germicidal, anti-inflammatory, and antidepressant properties. They also hold high concentrations of flavonoids, chemicals thought to boost the immune system. The plant (*wort* means "plant" in Old English) is named for St. John the Baptist because its yellow flowers are said to bloom on the anniversary of his execution. A woody perennial, its leaves are dotted with glands that produce a red oil when pinched. For visual characteristics of St.-John's-wort, see the Color Guide to Prescription Drugs and Herbs.

PREPARATIONS

Over the counter:
Available as dried leaves and flowers, tinctures, extract, oil, ointment, capsules, and prepared tea.

At home:

Tea: Add 1 to 2 tsp dried herb to 1 cup boiling water; steep covered for 15 minutes. Drink up to 3 cups a day.

Oil: Use a commercial preparation, or make by soaking the flowers in almond or olive oil until the oil turns bright red.

Ointment: Use a commercial preparation, or make by warming the leaves in hot petroleum jelly or a mixture of beeswax and almond oil.

Fresh: Apply crushed leaves and flowers to cleaned wounds.

Tincture: Add ¼ to 1 tsp to an 8-oz glass of water and drink daily.

Consult a qualified practitioner for the dosage appropriate for your specific condition.

Precautions

SPECIAL INFORMATION

- Consult a doctor or herbalist before using St.-John's-wort.
- Use of this herb by children for more than seven to 10 days should be done in conjunction with a healthcare practitioner.

POSSIBLE INTERACTIONS

Amino acids tryptophan and tyrosine; amphetamines; asthma inhalants; beer, coffee, wine; chocolate, fava beans, salami, smoked or pickled foods, and yogurt; cold or hay fever medicines; diet pills; narcotics; nasal decongestants: possible high blood pressure and nausea.

TARGET AILMENTS

Use externally for:

Wounds, including cuts, abrasions, burns; scar tissue

Take internally, in consultation with a herbalist or a doctor, for:

Depression

SIDE EFFECTS

SERIOUS

- High blood pressure; headaches; stiff neck
- Nausea; vomiting
- Worsening of sunburn in the fair-skinned; blistering after sun exposure.

Call your doctor immediately.

SUCRALFATE

VITAL STATISTICS

DRUG CLASS
Antiulcer Drugs

BRAND NAME
Carafate

OTHER DRUGS IN THIS CLASS
lansoprazole, omeprazole
Histamine H_2 Blockers: cimetidine, famotidine, nizatidine, ranitidine

GENERAL DESCRIPTION
Sucralfate is used primarily in the treatment and prevention of ulcers of the stomach and duodenum (first portion of the small intestine). It is also sometimes used to treat gastroesophageal reflux and gastrointestinal symptoms associated with the use of nonsteroidal anti-inflammatory drugs (NSAIDs) and aspirin.

The precise mechanisms by which sucralfate works are not clearly understood. However, the drug is believed to inhibit the digestive action of pepsin, one of the stomach's digestive juices. Sucralfate may also form a coating over ulcers, protecting them from the erosive effect of another digestive fluid, hydrochloric acid. Although sucralfate is often used alone, it is sometimes prescribed in conjunction with antacids for pain relief. For more information on side effects and possible drug interactions, see Antiulcer Drugs. For visual characteristics of the brand-name drug Carafate, see the Color Guide to Prescription Drugs and Herbs.

PRECAUTIONS

SPECIAL INFORMATION

- Sucralfate may interfere with the absorption of vitamins A, D, E, and K; if you are taking vitamin supplements, wait an hour before taking a dose of sucralfate.
- If you are also using antacids for relief from ulcer pain, take the antacid at least 30 minutes before or after taking sucralfate.
- Because this drug may cause dizziness or drowsiness, you may need to restrict your driving or your involvement in other potentially hazardous activities.
- Let your doctor know if you have had kidney or liver disease or any diseases that have caused obstruction of the gastrointestinal tract.

SUCRALFATE

POSSIBLE INTERACTIONS

Alcohol, caffeine, tobacco: avoid these substances that may irritate the ulcer.

Aluminum-containing antidiarrheal drugs, aspirin buffered with aluminum, and aluminum-containing vaginal douches: increased absorption of aluminum into the body, possibly to toxic levels.

Antacids: may keep sucralfate from working properly if taken within 30 minutes before or after sucralfate. Do not take aluminum-containing antacids at all; the combination may lead to a buildup of toxic levels of aluminum in the body.

Cimetidine and ranitidine: decreased effect of these drugs. Take them one to two hours before taking sucralfate.

Ciprofloxacin: decreased ciprofloxacin effect.

Digoxin: decreased digoxin effect.

Phenytoin: significantly decreased phenytoin effect. Do not take within two hours of taking sucralfate.

Tetracycline: decreased tetracycline effect.

Theophylline: decreased theophylline effect.

Warfarin: decreased warfarin effect.

Vitamins A, D, E, and K: decreased absorption of these vitamins.

TARGET AILMENTS

Duodenal ulcer

Gastric ulcer

Upper gastrointestinal bleeding associated with gastric ulcer or duodenal ulcer, or with gastritis

Gastroesophageal reflux

Gastrointestinal symptoms associated with the use of nonsteroidal anti-inflammatory drugs (NSAIDs) and aspirin

SIDE EFFECTS

NOT SERIOUS

- Constipation
- Mild back pain
- Diarrhea; nausea; vomiting
- Stomach cramping
- Dry mouth
- Rash or itching
- Dizziness
- Drowsiness

WITH THE EXCEPTION OF CONSTIPATION AND MILD BACK PAIN, THESE SYMPTOMS ARE RARE. SEE YOUR DOCTOR IF THESE SYMPTOMS PERSIST OR BECOME BOTHERSOME.

SULFAMETHOXAZOLE AND TRIMETHOPRIM

VITAL STATISTICS

DRUG CLASS
Antibiotics [Sulfonamides in Combination]

BRAND NAMES
Bactrim, Cotrim

GENERAL DESCRIPTION
Sulfamethoxazole, a sulfonamide antibiotic, is often combined with the antibiotic drug trimethoprim to increase the effectiveness of both medications. This combination is sometimes known as cotrimoxazole or TMP-SMZ.

Drugs in this antibiotic subclass are used against a wide variety of bacterial infections and are of two types: Bactericidal antibiotics kill bacteria by attacking bacterial cell walls. Bacteriostatic antibiotics prevent bacteria from reproducing, thus enabling the body's defenses to overcome the infection. Both component drugs in this sulfonamide antibiotic, which is a bacteriostatic drug, work by interfering with the ability of certain disease-causing bacteria to synthesize folic acid, thereby inhibiting the organisms' growth.

Antibiotics are not effective against fungal infections or against viruses, such as those that cause colds. But some illnesses with symptoms similar to colds and the flu, such as sinusitis or bronchitis, may be bacterial in origin and will respond to antibiotic treatment.

Because antibiotics target bacteria and not fungi, the drugs in this class can disturb the body's normal balance of fungi and bacteria. This imbalance may be manifested as a fungal superinfection, such as a yeast infection, or in symptoms of diarrhea or gastrointestinal disturbances. See Special Information *(right)* for advice on how to restore your body's normal balance of bacteria and fungi.

For visual characteristics of the brand-name drugs Bactrim and Cotrim, see the Color Guide to Prescription Drugs and Herbs.

Sulfamethoxazole and Trimethoprim

Precautions

SPECIAL INFORMATION

- Antibiotics kill not only harmful bacteria, but also "good" bacteria that keep unwanted fungi and intestinal organisms in check. Eating yogurt containing *Lactobacillus acidophilus* culture or taking acidophilus tablets may help restore the body's normal bacteria.
- Prolonged use of any antibiotic drug can lead to fungal infections, including candidiasis, or to bacterial infections such as pseudomembranous colitis.
- Pregnant and nursing women should avoid using this combination since it may interfere with folic acid metabolism in the fetus and infant, especially near birth.
- Cotrimoxazole may cause sensitivity to the sun or sunlamps. Limit your exposure while taking this drug.
- Cross-sensitivity reactions: If you are sensitive to thiazide diuretics, PABA, local anesthetics (benzocaine), or oral antidiabetic medicines, you may also have a sensitivity to cotrimoxazole. Advise your doctor of your sensitivity.
- Many people are sensitive to these drugs, so be sure to tell your doctor if you have severe allergies or bronchial asthma.
- To prevent reinfection, complete the full course of your prescription, even if you feel better before you've taken all the medicine.
- When taking these drugs, drink plenty of fluids to prevent formation of crystals in the urine.

Target Ailments

- Bronchitis (caused by *Hemophilus influenzae* or *Streptococcus pneumoniae*)
- Urinary tract infections
- Enterocolitis (caused by certain species of *Shigella*)
- Acute otitis media (in children)
- Prevention and treatment of pneumonia (*Pneumocystis carinii)* in people with compromised immune systems (including AIDS patients)
- Traveler's diarrhea
- Numerous other infections

SULFAMETHOXAZOLE AND TRIMETHOPRIM

POSSIBLE INTERACTIONS

This combination can interact with a number of drugs, especially those that affect the liver or blood. Consult your doctor before taking any other medication.

Anticoagulants (warfarin), anticonvulsants (hydantoin), oral antidiabetics, phenylbutazone (NSAID), or sulfinpyrazone (antigout): may interfere with action or metabolism of these drugs and could result in increased effects or toxicity. Your doctor may need to adjust the dosage.

Birth-control pills containing estrogen: may result in decreased contraceptive effectiveness and increased breakthrough bleeding.

Cyclosporine: decreased effectiveness of cyclosporine.

Digoxin: decreased digoxin effects.

Methotrexate: increased methotrexate effects.

SIDE EFFECTS

NOT SERIOUS

- Gastrointestinal problems (including diarrhea and nausea)
- Headache
- Dizziness
- Photosensitivity

LET YOUR DOCTOR KNOW IF THESE SYMPTOMS BECOME TROUBLESOME.

SERIOUS

- Allergic reactions (fever, itchy skin rash)
- Blood abnormalities causing fever, sore throat, unusual bleeding, bruising, tiredness, or weakness
- Liver problems, including jaundice
- Stevens-Johnson syndrome (fever, skin blisters or blisters and open sores on mucous membranes and genitals, weakness, joint pain)
- Urinary problems resulting in burning with urination, back pain
- Goiter
- Bluish fingernails, skin, or lips
- Difficulty in breathing

CALL YOUR DOCTOR IMMEDIATELY.

SULFONAMIDES IN COMBINATION

VITAL STATISTICS

DRUG CLASS
Antibiotics

GENERIC NAME
sulfamethoxazole and trimethoprim

GENERAL DESCRIPTION
Sulfonamides, a subclass of antibiotics, are synthetic derivatives of a compound that interferes with the ability of bacteria to produce folic acid, necessary for cell growth and development. While this doesn't immediately kill bacteria, it inhibits their growth and aids the body in its fight against infection. These drugs are often used in combinations to enhance the effectiveness of other medications and to offset possible bacterial resistance to sulfonamides.

Sulfamethoxazole is often combined with trimethoprim to obtain a broader spectrum of activity as well as increased drug effectiveness. For more information, including possible drug interactions, see Sulfamethoxazole and Trimethoprim; also see Antibiotics.

TARGET AILMENTS

Bronchitis; urinary tract infections; acute otitis media (in children); enterocolitis (caused by certain species of *Shigella*)

Prevention and treatment of pneumonia *(Pneumocystis carinii)* in people with compromised immune systems (including AIDS patients)

Traveler's diarrhea

PRECAUTIONS

SPECIAL INFORMATION
Antibiotics also affect "good" bacteria that keep unwanted fungi and intestinal organisms in check. Eating yogurt containing *Lactobacillus acidophilus* culture or taking acidophilus tablets may help restore the normal bacteria.

SIDE EFFECTS

NOT SERIOUS
- Gastrointestinal problems (including diarrhea and nausea); headache or dizziness; photosensitivity

LET YOUR DOCTOR KNOW IF THESE SYMPTOMS BECOME TROUBLESOME.

SERIOUS
- Allergic reactions (fever, itchy skin rash)
- Blood abnormalities causing fever, sore throat, unusual bleeding, bruising, tiredness, or weakness
- Liver problems, including jaundice; goiter
- Stevens-Johnson syndrome (fever, skin blisters or blisters and open sores on mucous membranes and genitals, weakness, joint pain)
- Urinary problems
- Bluish nails, skin, or lips
- Difficulty in breathing

CALL YOUR DOCTOR IMMEDIATELY.

Rx SULFONYLUREAS

VITAL STATISTICS

DRUG CLASS
Antidiabetic Drugs

GENERIC NAMES
glipizide, glyburide

GENERAL DESCRIPTION
A subclass of antidiabetic drugs, sulfonylureas (also known as oral hypoglycemics) are used to treat a form of non-insulin-dependent (Type 2) diabetes that cannot be controlled by diet and exercise alone. Sulfonylureas stimulate the release of existing insulin in people whose bodies are capable of producing insulin. These drugs do not lower blood sugar on their own but can work effectively when used in conjunction with a prescribed diet and exercise program. For more information about this class of drug, including additional precautions and possible drug interactions, see Oral Hypoglycemics. For information about other medications used to treat diabetes (including other oral medications classified as "antihyperglycemics," which work by a different mechanism from hypoglycemics), see the entries for Acarbose, Metformin, Troglitazone, Antidiabetic Drugs, and Insulin.

S

PRECAUTIONS

SPECIAL INFORMATION
- An overdose of these drugs can result in hypoglycemia (abnormally small concentrations of sugar in the blood). Signs of hypoglycemia include excessive hunger, cold sweats, shakiness, nervousness or anxiety, rapid pulse, headache, drowsiness, confusion, nausea, and cool, pale skin. Keep hard candy or fruit juice handy to raise your blood sugar level and counteract hypoglycemia. Call your doctor.
- Tell your doctor if you are allergic to sulfa drugs; you may also be allergic to sulfonylureas.

TARGET AILMENTS

Non-insulin-dependent (Type 2) diabetes

SIDE EFFECTS

NOT SERIOUS

- Constipation or diarrhea; nausea, vomiting, or stomach pain; heartburn
- Dizziness, mild drowsiness; headache
- Change in appetite
- Skin allergies; weakness; tingling of hands and feet

CALL YOUR DOCTOR IF THESE SYMPTOMS PERSIST.

SERIOUS

- Sore throat and unusual bleeding or bruising
- Water retention (edema)
- Weight gain
- Jaundice
- Abnormally light-colored stools; low-grade fever, fatigue, chills

CONTACT YOUR DOCTOR IMMEDIATELY. ALSO SEE THE OVERDOSE SYMPTOMS LISTED IN SPECIAL INFORMATION.

SULFUR

VITAL STATISTICS

GENERAL DESCRIPTION

Accounting for some 10 percent of the body's mineral content, sulfur is part of every cell, especially in the protein-rich tissues of hair, nails, muscle, and skin. It assists in metabolism as a part of vitamin B_1, biotin, and vitamin B_5; helps regulate blood sugar levels as a constituent of insulin; and helps regulate blood clotting. Sulfur is also known to convert some toxic substances into nontoxic ones that can then be excreted; for that reason it is used to treat poisoning from aluminum, cadmium, lead, and mercury.

Neither sulfur deficiency nor toxicity occurs naturally in humans.

RDA/EMDR

Not established.

NATURAL SOURCES

Any diet that provides sufficient protein is also providing adequate sulfur. Meat, fish, poultry, eggs, dairy products, peas, and beans are rich in both nutrients.

PRECAUTIONS

SPECIAL INFORMATION

Inorganic sulfur ingested in large amounts can be harmful, but excess organic sulfur from food is readily excreted.

TARGET AILMENTS

Toxic exposure

SIDE EFFECTS

NONE EXPECTED

SULPHUR

LATIN NAME
Sulphur

VITAL STATISTICS

GENERAL DESCRIPTION

The chemical element sulphur, or more commonly sulfur, is present in all living tissue. It was known to ancient societies, and in the Bible it is called brimstone. Among the various conditions to which it has been applied as a medication, for some 2,000 years, are skin disorders such as scabies. Commercially, sulfur is used in the production of dyes, fungicides, and gunpowder. Homeopathic physicians may prescribe dilute doses of the remedy *Sulphur* to treat conditions accompanied by irritability, intense itching, burning pains, and offensive odors. The homeopathic remedy is made from pure sulfur powder that is diluted with either milk sugar or a water-and-alcohol solution.

Like most homeopathic prescriptions, *Sulphur* was developed as a remedy by observation of the reactions of healthy individuals to doses of various strengths. The mental, emotional, and physical changes induced by *Sulphur* were then cataloged. When a patient exhibits a set of symptoms that matches the cataloged symptoms brought on by *Sulphur,* the homeopathic practitioner then prescribes it in an extremely dilute form. It is presumed that in this highly dilute dosage, *Sulphur* can counter the types of symptoms that are similar to the ones it induces when it is at full strength. For more information on homeopathic medicine, see page 14.

PREPARATIONS

Sulphur is available over the counter in various potencies, in both liquid and tablet form, at selected stores and pharmacies. Consult your homeopathic physician for more precise information.

PRECAUTIONS

SPECIAL INFORMATION

- Only the patient should touch the pills. If tablets are spilled, throw them away.
- The mouth should be clear of flavors 15 minutes before and after taking a remedy, and strong flavors and aromas should be avoided for the duration of treatment.

TARGET AILMENTS

Asthma that is worse at night and is accompanied by rattling mucus

Cough with chest pain

Morning diarrhea

Eye inflammation

Bursitis

Headache with burning pain

Indigestion

Joint pain

Anal itching with redness

Burning vaginal discharge

Eczema with intense itching and burning

SIDE EFFECTS

NONE EXPECTED

Rx SUMATRIPTAN

VITAL STATISTICS

DRUG CLASS
Antimigraine Drugs

BRAND NAME
Imitrex

GENERAL DESCRIPTION
Introduced in 1993, sumatriptan is an antimigraine drug used to treat classic migraine headaches (those preceded by the warning sensation known as an aura) as well as common migraines (those without an aura). The drug—originally sold only in injectable form but now also available as a tablet—provides fast relief from the intense pain associated with these types of headaches.

Sumatriptan, a vasoconstrictor, works by narrowing dilated blood vessels and reducing the amount of blood flowing through them. Swollen cranial blood vessels are believed to be a major cause of migraine headaches. Sumatriptan may also act as an anti-inflammatory; this action appears to further reduce the swelling. In addition, the medication relieves the nausea, vomiting, and intense light and sound sensitivity that frequently accompany migraines.

If you suffer from more than three migraine headaches per month, your doctor may suggest that you regularly take drugs that help prevent migraine attacks, such as beta-adrenergic blockers, calcium channel blockers, anti-inflammatory drugs, or antidepressants. If you have only one or two mild to moderate migraines per month, your doctor may recommend that you take vasoconstrictive drugs, anti-inflammatory medications, or opioid analgesics at the first sign of a headache.

PRECAUTIONS

SPECIAL INFORMATION
- Do not use this drug if you have ever had an allergic reaction to it.
- Do not use sumatriptan for the treatment of hemiplegic (restricted to one side of the head) or basilar (restricted to the base of the skull) migraine.
- Do not use this drug if you have uncontrolled high blood pressure (hypertension) or Prinzmetal's angina, or if you have had a heart attack or stroke.
- Inform your doctor and use this drug with caution if you are pregnant or nursing or if you have liver, kidney, or heart disease, coronary artery disease, heart arrhythmia, Raynaud's syndrome, or epilepsy; or are taking high blood pressure medications or other prescription or over-the-counter drugs, especially other migraine-relieving medications.
- Take at the first sign of a migraine. If your first dose fails to relieve your migraine, do not take a second dose without first checking with your doctor.

CONTINUED

SUMATRIPTAN

POSSIBLE INTERACTIONS

Alcohol: may cause excess sedation and make headaches worse.

Ergotamine: may increase the effects of sumatriptan. Allow at least 24 hours between taking ergotamine and sumatriptan.

Lithium, Monoamine oxidase (MAO) inhibitors, antidepressants: may result in excessive quantities of the neurotransmitter serotonin in the brain.

TARGET AILMENTS

Migraine headache

SIDE EFFECTS

NOT SERIOUS

- Tightness in the chest, jaw, or neck immediately after the drug is injected
- Pain, redness, or burning at the injection site
- Nausea or vomiting
- Dizziness or fainting
- Drowsiness
- Flushing, tingling, or numbness
- Excessive thirst
- Frequent urination

IF THESE PROBLEMS CONTINUE FOR MORE THAN AN HOUR, CONTACT YOUR DOCTOR.

SERIOUS

- Continuing pain or tightness in the chest
- Swelling of the face, lips, or eyelids
- Wheezing
- Changes in heart rate or blood pressure
- Skin rash
- Difficulty in swallowing or breathing
- Confusion

CONTACT YOUR DOCTOR IMMEDIATELY.

SUPERIOR SORE THROAT POWDER

VITAL STATISTICS

CHINESE NAME
Shuang Liao Hou Feng San

GENERAL DESCRIPTION
Superior Sore Throat Powder is a Chinese herbal formula used topically for sores in the mouth, including sore throat, mouth ulcers, toothache, sore gums, and canker sores. It comes in the form of a powder spray. With a practitioner's guidance, the formula can be used in the nose or ears for sinus or ear infections. It also soothes and helps heal skin conditions like boils and blisters. Many of the herbs in the formula get rid of "heat," a term used in Chinese medicine that in this case corresponds to inflammation and pain.

Chinese medicine takes a holistic approach to healthcare, fashioning remedies to treat the entire being as well as the specific parts or areas. Precise combinations of herbs are used to prevent and combat disease, which is thought to arise from disturbances in the flow of a bodily energy called chi (pronounced "chee") and blood, or from a lack of balance in the complementary states of yin and yang. A patent formula, Superior Sore Throat Powder is made by using a standardized combination of herbs and method of preparation.

INGREDIENTS
cow gallstones, borneol, licorice, indigo leaves, mother-of-pearl, coptis, sophora

PREPARATIONS
This formula is available in a spray bottle in many Chinese pharmacies and Oriental grocery stores.

PRECAUTIONS

WARNING
Use only for short periods of time and for no more than a week at a time.

TARGET AILMENTS
Sore throat and tonsillitis
Mouth ulcers or canker sores
Toothache or sore gums
Sinus infections
Carbuncles, boils, and skin blisters

SIDE EFFECTS

- This powder has a rather unpleasant bitter taste. Chinese medicine practitioners say that whether you taste them or not, the bitter herbs are precisely what gets rid of the inflammation.

Superoxide Dismutase

Vital Statistics

OTHER NAME
SOD

GENERAL DESCRIPTION
Superoxide dismutase, or SOD, is a naturally occurring antioxidant enzyme that contains minerals such as zinc, copper, and manganese. It protects the body's cells and keeps membranes, tissues, and muscles from hardening. Because of these qualities, SOD is thought to be useful in treating disorders that involve hardening of skin, tissues, and muscles. This category includes diseases such as scleroderma, rheumatoid arthritis, and other autoimmune disorders. Some animal research has suggested SOD can boost the immune system. Many human studies have shown SOD can restore tissue that has been hardened by radiation therapy. One study showed SOD could be effective in repairing radiation-damaged tissue several years after the damage occurred. And some research suggests SOD can help repair the heart muscle following a heart attack. SOD has also been found to protect against free radicals, irregular oxygen molecules that damage cells and tissues and contribute to the development of cancer.

Since orally administered SOD is destroyed in the intestines before it can reach the tissues, muscles, or joints, SOD in pill form is not effective. To be effective, SOD must be injected with a needle or by using liposomes, artificial membranelike structures that act as a delivery vehicle and are injected under the skin. SOD delivered through liposomes is called LIPSOD.

PREPARATIONS
Superoxide dismutase is sold in the United States in tablet form as a dietary supplement. Injectable forms are available only with medical supervision.

Precautions

WARNING
Injectable superoxide dismutase can cause life-threatening anaphylaxis. Symptoms include low blood pressure, paleness, severe itching, loss of consciousness, and coma.

TARGET AILMENTS
Anemia
Autoimmune diseases such as lupus, rheumatoid arthritis, and scleroderma
Vasculitis, including Behçet's disease and Kawasaki's disease
Cataracts (prevention)
Crohn's disease
Radiation-induced necrosis
Raynaud's syndrome

SIDE EFFECTS

SERIOUS

- Anaphylaxis

SEEK EMERGENCY HELP.

SYNTHROID

VITAL STATISTICS

DRUG CLASS
Thyroid Hormones

GENERIC NAME
levothyroxine

OTHER DRUGS IN THIS CLASS
thyroid USP

GENERAL DESCRIPTION
Synthroid is a brand name for levothyroxine, the drug of choice for thyroid replacement therapy because of its standard hormone content and predictable effect. Hormones produced by the thyroid gland regulate functions such as metabolism and protein synthesis, general body growth, and development of the bones and central nervous system. They also affect the heart rate. Thyroid hormone therapy usually must be maintained throughout the patient's life unless it is prescribed for a transient condition affecting thyroid function. Because these hormones are so critical to normal growth and development, children should be tested to ensure that their thyroid glands are functioning normally; those whose bodies are not producing sufficient quantities must be given supplemental thyroid hormones as soon as possible. Thyroid medications are sometimes used diagnostically to check for thyroid disease.

For visual characteristics, see the Color Guide to Prescription Drugs and Herbs.

PRECAUTIONS

SPECIAL INFORMATION
- Your doctor may tell you to continue using levothyroxine while you're pregnant or nursing. Although small amounts of this drug may cross the placenta or be present in breast milk, no studies have shown harm to the fetus or breast-feeding baby.
- Tell your doctor if you have cardiovascular disease, or if you have diabetes or other hormone problems, such as low pituitary gland secretions. Your doctor may decide not to use levothyroxine or to lower the dosage.
- Absorption of levothyroxine through the digestive tract may be affected by food. Take on an empty stomach (one hour before or two hours after a meal).
- The dosage for older people and for people with severe hypothyroidism or cardiovascular problems must be monitored closely. Dosages for older patients are usually lower than those prescribed for younger ones.
- In rare cases after long-term use at high dosages, levothyroxine may cause bone loss.

TARGET AILMENTS

Hypothyroidism (underactive or nonfunctioning thyroid) or as treatment following removal of thyroid gland

Goiter (enlargement of thyroid)

Some types of thyroid cancer, for prevention and treatment, especially after radiation therapy to the neck

CONTINUED

SYNTHROID

POSSIBLE INTERACTIONS

Anticoagulant and antiplatelet drugs (such as warfarin): increased anticlotting action. Your doctor may have to adjust the dosage of anticlotting drugs.

Antidepressants, including tricyclic antidepressants such as amitriptyline: increased action and side effects of both combined drugs, leading to heart-rhythm problems and other signs of excess stimulation.

Antidiabetic drugs (such as insulin): increased need for insulin or other diabetic drugs, perhaps leading to higher blood sugar levels. Your doctor may need to adjust your insulin dose.

Cholesterol-reducing drugs (such as cholestyramine): blocked or delayed absorption of levothyroxine, decreasing its effectiveness. Take levothyroxine one hour before or four to five hours after taking cholesterol-reducing drugs.

Heart-stimulating drugs (such as epinephrine or pseudoephedrine): increased effects of both combined drugs, potentially causing heart problems or an increased chance of levothyroxine overdose.

Other hormones (such as estrogen): may interfere with levothyroxine action, necessitating higher doses.

SIDE EFFECTS

NOT SERIOUS

- Changes in menstrual periods (short-term)
- Clumsiness
- Coldness
- Constipation
- Dry, puffy skin
- Headache
- Sleepiness, fatigue, or weakness
- Heart palpitations
- Muscle aches
- Weight gain
- Temporary hair loss in children

THESE PROBLEMS ARE RARE, BUT MAY OCCUR AT THE BEGINNING OF TREATMENT. CALL YOUR DOCTOR IF THEY PERSIST.

SERIOUS

- Allergic reactions such as skin rash or hives
- Severe persistent and ongoing headache
- Menstrual irregularity
- Changes in appetite
- Chest pain
- Irregular heartbeat; tremors
- Fever or sweating
- Nervousness; irritability
- Leg cramps
- Sensitivity to heat
- Weight loss

THESE PROBLEMS ARE RARE. IF YOU EXPERIENCE ANY OF THEM TELL YOUR DOCTOR RIGHT AWAY. YOUR DOCTOR MAY NEED TO ADJUST YOUR DOSAGE.

TABACUM

LATIN NAME
Nicotiana tabacum

VITAL STATISTICS

GENERAL DESCRIPTION

The remedy *Tabacum* comes from the tobacco plant, an annual herb native to the Americas. The plant is cultivated for its leaves, which are large and bitter tasting, and are prepared for use in smoking and chewing and as snuff. American Indians are believed to have been the first to smoke tobacco; the practice was later brought to Europe by Spanish explorers.

Although tobacco has not been employed principally as a medicine, it was used in the past in enemas to treat intestinal obstruction and as snuff to bring on sneezing, which was thought to be beneficial because it increases the secretion of mucus. However, its volatile oil, nicotine, is such a powerful poison that it has been used as an insecticide. The toxic effects of nicotine include nausea, vomiting, weakness, sweating, and palpitations.

The homeopathic remedy, used principally to treat extreme nausea and vomiting, is prepared from cut dry leaves, which are left for a time to soak in an alcohol solution.

Like most homeopathic prescriptions, *Tabacum* was developed as a remedy by observation of the reactions of healthy individuals to a series of doses of various strengths. The mental, emotional, and physical changes induced by *Tabacum* were then cataloged. When a patient exhibits a set of symptoms that matches the cataloged symptoms brought on by *Tabacum,* the homeopathic practitioner then prescribes it in an extremely dilute form. It is presumed that in this highly dilute dosage, *Tabacum* can counter symptoms that are similar to the ones it induces when it is at full strength. For more information on homeopathic medicine, see page 14.

PREPARATIONS

Tabacum is available over the counter in various potencies, in both liquid and tablet form, at selected stores and pharmacies. Consult your homeopathic physician for more precise information.

PRECAUTIONS

SPECIAL INFORMATION

- When a remedy is administered, no one but the patient should touch the pills. If tablets are spilled, throw them away.
- The mouth should be clear of flavors 15 minutes before and after taking a remedy, and strong flavors and aromas, such as coffee, camphor, and heavily scented perfumes, should be avoided for the duration of treatment.

TARGET AILMENTS

Extreme nausea with cold perspiration that is worse in a stuffy room; may be caused by pregnancy or motion sickness

Violent vomiting that is worse with movement and warmth and better in open air; may be caused by pregnancy or motion sickness

SIDE EFFECTS

NONE EXPECTED

T

TAMOXIFEN

VITAL STATISTICS

DRUG CLASS
Anticancer Drugs

BRAND NAME
Nolvadex

GENERAL DESCRIPTION
Tamoxifen is an antiestrogen drug used to prevent or delay the recurrence of breast cancer after primary therapy, including breast surgery, radiation therapy, and chemotherapy. In some breast cancers, the hormone estrogen can stimulate breast cancer growth. Tamoxifen works by preventing estrogen from acting on the estrogen-sensitive tissues and tumors of the breast. The drug may be given in conjunction with chemotherapy treatments after surgery or used alone to treat metastatic breast cancer.

PRECAUTIONS

WARNING
Using tamoxifen increases the risk of changes to the endometrium (the lining of the uterus), including hyperplasia, polyps, and endometrial cancer. Call your doctor right away if you experience abnormal vaginal bleeding, a possible symptom of endometrial cancer.

This drug appears to increase the risk of cataracts and retinopathy. Tell your doctor right away if you notice vision changes while using tamoxifen.

SPECIAL INFORMATION
- Do not use tamoxifen if you have had a serious adverse reaction to it.
- Tell your doctor if you have ever had thrombophlebitis, pulmonary embolism, impaired liver function, cataracts, a blood cell or bone marrow disorder, or abnormally high blood calcium levels. Your doctor may lower your dose of tamoxifen or prescribe a different drug.
- This drug may decrease your blood cell counts, so use with caution if you have significantly low levels of white blood cells or platelets. Your doctor may perform periodic blood tests.
- Maintain routine gynecologic care while taking tamoxifen. Report abnormal vaginal bleeding to your doctor.
- Do not use hormonal contraceptives with tamoxifen because they decrease tamoxifen's effects.
- Do not use tamoxifen during pregnancy or while breast-feeding, or become pregnant while using this drug.

TAMOXIFEN

POSSIBLE INTERACTIONS

Antacids and some antiulcer drugs (cimetidine, famotidine, and ranitidine): prematurely dissolve tamoxifen's enteric coating. Take these medications one to two hours before taking tamoxifen.

Anticancer drugs (bleomycin, daunorubicin, doxorubicin, fluorouracil, hydroxyurea, methotrexate, mitotane, mitoxantrone, procarbazine, and vincristine): increased risk of thromboembolism.

Anticoagulants (such as warfarin): increased anticoagulant effect.

Estrogen or oral contraceptives: decreased tamoxifen effect.

TARGET AILMENTS

Breast cancer (in women and men, although male breast cancer is rare)

SIDE EFFECTS

NOT SERIOUS

- Hot flashes
- Nausea or vomiting
- Skin rash or genital itching
- Increased flaring pain in tumor or bone
- Impotence and loss of libido in men

CONSULT YOUR DOCTOR IF THESE EFFECTS CONTINUE OR ARE BOTHERSOME.

SERIOUS

- Liver damage (no symptoms)
- Retinopathy, cataracts, or corneal changes
- Endometrial cancer, endometrial polyps, or endometrial hyperplasia (abnormal vaginal bleeding, pain or pressure in pelvis, change in vaginal discharge)
- Abnormally high blood calcium levels (confusion); low white blood cell count (fever, infections); low platelet count (bleeding)
- Thrombotic events, including pulmonary embolism (shortness of breath); deep vein thrombosis; superficial phlebitis

CALL YOUR DOCTOR PROMPTLY.

Tangerine Peel

LATIN NAME
Citrus reticulata

Vital Statistics

GENERAL DESCRIPTION

Sometimes called mandarin orange peel, this herb is prescribed for digestive disorders. Chinese medicine practitioners believe that the peel gets better as it ages, and its Chinese name, *chén pí,* can be translated into English as "aged peel." A mixture of aged tangerine peel and licorice has been used in a clinical study to treat mastitis (inflammation of the breast). Herbalists use the red part of tangerine peel (when dried, some parts are orange and others red) to control vomiting and belching. Chinese practitioners also prescribe young, or green, tangerine peel for breast and side pain and for hernia pain. The green peel has recently been used to raise blood pressure when it is too low. The best samples of the fruit are thin skinned, pliable, oily, and fragrant. Chinese herbalists characterize the herb as acrid, bitter, and warm.

Chinese medicine takes a holistic approach to healthcare, fashioning remedies to treat the entire being as well as the specific parts or areas. Single herbs may be used alone or in combination with other herbs to prevent and combat disease, which is thought to arise from disturbances in the flow of a bodily energy called chi (pronounced "chee") and blood, or from a lack of balance in the complementary states of yin and yang.

PREPARATIONS

Tangerine peel is available at any Chinese pharmacy or Asian food market, as well as at Western health food stores. It is also available in pill form.

Combinations: In a preparation with Asian ginseng, tangerine peel is used as a digestive stimulant. Chinese herbalists prescribe a mixture of tangerine peel, ripe bitter orange, and aucklandia for abdominal distention, fullness, and pain. And a preparation containing tangerine peel and pinellia root is used to treat a stifling feeling in the chest that makes deep breathing difficult, together with an excess of phlegm. For further information on appropriate preparations and doses, check with a herbal practitioner.

Precautions

WARNING

Do not use this herb if you have a dry cough or an excessively red tongue, or if you are spitting up blood.

TARGET AILMENTS
Take internally for:
Indigestion
Gas
Feeling of swelling, bloat, or fullness in the abdomen
Nausea and vomiting
Loose stools
Bringing up phlegm

SIDE EFFECTS

None expected

TARRAGON

LATIN NAME
Artemisia dracunculus

VITAL STATISTICS

GENERAL DESCRIPTION
This bushy perennial plant native to Asia has narrow bright green leaves and small flowers that do not yield seeds. Tarragon is believed to have been introduced into Europe by the Crusaders. It was used in the Middle Ages as an antidote to the bites and stings of poisonous snakes and insects and bites of rabid dogs. It also was used to fight the plague. The oil, which is colorless, has an aroma similar to anise.

Tarragon has antispasmodic, diuretic, stimulative, and mild laxative properties.

PREPARATIONS
The leaves are distilled to produce the essential oil. Dried tarragon leaves do not retain the healing properties of the fresh plant. The best way to preserve tarragon is to put fresh leaves in a bottle of white wine vinegar. After two weeks the vinegar will be ready to use.

Use a diffuser to scent a room, or add drops to a handkerchief and hold up to the nose as often as desired.

SIDE EFFECTS

MANY PEOPLE HAVE MILD REACTIONS TO A COMPONENT OF TARRAGON CALLED ESTRAGOLE (OR METHYL CHAVICOL). USE TARRAGON IN MODERATION AND WITH CARE.

PRECAUTIONS

WARNING
Tarragon is considered mildly toxic by some aromatherapists. It may also have carcinogenic properties. Avoid using tarragon oil during pregnancy.

SPECIAL INFORMATION
There are two varieties of tarragon: true, or French, tarragon, which is used in aromatherapy and in cooking; and false, or Russian, tarragon, which is of an inferior quality. The true tarragon plant is sterile and can be cultivated only by propagating the cuttings. Do not purchase tarragon seeds, which come from false tarragon.

TARGET AILMENTS
Menstrual and menopausal symptoms
Digestive ailments
Hiccups
Loss of appetite
Indigestion and gas
Shock
Anxiety and stress

TEA TREE

LATIN NAME
Melaleuca alternifolia

VITAL STATISTICS

GENERAL DESCRIPTION

Native to New South Wales, Australia, the tea tree gets its name from its use as a type of herbal tea, which is made from the leaves. The current knowledge of the plant's properties and uses comes from the Australian Aborigines, who have a long history of using tea tree. The oil has gained popularity as an ingredient in shampoo, mouthwashes, and body massage oil in the last two decades.

Tea tree is a powerful immunostimulant, increasing the immune system's ability to fight disease. Aromatherapists recommend having tea tree in a first-aid kit because of its antiseptic action against bacteria, fungi, and viruses. It is soothing to the skin and mucous membranes, and it is also effective as an insect repellent.

The tea tree or shrub has small, narrow leaves and yellow or purple flowers. It is closely related to the tree that produces the essential oil niaouli. Its tart oil ranges from colorless to pale yellow-green.

PREPARATIONS

The essential oil is distilled from the tea tree's leaves and twigs. The leaves need to be bruised so that they will release their oil.

STEAM INHALATIONS: For respiratory ailments add 6 drops oil to a bowl of water that has been boiled. With a towel over your head and the bowl, inhale for up to 5 minutes.

SKIN APPLICATIONS: Tea tree can be applied undiluted to the skin a drop at a time for small-sized skin problems. If irritation occurs, dilute by half or more with aloe gel. For acne, mix 2 drops oil in 2 tsp aloe gel.

BATHS OR SITZ BATHS: For vaginal and urinary problems add 5 to 10 drops oil to the water. To use tea tree as a douche, add 2 to 4 drops oil to the water used and shake well before application.

TARGET AILMENTS
Colds and flu
Tonsillitis (add 3 drops oil to ½ cup water and gargle)
Bronchitis
Sinusitis
Abscesses
Acne
Small burns, cuts, and wounds
Vaginal thrush; vaginitis
Bladder infections
Candida infection
Cold sores
Insect bites

SIDE EFFECTS

TEA TREE MAY CAUSE A SKIN REACTION IN SOME PEOPLE, DESPITE ITS HYPOALLERGENIC AND NONTOXIC CONSTITUTION.

Tea Tree Oil

LATIN NAME
Melaleuca spp.

Vital Statistics

GENERAL DESCRIPTION

The first Europeans to reach Australia made tea from the leaves of what then became known as the tea tree, which should not be confused with the common tea plant. For centuries before the Europeans arrived, native Australians were using the leaves of this tree as an antiseptic. Eventually the Europeans learned to use the leaves' volatile oil to treat cuts, abrasions, burns, insect bites, and other minor skin ailments. Modern studies show that the strong germicidal activity of tea tree oil is caused primarily by a single ingredient, terpineol. The oil, which smells like nutmeg, is extracted from the leaves by steam distillation. During World War II, tea tree oil was added to machine oils to reduce infection in the hands of workers during metal fabrication. The oils of some species of *Melaleuca* may irritate the skin and are not used. For visual characteristics of tea tree oil, see the Color Guide to Prescription Drugs and Herbs.

PREPARATIONS

Over the counter:

Available as oil and also as an additive to health and beauty products such as toothpaste, soap, and shampoo.

At home:

Apply fresh leaves directly to wounds.
Consult a qualified practitioner for the dosage appropriate for you and the specific condition being treated.

Precautions

SPECIAL INFORMATION

- People with sensitive skin should dilute tea tree oil with a bland oil, such as vegetable oil.
- Use of this herb by children for more than seven to 10 days should be done in conjunction with a healthcare practitioner.

POSSIBLE INTERACTIONS

Combining tea tree oil with other herbs may necessitate a lower dosage.

TARGET AILMENTS

Apply externally for:

Insect bites

Acne seen in teenagers, fungal infections such as athlete's foot, and other skin ailments

Minor vaginal infections (use as a douche)

Flea shampoos for pets

SIDE EFFECTS

NOT SERIOUS

LOCAL SKIN AND VAGINAL IRRITATION MAY DEVELOP IN SENSITIVE INDIVIDUALS. LET YOUR DOCTOR KNOW IF IT PERSISTS.

Temazepam

Vital Statistics

DRUG CLASS
Antianxiety Drugs [Benzodiazepines]

BRAND NAME
Restoril

OTHER DRUGS IN THIS SUBCLASS
alprazolam, clonazepam, diazepam, lorazepam, triazolam

GENERAL DESCRIPTION
A mild sedative and hypnotic, temazepam is prescribed for the short-term treatment of insomnia. Temazepam works by enhancing the action of a natural chemical in the brain that acts to depress certain areas of the central nervous system. The effects start after the first dose. Though temazepam can cause physical and psychological dependence, it is considered particularly useful because it has fewer toxicity problems, fewer side effects, and less abuse potential than other drugs used for the same purposes. For visual characteristics of temazepam and the brand Restoril, see the Color Guide to Prescription Drugs and Herbs.

Precautions

☠ ***WARNING***
Never combine alcohol with temazepam; the combination can cause dangerous central nervous system and respiratory depression. Do not abruptly stop taking temazepam. Sudden cessation can provoke withdrawal symptoms, including seizures; irritability; insomnia; confusion; mental depression; hypersensitivity to pain, noise, or light; and feelings of suspicion and distrust. Slowly reduce the dosage under your doctor's guidance.

SPECIAL INFORMATION
- Do not use this drug unless you can allow yourself seven or eight hours of sleep every night for the duration of the treatment. If you don't give the medication time to wear off, you may experience temporary amnesia, perhaps lasting several hours.
- Temazepam can impair your alertness, judgment, and coordination. Avoid driving and performing hazardous activities until you know how the drug affects you.
- Let your doctor know if you have narrow-angle glaucoma, a liver or kidney impairment, chronic respiratory disease, myasthenia gravis, depression, sleep apnea, or a history of drug abuse or addiction. Temazepam may make these conditions worse.
- This drug can cause sleep apnea in people with chronic respiratory disease, such as emphysema.
- Temazepam can cause physical and psychological dependence, sometimes after only one or two weeks, but usually after prolonged use.
- People with a history of drug or alcohol abuse are at a greater risk of psychological dependence on temazepam.
- Tolerance may increase with prolonged use; as your body adjusts to temazepam, the drug becomes less effective. Never increase the dose without consulting your doctor, because the risk of temazepam dependence increases with higher doses.
- Do not take temazepam if you are pregnant or breast-feeding.

TEMAZEPAM

POSSIBLE INTERACTIONS

Alcohol, anticonvulsants, antihistamines that cause drowsiness (clemastine, diphenhydramine), barbiturates, monoamine oxidase (MAO) inhibitors, opioids, tricyclic antidepressants: increased sedative effects, such as excessive mental (central nervous system) depression, sleepiness, and slow or shallow breathing. It is very important that you avoid taking temazepam in combination with any of these drugs.

Antacids: may slow the absorption of temazepam. Separate from the temazepam dose by an hour.

Beta blockers, cimetidine, disulfiram, erythromycin, ketoconazole, omeprazole, oral contraceptives, probenecid: may prolong the amount of time temazepam remains in your body, leading to increased temazepam effects and possible toxicity.

Clozapine: risk of profound hypotension (low blood pressure), slow or shallow breathing, cessation of breathing, and cardiac arrest leading to death.

Isoniazid: possible increased effect and toxicity of temazepam.

Levodopa: decreased levodopa effect.

Rifampin: possible decreased effect of temazepam.

Tobacco (smoking): decreased temazepam effects.

Valproic acid: increased temazepam effects, including mental depression.

Zidovudine: risk of zidovudine toxicity.

TARGET AILMENTS

Insomnia

SIDE EFFECTS

NOT SERIOUS

- Clumsiness or unsteadiness
- Lethargy
- Dry mouth
- Nausea
- Change in bowel habits
- Temporary amnesia (especially "traveler's amnesia" when taken to treat insomnia associated with jet lag)

TELL YOUR DOCTOR IF THESE SYMPTOMS PERSIST OR BECOME BOTHERSOME. CONTACT YOUR DOCTOR IF YOU ARE HAVING DIFFICULTY WITH YOUR MEMORY.

SERIOUS

- Drowsiness
- Dizziness or blurred vision
- Persistent or severe headache
- Confusion; changes in behavior (outbursts of anger, difficulty concentrating)
- Depression
- Hallucinations
- Uncontrolled movement of body or eyes
- Muscle weakness
- Chills or fever
- Sore throat
- Allergic reaction (rash or itching); jaundice; low blood pressure; anemia; low platelet count (unusual bruising or bleeding) (rare)

TELL YOUR DOCTOR ABOUT THESE SYMPTOMS RIGHT AWAY.

Terazosin

Vital Statistics

DRUG CLASS
$Alpha_1$-Adrenergic Blockers

BRAND NAME
Hytrin

OTHER DRUGS IN THIS CLASS
doxazosin

GENERAL DESCRIPTION
Introduced in 1987, terazosin is one of several $alpha_1$-adrenergic blocking agents used in the treatment of high blood pressure. It can be used alone or in conjunction with other drugs, such as beta-adrenergic blockers or diuretics, depending on the degree of hypertension. For more information, including possible drug interactions, see $Alpha_1$-Adrenergic Blockers.

TARGET AILMENTS

High blood pressure

Benign prostatic hyperplasia (benign enlargement of the prostate)

SIDE EFFECTS

Although rare, a slight (two- to three-pound) weight gain is possible with the use of this drug.

For additional side effects, see $Alpha_1$-Adrenergic Blockers.

Precautions

SPECIAL INFORMATION
- Avoid driving and hazardous tasks for 24 hours after the first dose, after a dosage increase, or after resumption of treatment.
- The effects of terazosin on pregnant women, nursing mothers, and children under 12 years of age are not yet known. Use only if directed by your physician.
- Before taking terazosin, tell your doctor if you have previously experienced an unusual or allergic reaction to doxazosin, prazosin, or terazosin (in which case you should not take terazosin) or have encountered dizziness, faintness, or lightheadedness with other drugs. Inform your doctor if you have a history of mental depression, stroke, or impaired circulation to the brain; coronary artery disease; impaired liver function or active liver disease; impaired kidney function; or any plans to undergo surgery in the near future.
- To minimize dizziness, take the first terazosin dose at bedtime. Dosages must be adjusted on an individual basis.
- Terazosin may affect some laboratory tests. Effects may include a mild decrease in white blood cell counts, certain cholesterol ratios, and blood sugar levels.
- The symptoms of prostate cancer are similar to those of benign prostate enlargement. Ask your doctor to test for prostate cancer before starting terazosin treatment.

Rx TERBUTALINE

VITAL STATISTICS

DRUG CLASS
Bronchodilators

BRAND NAMES
Brethaire, Brethine, Bricanyl

OTHER DRUGS IN THIS CLASS
Rx: albuterol, epinephrine, ipratropium, salmeterol, theophylline
OTC: ephedrine, epinephrine, theophylline

GENERAL DESCRIPTION
Introduced in 1974, terbutaline is prescribed to relieve the symptoms of bronchial asthma and the asthmalike symptoms of chronic bronchitis and emphysema. For more information, including additional possible interactions, see Bronchodilators. For the visual characteristics of the brand name drug Brethine, see the Color Guide to Prescription Drugs and Herbs.

PRECAUTIONS

WARNING
Your body can build up tolerance to bronchodilators used as inhalants, causing them to become less effective. If this happens, discontinue the drug and tell your doctor. Do not increase the dose. Increasing the dose can lead to serious, perhaps fatal bronchial constriction.

SPECIAL INFORMATION
- Women who are pregnant or breast-feeding should consult a doctor before using a bronchodilator.
- Inform your doctor if you have glaucoma, heart disease, hyperthyroidism, diabetes, or hypertension or are allergic to other bronchodilators.

POSSIBLE INTERACTIONS
Other antiasthmatic drugs: do not combine these drugs unless your doctor directs you to do so or unless your prescription contains a combination. Using two bronchodilators may increase the side effects, especially on the heart.

TARGET AILMENTS
Bronchial asthma; bronchitis; emphysema

SIDE EFFECTS

NOT SERIOUS
- Mild nausea; weakness; insomnia, nervousness; restlessness

CALL YOUR DOCTOR IF THESE EFFECTS BECOME BOTHERSOME.

SERIOUS
- Change in blood pressure; change in heartbeat (irregular or pounding, for example)
- Trembling; weakness
- Breathing problems
- Anxiety; nervousness
- Dizziness; lightheadedness
- Muscle cramps
- Nausea or vomiting
- Chest pain or discomfort (rare)

LET YOUR DOCTOR KNOW RIGHT AWAY IF YOU EXPERIENCE THESE SIDE EFFECTS.

Rx TERCONAZOLE

VITAL STATISTICS

DRUG CLASS
Antifungal Drugs [Vaginal Antifungal Drugs]

BRAND NAMES
Terazol 3, Terazol 7

OTHER DRUGS IN THIS SUBCLASS
Rx: clotrimazole, fluconazole, miconazole
OTC: clotrimazole, miconazole

GENERAL DESCRIPTION
The antifungal drug terconazole is available in vaginal creams and suppositories for the treatment of vaginal yeast infections (candidiasis). A common side effect of terconazole is headache, which afflicts about one-fourth of the women who use the medication. For more information, see Antifungal Drugs.

PRECAUTIONS

SPECIAL INFORMATION

- If you are pregnant or nursing, do not use a vaginal antifungal medication without consulting your doctor.
- Do not use this medication if you have a fever above 100°F; abdominal, shoulder, or back pain; or a malodorous vaginal discharge.
- Be sure to use this medication for the prescribed amount of time, even during menstruation or if your symptoms abate.
- If you are using a vaginal cream, protect your clothing from possible soiling by wearing panty liners or sanitary napkins.
- Avoid possible reinfection by wearing cotton rather than synthetic-fiber underwear.
- Refrain from sexual activity during treatment to avoid possible transmission and reinfection. Also, some vaginal antifungal preparations contain a vegetable oil base that might weaken latex condoms, diaphragms, or cervical caps.
- Douching may or may not be advised while using this medication; consult your doctor.
- If your symptoms do not show improvement within three to seven days, consult your doctor.
- If your symptoms return within two months, see your doctor; you may be pregnant or have a serious disorder, such as diabetes or an HIV infection.

TARGET AILMENTS

Yeast infections (candidiasis) of the vulva and vagina

SIDE EFFECTS

NOT SERIOUS

- Headache; mild abdominal or stomach cramps
- Irritation to the sexual partner's penis (rare)

CALL YOUR DOCTOR IF THESE SYMPTOMS CONTINUE OR ARE TROUBLESOME.

SERIOUS

- Vaginal burning, itching, or discharge
- Skin rash, hives, or other skin irritation

DISCONTINUE THE MEDICATION AND CONTACT YOUR DOCTOR.

Rx TERFENADINE

VITAL STATISTICS

DRUG CLASS
Antihistamines

BRAND NAMES
Seldane, Seldane-D

OTHER DRUGS IN THIS CLASS
Rx: astemizole, cetirizine, diphenhydramine, fexofenadine, loratadine, promethazine
OTC: brompheniramine, chlorpheniramine, clemastine, dexbrompheniramine, diphenhydramine, doxylamine, triprolidine

GENERAL DESCRIPTION
The first of the newer, nonsedating antihistamines, terfenadine is commonly used to treat the symptoms of seasonal allergies. It starts working in about an hour and reaches its peak effect in three to four hours. Terfenadine generally does not cause the drowsiness, jitters, insomnia, or dry mouth typical of other drugs of its kind. However, this drug can cause life-threatening cardiac problems when used in combination with certain antifungal and antibiotic drugs. Because of this, the Food and Drug Administration is considering removing the brand Seldane from the market; the drug fexofenadine is considered to be a safer alternative. See Antihistamines for more information, including possible side effects and additional possible interactions. For visual characteristics of the brand-name drugs Seldane and Seldane-D, see the Color Guide to Prescription Drugs and Herbs.

PRECAUTIONS

SPECIAL INFORMATION
- If your liver is impaired, terfenadine can build up in your body and provoke life-threatening heart problems. Depending on the severity of your liver condition, your doctor may prescribe a different antihistamine.
- Do not use terfenadine if you are breast-feeding.

POSSIBLE INTERACTIONS
Azithromycin, clarithromycin, erythromycin, itraconazole, ketoconazole, and troleandomycin: may interfere with the liver's metabolism of terfenadine, possibly causing life-threatening cardiac problems. WARNING: Do not take terfenadine in combination with any of these drugs.
Grapefruit juice: reported to interfere with the liver's metabolism of terfenadine, possibly causing life-threatening cardiac problems. WARNING: Do not take terfenadine with grapefruit juice.

TARGET AILMENTS

Nasal and respiratory allergies, including hay fever

Asthma induced by exercise (adjunct treatment)

SIDE EFFECTS
SEE ANTIHISTAMINES.

Rx TETRACYCLINES

VITAL STATISTICS

DRUG CLASS
Antibiotics

GENERIC NAMES
doxycycline, tetracycline

BRAND NAME
Sumycin (tetracycline)

GENERAL DESCRIPTION
Tetracyclines are natural or semisynthetic antibiotics developed from a particular strain of bacteria. The drugs work by inhibiting protein synthesis in certain disease-causing bacteria, including many that cause sexually transmitted diseases. Tetracyclines are also useful in treating many mosquito- and tick-borne diseases, such as Rocky Mountain spotted fever.

Tetracyclines are important for combating bacterial strains resistant to penicillin, or for use by patients who are sensitive or allergic to penicillin or other antibiotics. They are also useful for treating serious acne, which can cause lesions and scarring. Although their full actions in treating acne are not known, tetracyclines reduce concentrations of fatty acids in oil-gland secretions, suppress inflammation, and kill susceptible bacteria on the skin. These effects probably combine to reduce acne lesions.

For visual characteristics of the brand-name drug Sumycin, see the Color Guide to Prescription Drugs and Herbs.

PRECAUTIONS

SPECIAL INFORMATION
- Do not take these drugs with milk or dairy products. Take tetracyclines one to two hours before or two to three hours after consuming dairy products.
- Tetracyclines kill not only harmful bacteria but also "good" bacteria that keep unwanted fungi and intestinal organisms in check. Eating yogurt containing *Lactobacillus acidophilus* culture (or taking acidophilus tablets) may help restore the body's normal bacteria.
- Prolonged use of any antibiotic drug can lead to fungal infections, including candidiasis, or to bacterial infections such as pseudomembranous colitis.
- Tetracyclines should not be taken by pregnant or nursing women or by children under nine years of age. The drugs may cause permanent discoloration of teeth, underdevelopment of tooth enamel, and skeletal growth problems in the fetus, in nursing infants, and in young children who take them.
- Tetracyclines may cause liver toxicity or kidney problems in some individuals.
- Never take outdated tetracyclines or those that have changed in color, taste, or appearance; they may break down into toxic substances in the body.
- These drugs may cause increased sensitivity to the sun or to sunlamps. Limit your exposure while taking these medications.
- Most tetracyclines (except doxycycline) should be taken on an empty stomach.

Tetracyclines

POSSIBLE INTERACTIONS

Tell your doctor if you are taking lithium, insulin, digoxin, or an anticoagulant drug. Your dosage of these drugs may need to be adjusted.

Antacids, bicarbonate of soda, calcium, iron, laxatives, magnesium supplements: decreased absorption of tetracyclines. Take tetracyclines one to two hours before or two to three hours after taking these drugs.

Cholesterol-reducing drugs, such as cholestyramine: reduced absorption and effectiveness of tetracyclines. Allow several hours to pass between doses of tetracyclines and these drugs.

Cimetidine: decreased tetracycline absorption.

Estrogen-containing contraceptives or medications: reduced birth-control effect; possible pregnancy or breakthrough bleeding.

Penicillins: may interfere with tetracyclines, reducing effect of both drugs.

TARGET AILMENTS
Urinary tract infections; some sexually transmitted diseases (syphilis, gonorrhea, chlamydia)
Acne vulgaris (characterized by lesions and cysts)
Mosquito-borne diseases such as malaria, and tick-borne diseases such as Rocky Mountain spotted fever and Lyme disease
Skin and soft-tissue infections
Chronic bronchitis; pneumonia; sinusitis
Peptic ulcers

SIDE EFFECTS

NOT SERIOUS

- Lightheadedness; dizziness; gastrointestinal upsets (cramps, burning sensation in stomach, diarrhea, nausea, vomiting); photosensitivity
- Fungal infection of the mouth, genital, or rectal area; darkening or discoloration of the tongue (less common)

LET YOUR DOCTOR KNOW IF THESE SYMPTOMS PERSIST OR BECOME TROUBLESOME.

SERIOUS

- Discoloration of the teeth in infants or children; serious photosensitivity; apparent symptoms of diabetes (noticeable increase in volume of urine or frequency of urination, increased thirst, unusual tiredness or weakness)
- Liver or pancreas toxicity (yellowing of skin, abdominal pain, nausea, vomiting) (rare)

CALL YOUR DOCTOR IMMEDIATELY.

Rx THEOPHYLLINE

VITAL STATISTICS

DRUG CLASS
Bronchodilators

BRAND NAMES
Rx: Slo-Bid, Theo-Dur
OTC: Primatene Dual Action Formula, Primatene Tablets

GENERAL DESCRIPTION
Introduced in 1900, theophylline is an anti-asthmatic drug that acts by relaxing the muscles in the bronchial tubes as well as the blood vessels in the lungs. It is prescribed for symptoms of acute bronchial asthma, chronic bronchitis, and emphysema, and to help prevent bronchial-asthma episodes. Theophylline may be combined with other drugs such as ephedrine to provide additional relief of asthma symptoms, and with mild sedatives to relieve anxiety from asthma attacks. For more information, see Bronchodilators. For visual characteristics of the brand-name drug Theo-Dur, see the Color Guide to Prescription Drugs and Herbs.

PRECAUTIONS

SPECIAL INFORMATION
- Theophylline can cause adverse effects in individuals with liver disease, heart disease, seizures, peptic ulcers, or hypothyroidism. If you have any of these conditions do not use theophylline without your doctor's permission.
- Women who are pregnant or breast-feeding should consult a doctor before using a bronchodilator.
- Smoking may hasten theophylline's excretion; smokers may require higher doses.

POSSIBLE INTERACTIONS
Allopurinol, calcium channel blockers, cimetidine, ciprofloxacin, erythromycin, fluconazole, oral contraceptives, propranolol, troleandomycin: increased theophylline effect.
Carbamazepine, phenobarbital, phenytoin, rifampin: decreased theophylline effect.
Lithium: theophylline may decrease the effectiveness of lithium.
Zileuton: possible theophylline toxicity; theophylline dosage must be reduced significantly if these drugs are taken concurrently.

TARGET AILMENTS

Asthma

Chronic bronchitis

Emphysema

SIDE EFFECTS

NOT SERIOUS
- Mild nausea
- Insomnia; headache
- Nervousness

CALL YOUR DOCTOR IF THESE EFFECTS BECOME BOTHERSOME.

SERIOUS
- Heartburn or vomiting
- Changes in heartbeat (irregular or pounding)
- Trembling; seizures

DISCONTINUE USE AND TELL YOUR DOCTOR RIGHT AWAY IF YOU EXPERIENCE THESE SIDE EFFECTS.

THUJA

LATIN NAME
Thuja occidentalis

VITAL STATISTICS

GENERAL DESCRIPTION

The remedy *Thuja* comes from the leaves and green twigs of an evergreen tree that grows in moist soil in North America; it has been called, variously, western hemlock, white cedar, and tree of life. The twigs contain a substance that alters the concentration of salt, water, and electrolytes in the body. In past times, this plant was used to treat fever and intestinal worms and was used as an expectorant. Additionally, Native American herbalists used it to treat joint and other diseases. Modern-day herbalists use thuja for psoriasis and rheumatism and to treat warts.

The homeopathic *Thuja* is also employed commonly to treat warts. To prepare this remedy, the leaves and twigs are removed while the tree is in bloom, pounded, and then soaked in an alcohol solution.

Like most homeopathic prescriptions, *Thuja* was developed as a remedy by observation of the reactions of healthy individuals to doses of various strengths. The mental, emotional, and physical changes induced by *Thuja* were then cataloged. When a patient exhibits a set of symptoms that matches the cataloged symptoms brought on by *Thuja,* the homeopathic practitioner then prescribes it in an extremely dilute form. It is presumed that in this highly dilute dosage, *Thuja* can counter symptoms that are similar to the ones it induces when it is at full strength. For more information on homeopathic medicine, see page 14.

PREPARATIONS

Thuja is available over the counter in various potencies, in both liquid and tablet form, at selected stores and pharmacies. Consult your homeopathic practitioner for more precise information.

PRECAUTIONS

WARNING

Apart from its use to treat warts, *Thuja* should be taken only if prescribed by a homeopathic practitioner, because of its deep-acting nature.

SPECIAL INFORMATION

- When a remedy is administered, no one but the patient should touch the pills. If tablets are spilled, throw them away.
- The mouth should be clear of flavors 15 minutes before and after taking a remedy, and strong flavors and aromas, such as coffee, camphor, and heavily scented perfumes, should be avoided for the duration of treatment.

TARGET AILMENTS

Warts, especially on the chin, genitals, or anus, particularly those that grow in a cauliflower shape; painful or bleeding warts

Headaches related to overtiredness and stress, on left side of head and feeling like a nail pressing into the head

Joint inflammation and swelling aggravated by damp weather

SIDE EFFECTS

NONE EXPECTED

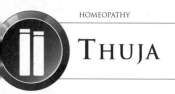

THYME

LATIN NAME
Thymus vulgaris

VITAL STATISTICS

GENERAL DESCRIPTION

This evergreen shrub native to the Mediterranean area has gray-green leaves. The garden variety has very fragrant clusters of mauve flowers. The oil's color can be white, red, or orange-brown, depending on the type of still and storage container.

Thyme has strongly stimulating, antiseptic, and antibacterial properties. It also has antispasmodic and digestive actions.

It has been used since ancient times. The Egyptians included it as an ingredient in embalming; Greeks and Romans drank it as a tea to aid digestion following banquets. It also was used as an antidote to bites from poisonous snakes. Soldiers from ancient times through the Crusades would bathe in thyme before battle, believing it to instill bravery.

PREPARATIONS

The essential oil is distilled from the leaves and flowering tops. For pain relief, thyme is helpful when used in the bath: add 5 to 10 drops oil and 2 tbsp bicarbonate of soda to reinforce the action of the oil. To make a massage oil, add 10 drops oil of thyme, 5 drops eucalyptus oil, and 2 drops wheat-germ oil to 1 tbsp soy oil.

Thyme used in aromatherapy inhalation may help laryngitis, coughing, asthma, depression, tiredness, colds, and flu. Use a diffuser to scent the air, or place a few drops in hot water or on a tissue.

Baths and skin application help to relieve skin problems, bladder infections, joint pain, depression, tiredness, backache, and flatulence.

PRECAUTIONS

WARNING

Buy thyme essential oil from a source other than eastern Europe. Thyme harvested in eastern Europe may contain high concentrations of radioactive fallout from the Chernobyl nuclear plant accident.

- Avoid during pregnancy.
- Avoid if you have high blood pressure.
- Do not use thyme oil internally. The oil is potentially toxic and can cause kidney damage.

TARGET AILMENTS
Laryngitis and coughing
Skin problems
Bladder infections
Joint pain; rheumatic aches and pains
Diarrhea and gas
Asthma
Depression and tiredness
Colds and flu
Backache and sciatica

SIDE EFFECTS

THYME ESSENTIAL OIL CAN BE IRRITATING TO MUCOUS MEMBRANES AND SKIN. USE IN MODERATION AND IN LOW DILUTIONS.

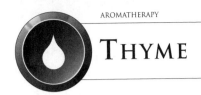

THYME

LATIN NAME
Thymus vulgaris

VITAL STATISTICS

GENERAL DESCRIPTION

Thyme, a popular cooking herb, can be therapeutic when used in medicinal amounts, although as with all herbs it should be taken upon the advice of a healthcare practitioner. The hardy herb yields leaves and blossoms that have long been used in preparations to ease coughs and promote healthy digestion.

Thyme has both relaxant and stimulant properties. In general, when the herb is used in small amounts it has a relaxing effect on the system, which can be helpful to relieve asthma and respiratory congestion, menstrual cramps, or indigestion. It is helpful for sore throat and cough associated with colds and flu.

The herb is valued as an antiseptic: Thymol, derived from thyme, is a common ingredient in mouthwash and sore throat remedies. A warm tea is helpful for headache, flatulence, and general debility associated with illness.

PREPARATIONS

Over the counter:

Available in dried bulk, in tincture, and as essential oil.

At home:

TEA: Pour 1 cup boiling water over 2 tsp dried herb; steep covered 10 minutes. Drink 1 to 3 cups per day.

TINCTURE: Take 1/8 to 1/2 tsp up to three times a day.

COMBINATIONS: For asthma, thyme may be combined with ephedra or lobelia. For whooping cough, combine with sundew, wild cherry, or anise. A bath with a decoction of thyme leaves and larch needles may help stimulate circulation.

Consult a qualified practitioner for the dosage appropriate for your specific condition.

PRECAUTIONS

WARNING

Do not use thyme if you are pregnant; it can cause miscarriage.

Young children should not be given medicinal quantities of thyme.

POSSIBLE INTERACTIONS

Combining thyme with other herbs may necessitate a lower dosage.

TARGET AILMENTS
Cough; sore throat; bronchitis
Asthma
Whooping cough
Colds and flu
Digestive problems

SIDE EFFECTS

NOT SERIOUS

- Headache or nausea
- Rash

SERIOUS

- Vomiting
- Diarrhea

THESE EFFECTS ARE FROM THE OIL ONLY. DISCONTINUE USE AND CONSULT YOUR DOCTOR.

Rx THYROID HORMONES

VITAL STATISTICS

GENERIC NAMES
levothyroxine, thyroid USP

GENERAL DESCRIPTION
Thyroid hormones are naturally or synthetically produced drugs—usually given orally—that are used to replace or supplement the normal secretions of the thyroid gland. Most preparations contain a mixture of several different thyroid hormones in varying ratios.

Hormones produced by the thyroid gland regulate functions such as metabolism and protein synthesis, general body growth, and development of the bones and central nervous system. They also affect the heart rate. Thyroid hormone therapy usually must be maintained throughout the patient's life unless it is prescribed for a transient condition affecting thyroid function.

Because these hormones are so critical to normal growth and development, children should be tested to ensure that their thyroid glands are functioning normally; those whose bodies are not producing sufficient quantities must be given supplemental thyroid hormones as soon as possible. Thyroid medications are sometimes used diagnostically to check for thyroid disease.

PRECAUTIONS

SPECIAL INFORMATION
- Your doctor may tell you to continue using thyroid hormones while you're pregnant or nursing. Although small amounts of these hormones may cross the placenta or be present in breast milk, no studies have shown harm to the fetus or breast-feeding baby.
- Tell your doctor if you have cardiovascular disease, or diabetes or other hormone problems such as low pituitary gland secretions. Your doctor may decide against thyroid hormones or lower the prescribed dosage.

TARGET AILMENTS
Hypothyroidism (underactive or nonfunctioning thyroid) or as treatment following removal of thyroid gland
Goiter (enlargement of thyroid)
Some types of thyroid cancer, especially after radiation therapy to the neck

POSSIBLE INTERACTIONS

Anticoagulant and antiplatelet drugs (such as warfarin): increased anticlotting action. Your doctor may have to adjust the dosage of anticlotting drugs.

Antidepressants, including tricyclic antidepressants such as amitriptyline: increased action and side effects of both combined drugs, leading to heart-rhythm problems and other signs of excess stimulation.

Antidiabetic drugs (such as insulin): increased need for insulin or other diabetic drugs, perhaps leading to higher blood sugar levels. Your doctor may need to adjust your insulin dose.

Cholesterol-reducing drugs (such as cholestyramine or colestipol): blocked or delayed absorption of thyroid hormones, decreasing their effectiveness. Take thyroid hormones one hour before or four to five hours after taking cholesterol-reducing drugs.

Food: decreases absorption and effectiveness of levothyroxine. Take the drug one hour before or two hours after meals.

Heart-stimulating drugs (such as epinephrine or pseudoephedrine): increased effects of both combined drugs, potentially causing heart problems or increased chance of thyroid hormone overdose.

Other hormones (such as estrogen): may interfere with thyroid hormone action, requiring higher doses.

SIDE EFFECTS

NOT SERIOUS

- Change in menstrual periods (short-term)
- Clumsiness
- Coldness
- Constipation
- Dry, puffy skin
- Headache
- Sleepiness
- Tiredness or weakness
- Heart palpitations
- Muscle aches
- Weight gain
- Temporary hair loss in children

THESE PROBLEMS ARE RARE BUT MAY OCCUR AT THE OUTSET OF TREATMENT. CALL YOUR DOCTOR IF THE PROBLEMS PERSIST.

SERIOUS

- Skin rash or hives
- Severe persistent and continuing headache
- Menstrual irregularity
- Changes in appetite
- Chest pain
- Irregular heartbeat; tremors
- Fever or sweating
- Nervousness; irritability
- Leg cramps
- Sensitivity to heat
- Weight loss

THESE PROBLEMS ARE RARE. IF YOU EXPERIENCE ANY OF THEM, CONTACT YOUR DOCTOR IMMEDIATELY. YOUR DOCTOR MAY ADJUST YOUR DOSAGE.

Rx THYROID USP

VITAL STATISTICS

DRUG CLASS
Thyroid Hormones

BRAND NAME
Armour Thyroid

GENERAL DESCRIPTION
Thyroid USP is a natural form of thyroid hormones obtained from the thyroid glands of domestic animals. It is not the most widely used drug for treating hypothyroidism (underactive thyroid) because it doesn't have a predictable hormone content; however, your doctor may prescribe it for you. The USP (United States Pharmacology) standards for the two active forms of thyroid hormone, T3 and T4, were recently revised. However, it is still difficult to determine the T4:T3 ratio in these glandular preparations, and the USP standards have not been fully implemented. For more information, including possible interactions with other drugs, see Thyroid Hormones.

PRECAUTIONS

SPECIAL INFORMATION
- Your doctor may tell you to continue using thyroid USP while you're pregnant or nursing. Although small amounts of thyroid may cross the placenta or be present in breast milk, no studies have shown harm to the fetus or breast-feeding baby.
- Tell your doctor if you have heart disease, high blood pressure, or diabetes or other hormone problems such as low pituitary gland secretions. Your doctor may decide against using thyroid USP or to lower the dosage.

TARGET AILMENTS

Hypothyroidism or as treatment following removal of the thyroid gland

Goiter (enlargement of thyroid)

Some types of thyroid cancer, especially after radiation therapy to the neck

SIDE EFFECTS

NOT SERIOUS

- Temporary hair loss
- Temporary changes in menstrual periods
- Clumsiness; coldness
- Constipation
- Dry, puffy skin
- Headache; sleepiness
- Weakness; muscle aches
- Heart palpitations
- Weight gain

THESE SYMPTOMS ARE RARE BUT MAY OCCUR AT THE BEGINNING OF TREATMENT. CALL YOUR DOCTOR IF THESE PROBLEMS PERSIST.

SERIOUS

- Allergic reactions (rash)
- Severe persistent headache
- Menstrual irregularity
- Weight loss
- Chest pain; irregular heartbeat; tremors; irritability
- Sensitivity to heat, sweating; leg cramps

CONTACT YOUR DOCTOR. YOUR DOSE MAY NEED TO BE ADJUSTED.

Tieh Ta Yao Gin

Vital Statistics

ENGLISH NAME
Traumatic Injury Medicine Essence

ALSO SOLD AS
Die Da Yao Jing

GENERAL DESCRIPTION
The Chinese medicine preparation *Tieh Ta Yao Gin* is a liniment used for many kinds of traumatic injury, including sports or martial arts injuries. The herbal formula increases blood circulation, which helps reduce bruising and swelling, relax the muscular tissue, and promote healing. It speeds the healing of sprains, fractures, and tears in the muscles and ligaments.

Chinese medicine takes a holistic approach to healthcare, fashioning remedies to treat the entire being as well as the specific parts or areas. Precise combinations of herbs are used to prevent and combat disease, which is thought to arise from disturbances in the flow of a bodily energy called chi (pronounced "chee") and blood, or from a lack of balance in the complementary states of yin and yang. A patent formula, *Tieh Ta Yao Gin* is made by using a standardized combination of herbs and method of preparation.

INGREDIENTS
dong quai, dragon blood resin, safflower, frankincense, myrrh, pseudoginseng, aloe, catechu

PREPARATIONS
This formula is available as a liquid in many Chinese pharmacies and Oriental grocery stores. It may also be found in martial arts stores.

Precautions

WARNING
Wash hands after applying, and be careful not to get in eyes.

SPECIAL INFORMATION
The liniment will stain clothes, but the stain can be removed with alcohol.

TARGET AILMENTS
Traumatic injuries
Bruises
Broken bones
Sprains and torn ligaments
Sports or martial arts injuries

SIDE EFFECTS
None expected

T

Rx TIMOLOL

VITAL STATISTICS

DRUG CLASS
Beta-Adrenergic Blockers

BRAND NAMES
Blocadren, Timolide, Timoptic (ophthalmic)

OTHER DRUGS IN THIS CLASS
atenolol, bisoprolol, metoprolol, nadolol, propranolol

GENERAL DESCRIPTION
Timolol belongs to a class of drugs that interfere with the action of certain parts of the nervous system, thereby slowing the heart rate and nerve impulses to the heart and other organs. This in turn results in lowered blood pressure and decreased angina. Among the first of the beta-blocking drugs to be developed, timolol is called a nonselective agent because it works in the whole body and can be used to treat a variety of medical conditions. In oral form, timolol is prescribed to help manage high blood pressure (hypertension), heart attack (myocardial infarction), and migraine headaches. In ophthalmic, or eye drop, form, the drug is used to control glaucoma and to prevent increased eye pressure during eye surgery.

T

PRECAUTIONS

See Beta-Adrenergic Blockers for more information, including side effects, precautions, and possible interactions of oral forms of timolol.

TARGET AILMENTS

Heart disease; angina (pain); heart attack (myocardial infarction); abnormal heart rhythms; high blood pressure (hypertension)

Migraine headaches

Schizophrenic and anxiety disorders

Glaucoma (ophthalmic form)

SIDE EFFECTS

OPHTHALMIC FORMS ONLY:

NOT SERIOUS

- Itching, stinging, or watering of the eye

CALL YOUR DOCTOR IF THIS EFFECT CONTINUES OR IS BOTHERSOME.

SERIOUS

- Redness of the eyes or inside the eyelids
- Blepharitis (inflammation of the eyelid)
- Conjunctivitis
- Keratitis (severe swelling, irritation, or inflammation of the cornea)
- Droopy upper eyelid
- Double or blurred vision, or other change in vision

TELL YOUR DOCTOR ABOUT THESE SYMPTOMS.

Rx TOBRAMYCIN

VITAL STATISTICS

DRUG CLASS
Antibiotics [Ophthalmic Antibiotics]

BRAND NAME
Tobrex

OTHER DRUGS IN THIS SUBCLASS
erythromycin

GENERAL DESCRIPTION
Tobramycin is an aminoglycoside antibiotic drug that works by killing bacteria. Tobramycin is administered by injection to treat severe systemic infections. When used for the eyes in solution or ointment form, tobramycin has fewer side effects and possible drug interactions than the injectable forms used for systemic problems.

PRECAUTIONS

SPECIAL INFORMATION
- Tell your doctor if you have ever had an allergic reaction to this or any similar medications. You may need different treatment.
- Prolonged use of ophthalmic antibiotics may result in a superinfection in the eye, with symptoms of a worsening infection. Discontinue and call your doctor.
- These drugs should not be used if you are pregnant or breast-feeding unless they are clearly needed.
- Tobramycin may slow the healing of corneal wounds.

POSSIBLE INTERACTIONS
None expected for ophthalmic forms. However, since systemic absorption through the eyes can occur, you should tell your doctor about any other medicine you are using.

TARGET AILMENTS

Eye infections due to strains of strep, staph, *Hemophilus influenzae,* and other bacteria

SIDE EFFECTS

NOT SERIOUS
- Blurred vision, slight burning, or stinging that occurs momentarily upon each application

SERIOUS
- Eye irritation that develops and persists after using this drug
- Itching, redness, or swelling

THESE MAY INDICATE AN ALLERGY OR A SUPERINFECTION. DISCONTINUE USE AND CALL YOUR DOCTOR RIGHT AWAY.

TOLNAFTATE

VITAL STATISTICS

DRUG CLASS
Antifungal Drugs

BRAND NAME
Tinactin

OTHER DRUGS IN THIS CLASS
Rx: clotrimazole, fluconazole, ketoconazole, miconazole, terconazole
OTC: clotrimazole, miconazole, undecylenate

GENERAL DESCRIPTION
Tolnaftate, available in topical aerosol, powder, cream, gel, or solution form, is used to treat several types of superficial fungal infections. It can also help prevent the development of some types of athlete's foot. Tolnaftate is not an effective treatment for bacterial or yeast infections (candidiasis). For more information, see Antifungal Drugs.

PRECAUTIONS

SPECIAL INFORMATION
- Do not use on children under age two or for diaper rash without consulting your doctor.
- Contact your doctor if your symptoms worsen or do not improve within 10 days.
- Do not allow the medication to come in contact with your eyes.
- Because it lacks antibacterial properties, tolnaftate is most effective for the dry, scaly type of athlete's foot.
- Although it may sting slightly when first applied, tolnaftate can be applied to broken skin.
- To prevent reinfection of fungal infections involving the feet or genitals, wear cotton rather than synthetic-fiber socks or underwear during treatment.
- Avoid wearing tight underwear if you have jock itch.

POSSIBLE INTERACTIONS
None expected.

TARGET AILMENTS

Jock itch

Body ringworm

White-brown skin patches (a ringworm infection known as tinea versicolor)

Athlete's foot

SIDE EFFECTS

NOT SERIOUS
- Skin may become slightly irritated at the site of application

IF THIS BECOMES BOTHERSOME, DISCONTINUE USE AND CONSULT YOUR DOCTOR.

TOPICAL ANTIBIOTICS

VITAL STATISTICS

GENERIC NAMES

Rx: chlorhexidine (for gums); mupirocin (for skin); combination of neomycin, polymyxin B, and hydrocortisone (antibiotic-corticosteroid for ears)

OTC: bacitracin, neomycin, polymyxin B

GENERAL DESCRIPTION

Topical antibiotics are used to prevent or clear up bacterial infections of the skin, ears, or gums. They should never be used interchangeably; drugs for the skin, for example, should not be applied to the ears or mouth. Each drug is effective against a specific group of bacteria. For self-treatment of minor skin wounds, it may therefore be useful to choose an over-the-counter product that combines two or more antibacterial ingredients.

Over-the-counter topical antibiotics are available in an ointment base that helps close and soothe wounds. In general, though, OTC drugs are used to guard against possible infections. Once a skin infection is under way, your doctor may prescribe a stronger medication.

PRECAUTIONS

SPECIAL INFORMATION

- Check with your doctor if you notice no improvement after using these medications for two or three days.
- Prolonged use of a prescription topical antibiotic may result in fungal superinfection.
- The use of topical antibiotics increases the risk of kidney damage or hearing loss in people with impaired kidney function who are already taking nephrotoxic medicines.
- If you are pregnant or nursing, check with your doctor before using.

POSSIBLE INTERACTIONS

Aminoglycosides: possible hypersensitivity reaction and toxicity, leading to permanent deafness if combined with neomycin, which is also an aminoglycoside.

Other possible interactions: see the entries for the generic drugs listed at left.

TARGET AILMENTS

Minor cuts, scrapes, and burns (bacitracin, neomycin, polymyxin B, to prevent bacterial infection)

Gingivitis (chlorhexidine)

Impetigo (mupirocin)

External ear canal infections (neomycin, polymyxin B, and hydrocortisone in combination)

SIDE EFFECTS

SEE THE ENTRIES FOR THE GENERIC DRUGS LISTED ABOVE, LEFT.

T

Rx TRAMADOL

VITAL STATISTICS

DRUG CLASS
Opioid Analgesics

BRAND NAME
Ultram

OTHER DRUGS IN THIS CLASS
codeine, hydrocodone, oxycodone, propoxyphene

GENERAL DESCRIPTION
A synthetic opioid analgesic, tramadol relieves pain by affecting the chemistry of the brain and nervous system. In general, opioid analgesics are used to treat temporary moderate-to-severe pain. As narcotics, opioid analgesics may cause physical and psychological dependence, especially if used for long periods of time. Tramadol, however, is not chemically related to the opiates and is possibly less likely than some other opioids to lead to respiratory depression, dependence, or symptoms of drug withdrawal.

PRECAUTIONS

☠ ***WARNING***
Tramadol can cause drowsiness, dizziness, and clumsiness. Restrict your activities as necessary. Do not drive or operate machinery until you know how tramadol affects you.

Long-term use can cause dependence, addiction, and withdrawal symptoms, although this appears much less likely than with other opioid analgesics.

An overdose of tramadol can be dangerous; contact a poison control center or seek emergency care if you've taken more than the amount prescribed.

SPECIAL INFORMATION
- Before taking tramadol, tell your doctor if you have a seizure disorder, kidney or liver disease, a history of drug dependence or abuse, including alcohol abuse, respiratory problems, or a history of hypersensitivity to opioids.
- Do not increase your dosage or frequency, or stop taking tramadol, without consulting your doctor.
- Tramadol has not been determined safe for use during pregnancy. Consult with your doctor if you are pregnant.
- Tramadol is not recommended for use by breast-feeding mothers, and its safety for children under age 16 has not been established.
- Discontinuing tramadol may produce symptoms of withdrawal; consult your doctor about any discomfort. Symptoms of withdrawal include fever, runny nose, or sneezing; diarrhea; goose flesh; unusually large pupils; nervousness or irritability; fast heartbeat.

TRAMADOL

- As for any opioid, seek emergency medical care if you overdose on tramadol. Symptoms of overdose include pinpoint pupils; slow, shallow, or troubled breathing, and slow heartbeat; extreme dizziness or weakness; confusion; convulsions.
- Do not drink alcoholic beverages while you are taking an opioid analgesic.

POSSIBLE INTERACTIONS

Alcohol, narcotics, phenothiazines, tranquilizers, or any other central nervous system depressants: increased sedative effect.

Anticholinergic drugs: opioid drugs may increase the effects of these drugs; risk of severe constipation and urinary retention (difficulty in urination with frequent urge to urinate).

Antidiarrheal drugs: risk of severe constipation.

Antihypertensives, diuretics: may lower blood pressure, causing orthostatic hypotension (dizziness related to change in body position).

Carbamazepine: can significantly decrease the effect of tramadol.

Metoclopramide: opioids render this drug less effective.

Monoamine oxidase (MAO) inhibitors, tricyclic antidepressants, and selective serotonin reuptake inhibitors (SSRIs): increased risk of seizures.

TARGET AILMENTS

Pain, moderate to moderately severe

SIDE EFFECTS

NOT SERIOUS

- Constipation; nausea; vomiting; loss of appetite; stomach pain; dry mouth; diarrhea; gas; heartburn
- Headache; drowsiness; malaise; clumsiness; dizziness
- Hot flashes, weakness, confusion, sweating, tiredness, flushing or redness of skin
- Nervousness; euphoria; trouble sleeping; difficulty performing tasks

CALL YOUR DOCTOR IF THESE SYMPTOMS PERSIST OR BECOME TROUBLESOME.

SERIOUS

- Breathing difficulty; seizure
- Constant urge to urinate or inability to urinate
- Blurred vision; balancing difficulty; faintness; fast heartbeat
- Skin reaction (itching, redness, swelling or blisters)
- Memory problems; hallucinations
- Dizziness or lightheadedness when rising from a sitting or lying position
- Sensations in hands and feet (burning, tingling, weakness, or trembling)

SEEK EMERGENCY TREATMENT IF YOU NOTICE ANY OF THESE SYMPTOMS.

TRANYLCYPROMINE

VITAL STATISTICS

DRUG CLASS
Antidepressants [Monoamine Oxidase (MAO) Inhibitors]

BRAND NAME
Parnate

OTHER DRUGS IN THIS SUBCLASS
isocarboxazid, phenelzine

GENERAL DESCRIPTION
Tranylcypromine, like other medications in the subclass of antidepressants known as monoamine oxidase (MAO) inhibitors, is used to treat depression, panic disorder with agoraphobia, and bulimia when other drugs have failed. See Monoamine Oxidase (MAO) Inhibitors for information on side effects and possible drug interactions.

TARGET AILMENTS

Major depression, especially if the condition has not responded to other drugs

Panic disorder

Prevention of vascular headache (including migraine) or tension headache

SIDE EFFECTS

See Monoamine Oxidase (MAO) Inhibitors.

PRECAUTIONS

WARNING
Tranylcypromine reacts with many drugs and foods. Following are some of the substances you should avoid when taking this drug: high-protein foods that are aged, fermented, or pickled, including (but not limited to) aged or processed cheeses; sour cream; alcohol, especially wine and beer (including alcohol-free wine and beer); pickled fish; dry sausages (salami); soy sauce; bean curd; yogurt; liver; figs; raisins; bananas; avocados; chocolate; papaya; meat tenderizers; and fava beans. Also avoid other antidepressant medications and caffeine. But beware: This is only a partial list. Talk to your doctor and pharmacist about other drugs and foods you should avoid.

SPECIAL INFORMATION
- Let your doctor know if you have diabetes, epilepsy, hypertension, hyperthyroidism, kidney or liver disease, or manic or suicidal tendencies, or if you have had a stroke.
- Let your doctor know if you have any history of angina or other heart disease.
- The full effects of tranylcypromine may not be felt until after several weeks of therapy.
- Use this drug during pregnancy or breastfeeding only if your doctor says that the benefits outweigh the risks.

Rx TRETINOIN

VITAL STATISTICS

DRUG CLASS
Antiacne Drugs

BRAND NAME
Retin-A (in various formulations)

GENERAL DESCRIPTION
Tretinoin, a derivative of vitamin A, is used topically to treat skin conditions such as acne. It is sometimes used in conjunction with other drugs, including benzoyl peroxide or antibiotics, to treat severe acne, although you should not combine it with other acne medications without your doctor's knowledge.

Although the exact mechanism by which tretinoin works has not been established, it is classified as a cell stimulant. The drug also appears to weaken the attachment of certain skin cells to each other. These actions cause skin and other cells to slough off the body's surface, possibly preventing plugs that block skin pores. Mild inflammation often accompanies its use. Acne may appear to worsen for up to a week after tretinoin is applied, because lesions just under the skin are made more prominent by the drug.

Tretinoin does not cure acne; your skin will return to its pretherapy state within three to six weeks after you stop taking the drug. Its effectiveness in reversing skin damage caused by exposure to ultraviolet radiation has not been confirmed.

Tretinoin may also be used to induce remission of acute promyelocytic leukemia.

PRECAUTIONS

WARNING
Absorption of tretinoin through the skin into the bloodstream is generally negligible, but this drug may produce side effects if absorbed in sufficient amounts. These include dizziness, headache, nausea, diarrhea, and ringing in the ears. Contact your doctor immediately if you have these symptoms.

SPECIAL INFORMATION
- If you are pregnant, consult your doctor before using this drug.
- To avoid irritation, be careful not to get any tretinoin in your eyes or in your mouth, nose, or other mucous membranes.
- You should not use tretinoin if your skin is inflamed by sunburn, windburn, cuts, or abrasions.
- Tretinoin may cause increased sensitivity to the sun and to ultraviolet radiation. Wear a sunscreen or cover affected skin when outdoors, and do not use a sunlamp.
- Tretinoin may cause increased sensitivity to cold or wind.
- You may wear nonmedicated cosmetics, but be sure to wash your skin thoroughly to remove any cosmetics before applying tretinoin.

TARGET AILMENTS

Acne (used alone or in combination with other drugs)

Skin disorders such as keratinization, keratosis, and flat warts

CONTINUED

TRETINOIN

POSSIBLE INTERACTIONS

Medicated, abrasive, or peeling acne products (such as benzoyl peroxide or medicated soaps): do not use with tretinoin except under a doctor's direction because the two medications may be incompatible; may also cause excessive irritation or drying of the skin.

Medicated cosmetics: may cause excessive irritation of the skin.

Minoxidil (topical agent for hair growth, especially in bald men or women): tretinoin increases the absorption of minoxidil and may increase its side effects, which include low blood pressure, heart-rhythm problems, and impotence. Let your doctor know if you are using minoxidil.

Perfumes or astringents containing alcohol: may cause excessive irritation or drying of the skin. Consult your doctor before using these products.

SIDE EFFECTS

NOT SERIOUS

- Warming or reddening of the skin
- Mild stinging or peeling of the skin

CONSULT YOUR DOCTOR IF THESE SYMPTOMS BECOME EXCESSIVE. HOWEVER, MILD INFLAMMATION AND PEELING OF THE SKIN MAY REPRESENT THE NORMAL ACTION OF THE DRUG AND MAY LESSEN WITH TIME.

SERIOUS

- Crusting, blistering, swelling, and darkening or lightening of the skin
- Severe reddening or burning of the skin

CONSULT YOUR DOCTOR, WHO MAY TELL YOU TO STOP USING THE DRUG OR TO USE IT LESS OFTEN, DEPENDING ON THE SEVERITY OF THE SYMPTOMS.

TRIAMCINOLONE

VITAL STATISTICS

DRUG CLASS
Corticosteroids

BRAND NAMES
Azmacort, Nasacort

OTHER DRUGS IN THIS CLASS
Rx: beclomethasone, betamethasone, fluticasone, methylprednisolone, mometasone furoate, prednisone
OTC: hydrocortisone

GENERAL DESCRIPTION
Triamcinolone is a potent adrenal corticosteroid, available in nasal spray and oral inhalant forms. The drug, introduced in 1985, is normally prescribed when a person's medical condition does not respond to other treatments. Oral inhalant forms of triamcinolone are used to treat bronchial asthma; they are intended to prevent, not relieve, acute asthma attacks. Triamcinolone may also be used as an anti-inflammatory drug for systemic diseases and as a topical agent for skin diseases.

In nasal spray form, triamcinolone is used to treat allergic rhinitis (nasal inflammation). It is also used for severe seasonal or perennial hay fever when decongestants are inadequate (although clearing your nasal passages with a decongestant spray before using triamcinolone may improve the drug's effectiveness). Some systemic absorption may occur with long-term use of triamcinolone. For more information, see Corticosteroids.

PRECAUTIONS

SPECIAL INFORMATION

- Ask your doctor about the risks and benefits of corticosteroid treatment if you have or have had any of the following conditions: HIV infection or AIDS, heart disease, hypertension, ulcerative colitis, diabetes, diverticulitis, gastritis or peptic ulcers, recent chickenpox or measles, candidiasis or other fungal infections, glaucoma, herpes simplex, liver or kidney disease, myasthenia gravis, osteoporosis, anastomoses, lupus, tuberculosis, recent intestinal problems, or any infection, such as a cold or flu.
- Corticosteroid nasal and oral sprays or inhalants may be absorbed into your system after prolonged use. Tell your doctor if you are taking any other medication, and watch for any significant side effects or possible drug interactions.
- One of the actions of corticosteroids is to suppress your immune system, thereby making you more susceptible to opportunistic infections. Corticosteroids can also mask symptoms of infection that occur while you are taking them; because the symptoms will not appear, an infection may worsen without your being aware of it.
- Prolonged use of corticosteroids can cause birth defects. Pregnant and nursing women should consult a doctor before using this drug.
- Check with your doctor before you stop using this drug. It may be necessary to reduce the dosage gradually to avoid serious consequences.
- Avoid using triamcinolone if you have a bacterial infection of the nose or status asthmaticus.

CONTINUED

TRIAMCINOLONE

POSSIBLE INTERACTIONS

Aminoglutethimide, antacids, barbiturates, carbamazepine, phenytoin, and rifampin: decreased effectiveness of corticosteroids.

Diuretics: decreased effectiveness of both combined drugs.

Growth hormones, isoniazid, potassium supplements, and salicylates: corticosteroids may decrease the effectiveness of these drugs.

Oral anticoagulants: corticosteroids may increase or decrease the effectiveness of oral anticoagulants.

Vaccines (live virus, other immunizations): corticosteroids may make you more susceptible to the injected virus.

TARGET AILMENTS

Hay fever (allergic rhinitis)

Nonallergic inflammation of the nasal passages

Severe asthma

SIDE EFFECTS

NOT SERIOUS

- White patches in mouth, throat, or nose
- Throat irritation; hoarseness
- Stuffy or runny nose
- Burning, dryness, or stinging inside the nose

SEE YOUR DOCTOR IF THESE SYMPTOMS PERSIST OR IF THERE IS NO IMPROVEMENT IN YOUR CONDITION IN THREE WEEKS.

SERIOUS

NONE EXPECTED WITH LOW-DOSE, SHORT-TERM USE.

TRIAMTERENE

VITAL STATISTICS

DRUG CLASS
Diuretics

BRAND NAMES
Dyazide, Dyrenium, Maxzide, Maxzide-25

OTHER DRUGS IN THIS CLASS
amiloride, bumetanide, furosemide, hydrochlorothiazide, indapamide, potassium chloride (adjunct therapy), spironolactone

GENERAL DESCRIPTION
Triamterene, among the drugs known as potassium-sparing diuretics, is prescribed for high blood pressure (hypertension), congestive heart failure, and liver problems associated with fluid retention. Because it prevents the excess excretion of potassium from the body, triamterene is frequently used in combination with nonpotassium-sparing diuretics, such as hydrochlorothiazide. See Diuretics for more information, including additional possible drug interactions. For information about a nonpotassium-sparing diuretic often used in combination with this drug, see Hydrochlorothiazide. For visual characteristics of the combination drug triamterene and hydrochlorothiazide, see the Color Guide to Prescription Drugs and Herbs.

PRECAUTIONS

WARNING
Taking diuretics in hot weather or while engaged in heavy exertion can cause a dangerous loss of fluids or minerals. Watch for signs of dehydration (fatigue, dizziness, headache, nausea).

SPECIAL INFORMATION
- Do not take potassium supplements (including salt substitutes) while on this medication. You should also avoid potassium-rich foods such as bananas.
- While you are taking this medicine, your skin may burn more readily when exposed to sunlight. To protect your skin, use a sunblocking lotion when outside and avoid prolonged exposure to the sun and sunlamps.
- When triamterene is suddenly discontinued after prolonged use, a rebound effect may occur, causing a rapid and potentially dangerous buildup of potassium in the body. Gradual discontinuation of this diuretic is important to prevent potassium toxicity.
- Because diuretics have both known and suspected effects on glucose (blood sugar)

TARGET AILMENTS

General edema (swelling caused by water retention)

Edema associated with various medical conditions, including congestive heart failure and cirrhosis of the liver

High blood pressure (hypertension)

CONTINUED

TRIAMTERENE

levels, people with diabetes or who have been diagnosed with borderline diabetes should have their blood sugar levels monitored closely.

- Tell your doctor if you have renal stones or gouty arthritis.
- Avoid using this drug if you are pregnant.
- Children are especially susceptible to adverse effects.

POSSIBLE INTERACTIONS

Lithium: increased risk of lithium toxicity.

Nonsteroidal anti-inflammatory drugs (NSAIDs), especially indomethacin: risk of kidney failure.

Other blood pressure drugs, including beta-adrenergic blockers and angiotensin-converting enzyme (ACE) inhibitors: increased blood potassium levels and possible toxicity.

SIDE EFFECTS

NOT SERIOUS

- Increased risk of sunburn
- Headache
- Blurred vision
- Diarrhea
- Dizziness or lightheadedness when getting up (orthostatic hypotension)

LET YOUR DOCTOR KNOW IF THESE SYMPTOMS CONTINUE OR BECOME TROUBLESOME.

SERIOUS

- Nausea or vomiting
- Fatigue or weakness
- Irregular or weak pulse
- Increased thirst, dry mouth, or sore throat
- Muscle pain or cramps
- Mood changes
- Mental confusion
- Bleeding in urine or stools (rare)
- Unusual bruising (rare)
- Skin rash; sensitivity to light (rare)

TELL YOUR DOCTOR IMMEDIATELY IF YOU EXPERIENCE ANY OF THESE SYMPTOMS. YOU MAY BE ADVISED TO LOWER YOUR DOSAGE AND INCREASE YOUR INTAKE OF FLUIDS AND MINERALS.

TRIAZOLAM

VITAL STATISTICS

DRUG CLASS
Antianxiety Drugs [Benzodiazepines]

BRAND NAME
Halcion

OTHER DRUGS IN THIS SUBCLASS
alprazolam, clonazepam, diazepam, lorazepam, temazepam

GENERAL DESCRIPTION
A sedative-hypnotic, triazolam is prescribed for the treatment of insomnia. Triazolam is more likely than most other benzodiazepines to cause short-term amnesia if you have to wake up and be alert before the drug's effects have worn off.

PRECAUTIONS

WARNING
Never combine alcohol with triazolam; the combination can cause dangerous central nervous system and respiratory depression.

On rare occasions, triazolam may cause the following side effects: jaundice, low blood pressure, anemia, or low platelet count (unusual bruising or bleeding). If you experience these effects, call your doctor right away.

SPECIAL INFORMATION
- Triazolam can impair your alertness, judgment, and coordination. Avoid driving and performing hazardous activities until you know how the drug affects you.
- Let your doctor know if you have narrow-angle glaucoma, a liver or kidney impairment, chronic respiratory disease, myasthenia gravis, depression, sleep apnea, or a history of drug abuse or addiction. Triazolam may exacerbate these conditions.
- Triazolam can cause sleep apnea in people with chronic respiratory disease, such as emphysema.
- Triazolam can cause physical and psychological dependence, sometimes after only one or two weeks, but usually after prolonged use.
- People with a history of drug or alcohol abuse are at a greater risk of psychological dependence on triazolam.
- Tolerance may increase with prolonged use; as your body adjusts to triazolam, the drug becomes less effective. Never increase the dose without consulting your doctor, because the risk of triazolam dependence increases with higher doses.
- Do not take triazolam if you are pregnant or breast-feeding.
- Do not abruptly stop taking triazolam. Sudden cessation can provoke withdrawal symptoms, including seizures; irritability; insomnia; confusion; mental depression; hypersensitivity to pain, noise, or light; and feelings of suspicion and distrust. Slowly reduce the dosage under your doctor's guidance.

CONTINUED

TRIAZOLAM

POSSIBLE INTERACTIONS

Alcohol, anticonvulsants, antihistamines that cause drowsiness (clemastine, diphenhydramine), barbiturates, MAO inhibitors, opioids, tricyclic antidepressants: increased sedative effects, such as excessive mental (central nervous system) depression, sleepiness, and slow or shallow breathing. It is very important that you avoid taking triazolam in combination with any of these drugs.

Antacids: may slow the absorption of triazolam. Separate from triazolam dose by an hour.

Beta-adrenergic blockers, cimetidine, disulfiram, erythromycin, ketoconazole, omeprazole, oral contraceptives, probenecid: may prolong the amount of time triazolam remains in your body, leading to increased triazolam effects and possible toxicity.

Clozapine: risk of profound hypotension (low blood pressure), slow or shallow breathing, cessation of breathing, and cardiac arrest leading to death.

Isoniazid: increased triazolam effect and possible toxicity.

Levodopa: decreased levodopa effect.

Rifampin: possible decreased effect of triazolam.

Tobacco (smoking): decreased triazolam effects.

Valproic acid: increased triazolam effects, including mental depression.

Zidovudine: risk of zidovudine toxicity.

TARGET AILMENTS

Insomnia

SIDE EFFECTS

NOT SERIOUS

- Clumsiness or unsteadiness
- Lethargy
- Dry mouth
- Nausea
- Change in bowel habits
- Temporary amnesia (especially "traveler's amnesia") when taken to treat insomnia associated with jet lag

TELL YOUR DOCTOR IF THESE SYMPTOMS PERSIST OR BECOME BOTHERSOME. CONTACT YOUR DOCTOR IF YOU ARE HAVING DIFFICULTY WITH YOUR MEMORY.

SERIOUS

- Drowsiness
- Dizziness or blurred vision
- Persistent or severe headache
- Confusion
- Depression
- Changes in behavior (outburst of anger, difficulty concentrating)
- Hallucinations
- Uncontrolled movement of body or eyes
- Muscle weakness
- Chills or fever
- Sore throat

TELL YOUR DOCTOR ABOUT THESE SYMPTOMS RIGHT AWAY.

Tricyclic Antidepressants (TCAs)

Vital Statistics

DRUG CLASS
Antidepressants

GENERIC NAMES
amitriptyline, doxepin, nortriptyline

GENERAL DESCRIPTION
An important group of antidepressant drugs, tricyclic antidepressants (TCAs) are widely used to treat depressive illnesses and, less often, to treat ulcers.

Precautions

WARNING
On rare occasions, antidepressant drugs may cause the following effects: allergic reactions, skin rash or spots, bruising or bleeding, jaundice, sore throat, fever, ringing in the ears. Call your doctor immediately if you notice these symptoms.

SPECIAL INFORMATION
- Before taking tricyclic antidepressants, let your doctor know if you are suffering from glaucoma, urinary retention, epilepsy, hyperthyroidism, or heart disease.
- Antidepressants may cause drowsiness. When taking these drugs, use care while driving, operating machinery, or performing tasks that require mental alertness.
- Antidepressants can trigger manic attacks in individuals with manic-depression. Be sure to tell your doctor if you have manic-depression.
- Antidepressants can affect blood sugar (glucose tolerance) tests by causing fluctuation in blood sugar levels.
- The full effects of an antidepressant drug may not occur for several weeks.
- If you are pregnant, nursing, or planning a pregnancy, check with your doctor before taking antidepressants.
- Do not stop taking this drug without consulting your doctor first. Sudden withdrawal may result in uncomfortable symptoms.

POSSIBLE INTERACTIONS

Alcohol, sedatives, and other drugs that depress the central nervous system: increased antidepressant effects, leading to problems such as respiratory depression or very low blood pressure; do not take alcohol while taking these drugs.

Anticoagulant drugs (such as warfarin): tricyclic antidepressants may increase the anticlotting activity.

Anticonvulsants: decreased effectiveness of anticonvulsants, making seizures more likely.

Antihistamines: increased antihistamine action, including any side effects; antihistamines may also increase the action of antidepressants, including any side effects.

Barbiturates, carbamazepine: decreased effectiveness of tricyclic antidepressants.

Cimetidine (antiulcer), quinidine: increased TCA effects.

Clonidine (blood pressure medication): may

TARGET AILMENTS
Major depressive disorders
Obsessive-compulsive disorders
Panic disorders
Enuresis (bedwetting)
Eating disorders

T

CONTINUED

TRICYCLIC ANTIDEPRESSANTS (TCAs)

decrease effect of clonidine and cause a dangerous increase in blood pressure.

Haloperidol (antipsychotic), oral contraceptives, phenothiazines (antipsychotic), levodopa (anti-Parkinsonism): increased levels of TCAs; dosage adjustments may be necessary.

MAO inhibitors: severe, possibly fatal reactions such as seizures, tremor, and coma because of additive effects of the drugs.

Other antidepressants: combining antidepressants will likely increase the action of one or both drugs, leading to increased side effects.

Thyroid medications: combining tricyclic antidepressants with thyroid drugs may increase the effects, including side effects, of both medications.

Tobacco (smoking): increased elimination of TCAs from the body, lessening their effectiveness.

SIDE EFFECTS

NOT SERIOUS

- Dizziness on changing position
- Drowsiness or insomnia
- Mild fatigue or weakness
- Dry mouth
- Headache
- Increased appetite or food cravings; weight gain
- Nausea or, less frequently, diarrhea
- Increased sweating
- Photosensitivity

LET YOUR DOCTOR KNOW IF THESE SYMPTOMS PERSIST OR BECOME TROUBLESOME.

SERIOUS

- Blurred vision
- Confusion; delirium; hallucinations
- Paralytic ileus (blockage of intestines, possibly indicated by abdominal pain or swelling, difficulty in breathing, and severe constipation)
- Difficulty in urination
- Eye pain from aggravated glaucoma
- Tremors
- Changes in heartbeat
- Nervousness or restlessness
- Parkinson's-like symptoms (shuffling walk, stiffness in the extremities)

TELL YOUR DOCTOR ABOUT THESE EFFECTS RIGHT AWAY. YOU MAY REQUIRE A DOSAGE ADJUSTMENT.

Rx TRIMOX

VITAL STATISTICS

DRUG CLASS
Antibiotics [Penicillins]

GENERIC NAME
amoxicillin

OTHER DRUGS IN THIS SUBCLASS
amoxicillin and clavulanate, ampicillin, penicillin V

GENERAL DESCRIPTION
Trimox is a brand name for the generic drug amoxicillin. Introduced in 1969, amoxicillin is a penicillin antibiotic commonly used to treat genitourinary tract infections, gonorrhea, otitis media, sinusitis, pharyngitis, and other bacterial infections caused by certain strains of staph, strep, and *E. coli*. For more information, see Penicillins. For visual characteristics, see the Color Guide to Prescription Drugs and Herbs.

TARGET AILMENTS
Genitourinary tract infections
Gonorrhea
Otitis media
Sinusitis
Pharyngitis

SIDE EFFECTS
SEE PENICILLINS.

PRECAUTIONS

WARNING
In some people, Trimox may cause an allergic reaction. Symptoms include skin rash, hives, intense itching, or difficulty breathing. Severe allergic reactions (anaphylactic shock) can be life threatening; call your doctor, 911, or your emergency number immediately.

SPECIAL INFORMATION
- Taking Trimox when you have mononucleosis may produce a skin rash.
- Take the full course of your prescription, even if you feel better before finishing the medicine; otherwise, the infection may return.
- Tell your doctor if you are allergic to cephalosporins; you may also be allergic to penicillins.
- If possible, avoid taking this drug if you are pregnant or breast-feeding.

POSSIBLE INTERACTIONS
Allopurinol: may cause a skin rash.
Bacteriostatic drugs (chloramphenicol, erythromycins, sulfonamides, tetracyclines): these medicines can interfere with the bacteria-killing action of Trimox.
Probenecid: decreases the kidneys' ability to excrete penicillins, possibly leading to penicillin toxicity.

TRIPHASIL

VITAL STATISTICS

DRUG CLASS
Estrogens and Progestins [Oral Contraceptives]

GENERIC NAMES
6 brown tablets: 0.05 mg levonorgestrel, 30 mcg ethinyl estradiol
5 white tablets: 0.075 mg levonorgestrel, 40 mcg ethinyl estradiol
10 light yellow tablets: 0.125 mg levonorgestrel, 30 mcg ethinyl estradiol

GENERAL DESCRIPTION
The brand-name drug Triphasil is an oral contraceptive used to prevent pregnancy. Triphasil combines a progestin drug (levonorgestrel) with an estrogen (ethinyl estradiol). This combination contraceptive works mainly by preventing ovulation. Triphasil also alters both the cervical mucus (making it more difficult for sperm to enter the uterus) and the uterine lining (preventing a fertilized egg from attaching to the uterus, as happens in a normal pregnancy).

Triphasil is available in 21- and 28-day regimens. Your period normally occurs during the seven days you don't take pills—if you're on the 21-day regimen—or while you take the seven placebo pills included in the 28-day regimen.

A triphasic contraceptive, Triphasil provides lower doses of estrogen and progestin by varying the dose ratios over a 21-day cycle. The lower dosage helps lessen any side effects. For side effects, possible interactions, and additional special information, see Estrogens and Progestins. For visual characteristics, see the Color Guide to Prescription Drugs and Herbs.

PRECAUTIONS

WARNING
Do not use Triphasil if you are pregnant or breast-feeding. If you suspect you are pregnant, discontinue use immediately to avoid harming the fetus.

Do not smoke if you are using oral contraceptives. The combination can increase the risk of heart-related side effects, including heart attack, stroke, and blood clots, especially in women over 35.

Oral contraceptives increase your risk of blood clots. Get medical attention immediately if you experience any of the following: severe pain in leg, chest, or abdomen; sudden headaches; changes in speech, vision, or breathing; weakness or numbness in extremities. These symptoms may indicate blood clots.

SPECIAL INFORMATION
Before taking Triphasil, let your doctor know if you are a smoker or have liver disease, gallbladder disease, a history of breast cancer, a history of depression, fibrocystic breast changes, endometriosis, uterine fibroids, diabetes, asthma, epilepsy, heart disease, high cholesterol, blood-clotting disorders, stroke, or high blood pressure. Your doctor will determine whether or not you should use these drugs.

TARGET AILMENTS
Triphasil is used primarily for birth control.

SIDE EFFECTS
SEE ESTROGENS AND PROGESTINS.

TROGLITAZONE

VITAL STATISTICS

DRUG CLASS
Antidiabetic Drugs [Oral Antihyperglycemics]

BRAND NAME
Rezulin

OTHER DRUGS IN THIS SUBCLASS
insulin; acarbose, metformin (Oral Antihyperglycemics); glipizide, glyburide (Oral Hypoglycemics)

GENERAL DESCRIPTION
Troglitazone, available since March 1997, is an oral antihyperglycemic drug. It is aimed primarily at patients with Type 2 diabetes who take insulin injections but still have abnormally high glucose (blood sugar) levels, or hyperglycemia.

Troglitazone is the first drug to target insulin resistance, the main cause of Type 2 diabetes, in which the body produces insulin but doesn't use it correctly, so that blood sugar levels become harmfully high. This drug is aimed at those who don't respond well to oral medication or insulin injections. In the presence of insulin, troglitazone improves the body's use of glucose by stimulating the uptake of glucose by muscle tissue. The drug also decreases glucose production in the liver.

TARGET AILMENTS

Type 2 diabetes mellitus

SIDE EFFECTS

NOT SERIOUS

- Reversible jaundice
- Weakness
- Anemia

CALL YOUR DOCTOR IF THESE SYMPTOMS PERSIST OR BECOME TROUBLESOME. AS WITH ALL NEW DRUGS, ADDITIONAL ADVERSE EFFECTS MAY BECOME EVIDENT WITH INCREASED USE.

SERIOUS

ALTHOUGH CLINICAL TRIALS SHOW THAT IT IS GENERALLY WELL TOLERATED, THIS DRUG IS TOO NEW TO HAVE A HISTORY OF SERIOUS SIDE EFFECTS.

T

CONTINUED

TROGLITAZONE

PRECAUTIONS

☠ ***WARNING***

Troglitazone works only in the presence of insulin, whether produced naturally by the pancreas or taken by injection. If you are taking insulin injections, be aware that troglitazone may increase the risk of hypoglycemia (low blood sugar) and require a reduction in your insulin dosage.

Do not use troglitazone if you have kidney or liver disease, or moderate to severe heart disease.

SPECIAL INFORMATION

- Before taking troglitazone, tell your doctor if you are a premenopausal, anovulatory woman, as troglitazone may cause a resumption of ovulation, thereby increasing the possibility of pregnancy.
- Troglitazone should be taken with meals. If you miss a dose at a meal, you may take it at the next meal. If you miss an entire day's dosage, you should not double the next day's dose.
- It is important to maintain your recommended dietary and exercise regimen while taking this medication.
- Be sure to have your blood glucose and glycosylated hemoglobin tested regularly and to have regular checkups with your doctor while taking this drug.
- If you develop a fever or infection, experience a trauma, or undergo surgery, you should inform your doctor, as these events may upset your glucose levels and necessitate a dosage adjustment.
- Troglitazone should not be used during pregnancy or by nursing mothers or pediatric patients.

POSSIBLE INTERACTIONS

Cholestyramine: greatly reduces the body's ability to absorb and use troglitazone.

Insulin: may increase risk for hypoglycemia.

Oral contraceptives containing ethinyl estradiol and norethindrone: reduced effectiveness of these drugs.

Terfenadine: reduced effectiveness of terfenadine.

TURMERIC

LATIN NAME
Curcuma longa

VITAL STATISTICS

GENERAL DESCRIPTION

The turmeric root, an ingredient of Indian curries for thousands of years, also has medicinal properties. Today in Ayurvedic (Hindu) medicine, turmeric is used for several puposes, including as a digestive aid. One of its active ingredients, curcumin, induces the flow of bile, which breaks down fats. Curcumin is also an anti-inflammatory agent and thus relieves the aches and pains associated with arthritis.

Turmeric also contains a volatile oil that functions as an external antibiotic, preventing bacterial infection in wounds. In traditional Chinese medicine turmeric is categorized as acrid, bitter, and warm. The turmeric plant is recognized by spongy, orange bulbs and yellow trumpet-shaped flowers.

Chinese medicine is a holistic system, fashioning remedies to treat the entire being as well as the specific parts or areas. Single herbs may be used alone or in combination with other herbs to prevent and combat disease, which is thought to arise from disturbances in the flow of a bodily energy called chi (pronounced "chee") and blood, or from a lack of balance in the complementary states of yin and yang.

PREPARATIONS

Over the counter:

Turmeric is available as powdered root, capsules, and liquid extract.

At home:

COMBINATIONS: For shoulder pain, mix turmeric with cinnamon twig and astragalus. Menstrual cramps and pain after childbirth may be alleviated with turmeric and cinnamon bark; for menstrual irregularity combine with dong quai. Turmeric is mixed with sesame or salad oil and applied externally to swollen areas.

PRECAUTIONS

SPECIAL INFORMATION

- If you are pregnant, consult your practitioner before using turmeric.
- If you are trying to conceive or if you have a history of fertility problems, consult your practitioner before using. One animal study indicated that the herb reduces fertility.
- If you have a blood-clotting disorder, consult your practitioner before using. Turmeric may have an anticoagulant effect.
- Use low-strength preparations for adults over 65 or children. Do not give to children under two years of age.

TARGET AILMENTS

Take internally for:

Shoulder pain

Menstrual cramps; pain after childbirth; menstrual irregularity

Apply externally for:

Skin infections

SIDE EFFECTS

NOT SERIOUS

- Heartburn
- Upset stomach

REDUCE DOSAGE OR DISCONTINUE. CONSULT YOUR PRACTITIONER.

TURMERIC

LATIN NAME
Curcuma longa

VITAL STATISTICS

GENERAL DESCRIPTION

The turmeric root, an ingredient of Indian curries for thousands of years, also has medicinal properties. Turmeric is used for several purposes, including as a digestive aid. One of its active ingredients, curcumin, induces the flow of bile, which in turn breaks down fats. Curcumin is also an anti-inflammatory agent and thus relieves the aches and pains associated with arthritis.

Turmeric also contains a volatile oil that functions as an external antibiotic, preventing bacterial infection in wounds. The turmeric plant is recognized by spongy, orange bulbs and yellow trumpet-shaped flowers. For visual characteristics of turmeric, see the Color Guide to Prescription Drugs and Herbs.

PREPARATIONS

Over the counter:

Turmeric is available as powdered root, capsules, and liquid extract.

At home:

DECOCTION: Steep covered 1 tsp turmeric powder in 1 cup milk for 15 to 20 minutes. Drink up to 3 cups a day.

Consult a qualified practitioner for the dosage appropriate for your specific condition.

SIDE EFFECTS

NOT SERIOUS

- Heartburn
- Upset stomach

REDUCE DOSAGE OR DISCONTINUE USE. CONSULT YOUR PRACTITIONER.

PRECAUTIONS

SPECIAL INFORMATION

- If you are pregnant, consult your practitioner before using turmeric.
- One animal study indicated that the herb reduces fertility. If you are trying to conceive or if you have a history of fertility problems, consult your practitioner before using.
- If you have a blood-clotting disorder consult your practitioner before using. Turmeric is thought to have an anticlotting effect.
- Use low-strength preparations for children, or adults over 65. Do not give to children under two years of age.
- Use of this herb by children for more than seven to 10 days should be done in conjunction with a healthcare practitioner.

POSSIBLE INTERACTIONS

Combining turmeric with other herbs may necessitate a lower dosage.

TARGET AILMENTS

Take internally for:

- Digestive disorders
- Fever
- Chest congestion
- Menstrual irregularity
- Aches and pains of arthritis

Apply externally for:

- Pain and swelling caused by trauma

Tu Zhung Feng Shi Wan

Vital Statistics

ENGLISH NAME
Eucommia Bark Wind Damp Pills

GENERAL DESCRIPTION
Tu Zhung Feng Shi Wan is a formula for muscle aches and pains in the lower half of the body. It has also been used for pain in the joints or lower back, especially pain that comes when the weather changes. It is used for sciatica and even gout. The herbs in the formula strengthen the tendons and bones, stimulate the circulation, and stop pain.

Chinese medicine takes a holistic approach to healthcare, fashioning remedies to treat the entire being as well as the specific parts or areas. Precise combinations of herbs are used to prevent and combat disease, which is thought to arise from disturbances in the flow of a bodily energy called chi (pronounced "chee") and blood, or from a lack of balance in the complementary states of yin and yang. A patent formula, *Tu Zhung Feng Shi Wan* is made by using a standardized combination of herbs and method of preparation.

INGREDIENTS
dong quai, eucommia, cinnamon bark, pubescent angelica root, codonopsis, loranthus, achyranthes, gentiana macrophylla root, ledebouriella, poria, Chinese wild ginger *(asari cum radice),* ligusticum

PREPARATIONS
This formula is available in pills in many Chinese pharmacies and Oriental grocery stores.

Precautions

WARNING
Do not use during pregnancy. Do not use if the aches are from a cold or flu.

TARGET AILMENTS
Low back pain and joint pains that are more pronounced with weather changes
Wandering joint pain
Sciatica
Gouty arthritis

SIDE EFFECTS
None expected

T

Rx TYLENOL WITH CODEINE

VITAL STATISTICS

DRUG CLASS
Analgesics [Opioid Analgesics]

OTHER DRUGS IN THIS SUBCLASS
hydrocodone, oxycodone, propoxyphene, tramadol

GENERAL DESCRIPTION
Tylenol with Codeine is the brand-name form of a combination medication containing acetaminophen and codeine. Codeine is a narcotic analgesic, acting on the central nervous system (the spinal cord and brain) to alter the perception of pain; acetaminophen acts at the site of the pain. Codeine also helps control coughing. For more information, see Opioid Analgesics.

PRECAUTIONS

SPECIAL INFORMATION

- Although codeine is less habit forming than most other opioid analgesics, drugs such as Tylenol with Codeine should be used with caution because codeine use can lead to addiction, both physical and psychological.
- Seek emergency medical care if you overdose on codeine. Symptoms include pinpoint pupils; slow, shallow, or troubled breathing; slow heartbeat; dizziness or weakness; confusion; convulsions.
- Do not drink alcoholic beverages while you are taking this drug.
- Because of the combination of analgesics in Tylenol with Codeine, read the label carefully before taking any other medication to avoid accidental overdose.

TARGET AILMENTS

Mild to severe pain, especially from acute trauma or surgery

Moderate to severe tension headaches

SIDE EFFECTS

NOT SERIOUS

- Dizziness or drowsiness
- Dry mouth
- Headache
- Nervousness
- Difficulty in urination
- Frequent urge to urinate
- Mild nausea, constipation

CONSULT YOUR DOCTOR IF THESE SYMPTOMS CONTINUE.

SERIOUS

- Slow or shallow breathing
- Somnolence
- Skin rash, hives or itching, or facial swelling
- Decrease in blood pressure or heart rate
- Fast heartbeat with increased sweating and shortness of breath
- Severe constipation, nausea, stomach pain, or vomiting

DISCONTINUE USE AND CALL YOUR DOCTOR IF YOU EXPERIENCE THESE SYMPTOMS.

Rx ULTRAM

VITAL STATISTICS

DRUG CLASS
Analgesics [Opioid Analgesics]

GENERIC NAME
tramadol

OTHER DRUGS IN THIS SUBCLASS
codeine, hydrocodone, oxycodone, propoxyphene

GENERAL DESCRIPTION
A synthetic opioid analgesic, the brand-name drug Ultram relieves pain by affecting the chemistry of the brain and nervous system. Ultram may be less likely than nonsteroidal anti-inflammatory drugs (NSAIDs) to cause gastrointestinal problems such as bleeding. It is not chemically related to the opiates and is possibly less likely than some other opioids to lead to dependence or symptoms of drug withdrawal.

For visual characteristics, see the Color Guide to Prescription Drugs and Herbs.

PRECAUTIONS

WARNING
Ultram can cause drowsiness and clumsiness. Restrict your activities as necessary. Do not drive or operate machinery until you know how Ultram affects you.

Long-term use may cause dependence, addiction, and withdrawal symptoms.

An overdose of Ultram can be dangerous; contact a poison control center or seek emergency care if you have taken more than the amount prescribed.

SPECIAL INFORMATION
- Before taking Ultram, tell your doctor if you have a seizure disorder; kidney or liver disease; a history of drug dependence or abuse including alcohol abuse; respiratory problems; or a history of hypersensitivity to opioids.
- Do not increase your dosage or frequency, or stop taking Ultram, without consulting your doctor.
- Ultram has not been determined safe for use during pregnancy. Consult with your doctor if you are pregnant.
- Ultram is not recommended for use by breast-feeding mothers, and its safety for children under the age of 16 has not been established.
- Discontinuing Ultram may involve symptoms of withdrawal; consult your doctor about any discomfort.

CONTINUED

ULTRAM

POSSIBLE INTERACTIONS

Alcohol, narcotics, phenothiazines, tranquilizers, or any other central nervous system depressants: increased sedative effect.

Carbamazepine: can significantly decrease the effect of Ultram.

Monoamine oxidase (MAO) inhibitors, tricyclic antidepressants, and selective serotonin reuptake inhibitors (SSRIs): increased risk of seizures.

TARGET AILMENTS

Pain that is moderate to moderately severe

SIDE EFFECTS

NOT SERIOUS

- Constipation; nausea or vomiting; loss of appetite; stomach pain; dry mouth; diarrhea; gas; heartburn; headache; drowsiness or malaise; clumsiness or dizziness; hot flashes; weakness or confusion; difficulty performing tasks; sweating; tiredness; flushing or redness of skin; nervousness or euphoria; trouble sleeping

CALL YOUR DOCTOR IF THESE SYMPTOMS PERSIST.

SERIOUS

- Breathing difficulty; seizure

SEEK EMERGENCY TREATMENT.

- Constant urge to urinate or inability to urinate
- Blurred vision; difficulty in balancing
- Faintness or fast heartbeat
- Skin reaction (itching, redness, swelling, or blisters)
- Memory problems or hallucinations
- Dizziness or lightheadedness when rising from a sitting or lying position
- Sensations in hands and feet (burning, tingling, weakness, or trembling)

CALL YOUR DOCTOR IMMEDIATELY.

UNDECYLENATE

VITAL STATISTICS

DRUG CLASS
Antifungal Drugs

BRAND NAMES
Desenex, Cruex, Fungoid Solution

OTHER DRUGS IN THIS CLASS
Rx: clotrimazole, fluconazole, ketoconazole, miconazole, terconazole
OTC: clotrimazole, miconazole

GENERAL DESCRIPTION
Undecylenate is the main ingredient in several over-the-counter topical antifungal treatments for superficial fungal infections such as ringworm of the body, feet (athlete's foot), and groin (jock itch). Although it does slow the growth and reproduction of fungal cells, it is not as effective as some other antifungal medicines and is no longer widely recommended for treating these infections. See Antifungal Drugs for more information. Also see Vaginal Antifungal Drugs for information about medications commonly used to treat vaginal yeast infections.

PRECAUTIONS

SPECIAL INFORMATION
- Undecylenate should not be used to treat children under two years except at the direction of your doctor.
- Wash and dry the affected area before applying, and cover the area thoroughly with the medication.
- Consult your doctor if no improvement is seen within four weeks.
- Avoid getting the medicine in your eyes.

POSSIBLE INTERACTIONS
None expected.

TARGET AILMENTS

Jock itch

Athlete's foot

Ringworm

SIDE EFFECTS

NOT SERIOUS
- Mild skin irritation

SERIOUS
- Severe skin irritation or hives

DISCONTINUE USE. CALL YOUR DOCTOR IF PROBLEMS PERSIST.

U

URTICA

LATIN NAME
Urtica urens

VITAL STATISTICS

GENERAL DESCRIPTION

Often called stinging nettle, species of *Urtica* are encountered widely throughout the world. The plants are covered with prickly hairs that irritate the skin on contact and further inflame by injecting a toxic fluid. At various times, parts of the nettle plant have been the source of an oil used in lamps, a dye, and a blood cleanser, and the stems were once used in manufacturing rope and paper. Modern European herbalists consider nettle a tonic that strengthens and detoxifies the body.

The homeopathic preparation *Urtica* is made from the fresh plant while in flower, which is pounded and steeped in alcohol. It is used principally to treat disorders that involve burning or scalding sensations. When a patient exhibits a set of symptoms that matches the cataloged symptoms brought on by *Urtica,* the homeopathic practitioner then prescribes it in an extremely dilute form. For more information on homeopathic medicine, see page 14.

PREPARATIONS

Urtica is available over the counter in various potencies, in both liquid and tablet form, at selected stores and pharmacies. Consult your homeopathic physician for more precise information.

SIDE EFFECTS

NONE EXPECTED

PRECAUTIONS

SPECIAL INFORMATION

- When a remedy is administered, no one but the patient should touch the pills. If tablets are spilled, throw them away.
- The mouth should be clear of flavors 15 minutes before and after taking a remedy, and strong flavors and aromas, such as coffee, camphor, and heavily scented perfumes, should be avoided for the duration of treatment.

TARGET AILMENTS
Pain of rheumatism, neuritis, or neuralgia
Skin that is itchy, blistered, or hot; hives worsened by warmth or exercise
Lack or overabundance of breast milk
Vaginal itching
Burns
Bites and stings
Food poisoning caused by bad shellfish
Hives caused by allergy to shellfish (if respiratory distress accompanies the reaction, get emergency medical care immediately)

USNEA

LATIN NAME
Usnea spp.

VITAL STATISTICS

GENERAL DESCRIPTION

Usnea, or larch moss, refers to a group of lichens, which are plants made up of algae and fungi that grow together in an interdependent relationship. Larch moss is found hanging from the larch and many other trees in the Northern Hemisphere. Sometimes called old-man's-beard for its shaggy appearance, it frequently appears in fruit orchards. The active ingredient, usnic acid, seems to have an antibiotic effect against the Gram-positive class of bacteria, which includes, for example, *Streptococcus.* It may also be effective against some fungi and protozoans.

Usnea is believed to work by disrupting the cell metabolism of bacteria and other simple organisms, although it does not damage human cells. Herbalists consider it an immune system stimulant and a muscle relaxant. Some other species of usnea, including at least four found in the western United States, are also used as herbal remedies and serve as food for some animals and people.

PREPARATIONS

Over the counter:

The dried herb is available in bulk, powder, or tincture.

At home:

TEA: Steep covered 2 to 3 tsp dried lichen or 1 to 2 tsp powder in 1 cup boiling water. Take three times daily.

Consult a qualified practitioner for the dosage appropriate for you and the specific condition being treated.

PRECAUTIONS

WARNING

Avoid if pregnant; usnea may stimulate uterine contractions. Dilute tincture before ingesting; high concentrations may cause digestive problems. Do not use for more than three consecutive weeks.

Use of this herb by children for more than seven to 10 days should be done in conjunction with a healthcare practitioner.

POSSIBLE INTERACTIONS

Combining usnea with other herbs may necessitate a lower dosage.

TARGET AILMENTS

Take internally for:

Colds, influenza, sore throats, and respiratory infections; gastrointestinal irritations

Apply externally for:

Skin ulcers and fungal infections such as athlete's foot; urinary tract infections such as urethritis and cystitis; vaginal infections (use as a douche)

SIDE EFFECTS

NOT SERIOUS

IF DIGESTIVE DISORDERS ARISE, REDUCE DOSAGE. CALL YOUR DOCTOR IF THESE SYMPTOMS PERSIST.

Uva Ursi

LATIN NAME
Arctostaphylos uva-ursi

Vital Statistics

GENERAL DESCRIPTION

The leaves of the uva ursi shrub have been used worldwide for urinary problems for at least 1,000 years. They contain arbutin, which is converted in the urinary tract to hydroquinone, a widely used antiseptic. They also contain tannin, an astringent useful in treating wounds, and allantoin, which soothes and accelerates tissue healing. Uva ursi, which literally means bearberry, is an ingredient in most herbal teas that are taken for urinary problems. For visual characteristics of uva ursi, see the Color Guide to Prescription Drugs and Herbs.

PREPARATIONS

Over the counter:

Available as dried leaves, tincture, or tea, alone or combined with other ingredients.

At home:

Tea: Simmer covered 1 to 2 tsp dried leaves per 8 oz hot water for 5 to 10 minutes. To counteract the effect of the tannin content, add peppermint or chamomile. Drink 3 cups a day.

Compress: Make a tea; strain and discard the herb. Soak a pad in the tea and apply.

Consult a practitioner for the dosage appropriate for you and your specific condition.

Precautions

SPECIAL INFORMATION

- Uva ursi's disinfectant properties work only in an alkaline environment. When taking this herb, avoid acidic foods, such as most fruit juices, sauerkraut, and vitamin C.
- Hydroquinone is toxic in high doses; use uva ursi only in recommended amounts.
- Pregnant women should not use uva ursi; it may stimulate uterine contractions.
- Use of this herb by children for more than seven to 10 days should be done in conjunction with a healthcare practitioner.

POSSIBLE INTERACTIONS

Combining uva ursi with other herbs may necessitate a lower dosage.

Target Ailments

Take internally for:

Mild urinary tract infections, such as urethritis and cystitis

Apply externally for:

Minor skin problems, such as cuts and abrasions; vaginitis (use as a douche)

SIDE EFFECTS

NOT SERIOUS

Uva ursi may produce dark green urine; this is harmless. The herb's high tannin content may cause stomach upset.

SERIOUS

Ringing in the ears, nausea, and convulsions were reported in a 1949 study involving very high doses of isolated hydroquinone. Prescribed doses of the whole herb are considered safe, but in case of such side effects, discontinue until you contact your doctor.

Vaginal Antifungal Drugs

Vital Statistics

DRUG CLASS
Antifungal Drugs

GENERIC NAMES
Rx: clotrimazole, fluconazole, miconazole, terconazole
OTC: clotrimazole, miconazole

GENERAL DESCRIPTION
Vaginal antifungal drugs are commonly prescribed for vaginal yeast infections. They work by damaging the membranes of fungal cells and inhibiting the enzyme activity essential for the cells' growth and reproduction. The drugs are available in the form of vaginal creams and suppositories. For more information, see entries for the generic drugs listed above. See also Antifungal Drugs.

Precautions

SPECIAL INFORMATION
- If you are pregnant or nursing, do not use a vaginal antifungal medication without consulting your doctor.
- Do not use if you have a fever above 100°F; abdominal, shoulder, or back pain; or a malodorous vaginal discharge.
- Be sure to use these medications for the prescribed amount of time, even during menstruation or if your symptoms abate.
- If you are using a vaginal cream, protect clothing from possible soiling by wearing panty liners or sanitary napkins.
- Avoid possible reinfection by wearing cotton rather than synthetic-fiber underwear.
- Refrain from sexual activity during treatment to avoid possible transmission and reinfection. Also, be aware that some vaginal antifungal preparations contain a vegetable oil base that might weaken latex condoms, diaphragms, or cervical caps.
- If your male partner has any penile discomfort, burning, irritation, or itchiness, he may require simultaneous treatment for infection. He should consult his doctor.
- Douching may or may not be advised while using this medication; consult your doctor.
- If your symptoms do not show improvement within three to seven days, consult your doctor.
- If your symptoms return within two months, see your doctor; you may be pregnant or have a serious disorder, such as diabetes or an HIV infection.

TARGET AILMENTS

Yeast infections (candidiasis) of the vulva and vagina

SIDE EFFECTS

NOT SERIOUS
- Headaches; mild abdominal or stomach cramps; irritation to the sexual partner's penis (rare)

CALL YOUR DOCTOR IF THESE SYMPTOMS CONTINUE OR ARE TROUBLESOME.

SERIOUS
- Vaginal burning, itching, or discharge; skin rash, hives, or other skin irritation

DISCONTINUE THE MEDICATION AND CONTACT YOUR DOCTOR.

VALACYCLOVIR

VITAL STATISTICS

DRUG CLASS
Antiviral Drugs

BRAND NAME
Valtrex

OTHER DRUGS IN THIS CLASS
acyclovir, zidovudine

GENERAL DESCRIPTION
A relatively new antiviral drug, valacyclovir is converted in the body to the active agent acyclovir, which blocks the formation of viral genetic material, stopping the virus from multiplying and spreading. It has been used to treat patients with herpes zoster (or shingles) and to relieve symptoms of recurrent genital herpes in people with a normal immune system.

In genital herpes, this drug decreases the amount of time patients are in pain. It is most effective if begun within 24 hours of the start of symptoms, and is given for five days. For patients with herpes zoster, valacyclovir relieves the acute pain and helps blisters heal faster. The drug is best started within two days of the appearance of a rash and is taken for seven days. The product is not intended for long-term use.

PRECAUTIONS

WARNING
Tell your doctor if you have any disease of the liver or kidneys. Valacyclovir is not recommended for use in patients with cirrhosis. Your doctor will lower your dosage if you have reduced kidney function. Also tell your doctor if your immune system is suppressed because of an illness or a drug you are taking.

Do not take this drug if you have advanced human immunodeficiency virus (HIV) or other immune problems or have received a bone marrow or renal transplant. Serious complications could result.

SPECIAL INFORMATION
- Do not take valacyclovir while nursing a baby. There is insufficient information to determine whether valacyclovir is safe to take during pregnancy.
- Because this drug may cause dizziness or weakness, restrict driving and other hazardous activities as needed.
- The safety and efficacy of valacyclovir in children has not been established.
- If you miss a dose of this medication, don't double the next dose. Take the missed dose when you remember if it is less than two hours late. If it is more than two hours late, wait for the next dose.

POSSIBLE INTERACTIONS
Valacyclovir can have adverse interactions with a wide variety of other medications; ask your doctor or pharmacist for more information.

TARGET AILMENTS

Herpes zoster

Recurrent genital herpes

SIDE EFFECTS

- Headache; nausea; vomiting; dizziness; fatigue; gastrointestinal disturbance

CALL YOUR DOCTOR IF THESE PROBLEMS PERSIST.

VALERIAN

LATIN NAME
Valeriana officinalis

VITAL STATISTICS

GENERAL DESCRIPTION

Valerian root has been used for more than 1,000 years for its calming qualities, and recent research has confirmed its efficacy and safety as a mild tranquilizer and sleep aid. For sufferers of insomnia, valerian has been found to hasten the onset of sleep, improve sleep quality, and reduce nighttime awakenings. Unlike barbiturates or benzodiazepines, prescribed amounts leave no morning grogginess and do not interfere with the vivid dreaming sleep known as REM sleep. It is not habit forming and produces no withdrawal symptoms when discontinued. The plant is a hardy perennial that reaches a height of about five feet. As the roots dry, they develop an unpleasant odor compared by one herbalist to that of dirty socks. Most people add sugar or honey to make valerian tea more palatable. For visual characteristics of valerian, see the Color Guide to Prescription Drugs and Herbs.

PREPARATIONS

Over the counter:

Valerian is widely available dried or as capsules, tinctures, and teas.

At home:

TEA: Steep covered 2 tsp dried, chopped root in 1 cup boiling water. Let stand covered 8 to 12 hours. Or simmer covered 2 tsp root in 8 oz water for 10 minutes. Drink 1 cup before bed.

Consult a qualified practitioner for the dosage appropriate for you and the specific condition being treated.

PRECAUTIONS

SPECIAL INFORMATION

- Do not take valerian with conventional tranquilizers or sedatives, because of possible additive effects.
- Paradoxically, valerian may produce excitability in some people.
- Because valerian is a sedative, avoid driving until you know how the herb affects you.

POSSIBLE INTERACTIONS

Combining valerian with other herbs may necessitate a lower dosage.

TARGET AILMENTS

Insomnia; anxiety, nervousness, anxiety-induced heart palpitations; headache; intestinal pains; menstrual cramps

SIDE EFFECTS

NOT SERIOUS

- Mild headache; upset stomach

REDUCE DOSAGE; LET YOUR DOCTOR KNOW IF PROBLEMS PERSIST.

SERIOUS

- More severe headache; restlessness; nausea; morning grogginess; blurred vision (using too much valerian)

CONTACT YOUR DOCTOR, WHO WILL PROBABLY TELL YOU TO TAKE LESS OR STOP USING THE HERB.

Valium

Vital Statistics

DRUG CLASS
Antianxiety Drugs [Benzodiazepines]

GENERIC NAME
diazepam

GENERAL DESCRIPTION
Valium is a brand name for the generic drug diazepam, which has been used since 1963 to reduce anxiety and nervous tension. Despite its history of being overprescribed, particularly in the years immediately following its introduction, Valium is effective in up to 80 percent of anxiety patients and is now considered one of the drugs of choice for treating mild to moderate anxiety. However, Valium should not be used for the stress and anxiety of everyday living.

Like other benzodiazepines, Valium is potentially habit forming, especially when used for extended periods of time or at high dosages. The drug may also be used to treat acute alcohol withdrawal and presurgery anxiety, and as an adjunct treatment for skeletal muscle spasms and seizure disorders. For visual characteristics of Valium, see the Color Guide to Prescription Drugs and Herbs.

TARGET AILMENTS
Anxiety and panic disorders
Alcohol withdrawal
Convulsions or seizures; skeletal muscle pain and spasticity; presurgery anxiety (as an adjunct)

Precautions

WARNING
Never combine alcohol with Valium; the combination can cause dangerous central nervous system and respiratory depression.

Do not abruptly stop taking Valium. Sudden cessation can provoke withdrawal symptoms, including seizures; irritability; insomnia; confusion; mental depression; hypersensitivity to pain, noise, or light; and feelings of suspicion and distrust. Slowly reduce the dosage under your doctor's guidance.

SPECIAL INFORMATION
- Valium can impair your alertness, judgment, and coordination. Avoid driving and performing hazardous activities until you know how the drug affects you.
- Let your doctor know if you have narrow-angle glaucoma, a liver or kidney impairment, chronic respiratory disease, myasthenia gravis, depression, sleep apnea, or a history of drug abuse or addiction. Valium may exacerbate these conditions.
- This drug can cause sleep apnea in people with chronic respiratory disease, such as emphysema.
- Valium can cause physical and psychological dependence, sometimes after only one or two weeks, but usually after prolonged use.
- People with a history of drug or alcohol abuse are at a greater risk of psychological dependence on Valium.

- Tolerance may increase with prolonged use; as your body adjusts to Valium, the drug becomes less effective. Never increase the dose without consulting your doctor, because the risk of Valium dependence increases with higher doses.
- Do not take Valium if you are pregnant or breast-feeding.

POSSIBLE INTERACTIONS

Alcohol, anticonvulsants, antihistamines that cause drowsiness (clemastine, diphenhydramine), barbiturates, MAO inhibitors, opioids, tricyclic antidepressants: increased sedative effects, such as excessive mental (central nervous system) depression, sleepiness, and slow or shallow breathing. It is very important that you avoid taking Valium in combination with any of these drugs.

Antacids: may slow the absorption of Valium. Separate from Valium dose by an hour.

Beta blockers, cimetidine, disulfiram, erythromycin, ketoconazole, omeprazole, oral contraceptives, probenecid: may prolong the amount of time Valium remains in your body, leading to increased Valium effects and possible toxicity.

Clozapine: risk of profound hypotension (low blood pressure), slow or shallow breathing, cessation of breathing, and cardiac arrest leading to death.

Isoniazid: increased Valium effect and possible toxicity.

Levodopa: decreased levodopa effect.

Phenytoin: possible phenytoin toxicity.

Rifampin: decreased Valium effect.

Tobacco (smoking): decreased Valium effects.

Valproic acid: increased Valium effects, including mental depression.

Zidovudine: risk of zidovudine toxicity.

SIDE EFFECTS

NOT SERIOUS

- Clumsiness or unsteadiness
- Lethargy
- Dry mouth
- Nausea
- Change in bowel habits
- Temporary amnesia (especially "traveler's amnesia" when taken to treat insomnia associated with jet lag)

TELL YOUR DOCTOR IF THESE SYMPTOMS PERSIST OR BECOME BOTHERSOME. CONTACT YOUR DOCTOR IF YOU ARE HAVING DIFFICULTY WITH YOUR MEMORY.

SERIOUS

- Drowsiness
- Dizziness or blurred vision
- Persistent or severe headache
- Confusion
- Depression
- Changes in behavior (outbursts of anger, difficulty concentrating)
- Hallucinations
- Uncontrolled movement of body or eyes
- Muscle weakness
- Chills or fever
- Sore throat

TELL YOUR DOCTOR ABOUT THESE SYMPTOMS RIGHT AWAY.

Valproic Acid

Vital Statistics

DRUG CLASS
Anticonvulsant Drugs

BRAND NAMES
Depakene, Depakote

OTHER DRUGS IN THIS CLASS
carbamazepine, phenytoin

GENERAL DESCRIPTION
Introduced in 1967, valproic acid is used in the control of epileptic seizures, primarily the simple and complex absence types (petit mal). It is also used alone or as an adjunct to other anticonvulsant drugs to treat other types of epilepsy. For visual characteristics of the brand-name drug Depakene, see the Color Guide to Prescription Drugs and Herbs. For more information, see Anticonvulsant Drugs.

Precautions

WARNING
Valproic acid overdose can be fatal: Seek emergency help. Overdose symptoms include restlessness, hand tremors, hallucinations, and deep coma.

SPECIAL INFORMATION
- Do not use valproic acid if you have had an allergic reaction to this drug, an active liver disease or significant liver function impairment, or a bleeding disorder.
- Tell your physician if you are taking anticoagulants, other anticonvulsants, or any other drugs (prescription or over-the-counter), especially those that depress the central nervous system, such as antihistamines, antidepressants, tranquilizers, barbiturates, narcotics, sedatives, pain medication, sleeping pills, or muscle relaxants.
- Before using this drug, tell your doctor if you have a history of brain, blood, liver, or kidney disease; are pregnant or planning a pregnancy; or are anticipating surgery or dental extraction.
- You can take valproic acid with food to reduce stomach upset. To prevent irritation of the mouth or throat, swallow the tablets or capsules whole, without chewing or breaking them.
- Older adults are more likely to develop side effects from this drug and should be treated with smaller dosages.

Valproic Acid

- Blood cell counts may show decreased white cells and platelets.
- Valproic acid may affect some laboratory tests, including liver function tests. Be sure to tell any healthcare practitioner who gives you a lab test that you are taking this medication.
- Do not stop taking this drug or switch brands without consulting your physician.

POSSIBLE INTERACTIONS

Alcohol, antidepressants, barbiturates, sedatives, tranquilizers, and other depressant drugs: increased depressive and sedative effects.

Anticoagulant and antiplatelet drugs, including aspirin: increased risk of bleeding.

Phenytoin and other anticonvulsants: concurrent use of phenytoin or another anticonvulsant with valproic acid may increase the risk of breakthrough seizures.

TARGET AILMENTS
Epileptic seizures, absence types
Epileptic seizures, other types
Prevention and treatment of bipolar disorder (manic-depression)

SIDE EFFECTS

NOT SERIOUS

- Loss of appetite
- Indigestion
- Mild nausea
- Vomiting and diarrhea
- Unusual weight loss or gain
- Skin rash
- Trembling arms and hands
- Change in menstrual periods
- Lethargy
- Drowsiness
- Dizziness
- Unsteadiness
- Emotional changes

CALL YOUR PHYSICIAN IF THESE OR OTHER SIDE EFFECTS PERSIST OR ARE BOTHERSOME.

SERIOUS

- Bizarre behavior
- Hallucinations
- Unusual bleeding or bruising
- Yellow eyes or skin
- Severe stomach cramps
- Double vision
- Spots in front of your eyes
- Jerky or rolling eye movements
- Swelling of the face
- Continual nausea or vomiting

SEEK MEDICAL CARE IMMEDIATELY.

VANADIUM

VITAL STATISTICS

GENERAL DESCRIPTION

The precise role of the trace mineral vanadium in human nutrition is little known but possibly essential. Limited evidence suggests that vanadium lowers blood sugar levels in some people and inhibits tumor development, and therefore may protect against diabetes and some forms of cancer. It also appears to contribute to cholesterol metabolism and hormone production.

Because the symptoms of vanadium deficiency are unknown, researchers assume that humans require only a small amount, which diet apparently provides.

RDA/EMDR

Not established.

NATURAL SOURCES

Vanadium exists in whole grains, nuts, root vegetables, liver, fish, and vegetable oils.

TARGET AILMENTS

Cancer

Diabetes

SIDE EFFECTS

NONE EXPECTED

Rx VANCENASE

VITAL STATISTICS

DRUG CLASS
Corticosteroids

GENERIC NAME
beclomethasone

OTHER DRUGS IN THIS CLASS
Rx: betamethasone, fluticasone, methylprednisolone, mometasone furoate, prednisone, triamcinolone
OTC: hydrocortisone

GENERAL DESCRIPTION
Vancenase is a brand name for nasal aerosol and nasal spray forms of the generic drug beclomethasone, a potent adrenal corticosteroid that acts to inhibit inflammation. Introduced in 1976, beclomethasone is normally prescribed when a person does not respond to other treatments. Concurrent use of bronchodilators in tablet, nasal spray, or oral inhalant form may increase the effects of beclomethasone.

As a nasal spray, beclomethasone is used to treat severe seasonal or perennial hay fever (allergic rhinitis) when decongestants are inadequate (although clearing your nasal passages with a decongestant spray before using beclomethasone may improve the drug's effect; do not use a nasal decongestant for more than three to five days). Some systemic absorption may occur with long-term use of beclomethasone. For more information, see Corticosteroids.

PRECAUTIONS

SPECIAL INFORMATION
- Beclomethasone should not be used for nonasthmatic lung diseases without the advice of your physician.
- Use with caution if you have a nasal disease; consult your doctor.
- Beclomethasone should be avoided by individuals who are hypersensitive to medication.
- Corticosteroid nasal and oral sprays may be absorbed into your system after prolonged use. Tell your doctor if you are taking any other medication, and watch for any significant side effects or possible drug interactions.
- It may take up to three weeks for this drug to deliver maximum benefits. If by then you notice no improvement in your condition, consult your physician.
- Ask your doctor about the risks and benefits of corticosteroid treatment if you have or have had any of the following conditions: HIV infection or AIDS, heart disease, hypertension, ulcerative colitis, diabetes, diverticulitis, gastritis or peptic ulcers, recent chickenpox or measles, candidiasis or other fungal infections, glaucoma, herpes simplex,

TARGET AILMENTS

Nasal inflammation, including seasonal and perennial allergic rhinitis

Nonallergic inflammation of the nasal passages

Nasal polyps (prevention after surgery)

CONTINUED

VANCENASE

liver or kidney disease, myasthenia gravis, osteoporosis, anastomoses, lupus, tuberculosis, recent intestinal problems, or any infection, such as a cold or flu.

- Prolonged use of corticosteroids can cause birth defects. Pregnant and nursing women should avoid these drugs.
- One of the actions of corticosteroids is to suppress your immune system, which can make you more susceptible to opportunistic infections. Corticosteroids can also mask symptoms of infection that occur while you are taking these drugs; because the symptoms will not appear, an infection may worsen without your being aware of it.
- Prolonged use of corticosteroids increases the risk of osteoporosis, cataracts, glaucoma, Cushing's syndrome (moon face), and diabetes. It can also reactivate tuberculosis.

POSSIBLE INTERACTIONS

Vaccines (live virus, other immunizations): beclomethasone may make you more susceptible to the injected virus.

SIDE EFFECTS

NOT SERIOUS

- Throat irritation
- Stuffy or runny nose
- Burning or dryness inside the nose

SEE YOUR DOCTOR IF THESE SYMPTOMS PERSIST OR IF THERE IS NO IMPROVEMENT IN YOUR CONDITION IN THREE WEEKS.

SERIOUS

- White patches or crusting in the nose
- Headache
- Nausea or vomiting
- Hives or skin rash

CONTACT YOUR DOCTOR IMMEDIATELY.

VASOTEC

VITAL STATISTICS

DRUG CLASS
Angiotensin-Converting Enzyme (ACE) Inhibitors

GENERIC NAME
enalapril

GENERAL DESCRIPTION
Vasotec is a brand name for the generic drug enalapril. Like other ACE inhibitors, this drug relaxes arterial walls, thereby lowering blood pressure and reducing the work load of the heart. For these reasons this drug, introduced in 1985, is used to treat high blood pressure (hypertension) and congestive heart failure. Enalapril is sometimes combined with the diuretic drug hydrochlorothiazide for increased blood-pressure-lowering action. For further information, see Angiotensin-Converting Enzyme (ACE) Inhibitors. For visual characteristics of Vasotec, see the Color Guide to Prescription Drugs and Herbs.

PRECAUTIONS

WARNING
Get medical attention immediately if you notice swelling of your face, tongue, or vocal cords or have difficulty swallowing or breathing; this reaction can be life threatening.

Do not take Vasotec during pregnancy; enalapril has caused birth defects and death of the fetus and newborn.

SPECIAL INFORMATION
- This drug causes an increase in blood levels of potassium. Do not use potassium-rich products, including salt substitutes and low-salt milk, without first consulting your doctor. The potassium in your blood could rise to dangerous levels, leading to heart-rhythm problems.
- Do not abruptly stop taking Vasotec. The dosage must be reduced gradually.

TARGET AILMENTS

High blood pressure

Congestive heart failure (in conjunction with digitalis preparations and diuretics)

SIDE EFFECTS

NOT SERIOUS
- Dry, persistent cough
- Headache or fatigue
- Nausea or diarrhea
- Loss of sense of taste
- Temporary rash, itching
- Dizziness on suddenly rising or changing position

CALL YOUR DOCTOR IF THESE EFFECTS BECOME BOTHERSOME.

SERIOUS
- Fainting; drowsiness
- Persistent skin rash
- Joint pain
- Numbness and tingling
- Abdominal pain, vomiting, or diarrhea
- Fever and sore throat
- Chest pain; palpitations
- Jaundice

CALL YOUR DOCTOR RIGHT AWAY.

VEETIDS

VITAL STATISTICS

DRUG CLASS
Antibiotics [Penicillins]

GENERIC NAME
penicillin V

OTHER DRUGS IN THIS SUBCLASS
amoxicillin, amoxicillin and clavulanate, ampicillin

GENERAL DESCRIPTION
Veetids is a brand name for the generic drug penicillin V. Introduced in 1953, penicillin V is commonly used to treat otitis media and infections of the respiratory tract, as well as skin infections. It may be prescribed to prevent endocarditis and rheumatic fever. This type of penicillin is not used to treat severe infections.

A subclass of antibiotic drugs, penicillins act by killing sensitive strains of growing bacteria. Penicillins are ineffective against fungi, viruses, and parasites. When discovered in 1928, "penicillin" referred to a single drug. Today, more than 20 penicillins—some derived from molds or bacteria, others produced synthetically—are used to treat a wide range of bacterial infections. Penicillins work by attacking a bacterium's cell wall. Because body cells have a membrane but no cell wall, these drugs can selectively destroy invading bacteria without harming body tissues.

For more information, see Penicillins. For visual characteristics of Veetids, see the Color Guide to Prescription Drugs and Herbs.

PRECAUTIONS

SPECIAL INFORMATION
- Take the full course of your prescription, even if you feel better before finishing the medicine; otherwise, the infection may return.
- Most penicillins are better absorbed if taken on an empty stomach. However, Veetids works equally well whether taken on a full or an empty stomach.
- Tell your doctor if you are allergic to cephalosporins; you may also be allergic to penicillins.
- Let your doctor know if you have impaired kidneys, gastrointestinal disease, or a history of bleeding disorders. Your doctor may need to adjust your dosage, monitor you more closely, or prescribe a different drug.
- Veetids also kills "good" intestinal bacteria that keep harmful fungi and intestinal bacteria in check. Eating yogurt containing *Lactobacillus acidophilus* culture or taking acidophilus tablets may help restore the body's normal bacteria.
- Prolonged use of any antibiotic drug can lead to fungal infections, including candidiasis, or to bacterial infections such as pseudomembranous colitis.
- If possible, avoid taking Veetids if you are pregnant or breast-feeding.

POSSIBLE INTERACTIONS

Allopurinol: may cause a skin rash.

Bacteriostatic drugs (chloramphenicol, erythromycins, sulfonamides, tetracyclines): these medicines can interfere with the bacteria-killing action of all penicillins.

Estrogen (oral contraceptives): decreased effectiveness in preventing pregnancy.

TARGET AILMENTS
Otitis media
Skin infections
Respiratory tract infections
Endocarditis
Rheumatic fever

SIDE EFFECTS

NOT SERIOUS

- Mild nausea
- Mild diarrhea
- Oral candidiasis (sore mouth or tongue)
- Vaginal candidiasis

TELL YOUR DOCTOR WHEN CONVENIENT.

SERIOUS

- Allergic reaction (skin rash, hives, intense itching, or difficulty breathing)
- Severe allergic reactions (anaphylactic shock)

CAN BE LIFE THREATENING; CALL YOUR DOCTOR, 911, OR YOUR EMERGENCY NUMBER IMMEDIATELY.

- Unusual bruising or bleeding
- Sore throat with fever
- Severe abdominal pain with diarrhea
- Seizures

CALL YOUR DOCTOR IMMEDIATELY.

VENLAFAXINE

VITAL STATISTICS

DRUG CLASS
Antidepressants

BRAND NAME
Effexor

GENERAL DESCRIPTION
Venlafaxine is closely related to the subclass of antidepressants known as selective serotonin reuptake inhibitors (SSRIs). This drug is prescribed to treat depression that interferes with daily functioning. It may also be used to treat obsessive-compulsive disorder. Venlafaxine restores normal levels of brain chemicals, particularly serotonin and norepinephrine, and helps restore a normal mood and normal thought processes. For visual characteristics of the brand-name drug Effexor, see the Color Guide to Prescription Drugs and Herbs. See Antidepressants for additional information.

PRECAUTIONS

SPECIAL INFORMATION

- Before taking this drug, tell your doctor if you have liver or kidney disease; high blood pressure; suicidal thoughts; allergies to other medicines; or a history of seizures.
- Monitor your blood pressure frequently while taking this drug.
- Avoid alcohol while taking venlafaxine.

POSSIBLE INTERACTIONS
Venlafaxine may interact with other antidepressants as well as with the following drugs: alcohol, narcotic analgesics such as morphine, sleep aids, antipsychotic drugs such as tranquilizers, anti-Parkinsonism drugs, and histamine H_2 blockers such as cimetidine. Talk with your doctor before taking any of these medications.

Monoamine oxidase (MAO) inhibitors: may cause severe, possibly fatal reactions such as seizures, coma, or death. Do not begin taking this drug within 14 days of discontinuing treatment with an MAO inhibitor; allow at least seven days between the last dose of venlafaxine and the first dose of an MAO inhibitor.

TARGET AILMENTS

Major depression

SIDE EFFECTS

NOT SERIOUS

- Sleepiness or insomnia
- Dizziness; sweating
- Nervousness; anxiety
- Nausea; dry mouth; vomiting; constipation or diarrhea
- Heartburn; weight loss

CALL YOUR DOCTOR IF THESE SYMPTOMS PERSIST OR BECOME BOTHERSOME.

SERIOUS

- Headache; sexual dysfunction; vision problems
- Changes in heartbeat or rapid heartbeat; increased blood pressure
- Agitation, mood changes; rash; ringing in the ears
- Urinary problems; extreme drowsiness; convulsions

CALL YOUR DOCTOR IMMEDIATELY.

Rx VENTOLIN

VITAL STATISTICS

DRUG CLASS
Bronchodilators

GENERIC NAME
albuterol

OTHER DRUGS IN THIS CLASS
Rx: epinephrine, ipratropium, salmeterol, terbutaline, theophylline
OTC: ephedrine, epinephrine, theophylline

GENERAL DESCRIPTION
Ventolin is a brand name for albuterol, an antiasthmatic drug that acts by relaxing the muscles surrounding the bronchial tubes. Ventolin is commonly prescribed for symptoms of acute bronchial asthma. The drug is also used to reduce the frequency and severity of recurrent asthma attacks and exercise-induced bronchospasms. Ventolin is available as an inhalant, and in syrup and tablet form. For more information, see Bronchodilators.

PRECAUTIONS

WARNING
Your body can build up tolerance to bronchodilator inhalants, causing them to become less effective. If this happens, discontinue the drug and tell your doctor. Do not increase the dose. Increasing the dose can lead to serious, perhaps fatal bronchial constriction. Overuse of albuterol can cause heart-rhythm irregularities.

SPECIAL INFORMATION
- Before you use albuterol, tell your doctor if you have cardiovascular disease, narrow-angle glaucoma, prostatic hypertrophy, or difficulty urinating.
- Women who are pregnant or breast-feeding should consult a doctor before using a bronchodilator.

POSSIBLE INTERACTIONS
Beta-adrenergic blockers: decreased effects of both drugs.
See Bronchodilators for other interactions.

TARGET AILMENTS

Bronchial asthma

Bronchospasms induced by exercise

SIDE EFFECTS

NOT SERIOUS
- Mild nausea or weakness
- Nervousness, restlessness, or insomnia

CALL YOUR DOCTOR IF THESE EFFECTS BECOME BOTHERSOME.

SERIOUS
- Changes in blood pressure or heartbeat (irregular or pounding, for example)
- Trembling; anxiety
- Breathing problems
- Dizziness; lightheadedness
- Muscle cramps
- Nausea or vomiting
- Chest pain or discomfort (rare)

LET YOUR DOCTOR KNOW RIGHT AWAY IF YOU EXPERIENCE THESE SIDE EFFECTS.

VERAPAMIL

VITAL STATISTICS

DRUG CLASS
Calcium Channel Blockers

BRAND NAMES
Calan SR, Isoptin SR, Verapamil SR, Verelan

OTHER DRUGS IN THIS CLASS
amlodipine, diltiazem, isradipine, nifedipine

GENERAL DESCRIPTION
Introduced in 1967, verapamil is prescribed for high blood pressure, angina, and heart-rhythm problems. It works by blocking the passage of calcium into muscle cells, thus decreasing the contraction of the heart and arteries, dilating the arteries, lowering blood pressure, and preventing some spasms of the coronary arteries. It is used alone or in combination with other heart and blood pressure medications. For visual characteristics of the brands Calan SR, Verapamil SR, and Verelan, see the Color Guide to Prescription Drugs and Herbs. For information on possible drug interactions, see Calcium Channel Blockers.

PRECAUTIONS

SPECIAL INFORMATION
- Recent findings have prompted warnings from some healthcare professionals about the safety of calcium channel blockers. Before using verapamil, be sure to discuss this matter thoroughly with your doctor. If you are already taking this drug, do not stop the medication without first consulting your doctor.
- Pregnant and nursing women should use verapamil only if it is clearly needed.
- Let your doctor know if you are suffering from low blood pressure (hypotension); heart, liver, or kidney disease; or congestive heart failure.
- Use with caution if you are also taking a beta blocker.
- Drinking grapefruit juice may increase blood levels of verapamil.

TARGET AILMENTS

Angina

Heart-rhythm problems

High blood pressure

SIDE EFFECTS

NOT SERIOUS
- Gastrointestinal upset (constipation, nausea, diarrhea)
- Headache
- Dizziness; lightheadedness
- Edema

CALL YOUR DOCTOR IF THESE EFFECTS BECOME TROUBLESOME.

SERIOUS
- Heart problems, such as congestive heart failure, heart-rhythm irregularities, or increased angina (heart pain)
- Low blood pressure
- Swelling of the lower extremities
- Allergic reactions, such as skin rash
- Bleeding or tender gums

CONTACT YOUR DOCTOR IMMEDIATELY.

Rx VICODIN

VITAL STATISTICS

DRUG CLASS
Analgesics

GENERIC NAME
hydrocodone and acetaminophen (combination)

OTHER BRAND NAMES
Anexia, Lortab, Zydone

GENERAL DESCRIPTION
The brand-name drug Vicodin combines hydrocodone with acetaminophen for the relief of moderate to moderately severe pain.

Hydrocodone, a painkiller and cough suppressant, is an opioid analgesic that acts on the central nervous system (the spinal cord and brain). It may cause physical and psychological dependence, especially if used for long periods of time.

Acetaminophen is a pain reliever as well as a fever reducer and is a good alternative to aspirin, particularly for people who are allergic to aspirin. It is not effective, however, in the reduction of inflammation.

For visual characteristics of Vicodin, see the Color Guide to Prescription Drugs and Herbs.

PRECAUTIONS

SPECIAL INFORMATION

- Adults should take Vicodin exactly as prescribed. The safety and effectiveness of this drug have not been established for children.
- Do not take Vicodin if you are sensitive to or have ever had an allergic reaction to hydrocodone or acetaminophen.
- Do not drive a car or operate dangerous machinery until you know how Vicodin affects you.
- Use caution in taking Vicodin if you have a head injury. Narcotics increase the pressure of fluid within the skull, which may be exaggerated in head injuries; they can also interfere with the treatment of people with head injuries.
- Before taking Vicodin, tell your doctor if you have any of the following: a severe liver or kidney disorder; an underactive thyroid; Addison's disease; an enlarged prostate; or urethral stricture.
- The narcotic hydrocodone may interfere with the diagnosis and treatment of abdominal conditions.
- Hydrocodone suppresses the cough reflex; be careful using Vicodin after surgery if you have lung disease.
- High doses of hydrocodone may produce troubled, irregular, or slowed breathing as well as drowsiness, mood changes, and mental clouding.
- Do not drink alcohol while taking Vicodin.
- Do not take Vicodin if you are pregnant or breast-feeding.
- Vicodin should be administered with caution in elderly or debilitated patients.

VICODIN

POSSIBLE INTERACTIONS

Alcohol: increased central nervous system depression. Possible liver toxicity.

Antianxiety drugs, antihistamines, antipsychotic drugs, antispasmodic drugs, tranquilizers, and other opioid analgesics: increased effects of these medications. Your dose may need to be reduced.

Monoamine oxidase (MAO) inhibitors: increased effects of these drugs or of Vicodin.

Tricyclic antidepressants: increased effects of these drugs or of Vicodin.

TARGET AILMENTS

Moderate to moderately severe pain

SIDE EFFECTS

NOT SERIOUS

- Constipation
- Dizziness; lightheadedness
- Drowsiness
- Nausea
- Sedation
- Skin rash
- Vomiting

CALL YOUR DOCTOR IF THESE EFFECTS PERSIST OR BECOME BOTHERSOME.

SERIOUS

- Breathing problems
- Cold and clammy skin
- Extreme sleepiness, leading to stupor or coma
- Heart arrhythmias
- Limp muscles
- Physical or psychological dependence

CALL YOUR DOCTOR IMMEDIATELY.

VITAMIN A

VITAL STATISTICS

OTHER NAMES
retinene, retinoic acid, retinol, retinyl palmitate

GENERAL DESCRIPTION
The first vitamin ever discovered, vitamin A is essential for good vision—especially in dim light—and for healthy skin, hair, and mucous membranes of the nose, throat, respiratory system, and digestive system. This vitamin is also necessary for the proper growth and development of bones and teeth. It stimulates the healing of wounds and is used to treat some skin disorders. Beta carotene, the precursor to vitamin A, is a carotenoid, a type of pigment found in plants. Your skin stores beta carotene, and your body metabolizes it to produce vitamin A as needed. Excess beta carotene, along with other carotenoids such as alpha carotene, acts as an antioxidant and supports immune function, so it increases your resistance to infection; it may help prevent some cancers and vision problems such as night blindness. Beta carotene may also help lower cholesterol levels and reduce the risk of heart disease.

RDA
Men: 5,000 IU (or 3 mg beta carotene)
Women: 4,000 IU (or 2.4 mg beta carotene)

NATURAL SOURCES
Vitamin A is present in orange and yellow vegetables and fruits such as dried apricots, sweet potatoes, and yams; dark green leafy vegetables such as broccoli, collard and mustard greens, and kale; chili peppers; whole milk, cream, and butter; and organ meats such as liver.

PRECAUTIONS

WARNING
Because it is fat soluble, vitamin A is stored in the body long term, and toxicity is possible if one uses high doses over a long period of time. Beta carotene does not have associated toxicity, even in high doses.

Pregnant women or women who may become pregnant should avoid supplementation. Doses over 10,000 IU during pregnancy may result in birth defects.

SPECIAL INFORMATION
Too much vitamin A can cause headaches; insomnia; restlessness; vision problems; nausea; dry, flaking skin; or an enlarged liver or spleen.

TARGET AILMENTS
Cancer
Heart disease
High cholesterol
Immune problems
Vision problems
Wounds
Viral illnesses
Vaginal candidiasis

SIDE EFFECTS
NONE EXPECTED AT RECOMMENDED LEVELS.

VITAMIN B COMPLEX

VITAL STATISTICS

GENERAL DESCRIPTION

As its name implies, vitamin B complex is a combination, or mixture, of eight essential vitamins. Although each is chemically distinct, the B vitamins coexist in many of the same foods and often work together to bolster metabolism, maintain healthy skin and muscle tone, enhance immune and nervous system function, and promote cell growth and division—including that of the red blood cells that help prevent anemia. Together they may also combat stress, depression, and cardiovascular disease.

RDA

See individual vitamin entries.

NATURAL SOURCES

Foods rich in B-complex vitamins include liver and other organ meats, fish, poultry, brewer's yeast, eggs, beans and peas, dark green leafy vegetables, whole-grain cereals, and dairy products.

PRECAUTIONS

☠ *WARNING*

A deficiency of one B vitamin often means that intake of all B vitamins is low. If your doctor suggests you need more B vitamins, take a daily multivitamin or B-complex supplement rather than individual B-vitamin supplements.

SPECIAL INFORMATION

- Most B vitamins are nontoxic unless taken in excessively large amounts.
- B vitamins, which are water soluble, are dispersed throughout the body and must be replenished daily; any excess is excreted in urine.
- People susceptible to vitamin B deficiency include pregnant women, nursing mothers, vegetarians, alcoholics, "sugarholics," the elderly, and people with malabsorption conditions or those who take certain antibiotics long term; the symptoms of deficiency include oily and scaly skin, upset stomach, headaches, anxiety, moodiness, and heart arrhythmias.
- Absorption of B vitamins can be decreased by magnesium supplements; those taking such supplements should ensure that their intake of B vitamins is adequate.

TARGET AILMENTS
Depression
Heart disease
Immune problems
Skin problems
Stress

SIDE EFFECTS

NONE EXPECTED

VITAMIN B_1 (THIAMINE)

VITAL STATISTICS

OTHER NAME
thiamine

GENERAL DESCRIPTION
Thiamine is sometimes called the energy vitamin because it is needed to metabolize carbohydrates, fats, and proteins and helps convert excess glucose into stored fat. Vitamin B_1 also ensures proper nerve-impulse transmission and contributes to maintaining normal appetite, muscle tone, and mental health. In the 1930s thiamine was discovered to be the cure for the crippling and potentially fatal disease beriberi. Now that rice, flour, and bread are generally enriched with thiamine, beriberi is relatively rare.

RDA
Men: 1.5 mg
Women: 1.1 mg

NATURAL SOURCES
A diet that regularly includes lean pork, milk, whole grains, peas, beans, peanuts, or soybeans generally provides enough thiamine.

PRECAUTIONS

WARNING
Alcohol suppresses thiamine absorption; for this reason and because they typically have poor diets, alcoholics are likely to be deficient in thiamine and other nutrients.

SPECIAL INFORMATION
- Athletes, laborers, pregnant women, and other people who burn great amounts of energy may require more than the adult RDA of thiamine.
- Mild deficiency may cause fatigue, loss of appetite, nausea, moodiness, confusion, anemia, and possibly heart arrhythmias. To increase thiamine levels, try changing your diet or taking a multivitamin instead of thiamine supplements.
- Large doses up to 100 mg of thiamine may alleviate itching from insect bites; otherwise, megasupplements are not known to be either harmful or helpful.
- Very large doses may cause nervousness, itching, flushing, or tachycardia in sensitive people.

TARGET AILMENTS
Anemia
Fatigue

SIDE EFFECTS
None expected

VITAMIN B2

VITAL STATISTICS

OTHER NAME
riboflavin

GENERAL DESCRIPTION
Like other members of the vitamin B complex, riboflavin helps produce energy from carbohydrates, fats, and proteins. Riboflavin also promotes healthy skin, hair, nails, and mucous membranes; aids the production of red blood cells, corticosteroids, and thyroid hormones; and is required for the proper function of the nerves, eyes, and adrenal glands. It is often used to treat acne, anemia, cataracts, and depression.

RDA
Men: 1.7 mg
Women: 1.3 mg
Pregnant women: 1.6 mg

NATURAL SOURCES
Lean organ meats, enriched bread and flour, cheese, yogurt, eggs, almonds, soybean products such as tofu, and green leafy vegetables—especially broccoli—are good sources. Store these foods in the dark, because vitamin B_2 breaks down in sunlight.

PRECAUTIONS

WARNING
Alcoholics and elderly people are susceptible to riboflavin deficiency: The signs include oily, dry, scaly skin rash; sores, especially on the lips and corners of the mouth; a swollen, red, painful tongue; sensitivity to light; and burning or red, itchy eyes.

SPECIAL INFORMATION
- Although vitamin B_2 supplements are available, they provide far more riboflavin than anyone needs. Diet changes are better, or take a multivitamin supplement. It is best to take the supplements with food, which increases their absorption tremendously compared with taking the tablets alone.
- A well-balanced diet provides most people with adequate riboflavin, although athletes and others who need a great deal of energy may require more than the RDA.

TARGET AILMENTS
Fatigue
Depression
Skin problems
Vision problems

SIDE EFFECTS
NONE EXPECTED

VITAMIN B_5

VITAL STATISTICS

OTHER NAME
pantothenic acid

GENERAL DESCRIPTION
The Greek term *pan* in *pantothenic acid* means "everywhere," indicating this vitamin's abundance. Along with other B vitamins, pantothenic acid is required for converting food into energy; building red blood cells; making bile; and synthesizing fats, adrenal gland steroids, antibodies, and acetylcholine and other neurotransmitters—chemicals that permit nerve transmission. Pantothenic acid in dexpanthenol lotions and creams relieves the pain of burns, cuts, and abrasions; reduces skin inflammation; and speeds wound healing.

Although a deficiency in this vitamin does not seem to occur with a normal diet and is likely only in the case of extreme starvation, deficiencies have been recorded in those with inadequate diets, producing symptoms of depression, insomnia, increased susceptibility to infection, irritability, and often adrenal fatigue.

A pantothenic acid supplement, calcium pantothenate, is available.

EMDR
4 mg to 7 mg

NATURAL SOURCES
Vitamin B_5 is abundant in organ meats, dark turkey meat, salmon, wheat bran, brewer's yeast, brown rice, lentils, nuts, beans, corn, peas, sweet potatoes, and eggs.

PRECAUTIONS

SPECIAL INFORMATION
Excess pantothenic acid may cause diarrhea.

TARGET AILMENTS
Immune problems
Wounds

SIDE EFFECTS
NONE EXPECTED

V

Vitamin B_6

Vital Statistics

OTHER NAME
pyridoxine

GENERAL DESCRIPTION
Vitamin B_6 encompasses a family of compounds that includes pyridoxine, pyridoxamine, and pyridoxal. This vitamin supports immune function, nerve-impulse transmission (especially in the brain), energy metabolism, and red blood cell synthesis. Prescribed as a drug, vitamin B_6 can sometimes alleviate carpal tunnel syndrome, infant seizures, and premenstrual syndrome.

RDA
Men: 2 mg
Women: 1.6 mg
Pregnant women: 2.2 mg

NATURAL SOURCES
Brown rice, lean meats, poultry, fish, bananas, avocados, whole grains, corn, and nuts are rich in vitamin B_6.

Precautions

☠ *WARNING*
Taking too much or too little vitamin B_6 can impair nerve function and mental health. If high levels (2,000 mg to 5,000 mg) are taken for several months, vitamin B_6 can become habit forming and may induce sleepiness as well as tingling, numb hands and feet. These symptoms will most likely disappear when the vitamin B_6 intake is reduced, and there is usually no permanent damage.

SPECIAL INFORMATION
- People most likely to be at risk for vitamin B_6 deficiency include anyone with a malabsorption problem such as lactose intolerance or celiac disease; diabetic or elderly people; and women who are pregnant, nursing, or taking oral contraceptives.
- Severe deficiency is rare. Mild deficiency may cause acne and inflamed skin, insomnia, muscle weakness, peripheral neuropathy or paresthesias that can mimic carpal tunnel syndrome, nausea, irritability, depression, and fatigue. For mild deficiency, a daily multivitamin supplement is usually recommended to boost low vitamin B_6 levels.

TARGET AILMENTS
Carpal tunnel syndrome
Depression
Fatigue
Immune problems
Premenstrual syndrome
Skin problems

SIDE EFFECTS
NONE EXPECTED

VITAMIN B_{12}

VITAL STATISTICS

OTHER NAME
cobalamin

GENERAL DESCRIPTION
Vitamin B_{12} is the largest and most complex family of the B vitamins; it includes several chemical compounds known as cobalamins. Cyanocobalamin, the stablest form, is the one most likely to be found in supplements. Like other B vitamins, B_{12} is important for converting fats, carbohydrates, and protein into energy, and assisting in the synthesis of red blood cells. It is critical for producing the genetic materials RNA and DNA as well as myelin, a fatty substance that forms a protective sheath around nerves.

Unlike other B vitamins, vitamin B_{12} needs several hours to be absorbed. Excess vitamin B_{12} is excreted in urine, even though a backup supply can be stored for several years in the liver. Vitamin B_{12} is considered nontoxic, even when taken at several times the RDA.

RDA
Adults: 2 mcg
Pregnant women: 2.2 mcg

NATURAL SOURCES
Vitamin B_{12} is not produced by plants but is supplied through animal products such as organ meats, fish, eggs, and dairy products.

TARGET AILMENTS
Anemia
Depression
Fatigue

PRECAUTIONS

SPECIAL INFORMATION
- High doses of folic acid (vitamin B_9) can decrease levels of B_{12}.
- Dietary deficiency is uncommon and is usually limited to alcoholics, strict vegetarians, and pregnant or nursing women—who should take supplements. More often, deficiency stems from an inability to absorb the vitamin, a problem that may occur for years before symptoms show; it tends to affect the elderly, those who have had stomach surgery, or people who have a disease of malabsorption, such as colitis.
- Signs of vitamin B_{12} deficiency include a sore tongue, weakness, weight loss, body odor, back pains, and tingling arms and legs. Severe deficiency leads to pernicious anemia, causing fatigue, a tendency to bleed, lemon yellow pallor, abdominal pain, stiff arms and legs, irritability, and depression.
- Without treatment, pernicious anemia can lead to permanent nerve damage and possibly death; the disease can be controlled, although not cured, with regular injections of B_{12}.
- Lack of calcium, vitamin B_6, or iron may also interfere with the normal absorption of vitamin B_{12}.

SIDE EFFECTS
NONE EXPECTED

Vitamin C

Vital Statistics

OTHER NAME
ascorbic acid

GENERAL DESCRIPTION
Vitamin C is well known for its ability to prevent and treat scurvy, a disease that causes swollen and bleeding gums, aching bones and muscles, and in some cases even death. Connective tissue throughout the body is made of collagen, which depends on vitamin C for its production. In this role, vitamin C helps heal wounds, burns, bruises, and broken bones. As a powerful antioxidant and immune system booster, vitamin C may alleviate the pain of rheumatoid arthritis, protect against atherosclerosis and heart disease, and help prevent some forms of cancer, and has the reputed potential (yet unproved) to prevent the common cold. More than the RDA may be needed under conditions of physical or emotional stress.

Because it is water soluble, excess vitamin C is excreted in the urine, so large amounts of it may usually be taken without fear of toxicity. Doses larger than 1,000 mg a day have been suggested for preventing cancer, infections including the common cold, and other ailments.

RDA
Adults: 60 mg
Pregnant women: 70 mg

NATURAL SOURCES
Sources of vitamin C include citrus fruits, rose hips, bell peppers, strawberries, broccoli, cantaloupes, tomatoes, and leafy greens.

Precautions

WARNING
In some people, large doses of vitamin C may induce such side effects as nausea, diarrhea, reduced selenium and copper absorption, excessive iron absorption, increased kidney stone formation, and a false-positive reaction to diabetes tests.

SPECIAL INFORMATION
- Vitamin C breaks down faster than any other vitamin, so it is best to eat fruits and vegetables when fresh and to cook them minimally or not at all.
- Slight vitamin C deficiency is fairly common, although severe deficiencies are rare in the United States today. Symptoms of deficiency include weight loss, fatigue, bleeding gums, easy bruising, reduced resistance to colds and other infections, and wounds and fractures that are slow to heal.

TARGET AILMENTS
Cancer
Heart disease
Immune problems
Wounds

SIDE EFFECTS
None expected

VITAMIN D

VITAL STATISTICS

OTHER NAMES
cholecalciferol, ergocalciferol

GENERAL DESCRIPTION
Vitamin D not only promotes healthy bones and teeth by regulating the absorption and balance of calcium and phosphorus but also fosters normal muscle contraction and nerve function. Vitamin D prevents rickets, a disease of calcium-deprived bone that results in bowlegs, knock-knees, and other bone defects. Vitamin D supplements may help treat psoriasis and slow or even reverse some cancers, such as myeloid leukemia.

RDA
Adults: 200 IU (5 mcg)
Children, adolescents, and pregnant women: 400 IU (10 mcg)

NATURAL SOURCES
Fatty fish such as herring, salmon, and tuna, followed by dairy products, are the richest natural sources of this nutrient. Few other foods naturally contain vitamin D, but 10 minutes in the midday summer sun enables the body to produce about 200 IU of it. Milk, breakfast cereals, and infant formulas are fortified with vitamin D.

PRECAUTIONS

WARNING
Vitamin D is fat soluble; excess amounts of it are stored in the body. Because of its potentially toxic effects, vitamin D should not be taken in supplements of more than 400 IU daily unless prescribed by a doctor.

SPECIAL INFORMATION
- In adults, vitamin D deficiency can cause nervousness and diarrhea, insomnia, muscle twitches, and bone weakening, and it may worsen osteoporosis.
- Too much vitamin D raises the calcium level in the blood, which in turn may induce headaches, nausea, loss of appetite, excessive thirst, muscle weakness, and even heart, liver, or kidney damage as calcium deposits accumulate in soft tissue.
- In some latitudes, people don't get enough sunshine and cannot make enough vitamin D for several months of the year; those people should ensure that they get enough through diet or through supplements in the amount of 400 IU to 800 IU per day. Supplements over 400 IU per day should be prescribed by a doctor, however.

TARGET AILMENTS
Cancer
Skin problems

SIDE EFFECTS
NONE EXPECTED

V

VITAMIN E

VITAL STATISTICS

OTHER NAME
alpha-tocopherol

GENERAL DESCRIPTION
Vitamin E encompasses a family of compounds called tocopherols, of which alpha-tocopherol is the most common. It is required for proper function of the immune system, endocrine system, and sex glands. As a powerful antioxidant, it prevents unstable molecules known as free radicals from damaging cells and tissues. In this capacity, vitamin E deters atherosclerosis, accelerates the healing of wounds, protects lung tissue from inhaled pollutants, may reduce risk for heart disease, and may prevent premature skin aging. Researchers suspect that vitamin E has other beneficial effects ranging from preventing cancer and cataracts to alleviating rheumatoid arthritis and a skin disorder associated with lupus.

Because of its many suggested therapeutic roles, vitamin E is popular as an oral supplement and an ingredient of skin-care products. Although it is fat soluble, vitamin E is considered nontoxic because it does no harm except in extremely high doses.

RDA
Women: 12 IU (8 mg)
Men and pregnant or nursing women:
15 IU (10 mg)

NATURAL SOURCES
Vegetable oils, nuts, dark green leafy vegetables, organ meats, seafood, eggs, and avocados are rich food sources of vitamin E.

PRECAUTIONS

SPECIAL INFORMATION
Symptoms of vitamin E deficiency, such as fluid retention and hemolytic anemia, are rare in adults but are sometimes seen in premature infants.

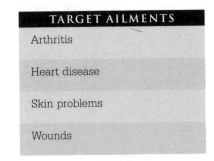

TARGET AILMENTS
Arthritis
Heart disease
Skin problems
Wounds

SIDE EFFECTS
NONE EXPECTED

VITAMIN K

VITAL STATISTICS

OTHER NAMES
menadione, phytonadione

GENERAL DESCRIPTION
Vitamin K is needed in a small but critical amount to form essential proteins, mainly for blood clotting but also for kidney function and bone metabolism. Vitamin K exists in two natural forms that require some dietary fat for absorption.

RDA
Men: 80 mcg
Women: 65 mcg

NATURAL SOURCES
Bacteria living in the intestines produce about half the body's needs; the rest comes from diet. Good food sources include spinach, cabbage, broccoli, turnip greens, or other leafy vegetables; beef liver; green tea; cheese; and oats.

PRECAUTIONS

WARNING
Megadoses higher than 500 mcg can be toxic or cause an allergic reaction and must be prescribed by a doctor.

Large doses of vitamin E may interfere with vitamin K's blood-clotting effects.

SPECIAL INFORMATION
- Vitamin K deficiency is extremely rare in adults but may occur in newborns until their intestinal bacteria begin producing the vitamin. To enhance a newborn's blood-clotting ability, the mother may take vitamin K supplements before delivery, and infants usually receive them after birth. Otherwise, supplements are neither necessary nor recommended.
- Excessive calcium can interfere with vitamin K absorption, leading to deficiency.

TARGET AILMENTS
Osteoporosis

SIDE EFFECTS
NONE EXPECTED

Warfarin

Vital Statistics

DRUG CLASS
Anticoagulant and Antiplatelet Drugs

BRAND NAME
Coumadin

OTHER DRUGS IN THIS CLASS
aspirin, dalteparin, dipyridamole, heparin

GENERAL DESCRIPTION
Warfarin inhibits blood clotting by blocking vitamin K, a central ingredient in the production of four blood-clotting factors. Warfarin is administered orally and can be extremely dangerous if not used properly. You must have periodic blood tests to monitor clotting time. See Anticoagulant and Antiplatelet Drugs for important information on serious side effects, such as hemorrhaging, and drug interactions.

TARGET AILMENTS

Prevents and treats blood clots

Reduces risk of myocardial infarction and blood-clot formation after myocardial infarction

SIDE EFFECTS

NOT SERIOUS
- Minor bleeding
- Mild skin rash

CALL YOUR DOCTOR IF THESE EFFECTS PERSIST OR BECOME BOTHERSOME.

Precautions

WARNING
Do not use without telling your physician if you have had a heart attack, uncontrolled high blood pressure, ulcers, or a stroke.

Pregnant women should not take warfarin because it can cause serious birth defects.

SPECIAL INFORMATION
- Nursing women should check with a physician before taking warfarin.
- Tell your doctor if you have or have had low blood pressure, an impaired kidney or liver, a bleeding disease or disorder, chest pains, allergies, asthma, colitis, diabetes, active tuberculosis, a recent childbirth, medical or dental surgery, spinal anesthesia, x-rays, a bad fall, heavy bleeding or heavy menstrual periods, diarrhea, or any other medical problem. Also, tell your doctor if you are using an intrauterine device (IUD) for birth control or a catheter.
- Tell your pharmacist, dentist, and physician that you are taking the medicine. You may be advised to carry a medication identification card.
- Avoid dangerous activities that might cause injuries. Be sure to report all falls and blows to your doctor. Internal bleeding may occur without symptoms.

POSSIBLE INTERACTIONS
A number of drugs can increase or decrease warfarin's effects. Tell your doctor about all prescription and over-the-counter drugs you are taking.

Vitamin K: counteracts warfarin. Avoid eating large quantities of foods rich in vitamin K, including green leafy vegetables, dairy products, bacon, beef liver, cabbage, cauliflower, and fish.

WHEAT GERM

VITAL STATISTICS

GENERAL DESCRIPTION

Wheat germ, the heart of the wheat berry, is the most healthful part of the grain. It contains vitamins B and E, protein, iron, calcium, copper, magnesium, zinc, and potassium.

Wheat germ is a good source of fiber, which can relieve constipation and may reduce the risk of developing colon and rectal cancer. A quarter cup contains 40 percent of the recommended daily allowance of vitamin E. In addition, including wheat germ as part of the daily diet has been found to lower levels of LDL, the so-called "bad" cholesterol.

Oil taken from wheat germ is also high in vitamin E. It can be ingested, or can be used externally to relieve sores or burns on the skin. Some research has suggested that octacosanol, an ingredient in wheat-germ oil, can help improve athletic performance and endurance. And some manufacturers have maintained that the presence of octacosanol makes wheat-germ oil a better source of vitamin E than other supplements, though such claims have been questioned by medical experts. While some early studies suggested that wheat-germ oil may have some beneficial effects in treating muscular dystrophy, more recent research disproved this theory.

Because it is such a good source of vitamin E, wheat germ may be helpful for many ailments and health conditions that appear to benefit from vitamin E supplementation.

PREPARATIONS

Available as flakes at grocery stores and health food stores. Also available in oil form. Wheat germ can become rancid, so it should be covered tightly and kept refrigerated.

TARGET AILMENTS

- High LDL cholesterol
- Heart disease
- Cancer
- Stroke
- Diabetes
- Fibrocystic breast disease
- Menopausal symptoms
- Other conditions that benefit from vitamin E supplementation

SIDE EFFECTS

NONE EXPECTED

WHITE WILLOW

LATIN NAME
Salix alba

VITAL STATISTICS

GENERAL DESCRIPTION

White willow, like other willows, is a natural source of salicin, a precursor of modern aspirin, and indeed it has been used for centuries worldwide as a pain reliever. Although all parts of the plant contain some salicin, the best source is the mature bark, either fresh or dried. Like other salicin-producing plants, white willow also reduces fever and inflammation, probably by suppressing the action of prostaglandins (hormonelike substances), which are produced by the body in response to injuries.

In addition to salicin, willow bark contains other compounds that the body metabolizes to salicylic acid and therefore acts more slowly and over a longer period than aspirin does.

PREPARATIONS

Over the counter:

Available as dried bark, tincture, tea, and capsules.

At home:

TEA: Simmer covered 1 to 2 tsp powdered bark in 1 cup water for 10 minutes; strain. Drink up to 3 cups a day. Mix with honey and lemon or another herbal tea to improve taste.

Consult a practitioner for the dosage appropriate for you and the specific condition.

PRECAUTIONS

WARNING

This herb should not be given to children unless prescribed by a healthcare practitioner knowledgeable about herbs or to those under 16 with a cold, influenza, or other viral illness. Using salicylates may cause Reye's syndrome, a potentially fatal condition.

Because it can worsen stomach ills, it should be used with caution by people with ulcers or other stomach problems.

POSSIBLE INTERACTIONS

Do not mix white willow with other salicylates, such as aspirin or wintergreen oil, because of the potential for additive side effects.

Combining white willow with other herbs may necessitate a lower dosage.

TARGET AILMENTS
Take internally for:
Arthritis; gout
Minor muscle strains
Menstrual cramps
Headache; fever; aches and pains
Apply externally for:
Sores and burns
Arthritis

SIDE EFFECTS

NOT SERIOUS

- Upset stomach
- Nausea
- Ringing in the ears

LOWER THE DOSAGE OR STOP USING WHITE WILLOW; CALL YOUR DOCTOR IF SYMPTOMS PERSIST.

WILD CHERRY BARK

LATIN NAME
Prunus serotina

VITAL STATISTICS

GENERAL DESCRIPTION

Native Americans used cherry bark for a number of ailments, and it became a popular remedy with the colonists as well. Today wild cherry bark is used by herbalists to treat coughs, colds, asthma, and bronchitis. It is also used as a mild sedative or tranquilizer.

PREPARATIONS

Over the counter:

Available as syrup, tincture, and dried bark.

At home:

DECOCTION: Pour 1 cup boiling water over 2 to 3 tsp dried bark. Simmer covered for 10 minutes. Drink up to 3 cups a day for no more than 10 days.

TINCTURE: Take 1/8 to 1/2 tsp up to three times a day for coughs for no more than 10 days.

COMBINATIONS: May be combined with many herbs.

Consult a practitioner for the dosage appropriate for your specific condition.

PRECAUTIONS

WARNING

Wild cherry leaves, bark, and pits contain a cyanide-like poison that can cause death. Do not exceed recommended dosage.

Pregnant women and nursing mothers should not use wild cherry bark preparations.

SPECIAL INFORMATION

- When used for coughs, if the cough does not go away within 10 days, consult your doctor.
- Do not give preparations containing wild cherry to children under two at all or to older ones for more than seven to 10 days except in conjunction with a healthcare practitioner. For children over two and for adults over 65, start with a low-strength dose and slowly increase.
- Use in medicinal amounts only in consultation with a doctor.

POSSIBLE INTERACTIONS

Combining wild cherry bark with other herbs may necessitate a lower dosage.

TARGET AILMENTS

Take internally for:

Coughs

Sluggish or weak digestion

Dyspepsia

Colds with coughs

Asthma

SIDE EFFECTS

NOT SERIOUS

- Stomach upset; diarrhea

USE LESS OR STOP USING.

SERIOUS

- Spasms; difficulty breathing or speaking

THESE EFFECTS MAY OCCUR IF RECOMMENDED DOSE IS EXCEEDED. STOP USING IMMEDIATELY AND CALL YOUR DOCTOR AT ONCE.

Wild Cranesbill

LATIN NAME
Geranium maculatum

Vital Statistics

GENERAL DESCRIPTION

Also known as alumroot or wild geranium, wild cranesbill is a fairly safe and effective herb for assorted gastrointestinal problems, including diarrhea and dysentery. It is thought to help strengthen mucous membranes and may help remedy excessive mucous discharges as well as bleeding associated with gastrointestinal problems. Some herbalists recommend it to help control menorrhagia (heavy menstrual flow) and diminish chronic vaginal discharge and inflammation. The herb contains tannins, resinous substances that can assist in wound healing, which may account for its use in treating such ailments as ulcers, hemorrhoids, and canker sores. The rhizome of wild cranesbill is harvested for medicinal use and is usually prepared as a decoction or tincture; it can also be made into an ointment for external use.

PREPARATIONS

Over the counter:
Available in capsules and tincture.

At home:

Tincture: Take 1/8 to 1/2 tsp three times a day.

Decoction: Place 1 to 2 tsp wild cranesbill in 1 cup cold water. Bring to boil and simmer covered for 10 to 15 minutes. Drink three times a day.

Combinations: To help control a heavy menstrual flow, combine equal parts wild cranesbill, shepherd's-purse, and liferoot tinctures; take as needed. For peptic ulcers, combine with marsh mallow or meadowsweet. For hemorrhoids, apply externally using a combination of powdered wild cranesbill and powdered yarrow mixed with cocoa butter.

Consult a qualified practitioner for the dosage appropriate for you and the specific condition being treated.

Precautions

SPECIAL INFORMATION

Use of this herb by children for more than seven to 10 days should be done in conjunction with a healthcare practitioner.

POSSIBLE INTERACTIONS

Combining wild cranesbill with other herbs may necessitate a lower dosage.

TARGET AILMENTS
Diarrhea
Dysentery
Menorrhagia
Gastritis

SIDE EFFECTS

None expected

W

Wild Yam

LATIN NAME
Dioscorea villosa

Vital Statistics

GENERAL DESCRIPTION

Used during the 18th and 19th centuries as a remedy for menstrual pain and complications associated with childbearing, wild yam is a perennial vine that entwines itself around fences and bushes. It is recognized by a slender reddish brown stem and drooping yellow flowers that bloom during the summer. Wild yam extract, taken from the root, contains an alkaloid substance that relaxes the muscles of the entire abdominal region. Consequently, it is prescribed to alleviate menstrual cramps and to relieve the nausea and muscle tension associated with pregnancy. Wild yam also contains steroidal saponins, believed to act as anti-inflammatory agents and used to reduce the swelling caused by rheumatoid arthritis. For visual characteristics of wild yam, see the Color Guide to Prescription Drugs and Herbs.

PREPARATIONS

Over the counter:

Wild yam is available as dried root, tincture, or capsules.

At home:

Tea: Simmer covered 1 to 2 tsp wild yam root with 1 cup water for 10 to 15 minutes. Drink three times daily.

Combinations: For intestinal colic, wild yam is combined with calamus, chamomile, and ginger. Rheumatoid arthritis is treated with a mix of wild yam and black cohosh. Herbalists use a combination of wild yam and cramp bark for menstrual cramps.

Consult a qualified practitioner for the dosage appropriate for you and the specific condition being treated.

Precautions

SPECIAL INFORMATION

- Wild yam is sometimes prescribed by herbalists for its supposed progesterone-like properties for women undergoing menopause. There is still a great deal of controversy, however, as to the effectiveness of this treatment. You should consult a practitioner before using wild yam as a progesterone supplement.
- This herb should not be used with children unless it is specifically prescribed by a healthcare practitioner who is knowledgeable about herbs.

POSSIBLE INTERACTIONS

Combining wild yam with other herbs may necessitate a lower dosage.

TARGET AILMENTS
Menstrual cramps
Nausea due to pregnancy
Morning sickness
Intestinal colic
Rheumatoid arthritis

SIDE EFFECTS

None expected

XIANG SHA YANG WEI PIAN

VITAL STATISTICS

ENGLISH NAME
Saussurea and Cardamom Stomach-Nourishing Tablets

ALSO SOLD AS
Hsiang Sha Yang Wei Pien

GENERAL DESCRIPTION
Xiang Sha Yang Wei Pian is used to treat people who have trouble with their digestion, often indicated by abdominal distention, burping, heartburn, nausea, diarrhea, and frequent tiredness. This formula may also be used to treat acute gastritis. Chinese practitioners believe that the herbs in this formula strengthen the digestive system, helping it work more effectively.

Chinese medicine takes a holistic approach to healthcare, fashioning remedies to treat the entire being as well as the specific parts or areas. Precise combinations of herbs are used to prevent and combat disease, which is thought to arise from disturbances in the flow of a bodily energy called chi (pronounced "chee") and blood, or from a lack of balance in the complementary states of yin and yang. A patent formula, *Xiang Sha Yang Wei Pian* is made by using a standardized combination of herbs and method of preparation.

INGREDIENTS
atractylodes, saussurea, amomum, cardamom, codonopsis, germinated barley sprouts, aged citrus peel, licorice, fermented herb mix

PREPARATIONS
This formula is available in pill form at many Chinese pharmacies and Oriental grocery stores.

TARGET AILMENTS

- Indigestion
- Heartburn
- Stomachache
- Nausea
- Diarrhea or loose stools
- Acute or chronic gastritis
- Gastric or duodenal ulcer symptoms

SIDE EFFECTS

NONE EXPECTED

XIAO CHAI HU WAN

VITAL STATISTICS

ENGLISH NAME
Minor Bupleurum Pills

GENERAL DESCRIPTION
A traditional Chinese formula, *Xiao Chai Hu Wan* is used when a person is ill with a cold or has flulike symptoms and cannot get quite well again, a condition the Chinese term as being stuck between the inside and the outside. Believed to strengthen the body and assist in pushing out disease, this formula may help alleviate low-grade fevers, fatigue, dizziness, and irritability. This formula may also help relieve fibromyalgia, described in Chinese medicine as tightness or distress that is caught in the muscles between the skin and the organs in the body.

Chinese medicine takes a holistic approach to healthcare, fashioning remedies to treat the entire being as well as the specific parts or areas. Precise combinations of herbs are used to prevent and combat disease, which is thought to arise from disturbances in the flow of a bodily energy called chi (pronounced "chee") and blood, or from a lack of balance in the complementary states of yin and yang. A patent formula, *Xiao Chai Hu Wan* is made by using a standardized combination of herbs and method of preparation.

INGREDIENTS
bupleurum, scutellaria, pinellia, fresh gingerroot, ginseng, honey-fried licorice, Chinese dates

PREPARATIONS
Available only from a practitioner of Oriental herbal medicine.

PRECAUTIONS

WARNING
Do not use if you have high blood pressure, severe headaches, or bleeding gums.

TARGET AILMENTS
Chronic fatigue syndrome
Epstein-Barr virus
Chronic low-grade fevers
Irritability and fatigue
Fibromyalgia
Hepatitis or jaundice
Malaria
Upper respiratory infection

SIDE EFFECTS

YOU MAY EXPERIENCE FEVER AND CHILLS WHEN YOU BEGIN TAKING THIS FORMULA.

Xiao Yao Wan

Vital Statistics

ENGLISH NAME
Rambling Powder Pills

ALSO SOLD AS
Hsiao Yao Wan—Bupleurum Sedative Pills

GENERAL DESCRIPTION
The formula *Xiao Yao Wan* is used to treat problems associated with constraint, a general condition that can manifest itself in a number of ways, including irritability, frustration, and as physical symptoms. In Chinese, the remedy's name means free and open flow, and it implies open-mindedness. *Xiao Yao Wan* is prescribed when a person's normal flow has been blocked, causing disruption. Symptoms of constraint include nausea, vomiting, diarrhea, and constipation.

Practitioners often prescribe *Xiao Yao Wan* for menstrual problems, such as irregular cycles or irregular menstrual flow, possibly with cramping, breast pain, and premenstrual syndrome (PMS). It is sometimes used to treat irritability, insomnia, and nightmares. And because *Xiao Yao Wan* treats disorders of the Liver system—which in Chinese medicine includes the eyes—this remedy may also be used for some eye problems.

Chinese medicine takes a holistic approach to healthcare, fashioning remedies to treat the entire being as well as the specific parts or areas. Precise combinations of herbs are used to prevent and combat disease, which is thought to arise from disturbances in the flow of a bodily energy called chi (pronounced "chee") and blood, or from a lack of balance in the complementary states of yin and yang. A patent formula, *Xiao Yao Wan* is made by using a standardized combination of herbs and method of preparation.

INGREDIENTS
bupleurum, dang gui, atractylodes, white peony root, poria, licorice, raw ginger, mint

PREPARATIONS
This formula is available in pill form in many Chinese pharmacies and Oriental grocery stores.

TARGET AILMENTS

- Chronic irritability or frustration
- Hepatitis
- Chronic gastritis; constipation; diarrhea; irritable bowel syndrome
- Peptic ulcers
- Painful or irregular menstrual periods
- Painful breasts
- Premenstrual syndrome (PMS)
- Insomnia or disturbed sleep
- Certain eye problems

SIDE EFFECTS
None expected

YARROW

LATIN NAME
Achillea millefolium

VITAL STATISTICS

GENERAL DESCRIPTION

Yarrow has been used to heal wounds since ancient times; the Greek hero of the Trojan War, Achilles, is said to have stopped the bleeding of his warriors' wounds by applying the crushed leaves of yarrow. Modern investigation has revealed many chemicals in yarrow that have anti-inflammatory and pain-relieving effects. The leaves, stems, and flower tops contain more than 10 different active ingredients, including salicylic acid, menthol, and camphor. Two major constituents, achilletin and achilleine, are thought to help blood coagulate, while thujone (also found in chamomile) has mild sedative properties. Because yarrow may have diuretic properties, it is sometimes used to treat menstrual bloating and high blood pressure. The somewhat bitter taste of yarrow tea can be relieved by adding sweeteners or other herbs.

A naturalized, three-foot-tall perennial from Eurasia, yarrow is widely planted in flower and herb gardens and found growing wild in most areas of the United States. For visual characteristics of yarrow, see the Color Guide to Prescription Drugs and Herbs.

PREPARATIONS

Over the counter:
Available as dried herb or tea.

At home:
TEA: Steep covered 1 to 2 tsp dried herb in 1 cup boiling water for 10 to 15 minutes. Drink hot up to 3 cups a day.
Consult a qualified practitioner for the dosage appropriate for you and the specific condition being treated.

PRECAUTIONS

SPECIAL INFORMATION

If you are allergic to ragweed, you may develop a rash from ingesting yarrow.

POSSIBLE INTERACTIONS

Combining yarrow with other herbs may necessitate a lower dosage.

TARGET AILMENTS

Take internally for:

Fever

Digestive disorders

Menstrual cramps

Anxiety; insomnia

High blood pressure

Apply externally for:

Minor wounds; bleeding

Vaginal irritations (use as a douche)

SIDE EFFECTS

NOT SERIOUS

- Rash or diarrhea

STOP USING THE HERB AND CONSULT YOUR DOCTOR.

YELLOW DOCK

LATIN NAME
Rumex crispus

VITAL STATISTICS

GENERAL DESCRIPTION

Native to Europe, this herb is now naturalized in the United States and is commonly found along roadsides and in fields and waste areas. Yellow dock is most valued for its gentle laxative properties. It stimulates bile production and is considered a blood purifier. Although the yellow roots and rhizomes are the portion used in herbal medicine, the lance-shaped, wavy-edged leaves are rich in vitamins C and A and may be eaten as cooked greens.

PREPARATIONS

Over the counter:
Available as tincture, capsules, and dried root.

At home:

DECOCTION: Place 2 to 3 tsp root in 1 cup water; bring to a boil; simmer covered for 10 to 15 minutes. Drink three times a day for no longer than two weeks.

TINCTURE: Take ⅛ to ½ tsp three times a day for no longer than two weeks. Long-term use as a tonic is permissible if taken under the supervision of a healthcare professional.

COMBINATIONS: May be combined with dandelion, burdock, and cleavers.

Consult a qualified practitioner for the dosage appropriate for you and the specific condition being treated.

PRECAUTIONS

SPECIAL INFORMATION

- If cooked and eaten, yellow dock greens should be boiled twice, each time in fresh water, to remove the excessive amount of oxalic acid they contain.
- Greens should not be eaten by people with gout or a history of kidney stones.
- Use of this herb by children for more than seven to 10 days should be done in conjunction with a healthcare practitioner.

POSSIBLE INTERACTIONS

Combining yellow dock with other herbs may necessitate a lower dosage.

TARGET AILMENTS

Take internally for:

Constipation; anemia; blood purification (as a liver tonic)

Rheumatic conditions

Enlarged lymph glands

Apply externally for:

Chronic skin conditions such as eczema and psoriasis

Skin eruptions; itchy skin

Ringworm and other fungal infections

SIDE EFFECTS

NOT SERIOUS

- Gastric disturbance
- Nausea; diarrhea

THESE EFFECTS MAY OCCUR IF LARGE DOSES ARE TAKEN.

YIN QIAO PIAN

VITAL STATISTICS

ENGLISH NAME
Honeysuckle and Forsythia Pills

ALSO SOLD AS
Yin Qiao Jie Du Pian, Yin Chiao Chieh Tu Pien

GENERAL DESCRIPTION
Yin Qiao Pian is the remedy most commonly prescribed for the beginning stage of a cold or flu. If taken early enough, it can often avert the illness or lessen its severity. The formula is used to treat a cold or flu that starts with a sore throat, a fever, and possibly a headache, and when the tongue has a yellow coating. *Yin Qiao Pian* strengthens the body's ability to ward off the illness. It is not especially effective after the cold has really taken hold.

This is probably the best known of all Chinese herbal formulas. Although the name appears on a variety of cold remedies, the ingredients may differ. Check the label and avoid any brands that contain caffeinium, paracetamolum, and chlorpheniraminum.

Chinese medicine takes a holistic approach to healthcare, fashioning remedies to treat the entire being as well as the specific parts or areas. Precise combinations of herbs are used to prevent and combat disease, which is thought to arise from disturbances in the flow of a bodily energy called chi (pronounced "chee") and blood, or from a lack of balance in the complementary states of yin and yang.

INGREDIENTS
honeysuckle, forsythia, burdock seeds, balloonflower root, mint, phragmites, licorice, lophatherum, schizonepeta, antelope horn, prepared soybean

PREPARATIONS
This formula is available in pill form at many Chinese pharmacies and Oriental grocery stores.

PRECAUTIONS

WARNING
This formula will not be effective if symptoms include excessive mucus or pronounced chills.

TARGET AILMENTS
Colds or upper respiratory infections (including flu)
Acute bronchitis
Beginning stage of measles
Sore throat, swollen glands, or tonsillitis
Conjunctivitis (pinkeye)

SIDE EFFECTS
NONE EXPECTED

YLANG-YLANG

LATIN NAME
Cananga odorata

VITAL STATISTICS

GENERAL DESCRIPTION

Native to the Philippines, ylang-ylang is a tropical tree with large, fragrant flowers on weeping branches. The flowers' scent is similar to that of narcissus.

Ylang-ylang has both stimulant and sedative properties. The oil, which is either clear or yellow, has a sweet, spicy aroma and is frequently used in perfumes and soaps. In Victorian times the oil was used in a popular hair treatment as a way to stimulate the scalp and promote hair growth. Today its uses are many and varied. Ylang-ylang is thought to help regulate the heart, for example, and is sometimes used as a secondary treatment for high blood pressure.

PREPARATIONS

The essential oil is distilled from the fresh flowers; smaller flowers produce more fragrant oil. Ylang-ylang is also solvent-extracted and sold as a concrete and an absolute.

Use ylang-ylang in the bath (add 5 to 10 drops to the bathwater) or as a massage oil; mix 10 drops ylang-ylang oil with 2 tbsp nut oil or aloe gel. These preparations can be used in nearly all appropriate applications of ylang-ylang oil. (For skin application, use only 5 drops of ylang-ylang oil in 2 tbsp aloe gel.)

A few drops placed on a tissue and inhaled can ease anxiety and nervousness. For the same effect, you can also use a diffuser to scent the air.

PRECAUTIONS

SPECIAL INFORMATION

Buy only from a reputable source. The oil is often adulterated with cocoa butter.

TARGET AILMENTS
Acne and oily skin
Depression
Insomnia
Impotence and low sex drive
Anxiety and stress
Hair loss
High blood pressure
Malaria, typhus, and other fevers
Fluid retention

SIDE EFFECTS

OVERUSE CAN CAUSE HEADACHE OR NAUSEA. DISCONTINUE OR USE LESS FREQUENTLY IF YOU EXPERIENCE THESE SYMPTOMS.

YUN NAN BAI YAO

VITAL STATISTICS

ENGLISH NAME
Yunnan (province) White Medicine

ALSO SOLD AS
Yun Nan Pai Yao

GENERAL DESCRIPTION
Yun Nan Bai Yao is quite a remarkable remedy, in that it stops bleeding without clotting the blood, and it keeps the blood from clotting without causing more bleeding. The formula is used to stanch all sorts of bleeding, both internal and external, as well as to treat surface bruises. It is often used in the treatment of certain menstrual problems, such as painful, heavily clotted periods; excessive menstrual flow; and hemorrhage after childbirth. Besides controlling blood flow, *Yun Nan Bai Yao* is said to ease pain and speed healing.

Chinese medicine takes a holistic approach to healthcare, fashioning remedies to treat the entire being as well as the specific parts or areas. Precise combinations of herbs are used to prevent and combat disease, which is thought to arise from disturbances in the flow of a bodily energy called chi (pronounced "chee") and blood, or from a lack of balance in the complementary states of yin and yang. A patent formula, *Yun Nan Bai Yao* is made by using a standardized combination of herbs and method of preparation.

INGREDIENTS
pseudoginseng in combination with other herbs (This formula was originally a family secret and is now a secret of the Chinese government.)

PREPARATIONS
This formula can be found in many Chinese pharmacies and Oriental grocery stores. It is sold in powder and capsule form. The powder is extremely bitter and is best used by sprinkling it on wounds. The capsules are easier to swallow. Included with the remedy is a small red pill that is to be taken if the wounds are severe, to help prevent shock.

PRECAUTIONS

WARNING
Do not use if you are pregnant.

While using this remedy, you should avoid eating fish, shellfish, lima beans, or cold or very sour food.

TARGET AILMENTS
Bleeding from open wounds
Trauma to soft tissue (sprains, strains, bruises)
Vomiting blood or intestinal bleeding; coughing up blood
Nosebleeds
Painful, clotted menstrual periods, excessive menstrual bleeding, postpartum hemorrhage
Postsurgical recovery

SIDE EFFECTS
NONE EXPECTED

ZANTAC

VITAL STATISTICS

DRUG CLASS
Antiulcer Drugs [Histamine H_2 Blockers]

GENERIC NAME
ranitidine

GENERAL DESCRIPTION
The brand-name drugs Zantac 150 and Zantac 300 are prescribed to treat ulcers of the stomach and duodenum (upper intestine). Zantac is also prescribed for Zollinger-Ellison syndrome, gastroesophageal reflux (in which stomach acid flows backward into the esophagus), and other conditions involving the overproduction of stomach acid.

The over-the-counter form, Zantac 75, is used not for ulcers but to relieve acid indigestion and heartburn. Although the OTC version is a lower dose of ranitidine than the prescription forms, essentially the same interactions apply, although the side effects are milder.

Belonging to the subclass of antiulcer drugs known as histamine H_2 blockers, Zantac works by blocking the effects of the chemical compound histamine in the stomach, thereby reducing the secretion of the digestive juice hydrochloric acid. For more information, including side effects and possible drug interactions, see Ranitidine and Antiulcer Drugs. For visual characteristics of Zantac 150, see the Color Guide to Prescription Drugs and Herbs.

PRECAUTIONS

SPECIAL INFORMATION
- Tell your doctor if you have a history of kidney or liver disease.
- If you are also using antacids for relief from ulcer pain, take the antacid at least two hours before or after taking Zantac.
- Because this drug may cause dizziness or drowsiness, you may need to restrict your driving or involvement in potentially hazardous activities.
- If you are pregnant or nursing, avoid Zantac.

POSSIBLE INTERACTIONS
See Ranitidine.

TARGET AILMENTS
Duodenal ulcer
Gastric ulcer
Zollinger-Ellison syndrome
Other conditions characterized by an overproduction of stomach acid
Gastroesophageal reflux disease
Erosive esophagitis (inflammation of the esophagus)
Acid indigestion and heartburn (OTC)

SIDE EFFECTS
SEE RANITIDINE.

Rx ZESTRIL

VITAL STATISTICS

DRUG CLASS
Angiotensin-Converting Enzyme (ACE) Inhibitors

GENERIC NAME
lisinopril

OTHER DRUGS IN THIS CLASS
benazepril, captopril, enalapril, fosinopril, quinapril, ramipril

GENERAL DESCRIPTION
Zestril is a brand name for the ACE inhibitor lisinopril. Introduced in 1988, Zestril relaxes arterial walls, lowering blood pressure. It is used in the management of hypertension (high blood pressure) and congestive heart failure. For further information, including possible drug interactions, see Angiotensin-Converting Enzyme (ACE) Inhibitors. For visual characteristics, see the Color Guide to Prescription Drugs and Herbs.

PRECAUTIONS

WARNING
Get medical attention immediately if you notice swelling of your face, tongue, or vocal cords or have difficulty swallowing or breathing; this reaction can be life threatening.

This drug should not be taken during pregnancy; it has been associated with death of the fetus and newborn.

SPECIAL INFORMATION
- Zestril increases blood potassium levels. Do not use potassium-rich products without first consulting your doctor. The potassium in your blood could rise to dangerous levels, leading to heart-rhythm problems.
- Do not abruptly stop taking this drug. Your doctor must reduce the dosage gradually.

TARGET AILMENTS

High blood pressure

Congestive heart failure (in conjunction with digitalis preparations and diuretics)

Heart attacks (used within 24 hours to improve survival)

SIDE EFFECTS

NOT SERIOUS
- Dry, persistent cough
- Headache; fatigue
- Nausea; mild diarrhea
- Loss of sense of taste
- Temporary skin rash

CALL YOUR DOCTOR IF THESE EFFECTS BECOME BOTHERSOME.

SERIOUS
- Fainting or dizziness
- Persistent skin rash
- Fever or chills; joint pain
- Numbness and tingling
- Abdominal pain, vomiting
- Chest pain or palpitations

CALL YOUR DOCTOR IMMEDIATELY.

ZHENG GU SHUI

VITAL STATISTICS

ENGLISH NAME
Bone-Correcting Water

GENERAL DESCRIPTION
Zheng Gu Shui is a liniment that is used for traumatic injury, including sprains and broken bones. It increases the circulation, which helps with bruising, pain, and swelling. It promotes the healing of bones, tendons, and ligaments. The broken bone must be set in order for this formula to be helpful.

Chinese medicine takes a holistic approach to healthcare, fashioning remedies to treat the entire being as well as the specific parts or areas. Precise combinations of herbs are used to prevent and combat disease, which is thought to arise from disturbances in the flow of a bodily energy called chi (pronounced "chee") and blood, or from a lack of balance in the complementary states of yin and yang. A patent formula, *Zheng Gu Shui* is made by using a standardized combination of herbs and method of preparation.

INGREDIENTS
pseudoginseng, angelica root, menthol crystal, camphor, camphor crystal, croton seeds, moghania, inula flower, alcohol

PREPARATIONS
Zheng Gu Shui is available as a bottled liquid in many Chinese pharmacies, Oriental grocery stores, and martial arts stores.

PRECAUTIONS

WARNING
Do not use internally.

SPECIAL INFORMATION
- Wash hands after using this liniment and be careful not to get it in the eyes.
- Do not use on open wounds.
- This formula is flammable, so keep it away from flames.

TARGET AILMENTS

Sprains and injury to ligaments and tendons

Bone fractures that have been set

Bruises

SIDE EFFECTS

NOT SERIOUS
- Allergic skin reaction (rash)

DISCONTINUE IF YOU EXPERIENCE THIS SYMPTOM.

Z

Zhi Bai Di Huang Wan

Vital Statistics

ENGLISH NAME
Anemarrhena Phellodenron Rehmannia Pills

ALSO SOLD AS
Zhi Bai Ba Wei Wan, Chih Pai Di Huang Wan, Chih Pai Pa Wei Wan

GENERAL DESCRIPTION
Zhi Bai Di Huang Wan is a formula used to treat ailments characterized in traditional Chinese medicine as "hot." It can be used for generalized "heat-related" symptoms such as night sweats, afternoon fevers, and menopausal hot flashes. It is also frequently used for "heat in the lower torso," a condition whose characteristic symptoms may include genital herpes, dark-colored urine, or frequent, painful urination. It is also used for certain kinds of chronic sore throat that a qualified practitioner of Chinese medicine would diagnose after a thorough examination of the tongue.

Chinese medicine takes a holistic approach to healthcare, fashioning remedies to treat the entire being as well as the specific parts or areas. Precise combinations of herbs are used to prevent and combat disease, which is thought to arise from disturbances in the flow of a bodily energy called chi (pronounced "chee") and blood, or from a lack of balance in the complementary states of yin and yang. A patent formula, *Zhi Bai Di Huang Wan* is made by using a standardized combination of herbs and method of preparation.

INGREDIENTS
rehmannia, Asian dogwood berries, dioscorea yam, alisma, tree peony root, poria, phellodendron, anemarrhena

PREPARATIONS
This formula is available in pill form in many Chinese pharmacies and Oriental grocery stores.

TARGET AILMENTS
Low-grade fevers and night sweats
Menopausal hot flashes
Urinary tract infection or irritation with frequent urination, pain, and burning
Genital herpes

SIDE EFFECTS
NONE EXPECTED

Z

ZHI WAN

VITAL STATISTICS

ENGLISH NAME
Hemorrhoid Pills

GENERAL DESCRIPTION
Zhi Wan is a hemorrhoid remedy that reduces swelling, inflammation, itching, and bleeding, and helps resolve infection and soften the hard lumps. This formula works at healing all the main symptoms of painful hemorrhoids.

Chinese medicine takes a holistic approach to healthcare, fashioning remedies to treat the entire being as well as the specific parts or areas. Precise combinations of herbs are used to prevent and combat disease, which is thought to arise from disturbances in the flow of a bodily energy called chi (pronounced "chee") and blood, or from a lack of balance in the complementary states of yin and yang. A patent formula, *Zhi Wan* is made by using a standardized combination of herbs and method of preparation.

INGREDIENTS
honeysuckle, safflower, hedgehog skin, pangolin scales, sophora, areca seeds, frankincense resin, myrrh, angelica root, unspecified substances

PREPARATIONS
This formula is available in pill form in many Chinese pharmacies and Oriental grocery stores.

TARGET AILMENTS

Hemorrhoids

SIDE EFFECTS

None expected

ZINC

VITAL STATISTICS

GENERAL DESCRIPTION

The mineral zinc is integral to the synthesis of RNA and DNA, the genetic material that controls cell growth, division, and function. In various proteins, enzymes, hormones, and hormonelike substances called prostaglandins, zinc contributes to many bodily processes, including bone development and growth; cell respiration; energy metabolism; wound healing; the liver's ability to remove toxic substances such as alcohol from the body; immune function; and the regulation of heart rate and blood pressure. An adequate zinc intake enhances the ability to taste, promotes healthy skin and hair, enhances reproductive functions, and may improve short-term memory and attention span. As an anti-inflammatory agent, zinc is sometimes used to treat acne, rheumatoid arthritis, and prostatitis. Taking supplemental zinc may boost resistance to infection, especially in the elderly, and stimulate wound healing.

Many American diets are slightly low in zinc. Young children, pregnant women, vegetarians, and elderly people are most susceptible to zinc deficiency. Loss of taste is usually the first warning; other symptoms are hair loss or discoloration, white streaks on the nails, dermatitis, loss of appetite, fatigue, and poor wound healing.

Zinc ointment, which contains zinc oxide, is the most common topical form, useful in skin disorders, burns, and other wounds.

RDA

Adults: 15 mg
Pregnant women: 30 mg

NATURAL SOURCES

Zinc is most easily obtained from lean meat and seafood, but it is also found in eggs, soybeans, peanuts, wheat bran, cheese, oysters, and other foods.

PRECAUTIONS

WARNING

Experts recommend increasing zinc levels by increasing the zinc-rich foods in your diet or by taking a multinutrient supplement that includes zinc chelate, zinc picolinate, or zinc aspartate, the three most easily absorbed forms. If zinc is used for more than three to six months to treat a chronic condition, it is essential to consult a nutritionist to avoid creating a mineral imbalance.

SPECIAL INFORMATION

- Zinc deficiency can retard growth in all children and stunt sexual development in boys.
- Ingesting extreme amounts of zinc daily can impair immune function and cause nausea, headaches, vomiting, dehydration, stomachaches, poor muscle coordination, fatigue, and possibly kidney failure.

TARGET AILMENTS
Immune problems
Skin problems
Wounds

SIDE EFFECTS
NONE EXPECTED

Zinc Oxide

Vital Statistics

BRAND NAME
Desitin

GENERAL DESCRIPTION
Zinc oxide is classified as a skin protectant. Skin protectants, in the form of dusting powders, lotions, ointments, and creams, have been used for centuries for temporary coverage, protection, and relief of burned, chafed, chapped, scraped, or otherwise irritated skin.

Zinc oxide is used to cover the skin to protect it from dryness and other harmful environmental stimuli. It is the sole or principal ingredient in a wide variety of over-the-counter preparations, particularly calamine, which is 98 percent zinc oxide.

Because of its cooling, slightly astringent, antiseptic, antibacterial, and protective actions, zinc oxide is considered particularly safe and effective in treating diaper rash and prickly heat in babies and in older persons who become incontinent. It protects chafed skin and seals out wetness.

In addition, preparations containing zinc oxide relieve the itching, discomfort, irritation, and burning of uncomplicated hemorrhoids and noncancerous anorectal disorders. They coat and protect the anorectal surface against chemically irritating bowel movements. They also prevent loss of moisture from anorectal surfaces, a major cause of irritation. Zinc oxide may be safely applied as a lotion, paste, or powder up to six times a day, or after bowel movements.

Used alone or in calamine, zinc oxide can also be applied externally or intrarectally as an astringent. In this capacity, it gathers irritating proteins from the skin or mucosal surface and covers them with a protective film.

Zinc oxide and calamine are applied externally to relieve the itching, pain, and discomfort of poison ivy, oak, and sumac.

Finally, this versatile drug can be used to relieve the discomfort of sunburn. When combined with titanium dioxide, zinc oxide is used as a topical sunscreen agent.

Precautions

SPECIAL INFORMATION
If the symptoms of hemorrhoids or anorectal disorders do not clear up completely within a week, consult a doctor. Rectal bleeding, mucous discharge, seepage of fecal matter, and protrusion of a hemorrhoid or of rectal tissue outside the anal canal are all potentially serious medical problems.

POSSIBLE INTERACTIONS
None expected.

TARGET AILMENTS
Diaper rash
Hemorrhoids (uncomplicated) or noncancerous anorectal disorders
Poison ivy, oak, and sumac
Sunburn (prevention and treatment)

SIDE EFFECTS
None expected

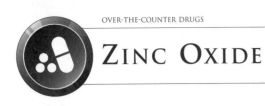

ZITHROMAX

VITAL STATISTICS

DRUG CLASS
Antibiotics [Erythromycins]

GENERIC NAME
azithromycin

GENERAL DESCRIPTION
Zithromax is a brand name for the antibiotic drug azithromycin, a derivative of erythromycin first introduced in 1991. Zithromax kills some bacteria outright and stops the growth and reproduction of others. For visual characteristics, see the Color Guide to Prescription Drugs and Herbs.

PRECAUTIONS

SPECIAL INFORMATION
- Tell your doctor if you are allergic to erythromycin, clarithromycin, or troleandomycin; you might also be allergic to Zithromax.
- Let your doctor know if you have impaired kidneys, an impaired liver, or a history of drug-induced colitis.
- Don't use Zithromax during pregnancy unless your doctor prescribes it. Avoid this drug if you are nursing.

POSSIBLE INTERACTIONS
Antacids containing aluminum, calcium, or magnesium: decreased Zithromax effect. Take Zithromax one hour before or two hours after taking antacids.
Anticoagulants: increased anticoagulant effect, risk of bleeding.
Astemizole, terfenadine: WARNING: There is a risk of life-threatening heart problems. Do not take astemizole or terfenadine if you are also taking Zithromax.
Carbamazepine, cyclosporine, digoxin, ergotamine, phenytoin, theophylline, triazolam: increased effects of these drugs, possible toxicity.

TARGET AILMENTS

Respiratory tract infections (including pharyngitis and sinusitis caused by strep); bronchitis; some types of pneumonia

Skin and soft-tissue infections

Chlamydial infections

SIDE EFFECTS

NOT SERIOUS
- Yeast infections
- Abdominal pain; mild diarrhea; nausea
- Dizziness; headache; fatigue

CONSULT YOUR DOCTOR IF THESE EFFECTS PERSIST.

SERIOUS
- Inflammation of the colon (diarrhea, cramps, vomiting, and fever)
- Kidney inflammation (fever, joint pain, rash)
- Anaphylactic reaction (severe itching, rash, or difficulty breathing)
- Swelling of the face, mouth, neck, hands, and feet

DISCONTINUE USE AND CONTACT YOUR DOCTOR IMMEDIATELY.

ZOCOR

VITAL STATISTICS

DRUG CLASS
Cholesterol-Reducing Drugs

GENERIC NAME
simvastatin

OTHER DRUGS IN THIS CLASS
cholestyramine, colestipol, fluvastatin, gemfibrozil, lovastatin, niacin, pravastatin

GENERAL DESCRIPTION
The brand-name drug Zocor was introduced in 1986. Zocor's generic ingredient, simvastatin, belongs to a subclass of cholesterol-reducing drugs known as HMG-CoA reductase inhibitors. These drugs alter the blood levels of cholesterol and other fats. They work by blocking a liver enzyme needed in the production of cholesterol. Simvastatin may also increase the blood level of high-density lipoproteins (HDLs), the so-called good cholesterol that seems to protect against heart disease. For more information, see Cholesterol-Reducing Drugs.

For visual characteristics, see the Color Guide to Prescription Drugs and Herbs.

PRECAUTIONS

SPECIAL INFORMATION
- If you become pregnant while taking Zocor, stop using it immediately and inform your doctor.
- Do not use this drug if you have had an allergic reaction to it in the past.
- Do not stop taking Zocor without first checking with your doctor; your blood cholesterol levels may increase again.
- Before undergoing emergency treatment or medical or dental surgery, be sure to tell your healthcare practitioner if you are taking this drug.

POSSIBLE INTERACTIONS
Erythromycin, immunosuppressants such as cyclosporine, niacin: increased risk of severe muscle disorder or kidney failure.
Digoxin: increased blood levels of digoxin.
Gemfibrozil: may affect the absorption and excretion of simvastatin; do not take concurrently.

TARGET AILMENTS

The major types of cholesterol disorders

SIDE EFFECTS

NOT SERIOUS
- Constipation
- Gas

CALL YOUR DOCTOR IF THESE EFFECTS PERSIST.

SERIOUS
- Fever
- Muscle aches
- Cramps

TELL YOUR DOCTOR IF YOU EXPERIENCE ANY OF THESE EFFECTS.

Zoloft

Vital Statistics

DRUG CLASS
Antidepressants [Selective Serotonin Reuptake Inhibitors (SSRIs)]

GENERIC NAME
sertraline

OTHER DRUGS IN THIS SUBCLASS
fluoxetine, paroxetine, venlafaxine

GENERAL DESCRIPTION
The brand-name drug Zoloft was introduced in 1986. Zoloft belongs to a subclass of antidepressants known as selective serotonin reuptake inhibitors (SSRIs) and works by altering levels of serotonin, an important brain chemical. This medication is prescribed for treatment of depression and obsessive-compulsive disorder. See Antidepressants for side effects and additional precautions.

TARGET AILMENTS

Major depressive disorders

Obsessive-compulsive disorder

SIDE EFFECTS

SEE ANTIDEPRESSANTS.

Precautions

SPECIAL INFORMATION

- The severity of any side effects may decrease with time (after two weeks) or with lowered dosages. If you have any questions about potential side effects, discuss them with your doctor.
- If you are pregnant, nursing, or planning a pregnancy, check with your doctor before taking sertraline.

POSSIBLE INTERACTIONS

Alcohol and other drugs that depress the central nervous system: increased effects of Zoloft, leading to problems such as respiratory depression or very low blood pressure.

Anticonvulsants: decreased effectiveness of anticonvulsants, making seizures more likely.

Antihistamines: increased antihistamine action, including any side effects; antihistamines may also increase the action of sertraline, including any side effects.

Digitalis preparations: using Zoloft with heart medications may increase blood levels of both the antidepressant and the heart drugs, increasing the risk of side effects.

Lithium: taking Zoloft with lithium could increase blood levels of lithium, leading to toxicity.

Monoamine oxidase (MAO) inhibitors: WARNING: severe, possibly fatal, reactions such as seizures, tremor, and coma because of additive effects of the drugs.

Other antidepressants: combining antidepressants will likely increase the action of one or both drugs, leading to increased side effects.

Rx ZOLPIDEM

VITAL STATISTICS

DRUG CLASS
Anti-Insomnia Drugs

BRAND NAME
Ambien

OTHER DRUGS IN THIS CLASS
antihistamines: diphenhydramine, doxylamine
benzodiazepines: lorazepam, temazepam, triazolam

GENERAL DESCRIPTION
Zolpidem, introduced in 1993, is the most commonly prescribed drug for the short-term (seven to 10 days) management of sleeping problems in adults. Its major advantages include a low incidence of adverse effects, rapid absorption and elimination, and minimal interference with normal sleep patterns, which includes the rapid eye movement (REM) stage.

A nonbenzodiazepine medication, zolpidem works by binding to a specific receptor in the brain to simulate normal sleep processes. Most users report few side effects, and little or no hangover effects, memory loss, or "rebound" insomnia when not using the drug.

The anti-insomnia drug class (sometimes called the sedative-hypnotic class) includes a large number of drugs used in the treatment of sleeping problems. Since insomnia is often related to psychological or physical disorders, the choice of medication will depend on the underlying condition. Certain benzodiazepines, a subclass of antianxiety drugs, are often prescribed for people in acute distress. Milder alternatives include the antihistamine drugs diphenhydramine and doxylamine, which are prescribed for short-term treatment of insomnia. Antipsychotic and antidepressant drugs with sedative effects are also used if warranted. For visual characteristics of the brand-name drug Ambien, see the Color Guide to Prescription Drugs and Herbs.

PRECAUTIONS

SPECIAL INFORMATION
- Do not take zolpidem if you have had an allergic reaction to this drug in the past.
- Before taking zolpidem, tell your doctor if any of the following conditions apply: You are pregnant, plan to become pregnant, or are nursing; you have a kidney or liver disease; you have sleep apnea; you have asthma, bronchitis, emphysema, or other chronic lung disease; you have a history of mental depression or disorder; you have a history of alcoholism or drug dependence.
- Zolpidem is most rapidly absorbed when taken on an empty stomach (at least two hours after eating).

Zolpidem

- Because zolpidem works so fast, it should be taken just before bedtime.
- Take zolpidem only if you have time to get a full night's sleep (seven or eight hours). Otherwise, the drug will not have time to wear off, and you may experience hangover effects, including drowsiness and memory problems.
- Older adults may be more sensitive to the drug's effects and side effects and may require a smaller dosage.
- Some people experience carryover effects from zolpidem the next day. If you haven't taken this drug before, wait to see how it affects you before driving, operating machinery, or doing anything that requires unimpaired coordination and clear vision.
- Long-term use of zolpidem may result in dependence. Withdrawal symptoms may occur when you stop taking the drug.

POSSIBLE INTERACTIONS

Alcohol and other central nervous system depressants (anesthetics, antidepressants, antihistamines, barbiturates, benzodiazepines, monoamine oxidase [MAO] inhibitors, muscle relaxants, narcotics or prescription pain medicines, tranquilizers): increased anti-insomniac and depressant effect.

Caffeine and nicotine: these are stimulants that can interfere with zolpidem's anti-insomniac effects.

TARGET AILMENTS

Insomnia (short-term)

SIDE EFFECTS

NOT SERIOUS

- Daytime drowsiness
- Dizziness or blurred vision
- Dry mouth
- Memory problems
- Abdominal or gastric pain
- Diarrhea
- Nausea
- Headache
- Unusual dreams
- Malaise

SEE YOUR DOCTOR IF THESE SYMPTOMS PERSIST OR BECOME BOTHERSOME.

SERIOUS

- Clumsiness
- Confusion
- Unsteadiness and falling
- Mental depression
- Skin rash
- Agitation or irritability
- Wheezing or difficulty in breathing
- Hallucinations
- Increased insomnia

CONTACT YOUR DOCTOR AS SOON AS POSSIBLE.

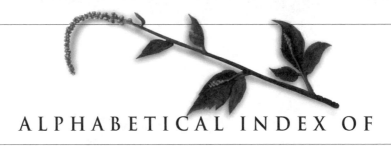

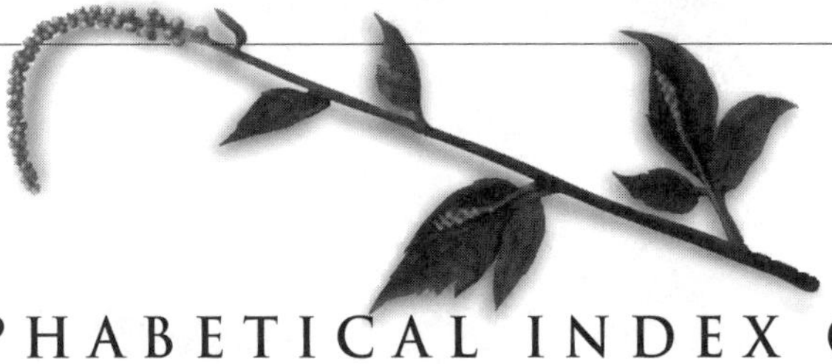

ALPHABETICAL INDEX OF NATURAL REMEDIES

All of the healing substances for each of the six natural therapies included in this book are listed here in alphabetical order, along with their target ailments. Use the page numbers to look up the entries for each remedy.

Aromatherapy

BASIL · 118
TARGET AILMENTS: Menopausal symptoms, anxiety, stress, fatigue, colds and flu, hay fever, insect bites, muscular aches and pains, rheumatism, menstrual cramps, bronchitis, sinusitis

BAY LAUREL · 120
TARGET AILMENTS: Digestive problems, loss of appetite, bronchitis, colds and flu, tonsillitis, scabies, lice, rheumatic aches, muscle and joint pain, arthritis, swollen lymph nodes

BERGAMOT · 131
TARGET AILMENTS: Mouth infections, sore throat, tonsillitis, flatulence, loss of appetite, colds and flu, cystitis, fever, depression, anxiety, stress

CAMPHOR · 177
TARGET AILMENTS: Acne and oily skin, arthritis, muscle and joint pains, rheumatism, sprains, bronchitis, colds and flu, fever

CHAMOMILE · 195
TARGET AILMENTS: Indigestion, menstrual problems, menopausal symptoms, skin inflammation, burns, sunburn, acne, boils, eczema, headache, anxiety, stress

CLARY SAGE · 231
TARGET AILMENTS: Anxiety, stress, depression, menstrual problems, menopausal symptoms, digestive cramps, burns, eczema and other skin problems, asthma, sore throat, excessive sweating

CYPRESS · 266
TARGET AILMENTS: Insomnia, varicose veins, cough, bronchitis, asthma, menstrual pain, menopausal symptoms, rheumatism, arthritis, diarrhea, excessive sweating

EUCALYPTUS · 322
TARGET AILMENTS: Fevers, colds and flu, sinus problems, coughing, bronchitis, boils, acne, cuts and sores, joint and muscle pain

EVERLASTING · 327
TARGET AILMENTS: Scarring, stretch marks, sunburn, acne, dermatitis, bruises, wrinkles, liver or spleen congestion, bronchitis, colds and flu, tendinitis, arthritis pain, muscle aches, sprains and strains

FRANKINCENSE · 354
TARGET AILMENTS: Asthma, bronchitis, coughing, anxiety, stress, colds and flu, cystitis, menstrual problems, gout, dermatitis, dry skin, stretch marks, scars, wrinkles

GERANIUM · 368
TARGET AILMENTS: Small wounds and burns, anxiety, stress, menopausal and menstrual symptoms, athlete's foot, eczema, shingles, sore throat, mouth ulcers, insect stings and bites, headaches, hemorrhoids

JASMINE ABSOLUTE · 429
TARGET AILMENTS: Migraine headache, depression, anxiety, stress, coughing, laryngitis, menstrual problems, irritated or dry skin, muscle spasms, sprains, low sex drive

LAVENDER · 453
TARGET AILMENTS: Headache, depression, stress, insomnia, muscular and joint pain, menstrual pain, digestive problems, nausea, colds and flu, athlete's foot, cuts and wounds, burns, sunburn, insect bites, acne, eczema, dermatitis

LEMON · 460
TARGET AILMENTS: Anxiety, depression, headache, insomnia, throat infections, high blood pressure, varicose veins, broken capillaries, palpitations, dandruff, eczema, psoriasis, premenstrual syndrome, irregular periods

LEMON-SCENTED EUCALYPTUS · 463
TARGET AILMENTS: Mosquito bites, skin irritations, athlete's foot, herpes sores, muscle tension, stress, asthma, laryngitis, colds and flu, sore throat

MYRRH · 529
TARGET AILMENTS: Eczema and other skin conditions, stretch marks, ringworm, athlete's foot, wounds, arthritis, bronchitis, mouth ulcers and gum problems, sore throat, colds and cough, diarrhea, yeast infections

NEROLI · 537
TARGET AILMENTS: Anxiety and stress, depression, insomnia, poor circulation, menstrual problems, broken capillaries, scars, stretch marks, wrinkles

NIAOULI · 541
TARGET AILMENTS: Allergies, bronchitis, colds and flu, minor wounds and burns, acne, boils, insect bites, muscle aches and pains, toothache, bladder infection

PALMAROSA · 576
TARGET AILMENTS: Flu, intestinal infections, digestive problems, anxiety, stress, anorexia, minor cuts and wounds, acne, dermatitis, oily or dry skin, cold sores, scars

PATCHOULI · 581
TARGET AILMENTS: Acne, athlete's foot, impetigo, cracked or chapped skin, cellulite, mature skin, dandruff, anxiety, stress, sexual problems, allergies, hemorrhoids

PEPPERMINT · 593
TARGET AILMENTS: Indigestion, nausea, headaches, neuralgia, muscle and joint pain, menstrual pain, bronchitis, sinus problems, colds and flu, motion sickness, shock, sore feet, mental fatigue

PINE · 613
TARGET AILMENTS: Anxiety, depression, nervous tension, skin disorders, arthritis, rheumatism, cystitis and other urinary problems, bronchitis, sinus problems, cough, flu, pneumonia

ROSE · 663
TARGET AILMENTS: Insomnia, anxiety, depression, nervous tension, low sex drive, loss of appetite, nausea, menstrual pain, cough, hay fever, sore throat, mouth ulcers, skin problems, eye and eyelid complaints

ROSEMARY · 665
TARGET AILMENTS: Indigestion, gas, constipation, liver problems, fluid retention, asthma, bronchitis, colds, flu, depression, rheumatism, arthritis, mental fatigue, poor memory, headache, hair loss, dandruff, low blood pressure, varicose veins, irregular menstrual periods, menstrual pain

TARRAGON · 729
TARGET AILMENTS: Menstrual and menopausal symptoms, digestive ailments, hiccups, loss of appetite, indigestion and gas, shock, anxiety, stress

TEA TREE · 730
TARGET AILMENTS: Colds and flu, tonsillitis, bronchitis, sinusitis, abscesses, acne, burns, cuts, wounds, vaginitis, bladder infections, yeast infections, cold sores, insect bites

THYME · 742
TARGET AILMENTS: Laryngitis, cough, skin problems, bladder infections, joint pain, rheumatic aches and pains, diarrhea, gas, asthma, depression, fatigue, colds and flu, backache, sciatica

YLANG-YLANG · 820
TARGET AILMENTS: Acne and oily skin, depression, insomnia, impotence, low sex drive, anxiety, stress, hair loss, high blood pressure, malaria, typhus, fevers, fluid retention

CONTINUED

Chinese Medicine

AGASTACHE • 26
TARGET AILMENTS: Nausea and vomiting, diarrhea and dysentery, morning sickness, swelling of the abdomen, reduced appetite, colds without fever

ANEMARRHENA • 56
TARGET AILMENTS: High fever and thirst accompanied by a rapid pulse; coughing that brings up thick, yellow phlegm; abnormally high sex drive and nocturnal emission; night sweats; low-grade fever; afternoon fever; certain types of dizziness and vertigo; ulcers in the mouth; bleeding gums

ANGELICA ROOT (PUBESCENS) • 58
TARGET AILMENTS: Acute and chronic pain in the lower back and legs that is sensitive to cold and damp weather, mild headache and toothache that respond to changes in the weather

APRICOT SEED • 98
TARGET AILMENTS: Coughing and wheezing, bronchitis or emphysema, asthma, constipation

ASTRAGALUS • 106
TARGET AILMENTS: Diarrhea, fatigue, lack of appetite, vomiting, chronic gastroenteritis, spontaneous sweating, abdominal pain and bleeding during pregnancy, edema (the accumulation of fluid in the body), reduced urination

ATRACTYLODES (WHITE) • 109
TARGET AILMENTS: General weakness and fatigue, loss of appetite, spontaneous perspiration, diarrhea, blood abnormalities or deficiencies that according to traditional Chinese medicine result from excessive bleeding

AUCKLANDIA • 111
TARGET AILMENTS: Diarrhea, lack of appetite, abdominal pain or distention, nausea, vomiting

BA ZHEN WAN • 121
TARGET AILMENTS: Fatigue with pale complexion, weakness following blood loss, dizziness or lightheadedness, postpartum fatigue, lack of menstruation, irregular menstruation

BEZOAR ANTIDOTAL TABLETS • 135
TARGET AILMENTS: Sore throat, tongue or mouth ulcers, toothache, tonsillitis or pharyngitis with fever, earache with fever, conjunctivitis, sores, carbuncles, boils

BIOTA • 139
TARGET AILMENTS: Bleeding disorders such as vomiting or coughing up blood, coughing that fails to bring up phlegm, bleeding gums, blood in the stool or urine, uterine bleeding, burns

BI YAN PIAN • 144
TARGET AILMENTS: Chronic or acute rhinitis, nasal sinusitis, hay fever and other allergies, pain in the forehead or cheekbones with congestion

BUPLEURUM • 160
TARGET AILMENTS: Low-grade fevers; malaria and malaria-like disorders; alternating chills and fever, typically accompanied by a bitter taste in the mouth, pain in the side, irritability, vomiting, or difficulty in breathing; prolapse of the uterus; dizziness and vertigo combined with pain in the chest and tenderness in the side or breast, often accompanied by irritability; nausea; indigestion

BU ZHONG YI QI WAN • 164
TARGET AILMENTS: Fatigue; chronic fatigue; chronic bronchitis or shortness of breath; prolapses of uterus, rectum, or stomach; urinary incontinence; some kinds of chronic diarrhea; some instances of excessive menstrual periods or spotting between periods

CHIEN CHIN CHIH TAI WAN • 202
TARGET AILMENTS: White vaginal discharge, painful menstrual periods, irregular menstrual periods, amenorrhea (lack of menstruation)

CHINESE FOXGLOVE ROOT • 204
TARGET AILMENTS: Lightheadedness; palpitations; low back pain and weak knees; weak, stiff joints; premature graying of hair; blurred vision or "floaters" in vision; hearing loss or tinnitus (ringing in the ears); insomnia or the inability to be still and restful; chronic low-grade fever; night sweats; hot flashes; constipation with dry, hard stools; irregular menstruation or uterine bleeding, especially after childbirth

CHINESE MOTHERWORT · 205
TARGET AILMENTS: Irregular menstruation or light menstrual flow; premenstrual abdominal pain; uterine fibroids; postpartum abdominal pain; infertility; difficulty in urinating; edema (swelling), particularly if accompanied by blood in the urine

CHINESE YAM · 206
TARGET AILMENTS: Weak digestion with diarrhea and fatigue, reduced appetite, frequent urination, excessive vaginal discharge, chronic coughing and wheezing, symptoms that accompany diabetes (such as weight loss, excessive urination)

CHING WAN HUNG · 207
TARGET AILMENTS: Burns from steam, hot water, flame, hot oil, chemicals, radiation therapy, and sunburn; hemorrhoids

CHIN SO KU CHING · 208
TARGET AILMENTS: Urinary incontinence, nocturnal emission, impotence, tinnitus (ringing in the ears), weakness of the lower back

CHRYSANTHEMUM FLOWER · 217
TARGET AILMENTS: Headaches, dizziness, hearing problems, hypertension (high blood pressure), conjunctivitis, red or dry eyes, blurred vision, spots in front of the eyes

CHUAN QIONG CHA TIAO WAN · 218
TARGET AILMENTS: Headache with weather changes, headache with sinusitis, headache with chills, fever and stuffy nose

CICADA · 219
TARGET AILMENTS: Swollen, sore throat with loss of voice; skin rash, particularly during the early stage of measles or chickenpox; red, painful, swollen eyes and blurred vision; high fever in childhood illnesses such as measles, which can cause convulsions, spasms, delirium, and terrifying nightmares in children

CIMICIFUGA · 222
TARGET AILMENTS: Skin rashes, including those of measles; headache accompanying measles; sore teeth and gums; canker sores; sore throats; prolapse of the uterus, rectum, or bladder

CINNAMON BARK · 223
TARGET AILMENTS: Poor digestion, diarrhea with undigested food, lack of appetite, abdominal spasms, excessive urination, impotence, lack of sexual desire, menstrual pain, lack of menstruation, infertility, wheezing from asthma caused by exposure to cold

CINNAMON TWIG · 224
TARGET AILMENTS: Colds, influenza, and low-grade fever accompanied by chills; arthritis; rheumatism; gynecological problems, such as painful menstruation or uterine fibroids

CLEAN AIR PILLS · 232
TARGET AILMENTS: Cough with thick sputum, pneumonia, bronchitis, thick sinus congestion, heavy fullness in the chest

CNIDIUM SEEDS · 239
TARGET AILMENTS: Impotence; female infertility; itchy skin; eczema; scabies, ringworm, or itchy, weeping skin lesions, especially in the genital area; vaginal discharge

CODONOPSIS ROOT · 243
TARGET AILMENTS: Diabetes; chronic cough and shortness of breath; prolapsed uterus, stomach, or rectum; lack of appetite, fatigue, and tired limbs; diarrhea and vomiting; excessive thirst

COIX · 246
TARGET AILMENTS: Urinary difficulty marked by edema (retention of body fluids), carbuncles, lung or intestinal abscesses, diarrhea, coated tongue (symptomatic of digestive problems), arthritic pains from weather changes, fever accompanied by inadequate urination, plantar warts

COPTIS · 254
TARGET AILMENTS: High fever with irritability, disorientation, or delirium; dysentery with hot, burning diarrhea; nosebleeds or bright red blood in the urine, stool, or vomit; bad breath or belching with bad odor; toothache; swollen gums; ulcers of the tongue and mouth; red, painful eyes

CORNUS · 255
TARGET AILMENTS: Excessive urination, incontinence, impotence, and other symptoms related to kidney and bladder problems; excessive sweating; lightheaded-

ness with weakness of the back and knees; excessive menstrual bleeding or prolonged menstruation

CORYDALIS • 258
TARGET AILMENTS: Abdominal pain, chest pain, pain resulting from traumatic injuries, menstrual pain, rheumatism pain, arthritis pain

CUSCUTA • 263
TARGET AILMENTS: Impotence, nocturnal emission, premature ejaculation, prostate problems, frequent urination, incontinence, diarrhea with lack of appetite, habitual or threatened miscarriage, backache from muscular weakness, dizziness, tinnitus (ringing in the ears), blurred vision

CYPERUS • 265
TARGET AILMENTS: Irregular menstruation, menstrual cramps, digestive problems such as gas and bloating, depression, moodiness, instability

DANDELION • 269
TARGET AILMENTS: Hepatitis; jaundice and other liver conditions; poor lactation in nursing mothers; painful and difficult urination; red, painful, swollen eyes; abscesses; boils, carbuncles, and sores, particularly on the breast

DONG QUAI • 294
TARGET AILMENTS: Menstrual irregularity, lack of menstruation, painful or insubstantial menstruation, stabbing pain, pain caused by traumatic injury, poor blood circulation, pale complexion, possible anemia, carbuncles that according to traditional Chinese medicine arise from stagnant blood, abscesses, sores, lightheadedness, blurred vision, heart palpitations

DU HUO JI SHENG WAN • 301
TARGET AILMENTS: Arthritis (rheumatoid arthritis and osteoarthritis); chronic low back pain; chronic lower body pain, stiffness, or numbness; joint pain that comes with cold, damp weather

EPHEDRA • 309
TARGET AILMENTS: Fever and chills, coughing, wheezing, nasal and chest congestion, indigestion or stomachache

ER CHEN WAN • 313
TARGET AILMENTS: Upper respiratory tract infection, chronic bronchitis, Ménière's disease, chronic gastritis or ulcer, goiter or lymph node swellings, fatty tumors

EUCOMMIA BARK • 324
TARGET AILMENTS: Weak muscles and bones, especially in the back and knees, accompanied by poor circulation; low back pain and soreness, accompanied by frequent urination; mild abdominal pain or slight vaginal bleeding during pregnancy; prevention of miscarriage and stabilization of pregnancy; back pain in pregnant women; dizziness and lightheadedness caused by high blood pressure

EVODIA FRUIT • 328
TARGET AILMENTS: Diarrhea with undigested food, especially morning diarrhea; headaches with vomiting; nausea accompanied by lack of appreciation for the taste of food; pain in the upper abdomen; hernia; indigestion; high blood pressure; sores of the mouth or tongue

FIELD MINT • 340
TARGET AILMENTS: Rashes in the early stages, sore throat, red eyes, headache, emotional instability, gynecological problems, childhood convulsions

FRITILLARIA AND LOQUAT SYRUP • 355
TARGET AILMENTS: Dry cough, cough associated with asthma, smoker's cough

GAN MAO LING • 358
TARGET AILMENTS: Colds or flu; flu with body aches; swollen glands in throat (with flulike symptoms); high fever, with or without chills

GANODERMA • 359
TARGET AILMENTS: Nervousness, insomnia, dizziness, asthma, allergy-related chronic bronchitis, weakened immune system, tumors, ulcers, poor blood circulation, mushroom poisoning

GARDENIA • 360
TARGET AILMENTS: Irritability; restlessness; insomnia; delirious speech; painful urination; sores of the nose, eyes, or mouth; jaundice (damp heat conditions); nosebleeds, vomiting blood, blood in the urine or stool ("hot bleeding")

GARLIC • 361
TARGET AILMENTS: Digestive disorders, diarrhea, food poisoning from shellfish, conditions that require an enema, colds, coughs, rheumatoid arthritis, hookworm, roundworm, ringworm of the scalp, carbuncles, swelling, pinworm, athlete's foot

GASTRODIA • 363
TARGET AILMENTS: Headaches, including migraines; dizziness; childhood convulsions; epilepsy

GENTIANA • 367
TARGET AILMENTS: Hepatitis, jaundice and other liver disorders, sexually transmitted diseases, vaginal discharge, inflammation of the pelvis, pain or swelling in the genital area, convulsions

GINGER • 369
TARGET AILMENTS: Vomiting, abdominal pain, menstrual irregularity, coughs, first- and second-degree burns

GINSENG, ASIAN • 373
TARGET AILMENTS: Symptoms of shock, profuse sweating, ice-cold extremities, shortness of breath, fever, thirst, irritability, diarrhea, vomiting, distention of the abdomen

GRAINS-OF-PARADISE FRUIT • 384
TARGET AILMENTS: Nausea and vomiting; abdominal pain, diarrhea, indigestion, gas, or loss of appetite; morning sickness; pain and discomfort during pregnancy; urinary incontinence

HONEYSUCKLE FLOWER • 393
TARGET AILMENTS: Sores and inflammation, particularly of the breast, throat, and eyes; heat rash; boils; fevers; colds; flu; salmonella and other microbial infections; intestinal abscesses; painful urination and dysentery

HSIAO KEH CHUAN • 397
TARGET AILMENTS: Cough with copious phlegm, asthma, bronchitis

HUANG LIEN SHANG CHING PIEN • 398
TARGET AILMENTS: Fever, ear infections, mouth ulcers, sore gums or throat, conjunctivitis (pinkeye), toothache, tonsillitis or swollen glands in the neck, sores or boils, acute bronchitis, early stages of pneumonia, constipation

HUO HSIANG CHENG CHI PIAN • 401
TARGET AILMENTS: Acute diarrhea; acute gastroenteritis, or intestinal flu; morning sickness; motion sickness with nausea; cholera

KAI KIT PILLS • 431
TARGET AILMENTS: Painful and difficult urination due to chronically enlarged prostate gland

KING TO'S NATURAL HERB LOQUAT FLAVORED SYRUP • 443
TARGET AILMENTS: Cough, sinus congestion, acute bronchitis, emphysema

LICORICE • 468
TARGET AILMENTS: Cough, colds, and sore throat; asthma and wheezing; poor digestion; ulcers; abdominal pains and spasms; carbuncles and sores

LIGUSTICUM • 470
TARGET AILMENTS: Painful, irregular, or absent menstrual periods; difficult labor; pain and soreness in the chest area; headache and dizziness

LIU WEI DI HUANG WAN • 474
TARGET AILMENTS: Night sweats or afternoon fevers; fatigue from chronic overwork; weakness of the lower back and legs; diabetes (yin-deficient type, according to traditional Chinese medicine); hyperthyroidism; symptoms of tuberculosis and AIDS; some kinds of weakened eyesight; some kinds of tinnitus or hearing loss; some chronic kidney problems

LONG DAN XIE GAN WAN • 477
TARGET AILMENTS: Conjunctivitis or red, painful eyes; otitis media; herpes; shingles; some migraine headaches; hepatitis with jaundice; acute gallstone attack; cystitis; urethritis; vaginal discharge; itchy, swollen genitals; some kinds of bad temper; hyperthyroidism or Graves' disease

LYCIUM FRUIT • 489
TARGET AILMENTS: Night blindness; tinnitus (ringing in the ears); dizziness; blurred vision; consumptive coughs; diabetes; sore back, knees, and legs; impotence and nocturnal emission

MAGNOLIA FLOWER • 495
TARGET AILMENTS: Nasal congestion, nasal discharge, sinus headaches, other sinus disorders

CONTINUED

MINOR BLUE DRAGON PILLS • 515
TARGET AILMENTS: Acute bronchitis, coughing with phlegm, asthma or wheezing, influenza

MUGWORT LEAF • 525
TARGET AILMENTS: Excessive menstrual bleeding, menstrual cramps, uterine bleeding, vaginal pain and bleeding during pregnancy, threatened miscarriage, pain relief, itchy lesions

NOTOGINSENG ROOT • 556
TARGET AILMENTS: Internal bleeding such as nosebleeds and blood in the stool and urine; coughing up blood; bleeding from injuries; swelling and pain of fractures, falls, contusions, and sprains; cuts; gunshot wounds

PEONY • 591
TARGET AILMENTS: Menstrual pain, irregular periods, premenstrual syndrome, irritability, cramping pain in limbs or abdomen, cramps with diarrhea, weakness with excessive sweating or loss of fluids

PILL CURING • 612
TARGET AILMENTS: Nausea, vomiting, abdominal pain and distention, diarrhea, motion sickness, gastroenteritis with fever and headache

PINELLIA • 614
TARGET AILMENTS: Cough with mucus and congestion; phlegmlike nodules (such as swollen lymph glands, goiter, sebaceous cysts); certain types of nausea and vomiting, including morning sickness; cloudy thinking, feeling, or perceiving

PING CHUAN WAN • 615
TARGET AILMENTS: Chronic bronchitis, emphysema, cough from lung weakness, shortness of breath from weakness

PLATYCODON • 617
TARGET AILMENTS: Cough, abscess of the throat or lung, sore throat or hoarseness

POLYGONUM • 620
TARGET AILMENTS: Dizziness and blurred vision; chronic fatigue; insomnia; prematurely gray hair; nocturnal emission; vaginal discharge; carbuncles, sores, abscesses, scrofula (a form of tuberculosis in the neck), goiter, and neck lumps; constipation; sore knees and back

PO SUM ON MEDICATED OIL • 624
TARGET AILMENTS: Joint pain (when joint is not red), pain from injury, toothache, cough

PROSTATE GLAND PILLS • 642
TARGET AILMENTS: Prostate infection or swelling, dribbling urine (in men), painful urination (in men), painful testicles, urinary tract infection

SAFFLOWER FLOWER • 669
TARGET AILMENTS: Delayed menstruation, poor blood circulation, blood clots, stabbing chest pain, burns, bruises and other injuries to the skin, sores and carbuncles, measles in its early stages

SANG JU YIN PIAN • 673
TARGET AILMENTS: Early stage of a cold or flu with symptoms such as headache, chest or nose congestion, sneezing, watery eyes, sore throat, fever

SAN SHE DAN CHUAN BEI YE • 674
TARGET AILMENTS: Cough with phlegm, bronchitis, emphysema, asthma with lots of phlegm

SARGASSUM SEAWEED • 675
TARGET AILMENTS: Nodules in the neck, including goiter and other thyroid disorders; scrofula (a form of tuberculosis); inadequate urination; edema (retention of body fluids); pain from hernia; swollen, painful testes

SCALLION • 678
TARGET AILMENTS: Chills and fevers, nasal congestion, abdominal pain and distention, sores and abscesses

SCHISANDRA • 679
TARGET AILMENTS: Chronic coughs and wheezing, asthma, allergic skin reactions, irritated skin, excessive sweating, insomnia, irritability, forgetfulness, dream-disturbed sleep, general lethargy, irregular heartbeat with coughing and thirst, palpitations, shortness of breath, nocturnal emission, vaginal discharge, frequent urination

SESAME OIL • 687
TARGET AILMENTS: Constipation, certain types of blurred vision, tinnitus (ringing in the ears), dizziness, recuperation after a severe illness—to help restore the vitality that serious illness depletes

SHI LIN TONG PIAN • 692
TARGET AILMENTS: Frequent and scanty urination, kidney stones or gallstones (if small), urinary tract infection (with or without bleeding), liver disease with swelling, kidney disease with edema (swelling)

SHI QUAN DA BU WAN • 693
TARGET AILMENTS: Fatigue with coldness, pale tongue, pale complexion

SKULLCAP • 697
TARGET AILMENTS: Diarrhea, dysentery, upper respiratory tract infections with fever, urinary tract infections, jaundice, hepatitis, nervous tension, irritability, headache, insomnia, epilepsy and other seizures, red face or eyes, coughing up or vomiting blood, nosebleeds, blood in the stool, abdominal pain and vaginal bleeding, threatened miscarriage during pregnancy, premenstrual stress

SUPERIOR SORE THROAT POWDER • 721
TARGET AILMENTS: Sore throat and tonsillitis, mouth ulcers or canker sores, toothache or sore gums, sinus infections, carbuncles, boils, skin blisters

TANGERINE PEEL • 728
TARGET AILMENTS: Indigestion; gas; feeling of swelling, bloat, or fullness in the abdomen; nausea and vomiting; loose stools; bringing up phlegm

TIEH TA YAO GIN • 747
TARGET AILMENTS: Traumatic injuries, bruises, broken bones, sprains and torn ligaments, sports or martial arts injuries

TURMERIC • 769
TARGET AILMENTS: Shoulder pain, menstrual cramps, pain after childbirth, menstrual irregularity, skin infections

TU ZHUNG FENG SHI WAN • 771
TARGET AILMENTS: Low back pain and joint pains that are more pronounced with weather changes, wandering joint pain, sciatica, gouty arthritis

XIANG SHA YANG WEI PIAN • 814
TARGET AILMENTS: Indigestion, heartburn, stomachache, nausea, diarrhea or loose stools, acute or chronic gastritis, gastric or duodenal ulcer symptoms

XIAO CHAI HU WAN • 815
TARGET AILMENTS: Chronic fatigue syndrome, Epstein-Barr virus, chronic low-grade fevers, irritability and fatigue, fibromyalgia, hepatitis or jaundice, malaria, upper respiratory tract infection

XIAO YAO WAN • 816
TARGET AILMENTS: Chronic irritability or frustration, hepatitis, chronic gastritis, constipation, diarrhea, irritable bowel syndrome, peptic ulcers, painful or irregular menstrual periods, painful breasts, premenstrual syndrome (PMS), insomnia or disturbed sleep, certain eye problems

YIN QIAO PIAN • 819
TARGET AILMENTS: Colds or upper respiratory tract infections (including flu), acute bronchitis, beginning stage of measles, sore throat, swollen glands, tonsillitis, conjunctivitis (pinkeye)

YUN NAN BAI YAO • 821
TARGET AILMENTS: Bleeding from open wounds; trauma to soft tissue (sprains, strains, bruises); vomiting blood; intestinal bleeding; coughing up blood; nose bleeds; painful, clotted menstrual periods; excessive menstrual bleeding; postpartum hemorrhage; postsurgical recovery

ZHENG GU SHUI • 824
TARGET AILMENTS: Sprains and injury to ligaments and tendons, bone fractures that have been set, bruises

ZHI BAI DI HUANG WAN • 825
TARGET AILMENTS: Low-grade fevers and night sweats; menopausal hot flashes; urinary tract infection or irritation with frequent urination, pain, and burning; genital herpes

ZHI WAN • 826
TARGET AILMENTS: Hemorrhoids

CONTINUED

Homeopathy

ACONITE • 24
TARGET AILMENTS: Angina, arrhythmia, anxiety, arthritis, asthma, bronchitis, colds and flu, croup, fever, eye inflammation, laryngitis, sore throat, otitis media, toothache

ALLIUM CEPA • 36
TARGET AILMENTS: Colds, coughs, watery and inflamed eyes, hay fever, neuralgia, earache

ANTIMONIUM TARTARICUM • 89
TARGET AILMENTS: Cold sweat, especially at night, bronchitis, chickenpox, measles, difficulty breathing, nausea, pneumonia, cough

APIS • 95
TARGET AILMENTS: Bites and stings, conjunctivitis, edema, headache, swollen joints, mumps

ARNICA • 99
TARGET AILMENTS: Blood blisters, broken bones, sprains, strains, bruises, rheumatism, toothache, groin strain

ARSENICUM ALBUM • 100
TARGET AILMENTS: Angina; anxiety disorders and panic attacks; asthma; hay fever; burns; chronic skin problems; fever and chills; headache; dry, hacking coughs; colds; colitis; indigestion; food poisoning; Crohn's disease; flu; insomnia

BELLADONNA • 125
TARGET AILMENTS: Colds, flu, sore throat, earache, fever and chills, arthritis, bursitis, gallstones, acute diverticulitis, colic, measles, mumps, neuralgia, sunstroke, varicose veins, toothache, teething pains, painful menstrual periods, breast-feeding complications

BRYONIA • 155
TARGET AILMENTS: Arthritis, backache, bursitis, colds with chest congestion, painful coughs, sore throat, flu, severe headaches, dizziness, nausea, vomiting, constipation, gastritis, acute diverticulitis, stomach flu, breast-feeding complications

CALCAREA CARBONICA • 167
TARGET AILMENTS: Lower back pain, broken bones, sprains, muscle cramps, constipation, chronic ear infections, eye inflammation, headaches, insomnia brought on by anxiety, eczema, allergies, asthma, teething problems, gastritis, gallstones, childhood diarrhea, menstrual problems, palpitations, arthritis

CALCAREA PHOSPHORICA • 168
TARGET AILMENTS: Anemia, broken bones, colds, cough with yellow mucus, exhaustion, headache, painful teething, joint pain, menstrual cramps

CANTHARIS • 180
TARGET AILMENTS: Bladder infections, sunburn, second-degree burns

CARBO VEGETABILIS • 185
TARGET AILMENTS: Cough, bronchitis, common cold, exhaustion, food poisoning, gas, headache, indigestion, sluggishness, stomach bloating

CAUSTICUM • 190
TARGET AILMENTS: Bedwetting, blisters, constipation, hoarseness, indigestion, joint pain, sore throat, scalds, third-degree burns

CHAMOMILLA • 197
TARGET AILMENTS: Irritability, toothache, painful menstrual periods, earaches, teething pain, difficulty getting to sleep

CHINA • 203
TARGET AILMENTS: Anemia, diarrhea, exhaustion, gas, headache, hepatitis, indigestion, malaria, stomach bloating, vomiting

COCCULUS • 241
TARGET AILMENTS: Severe nausea, hot flashes, exhaustion, numbness

COFFEA • 245
TARGET AILMENTS: Excitability, oversensitivity, headache, insomnia, toothache

COLOCYNTHIS • 250
TARGET AILMENTS: Anger and indignation, irritability, menstrual cramps, severe abdominal pain with nausea and vomiting, diarrhea, headache, sciatica, gout, rheumatism

DROSERA • 300
TARGET AILMENTS: Cough, whooping cough, sore throat

DULCAMARA • 302
TARGET AILMENTS: Colds, cough, diarrhea, cystitis, hives, warts, ringworm, backache, joint pain, weakness

EUPHRASIA • 325
TARGET AILMENTS: Red, swollen eyelids; watery eyes; conjunctivitis; intolerance of bright light; colds; cough; hay fever; measles; painful menstrual periods; prostatitis; constipation

FERRUM PHOSPHORICUM • 337
TARGET AILMENTS: Hacking coughs with chest pain, headaches, fevers, ear infections, incontinence, rheumatic joints, anemia, fatigue, nosebleeds, sore throat, vomiting, diarrhea, palpitations

GELSEMIUM • 364
TARGET AILMENTS: Anxiety, flu, headache, measles, sore throat, fever

HEPAR SULPHURIS • 390
TARGET AILMENTS: Abscesses; colds, sore throat, and earache; inflamed, slow-healing wounds; aching joints; cough; hoarseness; asthma; emphysema; croup; genital herpes; constipation

HYPERICUM • 411
TARGET AILMENTS: Backache, insect bites and stings

IGNATIA • 415
TARGET AILMENTS: Anxiety, dry coughs, sore throat, tension headaches, indigestion, insomnia, irritable bowel syndrome, painful hemorrhoids, grief, shock, depression

IPECAC • 422
TARGET AILMENTS: Asthma, colic, diarrhea, cough, flu, gastroenteritis, menstrual problems, motion sickness, persistent nausea, vomiting

KALI BICHROMICUM • 432
TARGET AILMENTS: Bronchitis, colds, croup, sinusitis, indigestion, joint pain

LACHESIS • 446
TARGET AILMENTS: Cough, croup, earache, sore throat, indigestion, throbbing headache, insomnia, hot flashes, heart arrhythmias, hemorrhoids, sciatica

LEDUM • 459
TARGET AILMENTS: Animal bites or insect stings, bruises, deep cuts or puncture wounds, gout, aching joints

LYCOPODIUM • 490
TARGET AILMENTS: Backache, bedwetting, cold, constipation, coughs, cystitis, headache, gout, indigestion, abdominal cramps, gas, heartburn, joint pain, sciatica, sore throat, eczema

MAGNESIA PHOSPHORICA • 491
TARGET AILMENTS: Headache, dizziness, involuntary muscle spasms, neuralgia, toothache, teething pains, sciatica, earache, writer's cramp, abdominal pain, gas, menstrual cramps, colic in infants

MERCURIUS VIVUS • 502
TARGET AILMENTS: Abscesses, backache, chickenpox, colds, cystitis, painful diarrhea, flu, earache with discharge, eye inflammation, indigestion, mouth ulcers, sore throat, toothache

NATRUM MURIATICUM • 534
TARGET AILMENTS: Anemia, backache, cold sores, colds, constipation, depression, eczema, fevers and chills, genital herpes, hay fever, indigestion, menstrual irregularity, migraine headaches

NUX VOMICA • 558
TARGET AILMENTS: Colds, stomach cramps from overeating, indigestion, constipation, cystitis, fever and chills, gas and gas pains, hangovers, headache, insomnia, irritable bowel syndrome, menstrual cramps with heavy flow, nausea, morning sickness, sinusitis, stomach flu, vomiting brought on by overeating or eating rich foods

PETROLEUM • 597
TARGET AILMENTS: Motion sickness; forgetfulness; irritability; pain and itching on feet, hands, and toes; diarrhea; headache; nausea

PHOSPHORUS • 609
TARGET AILMENTS: Bronchitis, pneumonia, coughs, eyestrain, gastritis, nosebleeds, indigestion, stomach ulcers, kidney infections, nasal polyps, hepatitis, anemia, hemorrhage, diarrhea, menstrual problems

CONTINUED

PHYTOLACCA • 611
TARGET AILMENTS: Breast abscess, infection, and cracked nipples in nursing mothers; mumps; sore throat; painful teething; pains where tendons attach to bones

PODOPHYLLUM • 619
TARGET AILMENTS: Diarrhea

PULSATILLA • 650
TARGET AILMENTS: Bedwetting, breast infections, chickenpox, conjunctivitis, coughs, headaches, eye inflammation, fever with chills, hay fever, incontinence, indigestion, aching joints, urethritis in men, late menstrual periods, otitis media, sciatica, sinusitis, varicose veins, depression

RHUS TOXICODENDRON • 658
TARGET AILMENTS: Arthritis, backache, bursitis, carpal tunnel syndrome, eye inflammation, genital herpes, hamstring injury, flu, headache, hives, joint pain from overexertion, impetigo, poison ivy, sprains with stiffness, toothache

RUMEX • 667
TARGET AILMENTS: Cough

RUTA • 668
TARGET AILMENTS: Carpal tunnel syndrome, eyestrain, sciatica, groin strain, sprains, tennis elbow, injuries of tendons and cartilage

SEPIA • 685
TARGET AILMENTS: Backaches, violent fits of coughing, cold sores, genital herpes, exhaustion, hair loss, gas, headaches with throbbing pain, sinusitis, urinary incontinence, hot flashes, menstrual cramps, motion sickness, nausea associated with pregnancy, brown spots on skin

SILICA • 694
TARGET AILMENTS: Athlete's foot, constipation, wounds, earache, weak fingernails, headache, abscesses, swollen glands in the neck, gum infections, hemorrhoids, breast cysts

SPONGIA • 708
TARGET AILMENTS: Colds and coughs, asthma

SULPHUR • 718
TARGET AILMENTS: Asthma, cough, diarrhea, eye inflammation, bursitis, headache, indigestion, joint pain, anal itching, burning vaginal discharge, eczema

TABACUM • 725
TARGET AILMENTS: Nausea or vomiting caused by pregnancy or motion sickness

THUJA • 741
TARGET AILMENTS: Warts, headache, inflammation and swelling of joints

URTICA • 776
TARGET AILMENTS: Rheumatism; neuralgia; burns; insect bites and stings; itchy, blistered, or hot skin; lack or overabundance of breast milk; vaginal itching

Nutritional Supplements

BEE POLLEN • 124
TARGET AILMENTS: Stress, fatigue, depression, bowel problems, cancer, heart ailments, arthritis

BIOFLAVONOIDS (VITAMIN P) • 138
TARGET AILMENTS: Abnormal bruising, inflammation, allergy, eye disorders, asthma

BLUE-GREEN ALGAE • 149
TARGET AILMENTS: Obesity, fatigue

BREWER'S YEAST • 151
TARGET AILMENTS: Eczema, nervousness, fatigue, heart problems, diabetes, constipation

BROMELAIN • 152
TARGET AILMENTS: Back pain, arthritis, inflammation, sinusitis, menstrual cramps, poor digestion

CHARCOAL, ACTIVATED • 198
TARGET AILMENTS: Diarrhea, gout, gas and gas pains, poisoning and drug overdose, hangover, hiccups

CHITOSAN • 209
(MARINE FIBER)
TARGET AILMENTS: High cholesterol, constipation, obesity, high blood pressure

CHONDROITIN SULFATE • 215
TARGET AILMENTS: Joint problems, weak cartilage, headache, respiratory ailments, allergies, arthritis, bursitis

COENZYME Q10 • 244
TARGET AILMENTS: Allergies, asthma, Alzheimer's disease, cancer, candidiasis, cardiovascular disease, congestive heart failure, cardiomyopathy, angina pectoris, diabetes mellitus, hypertension, muscular dystrophy, obesity, periodontal disease, respiratory disease, schizophrenia

DGL • 276
(DEGLYCYRRHIZINATED LICORICE)
TARGET AILMENTS: Peptic ulcers, mouth sores

DHEA • 277
(DEHYDROEPIANDROSTERONE)
TARGET AILMENTS: Depression, mood swings, heart disease, obesity, memory loss, weak bones, autoimmune disorders

DMSO • 292
(DIMETHYL SULFOXIDE)
TARGET AILMENTS: Interstitial cystitis

EDTA • 305
(ETHYLENEDIAMINETETRAACETIC ACID)
TARGET AILMENTS: Lead poisoning, atherosclerosis, angina, high blood pressure, circulatory problems, Alzheimer's disease

FIBER, DIETARY • 339
TARGET AILMENTS: High cholesterol, constipation, hemorrhoids, diverticulitis, obesity, heart disease, non-insulin-dependent (Type 2) diabetes, cancers of the colon and breast

GLANDULARS • 375
TARGET AILMENTS: Problems involving the thyroid, pancreas, liver, thymus, spleen, testes, ovary, pituitary gland, and adrenal cortex

GLUCOSAMINE SULFATE • 379
TARGET AILMENTS: Joint pain, joint stiffness, osteoarthritis

INDOLE-3-CARBINOL • 418
TARGET AILMENTS: Breast cancer (prevention)

LACTOBACILLUS ACIDOPHILUS • 447
TARGET AILMENTS: Canker sores, constipation, diarrhea, indigestion, gas, lactose intolerance, postantibiotic therapy, spastic colon, yeast infections, urinary tract infections

L-CARNITINE • 457
TARGET AILMENTS: High cholesterol; atherosclerosis; heart, liver, or kidney disease; obesity or anorexia nervosa; diabetes; muscular dystrophy

LECITHIN • 458
TARGET AILMENTS: Dizziness, fatigue, headache, liver disorders, high cholesterol, bipolar depression, insomnia, memory loss, Alzheimer's disease

L-LYSINE • 475
TARGET AILMENTS: Herpes, shingles, cold sores, sports injuries

MELATONIN • 499
TARGET AILMENTS: Jet lag, insomnia, stress, seasonal affective disorder, cancer (adjunct therapy)

OMEGA-3 FATTY ACIDS • 561
TARGET AILMENTS: Heart disease, high cholesterol, arthritis, colitis, psoriasis, atopic dermatitis (eczema), lupus, mulitple sclerosis, cancer

PAPAIN • 577
TARGET AILMENTS: Celiac disease, poor digestion, constipation, food allergies

PROANTHOCYANIDIN
(GRAPE-SEED EXTRACT) • 636
TARGET AILMENTS: Allergies that respond to antihistamines, arthritis, bruises, gum disease, phlebitis, ulcers, varicose veins and other vascular problems

CONTINUED

SHARK CARTILAGE · 688
TARGET AILMENTS: Joint pain, stiffness, swelling

SOYBEAN MILK · 704
TARGET AILMENTS: High cholesterol; lactose intolerance; osteoporosis; breast, ovarian, and endometrial cancers (risk reduction)

SUPEROXIDE DISMUTASE · 722
TARGET AILMENTS: Anemia; autoimmune diseases such as lupus, rheumatoid arthritis, and scleroderma; vasculitis, including Behçet's disease and Kawasaki's disease; cataracts (prevention); Crohn's disease; radiation-induced necrosis; Raynaud's syndrome

WHEAT GERM · 809
TARGET AILMENTS: High LDL cholesterol, heart disease, cancer, stroke, diabetes, fibrocystic breast disease, menopausal symptoms, other conditions that benefit from vitamin E supplementation

Vitamins and Minerals

BIOTIN (VITAMIN B_7, VITAMIN H) · 140
TARGET AILMENTS: Immune problems, skin problems

CALCIUM · 171
TARGET AILMENTS: Osteoporosis in adults; rickets in children; colorectal cancer (when taken with vitamin D and if prescribed by a doctor); regulation of blood pressure; reduction of risk of heart disease

CHLORIDE · 211
TARGET AILMENTS: Hypochlorhydria; dehydration

CHROMIUM · 216
TARGET AILMENTS: Diabetes, heart disease, hypoglycemia, alcoholism

COBALT · 240
TARGET AILMENTS: Anemia

COPPER · 253
TARGET AILMENTS: Cancer, heart disease, immune problems

FLUORIDE · 344
TARGET AILMENTS: Osteoporosis, tooth decay

FOLIC ACID (VITAMIN B_9) · 352
TARGET AILMENTS: Cancer, heart disease, immune problems, skin problems

IODINE · 421
TARGET AILMENTS: Goiter, skin problems

IRON · 424
TARGET AILMENTS: Anemia, fatigue

MAGNESIUM · 492
TARGET AILMENTS: Heart disease, menstrual problems, muscle cramps

MANGANESE · 496
TARGET AILMENTS: Sprains, strains, inflammation, diabetes

MOLYBDENUM · 519
TARGET AILMENTS: Tooth decay

NIACIN (VITAMIN B_3) · 540
TARGET AILMENTS: The major types of cholesterol disorders, particularly those in which high levels of blood fats have been linked to an increased risk of heart disease

PHOSPHORUS · 610
TARGET AILMENTS: Fatigue, fractures (prevention)

POTASSIUM (VARIOUS COMBINATIONS) · 625
TARGET AILMENTS: Heart disease, high blood pressure

SELENIUM · 682
TARGET AILMENTS: Arthritis, cancer, heart disease, immune problems

SODIUM · 702
TARGET AILMENTS: High blood pressure (reduction of sodium in the diet)

SULFUR • 717
TARGET AILMENTS: Toxic exposure

VANADIUM • 786
TARGET AILMENTS: Cancer, diabetes

VITAMIN A (RETINOL) • 797
TARGET AILMENTS: Cancer, heart disease, high cholesterol, immune problems, vision problems, wounds, viral illnesses, vaginal candidiasis

VITAMIN B COMPLEX • 798
TARGET AILMENTS: Depression, heart disease, immune problems, skin problems, stress

VITAMIN B_1 (THIAMINE) • 799
TARGET AILMENTS: Anemia, fatigue

VITAMIN B_2 (RIBOFLAVIN) • 800
TARGET AILMENTS: Fatigue, depression, skin problems, vision problems

VITAMIN B_5 (PANTOTHENIC ACID) • 801
TARGET AILMENTS: Immune problems, wounds

VITAMIN B_6 (PYRIDOXINE) • 802
TARGET AILMENTS: Carpal tunnel syndrome, depression, fatigue, immune problems, PMS, skin problems

VITAMIN B_{12} (COBALAMIN) • 803
TARGET AILMENTS: Anemia, depression, fatigue

VITAMIN C (ASCORBIC ACID) • 804
TARGET AILMENTS: Cancer, heart disease, immune problems, wounds

VITAMIN D (CHOLECALCIFEROL, ERGOCALCIFEROL) • 805
TARGET AILMENTS: Cancer, skin problems

VITAMIN E • 806
TARGET AILMENTS: Arthritis, heart disease, skin problems, wounds

VITAMIN K (MENADIONE, PHYTONADIONE) • 807
TARGET AILMENTS: Osteoporosis

ZINC • 827
TARGET AILMENTS: Immune problems, skin problems, wounds

Western Herbs

ALFALFA • 34
TARGET AILMENTS: Bladder inflammation, bloating, indigestion, constipation, halitosis

ALOE • 39
TARGET AILMENTS: Digestive disorders, stomach ulcers, constipation, minor burns, sunburn, infection in wounds, insect bites, acne, skin irritation, bruising, chickenpox, poison ivy, irritated eyes

ANISE • 61
TARGET AILMENTS: Cough, bronchitis, indigestion, gas

ASHWAGANDA • 101
TARGET AILMENTS: Muscle weakness, multiple sclerosis, rheumatism, fatigue, infertility, sterility, indigestion, heart disease, hay fever, carbuncles, sores, inflammation, swelling, ringworm

ASTRAGALUS • 107
TARGET AILMENTS: Chronic colds and flu, AIDS, cancer, chronic fatigue

BARBERRY • 117
TARGET AILMENTS: Jaundice, hepatitis, anemia, heartburn, hangover, constipation, swollen spleen, gallstones, sore throat, conjunctivitis, skin infections

BAYBERRY • 119
TARGET AILMENTS: Dysentery, diarrhea, fever, nasal congestion, sore throat, poor circulation, varicose veins, hemorrhoids

CONTINUED

CRAMP BARK • 261
TARGET AILMENTS: Muscular cramps, menstrual cramps, menopausal problems

DAMIANA • 268
TARGET AILMENTS: Nervous indigestion, hormone imbalance, impotence, testosterone deficiency, depression, anxiety, weakness

DANDELION • 270
TARGET AILMENTS: Poor digestion, gallbladder problems, liver inflammation, water retention

DEVIL'S CLAW • 273
TARGET AILMENTS: Arthritis, gout, liver dysfunction, gallbladder disorders, digestive problems, diabetes, skin lesions and boils

ECHINACEA • 304
TARGET AILMENTS: Colds and flu, mononucleosis, ear infections, septicemia, bladder infections, cuts, burns, wounds, abscesses, boils, insect bites and stings, hives, eczema, herpes

ELDER • 306
TARGET AILMENTS: Colds and flu, cough, rheumatism, hay fever, sinusitis, neuralgia, rash, eczema, dry skin, chilblains, bruises, sprains, wounds, conjunctivitis

ELECAMPANE • 307
TARGET AILMENTS: Cough, colds, bronchitis, asthma, emphysema, digestive problems, parasites

EPHEDRA • 310
TARGET AILMENTS: Colds, flu, nasal and chest congestion, asthma, hay fever

EUCALYPTUS • 323
TARGET AILMENTS: Arthritis, rheumatism, minor cuts and scrapes, asthma, colds, flu, bronchitis, whooping cough

EVENING PRIMROSE OIL • 326
TARGET AILMENTS: PMS, arthritis, dry eyes, multiple sclerosis, hypertension, eczema, brittle hair and nails

EYEBRIGHT • 330
TARGET AILMENTS: Eye irritations from hay fever, allergies, or colds; conjunctivitis; nasal congestion; cough

FENNEL • 335
TARGET AILMENTS: Digestive problems, colic, gas, diarrhea, insufficient milk in nursing mothers, muscle pain, rheumatism, conjunctivitis

FENUGREEK • 336
TARGET AILMENTS: Digestive disorders, sore throats and coughs, lactation problems of nursing mothers, boils, rashes, cuts, arthritis pain

FEVERFEW • 338
TARGET AILMENTS: Migraine headache

FLAXSEED • 342
TARGET AILMENTS: Constipation, digestive disorders, gallbladder problems, inflammation, arthritis, burns, boils

GARLIC • 362
TARGET AILMENTS: Colds, coughs, flu, high cholesterol, high blood pressure, atherosclerosis, digestive disorders, bladder infection, liver and gallbladder problems, athlete's foot, skin infections

GENTIAN • 366
TARGET AILMENTS: Digestive disorders, loss of appetite, arthritis, constipation

GINGER • 370
TARGET AILMENTS: Motion sickness, morning sickness, digestive disorders, menstrual cramps, colds, flu, arthritis, high cholesterol, high blood pressure

GINKGO • 371
TARGET AILMENTS: Vertigo, Alzheimer's disease, tinnitus, phlebitis, leg ulcers, cerebral atherosclerosis, diabetic vascular disease, Raynaud's syndrome, headaches, depression, stroke, heart attacks

GINSENG, AMERICAN • 372
TARGET AILMENTS: Depression, fatigue, stress, colds, inflammation, damaged immune system

GINSENG, SIBERIAN • 374
TARGET AILMENTS: Depression, fatigue, stress, colds, inflammation, damaged immune system

GOLDENSEAL • 382
TARGET AILMENTS: Infectious diarrhea, gastritis, ulcers, gallstones, jaundice, sinusitis, ear infections, laryngi-

CONTINUED

tis, sore throat, infected gums, postpartum uterine bleeding, vaginal yeast infections, eczema, fungal infections, dermatitis

GOTU KOLA • 383
TARGET AILMENTS: Poor circulation in the legs, edema, burns, skin injuries, psoriasis

HAWTHORN • 388
TARGET AILMENTS: High blood pressure, clogged arteries, heart palpitations, angina, inflammation of the heart muscle, insomnia, nervous conditions, sore throat

HIBISCUS • 391
TARGET AILMENTS: Constipation, bladder infection, mild nausea, sunburn

HOPS • 394
TARGET AILMENTS: Insomnia, anxiety, tension headache, indigestion, neuralgia

HOREHOUND • 395
TARGET AILMENTS: Cough, colds, bronchitis, fever, whooping cough

HORSETAIL • 396
TARGET AILMENTS: Bladder and urinary tract infections, prostatitis, kidney stones, rheumatism, arthritis, wounds, inflammation

HYSSOP • 412
TARGET AILMENTS: Cough, colds, bronchitis, indigestion, gas, anxiety, hysteria, petit mal seizures, cold sores, genital herpes, burns, wounds, skin irritations

JUNIPER • 430
TARGET AILMENTS: Bladder infections, digestive problems, high blood pressure, arthritis, gout

KAVA • 433
TARGET AILMENTS: Urinary disorders, prostate inflammation, gout, rheumatism, insomnia, fatigue, depression, muscle spasms

KELP • 437
TARGET AILMENTS: Goiter, hypothyroidism, radiation exposure

KOLA • 445
TARGET AILMENTS: Depression, migraine headache, poor appetite, diarrhea caused by nervousness, motion sickness, fluid retention, asthma

LAVENDER • 454
TARGET AILMENTS: Insomnia, depression, headache, poor digestion, nausea, gas, colic, burns, wounds, eczema, acne, candidiasis, ringworm, rheumatism

LEMON BALM • 461
TARGET AILMENTS: Depression, digestive disorders, headache, neuralgia, insomnia, high blood pressure, fever, colds, flu, herpes sores, eczema

LEMONGRASS • 462
TARGET AILMENTS: Diarrhea, stomachache, headache, fever, flu, athlete's foot, acne, circulatory problems

LICORICE • 469
TARGET AILMENTS: Cough, sore throat, constipation, heartburn, colic, stomach ulcers, arthritis, hepatitis, cirrhosis, skin ulcers, herpes sores

LINDEN • 471
TARGET AILMENTS: Fever, colds, flu, insomnia, headache

LOBELIA • 476
TARGET AILMENTS: Pneumonia, asthma, bronchitis, insect bites, poison ivy, fungal infections, muscle strain

MARSH MALLOW • 497
TARGET AILMENTS: Sore throat, cough, colds, flu, sinusitis, upset stomach, stomach ulcers, bladder infection, kidney stones, boils, cuts, burns, varicose veins, dental abscesses, gingivitis

MEADOWSWEET • 498
TARGET AILMENTS: Headache, pain, inflammation, muscle aches, arthritis, cramps, colds, flu, nausea, heartburn

MILK THISTLE • 514
TARGET AILMENTS: Cirrhosis, hepatitis, psoriasis

MISTLETOE • 518
TARGET AILMENTS: High blood pressure, cancer

MOTHERWORT • 524
TARGET AILMENTS: Delayed menstruation, premenstrual syndrome, menopausal problems, rapid heartbeat

MULLEIN • 526
TARGET AILMENTS: Bronchitis, flu, asthma, stomach cramps, diarrhea, tumors, hemorrhoids, ear problems

MYRRH • 530
TARGET AILMENTS: Gum disease, pharyngitis, sinusitis, colds, asthma, boils, congestion, coughs, wounds

NETTLE • 538
TARGET AILMENTS: Arthritis, gout, hay fever, eczema, vaginal yeast infections, hemorrhoids, diarrhea, chronic cystitis, hypertension, congestive heart failure

NUTMEG • 557
TARGET AILMENTS: Digestive disorders, insomnia

OATS • 559
TARGET AILMENTS: Depression, anxiety, insomnia, high cholesterol, indigestion, eczema, dry skin

OREGON GRAPE • 568
TARGET AILMENTS: Skin diseases, liver diseases, anemia, constipation, indigestion, nausea

PARSLEY • 579
TARGET AILMENTS: Indigestion, urinary tract infections, irregular menstruation, PMS

PASSIONFLOWER • 580
TARGET AILMENTS: Insomnia, anxiety, stress, neuralgia, shingles, menstrual cramps, Parkinson's disease, epilepsy, asthma, addictions

PAU D'ARCO • 582
TARGET AILMENTS: Bacterial, fungal, viral, and parasitic infections; indigestion

PENNYROYAL • 588
TARGET AILMENTS: Colds, coughs, PMS, menstrual cramps, gas, indigestion, anxiety

PEPPERMINT • 594
TARGET AILMENTS: Cramps, stomach pain, gas, nausea associated with migraine headaches, morning sickness, travel sickness, insomnia, anxiety, fever, colds, flu, itchy or inflamed skin

PLANTAIN • 616
TARGET AILMENTS: Diarrhea, cough, bronchitis, kidney and bladder infection, urinary incontinence, hemorrhoids, itchy, inflamed skin, cuts, snake and insect bites

PLEURISY ROOT • 618
TARGET AILMENTS: Colds, flu, bronchitis, indigestion

PSYLLIUM • 648
TARGET AILMENTS: Ulcers, colitis, constipation, diarrhea, hemorrhoids

RED CLOVER • 655
TARGET AILMENTS: Cough, bronchitis, whooping cough, indigestion, menopausal symptoms, eczema, psoriasis

RED RASPBERRY • 656
TARGET AILMENTS: Morning sickness, threatened miscarriage, complications during labor, diarrhea, mouth ulcers, bleeding gums

ROSE HIP • 664
TARGET AILMENTS: Colds and flu

ROSEMARY • 666
TARGET AILMENTS: Indigestion, upper respiratory infection and congestion, tension, muscle pain, sprains, rheumatism, neuralgia, skin infections

SAFFRON • 670
TARGET AILMENTS: High cholesterol, high blood pressure, atherosclerosis, indigestion, delayed menstruation

SAGE • 671
TARGET AILMENTS: Indigestion, gas, nausea, night sweats of menopause, mouth and throat infections, infected wounds, insect bites

SASSAFRAS • 676
TARGET AILMENTS: Skin irritations such as acne, boils, poison ivy and poison oak

SAW PALMETTO • 677
TARGET AILMENTS: Benign prostatic hyperplasia (enlargement of the prostate gland), nasal congestion, bronchitis, coughs due to colds

SENNA • 683
TARGET AILMENTS: Constipation

SHEEP SORREL • 690
TARGET AILMENTS: Constipation; diarrhea; mouth, throat,

CONTINUED

and stomach ulcers; excessive menstruation; itchy skin rashes such as hives and poison ivy

SHIITAKE • 691
TARGET AILMENTS: High cholesterol, depressed immune system, chronic fatigue syndrome, some forms of cancer

SKULLCAP • 698
TARGET AILMENTS: Nervous tension, headaches and muscle aches, insomnia, drug or alcohol withdrawal, PMS

SLIPPERY ELM • 699
TARGET AILMENTS: Wounds, cuts, cough and sore throat, digestive complaints, ulcers, colitis

SPEARMINT • 705
TARGET AILMENTS: Upset stomach; stomach spasms or cramps; gas; heartburn; morning sickness; nasal, sinus, and chest congestion; colds; headache; sore mouth or throat; muscle pain

ST.-JOHN'S-WORT • 709
TARGET AILMENTS: Cuts, abrasions, burns, scar tissue, depression

TEA TREE OIL • 731
TARGET AILMENTS: Insect bites, acne, fungal infections, athlete's foot, skin ailments, minor vaginal infections

THYME • 743
TARGET AILMENTS: Cough, colds, sore throat, bronchitis, asthma, flu, digestive problems

TURMERIC • 770
TARGET AILMENTS: Digestive disorders, fever, chest congestion, menstrual irregularity, arthritis, pain and swelling caused by trauma

USNEA • 777
TARGET AILMENTS: Colds, flu, sore throat, respiratory infections, gastrointestinal irritations, skin ulcers, athlete's foot, urinary tract infections, vaginal infections

UVA URSI • 778
TARGET AILMENTS: Urinary tract infections, minor cuts and abrasions, vaginitis

VALERIAN • 781
TARGET AILMENTS: Insomnia, anxiety, nervousness, headache, intestinal pains, menstrual cramps

WHITE WILLOW • 810
TARGET AILMENTS: Arthritis, gout, minor muscle strains, menstrual cramps, headache, fever, aches, pains, sores, burns

WILD CHERRY BARK • 811
TARGET AILMENTS: Cough, slow digestion, asthma

WILD CRANESBILL • 812
TARGET AILMENTS: Diarrhea, dysentery, menorrhagia, gastritis

WILD YAM • 813
TARGET AILMENTS: Menstrual cramps, morning sickness, rheumatoid arthritis

YARROW • 817
TARGET AILMENTS: Fever, digestive disorders, menstrual cramps, anxiety, insomnia, high blood pressure, minor wounds, bleeding, vaginal irritation

YELLOW DOCK • 818
TARGET AILMENTS: Constipation, anemia, rheumatism, skin diseases

BRAND NAME INDEX

Drugs in boldface are illustrated in the Color Guide to Prescription Drugs and Herbs, following page 432.

CONTINUED

GENERAL INDEX

A

B

CONTINUED

C

D

E

CONTINUED

I

J

K

CONTINUED

L

M

N

CONTINUED

O

P

CONTINUED

T

CONTINUED

U

V

W

X

Y

Z

BIBLIOGRAPHY

AROMATHERAPY

BOOKS:

The Alternative Advisor: The Complete Guide to Natural Therapies and Alternative Treatments. Alexandria, Va.: Time-Life Books, 1997.

Lawless, Julia. *The Encyclopaedia of Essential Oils.* Rockport, Mass.: Element Books, 1992.

Price, Shirley. *Aromatherapy for Common Ailments.* London: Gaia Books, 1991.

Ryman, Danièle. *Aromatherapy: The Complete Guide to Plant and Flower Essences for Health and Beauty.* New York: Bantam Books, 1993.

CHINESE MEDICINE

BOOKS:

Bensky, Dan, and Randall Barolet (comps. and trans.). *Chinese Herbal Medicine: Formulas and Strategies.* Seattle: Eastland Press, 1990.

Fratkin, Jake. *Chinese Herbal Patent Formulas: A Practical Guide.* Portland, Oreg.: Institute for Traditional Medicine and Preventative Health Care, 1986.

The Medical Advisor: The Complete Guide to Alternative and Conventional Treatments. Alexandria, Va.: Time-Life Books, 1996.

Naeser, Margaret A. *Outline Guide to Chinese Herbal Patent Medicines in Pill Form.* Boston: Boston Chinese Medicine, 1990.

Zhu, Chun-Han. *Clinical Handbook of Chinese Prepared Medicines.* Brookline, Mass.: Paradigm Publications, 1989.

HOMEOPATHY

BOOKS:

Gould, George M. *Blakiston's Gould Medical Dictionary* (4th ed.). New York: McGraw-Hill, 1984.

Castro, Miranda. *The Complete Homeopathy Handbook: A Guide to Everyday Health Care.* New York: St. Martin's Press, 1991.

Cummings, Stephen, MD, and Dana Ullman. *Everybody's Guide to Homeopathic Medicines.* New York: Putnam, Jeremy P. Tarcher/Perigee, 1991.

Lockie, Andrew, MD. *The Family Guide to Homeopathy.* New York: Simon & Schuster, Fireside Books, 1993.

The Medical Advisor: The Complete Guide to Alternative and Conventional Treatments. Alexandria, Va.: Time-Life Books, 1996.

OTHER SOURCES:

Hoffman, David L. "Therapeutic Herbalism: A Correspondence Course in Phytotherapy." Unpublished course materials. N.p., n.d.

NUTRITIONAL SUPPLEMENTS

BOOKS:

The Alternative Advisor: The Complete Guide to Natural Therapies and Alternative Treatments. Alexandria, Va.: Time-Life Books, 1997.

Balch, James F., MD, and Phyllis A. Balch. *Prescription for Nutritional Healing.* Garden City Park, N.Y.: Avery Publishing Group, 1990.

The Complete Book of Natural and Medicinal Cures. Emmaus, Pa.: Rodale Press, 1994.

Feltman, John (ed.). *The Prevention How-To Dictionary of Healing Remedies and Techniques.* Emmaus, Pa.: Rodale Press, 1992.

Garrison, Robert H., Jr., and Elizabeth Somer. *The Nutrition Desk Reference* (rev. ed.). New Canaan, Conn.: Keats Publishing, 1990.

Griffith, H. Winter, MD. *Complete Guide to Vitamins, Minerals, Nutrients, and Supplements.* Tucson, Ariz.: Fisher Books, 1988.

Haas, Elson M., MD. *Staying Healthy with Nutrition: The Complete Guide to Diet and Nutritional Medicine.* Berkeley, Calif.: Celestial Arts, 1992.

Hendler, Sheldon Saul, MD. *The Doctors' Vitamin and Mineral Encyclopedia.* New York: Simon & Schuster, 1990.

The Medical Advisor: The Complete Guide to Alternative and Conventional Treatments. Alexandria, Va.: Time-Life Books, 1996.

Murray, Michael T., and Joseph E. Pizzorno. *An Encyclopedia of Natural Medicine.* Rocklin, Calif.: Prima Publishing, 1991.

The PDR Family Guide to Nutrition and Health. Montvale, N.J.: Medical Economics, 1995.

Physician's Drug Handbook (6th ed.). Springhouse, Pa.: Springhouse Corporation, 1995.

Werbach, Melvyn R., MD.: *Nutritional Influences on Illness: A Sourcebook of Clinical Research* (2d ed.). Tarzana, Calif.: Third Line Press, 1993.

Nutritional Influences on Mental Illness: A Sourcebook of Clinical Research. Tarzana, Calif.: Third Line Press, 1991.

PERIODICALS:

"Can Pond Scum Really Keep You Healthy?" *University of California at Berkeley Wellness Letter,* January 1997.

Gazella, Karolyn A. "New Information on DHEA." *Health Counselor,* n.d.

Osborn, Blaire, and Linda Werling. "Evaluating the Sleep-Inducing Properties of Melatonin." *Alternative and Complementary Therapies,* November/December 1996.

Quillin, Patrick. "Nutrition Tip of the Season." *Healthy Thoughts Gazette,* Winter 1997.

Sahelian, Ray. "Questions and Answers about DHEA." *Health Counselor,* n.d.

Skolnick, Andrew A. "Scientific Verdict Still Out on DHEA." *Journal of the American Medical Association,* November 6, 1996.

OTHER SOURCES:

American Institute for Cancer Research. "Listing of 1995 AICR Research Grants." Pamphlet. Washington, D.C.: American Institute for Cancer Research, 1996.

Clouatre, Dallas, and Alan E. Lewis. "Melatonin and the Biological Clock." Booklet. New Canaan, Conn.: Keats Publishing, 1996.

Hansen, Clark. "Grape Seed Extract." Booklet. New York: Healing Wisdom Publications, 1995.

Johnston, Ingeborg M., and James R. Johnston. "Flaxseed (Linseed) Oil and the Power of Omega-3." Pamphlet. New Canaan, Conn.: Keats Publishing, 1990.

Walker, Morton. "EDTA Chelation and Clear Arteries: Putting IV Cardiac Therapy into a New Perspective." Paper presented at a meeting in Aruba, Netherlands Antilles, for the 5th International Symposium, Members of Region Two, American Society of Extra-Corporeal Technology, November 6-10, 1996.

OVER-THE-COUNTER AND PRESCRIPTION DRUGS

BOOKS:

Griffith, H. Winter, MD. *Complete Guide to Prescription and Nonprescription Drugs.* New York: Berkeley Publishing Group, Body Press/Perigee, 1996.

Lemcker, D. P., et al. *Primary Care of Women.* Norwalk, Conn.: Appleton & Lange, 1995.

The Medical Advisor: The Complete Guide to Alternative and Conventional Treatments. Alexandria, Va.: Time-Life Books, 1996.

The PDR Family Guide to Prescription Drugs (3d ed.). Montvale, N.J.: Medical Economics, 1995.

Physicians' Desk Reference, 51 Edition. Montvale, N.J.: Medical Economics, 1997.

Physicians' Desk Reference for Nonprescription Drugs (17th ed.). Montvale, N.J.: Medical Economics, 1996.

Physician's Drug Handbook (6th ed.). Springhouse, Pa.: Springhouse, 1995.

Rybacki, James J., PharmD., and James W. Long, MD. *The Essential Guide to Prescription Drugs* (1997 ed.). New York: HarperCollins, 1996.

Silverman, Harold M. *The Pill Book* (6th ed.). New York: Bantam Books, 1994.

USP DI–Volume 1: Drug Information for the Health Care Professional (17th ed.). Rockville, Md.: United States Pharmacopeial Convention, 1997.

Zimmerman, David R. *Zimmerman's Complete Guide to Nonprescription Drugs* (2d ed.). Detroit: Visible Ink Press, 1993.

PERIODICALS:

Fackelmann, Kathleen. "Marijuana on Trial: Is Marijuana a Dangerous Drug or a Valuable Medicine?" *Science News,* March 22, 1997.

Hussar, Daniel A. "New Drugs of 1995." *Journal of the American Pharmaceutical Association,* March 1996.

Mikuriya, Tod. "Critique: Marijuana and Health: Report of a Study by a Committee of the Institute of Medicine Division of Health Sciences Policy, National Academy of Science." *National Academy Press,* 1982.

"NIH Panel Says More Study Is Needed to Assess Marijuana's Medicinal Use." *Journal of the American Medical Association,* March 19, 1997.

"Pharmacists' Favorite OTCs of '95." *American Druggist,* June 1996.

"The Top 200 Drugs." *American Druggist,* February 1997.

OTHER SOURCES:

"Allegra™ (fexofenadine hydrochloride) Capsules." Product description. Hoechst Marion Roussel, 1997.

"How Rezulin Fits into Your Diabetes Control Plan." Brochure. Parke-Davis, Morris Plains, N.J., n.d.

"Low molecular weight heparin

CONTINUED

(dalteparin) in unstable coronary artery disease." Express Report from the 48th Annual Meeting of the Canadian Cardiovascular Society, Toronto, Ont., Oct. 24-28, 1995.

"Tramadol for Pain." Reprint. *Medical Sciences Bulletin,* April 1995. Available PharmInfoNet: http://pharminfo.com

WESTERN HERBS

BOOKS:

Castleman, Michael. *The Healing Herbs: The Ultimate Guide to the Curative Power of Nature's Medicines.* Emmaus, Pa.: Rodale Press, 1991.

The Complete Book of Natural and Medicinal Cures. Emmaus, Pa.: Rodale Press, 1994.

Foster, Steven, and James A. Duke. *A Field Guide to Medicinal Plants: Eastern and Central North America* (Peterson Field Guide Series). Boston: Houghton Mifflin, 1990.

Green, James. *The Male Herbal Health Care for Men and Boys.* Freedom, Calif.: Crossing Press, 1991.

Hoffman, David L. *The Complete Illustrated Holistic Herbal: A Safe and Practical Guide to Making and Using Herbal Remedies.* Shaftesbury, Dorset, England: Element Books, 1996.

Lawless, Julia. *The Encyclopaedia of Essential Oils.* Rockport, Mass.: Element Books, 1992.

Little, Elbert L. *The Audubon Society Field Guide to North American Trees.* New York: Alfred A. Knopf, 1980.

Mabey, Richard, et al. (eds.). *The New Age Herbalist: How to Use Herbs for Healing, Nutrition, Body Care, and Relaxation.* New York: Macmillan, 1988.

The Medical Advisor: The Complete Guide to Alternative and Conventional Treatments. Alexandria, Va.: Time-Life Books, 1996.

Mindell, Earl. *Earl Mindell's Herb Bible.* New York: Simon & Schuster, 1992.

Ody, Penelope. *The Complete Medicinal Herbal.* London: Dorling Kindersley, 1993.

Polunin, Miriam, and Christopher Robbins. *The Natural Pharmacy.* New York: Collier Books, Macmillan, 1992.

Price, Shirley. *Aromatherapy for Common Ailments.* London: Gaia Books, 1991.

Ryman, Danièle. *Aromatherapy: The Complete Guide to Plant and Flower Essences for Health and Beauty.* New York: Bantam Books, 1993.

Schar, Douglas. *Thirty Plants That Can Save Your Life!* Washington, D.C.: Elliott & Clark Publishing, 1993.

Tierra, Michael, MD. *Planetary Herbology: An Integration of Western Herbs into the Traditional Chinese and Ayurvedic Systems.* Twin Lakes, Wis.: Lotus Press, 1992.

Tyler, Varro E. *The Honest Herbal: A Sensible Guide to the Use of Herbs and Related Remedies* (3d ed.). New York: Pharmaceutical Products Press, Haworth Press, 1993.

Weiner, Michael A., MD. *The Herbal Bible: A Family Guide to Herbal Home Remedies.* San Rafael, Calif.: Quantum Books, 1992.

PERIODICALS:

Babal, Ken. "Cat's Claw: Healing Herb from the Amazon." *Health Store News,* December/January 1996.

Riggs, Maribeth. "Herbal Bitters: If They Taste Horrible, They're Good for You." *Herb Quarterly,* Fall 1995.

Sanchez, Don. "Cat's Claw." *New Editions HealthWorld,* December 1995.

Steinberg, Phillip N.:
"Amazon Medicine: A Vine from the Rain Forest That's Loaded with Healing Chemicals." *Natural Health,* May/June 1996.
"Cat's Claw *(Uña de Gato)*—A Wondrous Herb from the Amazon Rainforest." *Herb Quarterly,* Winter 1994.
"Cat's Claw: Medicinal Properties of This Amazon Vine." *Nutrition Science News,* n.d.

Yarnell, Eric, and Lisa Meserole. "Toxic Botanicals." *Alternative and Complementary Therapies,* February 1997.

OTHER SOURCES:

Hoffman, David L. "Therapeutic Herbalism: A Correspondence Course in Phytotherapy." Unpublished course materials. N.p., n.d.

Lee, Barbara. "Cat's Claw and Aloe Vera Combination: Two Botanicals for Today's Health Problems." http://www.cats-claw.com/cc_aloe.htm

Smith, Ed. "Therapeutic Herb Manual: The Therapeutic Administration of Liquid Herbal Extracts (Vol. 2)." Pamphlet. N.p., n.d.

"Standardized Extract: Cat's Claw *(Uncaria tomentosa):* Powerful New Formula Aids the Fight for Better Health." http://www.cats-claw.com/stand_x.htm

PICTURE CREDITS

FRONT COVER AND SPINE :
Jerry Pavia, The Virtual Garden ©1997, Time Life Inc.—Robin Reid.

BACK COVER:
Jerry Pavia, The Virtual Garden ©1997, Time Life Inc.—Robin Reid —Time-Life Inc.—art by Totally Incorporated.

BOOK:
The sources for the illustrations are listed below.
Illustrations of Western herbs created by Totally Incorporated.
Photographs of prescription drugs by Robin Reid, courtesy of Rite Aid Pharmacy.

ACKNOWLEDGMENTS

The editors wish to thank the following individuals and institutions for their valuable assistance in the preparation of this volume:

American Association of Poison Control Centers, Washington, D.C.; Lucille Arcouet, National Education Coordinator, Nelson Bach USA, Wilmington, Mass.; Roger Beem, General Nutrition Center, Alexandria, Va.; Dennis Bowen, Rite Aid Corporation, Beltsville, Md.; Stanley Cohen, School of Pharmacy, University of Pittsburgh, Pittsburgh, Pa.; Geoff Cook, Novartis Pharmaceutical Corp., East Hanover, N.J.; Sarah Datz, Rite Aid Corporation, Camp Hill, Pa.; Lester Grinspoon, MD, Harvard Medical School, Cambridge, Mass.; Laura Mahecha, Kline & Company, Inc., Fairfield, N.J.; Sydney Vallentyne, St. John's Herb Garden, Inc., Bowie, Md.; Janice Zoeller, *American Druggist,* New York, N.Y.; Kenneth G. Zysk, PhD, New York, N.Y.

POISON CONTROL CENTERS NATIONWIDE

AMERICAN ASSOCIATION OF POISON CONTROL CENTERS

3201 New Mexico Ave., N.W. • Suite 310 • Washington, D.C. 20016

ALABAMA		
Alabama Poison Center, Tuscaloosa	408-D Paul Bryant Drive, East Tuscaloosa, AL 35401	**(800) 462-0800 (AL only)** **(205) 345-0600**
Regional Poison Control Center	The Children's Hospital of Alabama 1600 - 7th Ave., South Birmingham, AL 35233-1711	**(800) 292-6678 (AL only)** **(205) 939-9201** **(205) 933-4050**
ARIZONA		
Arizona Poison and Drug Information Center	Arizona Health Sciences Center 1501 N. Campbell Ave. Tucson, AZ 85724	**(800) 362-0101 (AZ only)** **(520) 626-6016**
Samaritan Regional Poison Center	Good Samaritan Regional Medical Center, Ancillary-1 1111 E. McDowell Road Phoenix, AZ 85006	**(602) 253-3334**
CALIFORNIA		
California Poison Control System—Fresno Division (Central California)	Valley Children's Hospital 3151 N. Millbrook IN31 Fresno, CA 93703	**(800) 876-4766 (CA only)** **(209) 445-1222**
California Poison Control System—San Francisco Division	San Francisco General Hospital 1001 Potrero Ave., Bldg. 80 San Francisco, CA 94110	**(800) 876-4766 (CA only)** **(415) 502-8600**
California Poison Control System—San Diego Division	UCSD Medical Center 200 West Arbor Drive San Diego, CA 92103-8925	**(800) 876-4766 (CA only)**
California Poison Control System—Sacramento Division	UCDMC—HSF Rm. 1024 2315 Stockton Blvd. Sacramento, CA 95817	**(800) 876-4766 (CA only)**
COLORADO		
Rocky Mountain Poison and Drug Center	8802 E. 9th Ave. Denver, CO 80220-6800	**(800) 332-3073 (CO only)** **(303) 629-1123**
CONNECTICUT		
Connecticut Regional Poison Center	University of Connecticut Health Center 263 Farmington Ave. Farmington, CT 06030	**(800) 343-2722 (CT only)** **(860) 679-3056**
DISTRICT OF COLUMBIA		
National Capital Poison Center	3201 New Mexico Ave., N.W., Suite 310 Washington, D.C. 20016	**(202) 625-3333** **(202) 362-8563 (TTY)**

FLORIDA		
Florida Poison Information Center—Miami	University of Miami School of Medicine Department of Pediatrics P.O. Box 016960 (R-131) Miami, FL 33101	**(800) 282-3171 (FL only)**
Florida Poison Information Center—Jacksonville	University Medical Center University of Florida Health Science Center—Jacksonville 655 West 8th Street Jacksonville, FL 32009	**(800) 282-3171 (FL only)** **(904) 549-4480**
The Florida Poison Information Center—Tampa	Tampa General Hospital P.O. Box 1289 Tampa, FL 33601	**(800) 282-3171 (FL only)** **(813) 253-4444 (Tampa)**
GEORGIA		
Georgia Poison Center	Grady Memorial Hospital 80 Butler Street S.E. P.O. Box 26066 Atlanta, GA 30335-3801	**(800) 282-5846 (GA only)** **(404) 616-9000**
INDIANA		
Indiana Poison Center	Methodist Hospital of Indiana 1701 N. Senate Blvd. P.O. Box 1367 Indianapolis, IN 46206-1367	**(800) 382-9097 (IN only)** **(317) 929-2323**
KENTUCKY		
Kentucky Regional Poison Center	Kosair Children's Hospital Medical Towers South, Suite 572 P.O. Box 35070 Louisville, KY 40232-5070	**(800) 722-5725 (KY only)** **(502) 589-8222**
LOUISIANA		
Louisiana Drug and Poison Information Center	Northeast Louisiana University Sugar Hall Monroe, LA 71209-6430	**(800) 256-9822 (LA only)** **(318) 362-5393**
MARYLAND		
Maryland Poison Center	20 N. Pine Street Baltimore, MD 21201	**(800) 492-2414 (MD only)** **(410) 706-7701**
National Capital Poison Center (D.C. suburbs only)	3201 New Mexico Ave., N.W., Suite 310 Washington, D.C. 20016	**(202) 625-3333** **(202) 362-8563 (TTY)**
MASSACHUSETTS		
Massachusetts Poison Control System	300 Longwood Ave. Boston, MA 02115	**(800) 682-9211 (MA only)** **(617) 232-2120**

MICHIGAN		
Poison Control Center	Children's Hospital of Michigan 4160 John R., Suite 425 Detroit, MI 48201	**(800) 764-7661** **(313) 745-5711**
MINNESOTA		
Hennepin Regional Poison Center	Hennepin County Medical Center West Metro Center 701 Park Ave. Minneapolis, MN 55415	**(612) 347-3141** **Petlines:** **(612) 337-7387** **(612) 337-7474 (TDD)**
Minnesota Regional Poison Center	8100 - 34th Ave., South P.O. Box 1309 East Metro Center Minneapolis, MN 55440-1309	**(800) 222-1222 (Greater Minnesota)** **(612) 221-2113**
MISSOURI		
Cardinal Glennon Children's Hospital Regional Poison Center	1465 S. Grand Blvd. St. Louis, MO 63104	**(800) 366-8888 (MO only)** **(314) 772-5200**
MONTANA		
Rocky Mountain Poison and Drug Center	8802 East 9th Ave. Denver, CO 80220	**(800) 525-5042 (MT only)**
NEBRASKA		
The Poison Center	8301 Dodge Street Omaha, NE 68114	**(800) 955-9119 (NE & WY)** **(402) 390-5555 (Omaha)**
NEW JERSEY		
New Jersey Poison Information and Education System	201 Lyons Ave. Newark, NJ 07112	**(800) 764-7661 (NJ only)**
NEW MEXICO		
New Mexico Poison and Drug Information Center	University of New Mexico Health Sciences Library, Rm. 125 Albuquerque, NM 87131-1076	**(800) 432-6866 (NM only)** **(505) 272-2222**
NEW YORK		
Central New York Poison Control Center	SUNY Health Science Center 750 E. Adams Street Syracuse, NY 13203	**(800) 252-5655 (NY only)** **(315) 476-4766**
Finger Lakes Regional Poison Center	University of Rochester Medical Center 601 Elmwood Avenue Box 321, Room G-3275 Rochester, NY 14642	**(800) 333-0542 (NY only)** **(716) 275-3232**
Hudson Valley Regional Poison Center	Phelps Memorial Hospital Center 701 North Broadway North Tarrytown, NY 10591	**(800) 336-6997 (NY only)** **(914) 366-3030**

NEW YORK continued		
Long Island Regional Poison Control Center	Winthrop University Hospital 259 First Street Mineola, NY 11501	**(516) 542-2323**
New York City Poison Control Center	N.Y.C. Department of Health 455 First Ave., Room 123 New York, NY 10016	**(212) 340-4494 (212) P-O-I-S-O-N-S (212) 689-9014 (TDD)**
NORTH CAROLINA		
Carolinas Poison Center	1012 S. Kings Drive, Suite 206 P.O. Box 32861 Charlotte, NC 28232-2861	**(800) 84-TOXIN (NC only) 1-(800) 848-6946 (704) 355-4000**
OHIO		
Central Ohio Poison Center	700 Children's Drive Columbus, OH 43205-2696	**(800) 682-7625 (OH only) (614) 228-1323 (614) 228-2272 (TTY)**
Cincinnati Drug & Poison Information Center and Regional Poison Control System	P.O. Box 670144 Cincinnati, OH 45267-0144	**(800) 872-5111 (OH only) (513) 558-5111**
OREGON		
Oregon Poison Center	Oregon Health Sciences University 3181 S.W. Sam Jackson Park Road, CB 550 Portland, OR 97201	**(800) 452-7165 (OR only) (503) 494-8968**
PENNSYLVANIA		
Central Pennsylvania Poison Center	University Hospital Milton S. Hershey Medical Center Hershey, PA 17033	**(800) 521-6110 (Central PA only) (717) 531-6111**
The Poison Control Center	3600 Sciences Center, Suite 220 Philadelphia, PA 19104-2641	**(800) 722-7112 (215) 386-2100**
Pittsburgh Poison Center	3705 Fifth Ave. Pittsburgh, PA 15213	**(412) 681-6669**
RHODE ISLAND		
Rhode Island Poison Center	593 Eddy Street Providence, RI 02903	**(401) 444-5727**
TENNESSEE		
Middle Tennessee Poison Center	The Center for Clinical Toxicology, Vanderbilt University Medical Center 11651 - 21st Ave., South 501 Oxford House Nashville, TN 37232-4632	**(800) 288-9999 (TN only) (615) 936-2034**

CONTINUED

TEXAS		
Central Texas Poison Center	Scott & White Memorial Hospital 2401 S. 31st Street Temple, TX 76508	**(800) 764-7661 (TX only)** **(817) 724-7401**
North Texas Poison Center	5201 Harry Hines Blvd. P.O. Box 35926 Dallas, TX 75235	**(800) 764-7661 (TX only)**
Southeast Texas Poison Center	The University of Texas Medical Branch 301 University Ave. Galveston, TX 77550-2780	**(800) 764-7661 (TX only)** **(409) 765-1420**
UTAH		
Utah Poison Control Center	410 Chipeta Way, Suite 230 Salt Lake City, UT 84108	**(800) 456-7707 (UT only)** **(801) 581-2151**
VIRGINIA		
Blue Ridge Poison Center	University of Virginia Medical Center Box 67, Blue Ridge Charlottesville, VA 22901	**(800) 451-1428** **(804) 924-5543**
National Capital Poison Center (Northern Virginia only)	3201 New Mexico Ave., N.W., Suite 310 Washington, D.C. 20016	**(202) 625-3333** **(202) 362-8563 (TTY)**
WASHINGTON		
Washington Poison Center	155 N.E. 100th Street, Suite E400 Seattle, WA 98125	**(800) 732-6985 (WA only)** **(800) 572-0638 (TDD only)** **(206) 526-2121**
WEST VIRGINIA		
West Virginia Poison Center	3110 MacCorkle Ave., S.E. Charleston, WV 25304	**(800) 642-3625 (WV only)** **(304) 348-4211**
WYOMING		
The Poison Center	8301 Dodge Street Omaha, NE 68114	**(800) 955-9119 (NE & WY)** **(402) 390-5555 (Omaha)**